1001
LOW-CARB
RECIPES

**Hundreds of Delicious Recipes from Dinner to Dessert That
Let You Live Your Low-Carb Lifestyle and Never Look Back**

Dana Carpender

Bestselling author *500 Low-Carb Recipes*

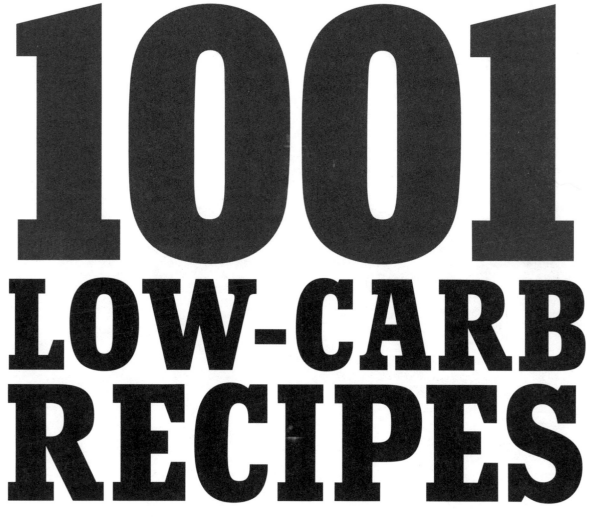

1001 LOW-CARB RECIPES

Hundreds of Delicious Recipes from Dinner to Dessert That
Let You Live Your Low-Carb Lifestyle and Never Look Back

Dana Carpender

Bestselling author *500 Low-Carb Recipes*

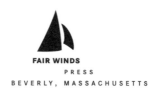

FAIR WINDS
PRESS
BEVERLY, MASSACHUSETTS

© 2010 Fair Winds Press
Text © 2010 Dana Carpender

First published in the USA in 2010 by
Fair Winds Press, a member of
Quarto Publishing Group USA Inc.
100 Cummings Center
Suite 406-L
Beverly, MA 01915-6101
www.fairwindspress.com

18 17 16 15 14   15 16 17

ISBN-13: 978-1-59233-414-8
ISBN-10: 1-59233-414-8

Library of Congress Cataloging-in-Publication Data available

Cover design by Kathie Alexander

Printed and bound in the U.S.A.

Contents

INTRODUCTION

What's the hardest thing about your low-carb diet? And what's the most common reason that people abandon their low-carb way of eating and all the health benefits and weight loss that come with it? It's boredom. After a few weeks of scrambled eggs and bacon for breakfast, a hamburger with no bun for lunch, and a steak—no baked potato—for dinner, day after day, people get fed up and quit. They just can't face a life of food monotony. Does this sound familiar?

If you've been getting bored with your low-carb diet, this is the book for you. You'll find dozens of exciting ways to vary a hamburger, a steak, pork chops, chicken, and even fish. You'll find a wide variety of side dishes and salads.

You'll find snacks and party foods that you can eat without feeling like you're depriving yourself. You'll even find recipes for bread—really, truly bread—not to mention muffins, waffles, and pancakes. In short, this book has recipes for all sorts of things you never *dreamed* you could have on a low-carb diet.

Did I come up with these recipes for you? Heck, no! I came up with these recipes for *me*.

Who am I? I'm a person who, through circumstances that surely could have happened to anyone, has spent the past several years writing about low-carbohydrate dieting. In fact, I spent so much time answering questions for the curious that I finally wrote a book, *How I Gave Up My Low Fat Diet and Lost Forty Pounds!* To supplement the book, I started an "e-zine"—an Internet newsletter—for low-carb dieters, called *Lowcarbezine!* So for the past few years, through the wonders of the Internet, I've been writing and developing recipes for a growing audience of low-carb dieters around the world.

I've always loved to cook, and I've always been good at it. My friends long ago dubbed me "The God of Food." So when low-fat, high-carb mania hit in the 1980s, I learned how to make a killer low-fat fettuccine Alfredo, curried chicken and mixed grain pilau, black beans and rice, blue corn pancakes, low-fat cheesecake—you name it.

And I got fat—really fat and sick and tired. Thank heavens, in 1995 I got smart and tried going low carb, instead. Within two days my energy levels skyrocketed and my clothes were looser. It was overwhelmingly clear that this was the way my body wanted to be fed and that this was the way of eating that would make me well. I had set my foot upon a path from which there was no turning back; I was low carb for life.

The only thing that nearly derailed me was a terrible sense of Kitchen Disorientation. I had to discard the vast majority of my recipes when I dropped the grains, beans, potatoes, and sugar from my diet. For the very first time in my life, I'd walk into my kitchen and have no idea what to cook—and I had always known what to cook and how to put together a menu. It really was pretty scary, and it certainly was depressing. But I set out to become as good a low-carb cook as I had been a low-fat cook.

What you hold in your hands is the end result of years and years of trial and error, of learning what works and what doesn't and of experimenting to find out which substitutes are yummy and which are just plain lame.

This is not, for the most part, a gourmet cookbook, which means that the recipes you find here are recipes you'll actually use. You'll find a lot of fairly simple recipes and a few more complex ones for special occasions. There's lots of family fare here—pork chops, meat loaf, burgers, and chicken. You'll find lots of meals you can cook on the stove top in a simple skillet and plenty of salads you can make ahead and stash in the refrigerator, ready to be pulled out and served when you dash in the door at a quarter-to-dinner-time. You'll find many one-dish meals that are protein and vegetables combined, from main dish salads to thick, hearty soups to casseroles. You'll also find ethnic flavors from around the world right alongside comfort foods you won't believe are low carb!

Why Is There Such a Wide Range of Carb Counts in the Recipes in This Book?

If carbs are your problem, then they're going to be your problem tomorrow, next week, next year, and even when you're old and gray. You cannot think in terms of going on a low-carb diet, losing your weight, and then going off your diet—you'll gain back every ounce just as sure as you're born. You'll also go back to blood-sugar swings, energy crashes, and nagging, insatiable hunger, not to mention all the health risks of hyperinsulinemia. In short, you are in this for life.

So if you are to have any hope of doing this forever, you're going to need to enjoy your food. You're going to need variety, flavor, color, and interest. You're going to need festive dishes, easy dishes, and comfort foods—a whole world of things to eat.

Because of this, I've included everything from very low-carb dishes, suitable for folks in the early, very low-carb "induction" stage of their diet, to "splurge" dishes, which would probably make most of us gain weight if we ate them every day but which still have far fewer carbs than their "normal" counterparts.

There's another reason for the range of carb counts: Carbohydrate intolerance comes in degrees, and different people can tolerate different daily carbohydrate intakes. Some of you, no doubt, need to stay in that 20-grams-a-day-or-less range, whereas many others—lucky souls—can have as much as 90 to 100 grams a day and stay slim. This cookbook is meant to serve you all.

Only you can know, through trial and error, how many grams of carbs you can eat in a day and still lose weight. It is up to you to pick and choose among the recipes in this book while keeping an eye on the carbohydrate counts provided. That way, you can put together menus that will please your palate and your family while staying below that critical carb level.

However, I do have this to say: Always, always, always the heart and soul of your low-carbohydrate diet should be meat, fish, poultry, eggs, healthy fats, and low-carb vegetables. This book will teach you a boggling number of ways to combine these things, and you should try them all. Don't just find one or two recipes that you like and make them over and over. Try at least one new recipe every week; that way, within a few months you'll have a whole new repertoire of familiar low-carb favorites!

You will, as I just mentioned, find recipes in this book for what are best considered low-carb treats. Do not take the presence of a recipe in this book to mean that it is something that you can eat every day, in unlimited quantities, and still lose weight. I can tell you from experience that even low-carb treats, if eaten frequently, will put weight on you. Recipes for breads, cookies, muffins, cakes, and the like are here to give you a satisfying, varied diet that you can live with for life, but they should not become the new staples of your diet. *Do not try to make your low-carbohydrate diet resemble your former Standard American Diet.* That's the diet that got you in trouble in the first place, remember?

One other thought: It is entirely possible to have a bad reaction to a food that has nothing to do with its carbohydrate count. Gluten, a protein from wheat that is essential for baking low-carb bread, causes bad reactions in a fair number of people. Soy products are problematic for many folks, as are nuts. Whey protein, used extensively in these recipes, contains lactose, which some people cannot tolerate. And surely you've heard of people who react badly to artificial sweeteners of one kind or another. I've also heard from diabetics who get bad blood-sugar spikes from eating even small quantities of onions or tomatoes.

Yet all of these foods are just fine for many, many low-carb dieters, and there is no way I can know which foods may cause a problem for which people. All I can tell you is to pay attention to your body. If you add a new food to your diet and you gain weight (and you're pretty certain it's not tied to something else, like a new medication), or you find yourself unreasonably hungry, tired, or "off" despite having stayed within your body's carbohydrate tolerance, you may want to consider avoiding that food. One man's meat is another man's poison, and all that.

What's a "Usable Carb Count"?

You may or may not be aware of the concept of the usable carb count, sometimes called the "effective carb count"; some low-carb books utilize this principle, whereas others do not. If you're not familiar with the concept, here it is in a nutshell:

Fiber is a carbohydrate and is, at least in American nutritional breakdowns, included in the total carbohydrate count. However, fiber is a form of carbohydrate made of molecules so big that you can neither digest nor absorb them. Therefore fiber, despite being a carbohydrate, will not push up your blood sugar and will not cause an insulin release. Even better, by slowing the absorption of the starches and sugars that occur with it, fiber actually lessens their bad influence. This is very likely the reason that high-fiber diets appear to be so much better for you than "American Normal."

For these reasons, many (if not most) low-carb dieters now subtract the grams of fiber in a food from the total grams of carbohydrate to determine the number of grams of carbohydrates that are actually a problem. These are the "usable" carbs, or the "effective carb count." These nonfiber grams of carbohydrates are what we count and limit. Not only does this approach allow us a much wider variety of foods, especially lots more vegetables, but it actually encourages us to add fiber to things such as baked goods. I am very much a fan of this approach, and therefore I give the usable carbohydrate count for these recipes. However, you will also find the breakdown of the total carb count and the fiber count.

Using This Book

I can't tell you how to plan your menus. I don't know if you live alone or have a family, if you have hours to cook or are pressed for time every evening, or what foods are your favorites. I can, however, give you a few pointers on what you'll find here that may make your meal planning easier.

There are a lot of one-dish meals in this book—main dish salads, skillet suppers that include both meat and vegetables, and hearty soups that are a full meal in a bowl. I include these because they're some of my favorite foods, and to my mind, they're about the simplest way to eat. I also think they lend a far greater variety to low-carb cuisine than is possible if you're trying to divide up your carbohydrate allowance for a given meal among three or four different dishes. If you have a carb-eating family, you can appease them by serving something on the side, such as whole wheat pitas split in half and toasted, along with garlic butter, brown rice, a baked potato, or some noodles. (Of course, I don't recommend that you serve them something like canned biscuits, Tater Tots, or Minute Rice, but that shouldn't surprise you.)

When you're serving these one-dish meals, remember that most of your carbohydrate allowance for the meal is included in that main dish. Unless you can tolerate more carbohydrates than I can, you probably don't want to serve a dish with lots of vegetables in it with even more vegetables on the side. Remember, it's the total usable carb count you have to keep an eye on. Complement simple meat dishes—such as roasted chicken, broiled steak, or pan-broiled pork chops—with the more carbohydrate-rich vegetable side dishes.

There's one other thing I hope this book teaches you to do, and that's break out of your old ways of looking at food. There's no law insisting that you eat eggs only for breakfast, have tuna salad for lunch every day, and serve some sort of meat and two side dishes for dinner. Are you short on both time and money? Serve eggs for dinner a couple of nights a week; they're fast, cheap, and unbelievably nutritious. Are you planing a family video night or game night? Skip dinner and make two or three healthy snack foods to nibble on. You just can't face another fried egg at breakfast? Throw a pork chop or a hamburger on the electric tabletop grill and you've got a fast and easy breakfast. Are you sick of salads for lunch? Take a protein-rich dip in a snap-top container and some cut up vegetables to work with you.

Helpful General Hints

- If you're not losing weight, go back to counting every carb. Remember that snacks and beverages count, even if they're made from recipes in this book. A 6-gram muffin may be a lot better for you and your waistline than a convenience store muffin, but it's still 6 grams, and it counts! Likewise, don't lie to yourself about portion sizes. If you make your cookies really big, so that you only get two dozen instead of four dozen from a recipe, the carb count per cookie doubles, and don't you forget it.

- Beware of hidden carbohydrates. It's important to know that the government lets food manufacturers put "0 grams of carbohydrates" on the label if a food has less than 0.5 gram per serving and "less than 1 gram of carbohydrate" if a food has between 0.5 gram and 0.9 gram. Even some diet sodas contain trace amounts of carbohydrates! These amounts aren't much, but they do add up if you eat enough of them. So if you're having trouble losing, count foods that say "0 grams" as 0.5 gram and foods that say "less than 1 gram" as 1 gram.

- Remember that some foods you may be thinking of as carb-free actually contain at least traces of carbohydrates. Eggs contain about 0.5 gram apiece, shrimp have 1 gram per 4-ounce portion, natural cheeses have about 1 gram per ounce, and heavy cream has about 0.5 gram per tablespoon. And coffee has more than 1 gram in a 10-ounce mug before you add cream and sweetener. (Tea, on the other hand, is carb-free.) If you're having trouble losing weight, get a food counter book and use it, even for foods you're sure you already know the carb counts of.

1

Ingredients You Need to Know About

Black Soy Beans

Most beans and other legumes are too high in carbohydrate for many low-carb dieters, but there is one exception: Black soy beans have a very low usable carb count, about 1 gram per serving, because most of the carb in them is fiber. Several recipes in this book call for canned black soy beans. Many natural food stores carry the Eden brand; if yours doesn't, I'll bet they could special-order them for you. Natural food stores tend to be wonderful about special orders.

If you can't find canned black soy beans, you may be able to find them dry and uncooked; if so, you'll have to soak them and then cook them for a very long time until they soften—soy beans can be stubborn. I'd recommend using your slow cooker.

I would also recommend not eating soy bean recipes several times a week. I know that soy has a reputation for being the Wonder Health Food of All Existence, but there are reasons to be cautious. Soy has been known for decades now to be hard on the thyroid, and if you're trying to lose weight and improve your health, a slow thyroid is the last thing you need. More alarmingly, there was a study done in Hawaii in 2000 that showed a correlation between the amount of tofu subjects ate in middle age and their rate and severity of cognitive problems in old age. Since scientists suspect the problem lies with the soy estrogens that have been so highly touted, any unfermented soy product, including our canned soy beans, is suspect.

This doesn't mean we should completely shun soy beans and soy products, but it does mean we need to approach them with caution and eat them in moderation. Since many low-carb specialty products are soy-heavy, you'll want to pay attention there, too.

Personally, I try to keep my soy consumption to 1 serving a week or less.

Eggs

There are a few recipes in this book that call for raw eggs, an ingredient currently frowned upon by nutritional "officialdom" because of the risk of salmonella. However, I have it on pretty good authority that only 1 out of every 16,000 uncracked, properly refrigerated eggs is actually contaminated. As one woman with degrees in public health and food science put it, "The risk is less than the risk of breaking your leg on any given trip down the stairs." So I use raw eggs now and again without worrying about it, and we've never had a problem around here.

However, this does not mean that there is no risk. You'll have to decide for yourself whether this is something you should worry about. I generally use very fresh eggs from local small farmers, which may well be safer than eggs that have gone longer distances, and thus have a higher risk of cracking or experiencing refrigeration problems.

One useful thing to know about eggs: Although you'll want very fresh eggs for frying and poaching, eggs that are at least several days old are better for hard boiling. They're less likely to stick to their shells in that maddening way we've all encountered. So if you like hard-boiled eggs (and they're certainly one of the most convenient low-carb foods), buy a couple of extra cartons of eggs and let them sit in the refrigerator for at least three or four days before you hard boil them.

Fats and Oils

Bland Oils

Sometimes you want a bland oil in a recipe, something that adds little or no flavor of its own. In that case, I recommend peanut, sunflower, or canola oil. These are the oils I mean when I simply specify "oil" in a recipe. Avoid highly polyunsaturated oils such as safflower; they deteriorate quickly both from heat and from contact with oxygen, and they've been associated with an increased risk of cancer.

Butter

When a recipe says butter, use butter, will you? Margarine is nasty, unhealthy stuff, full of hydrogenated oils, trans fats, and artificial everything. It's terrible for you. So use the real thing. If real butter strains your budget, watch for sales and stock up; butter freezes beautifully. Shop around, too. In my town I've found stores that regularly sell butter for anywhere from $2.25 a pound to $4.59 a pound. That's a big difference, and one worth going out of my way for.

Coconut Oil

Coconut oil makes an excellent substitute for hydrogenated vegetable shortening (Crisco and the like), which you should shun. You may find coconut oil at natural food stores or possibly in Oriental food stores. One large local grocery store carries it in the "ethnic foods" section with Indian foods. My natural food store keeps coconut oil with the cosmetics. They're still convinced that saturated fats are terrible for you, so they don't put it with the foods, but some folks use it for making hair dressings and soaps. Coconut oil is solid at room temperature, except in the summer, but it melts at body temperature. Surprisingly, it has no coconut flavor or aroma; you can use it for sautéing or in baking without adding any "off" flavor to your recipes.

Olive Oil

It surely will come as no surprise to you that olive oil is a healthy fat, but you may not know that there are various kinds. Extra-virgin olive oil is the first pressing. It is deep green, with a full, fruity flavor, and it makes all the difference in salad dressings. However, it's expensive and also too strongly flavored for some uses. I keep a bottle of extra-virgin olive oil on hand, but I use it exclusively for salads.

For sautéing and other general uses, I use a grade of olive oil known as "pomace." Pomace is far cheaper than extra-virgin olive oil, and it has a milder flavor. I buy pomace in gallon cans at the same Middle Eastern grocery store where I buy my low-carb specialty products. These gallon cans are worth looking for because they're the cheapest way to buy the stuff. If you can't find gallon cans of pomace, feel free to buy whatever cheaper, milder-flavored type of olive oil is available at your grocery store.

Be aware that if you refrigerate olive oil it will become solid. This is no big deal—it will be fine once it warms up again. If you need it quickly, you can run the bottle under warm water. Or if the container has no metal and will fit in your microwave, microwave it for a minute or so on low power.

Flour Substitutes

As you are no doubt aware, flour is out, for the most part, in low-carb cooking. Flour serves a few different purposes in cooking, from making up the bulk of most baked goods and creating stretchiness in bread dough to thickening sauces and "binding" casseroles. In low-carb cooking, we use different ingredients for these various purposes. Here's a rundown of flour substitutes you'll want to have on hand for low-carb cooking and baking:

Brans

Because fiber is a carbohydrate that we neither digest nor absorb, brans of one kind or another are very useful for bulking up (no pun intended!) low-carb baked goods. I use different kinds in different recipes. You'll want to have at least wheat bran and oat bran on hand; both of these are widely available. If you can also find rice bran, it's worth picking up, especially if you have high cholesterol. Of all the kinds of bran tested, rice bran was most powerful for lowering high blood cholesterol.

Ground Almonds and Hazelnuts

Finely ground almonds and hazelnuts are wonderful for replacing some or all of the flour in many recipes, especially cakes and cookies. Packaged almond meal is becoming easier to find; the widely distributed Bob's Red Mill brand makes one. It's convenient stuff, and you certainly may use it in any of the recipes that call for almond meal. If you can purchase hazelnut meal locally, it should also work fine in these recipes.

However, I prefer to make my own almond and hazelnut meal by grinding the shelled nuts in my food processor using the S-blade. It takes only a minute or so to reduce them to the texture of corn meal, after which I store the meal in a tightly lidded container. Why do I bother? Because the carb count is lower. How on earth can that be? Because I grind my nuts with the brown skins still on them, while commercial nut meal is made from almonds and hazelnuts that are "blanched"—have the skins removed. Since the skins are practically pure fiber, the fiber count of my homemade meal is higher, and the usable carb count per cup is accordingly lower. The carb counts in this book reflect my homemade, high-fiber meal; if you use purchased meal you'll want to revise your estimated carb count a gram or two higher per serving.

It's good to know that both almonds and hazelnuts actually expand a little during grinding. This surprised me because I thought they'd compress a bit. Figure that between ⅔ and ¾ of a cup of either of these nuts will become 1 cup when ground.

Guar and Xanthan Gums

These sound just dreadful, don't they? But they're in lots of your favorite processed foods, so how bad can they be? If you're wondering what the heck they are, here's the answer: They're forms of water-soluble fiber, extracted and purified. Guar and xanthan are both flavorless white powders; their value to us is as low-carb thickeners. Technically speaking, these are carbs, but they're all fiber, so don't worry about using them.

You'll find guar or xanthan used in small quantities in a lot of these recipes. Don't go dramatically increasing the quantity of guar or xanthan to get a thicker product, because in large quantities they make things gummy, and the texture is not terribly pleasant. But in these tiny quantities they add oomph to sauces and soups without using flour. You can always leave the guar or xanthan out if you can't find it; you'll just get a somewhat thinner result.

You'll notice that I often tell you to put the guar or xanthan through the blender with whatever liquid it is that you're using. This is because it is very difficult to simply whisk guar into a sauce and not get little gummy lumps in your finished sauce or soup, and the blender is the best way to thoroughly combine your ingredients.

If you don't own or don't want to use a blender, put your guar or xanthan in a salt shaker, and sprinkle it, bit by bit, over your sauce, stirring madly all the while with a whisk. The problem here, of course, is there's no way to know exactly how much you're using, so you'll just have to stop when your dish reaches the degree of thickness you like. Still, this can be a useful trick.

Your natural food store may well be able to order guar or xanthan for you (I slightly prefer xanthan, myself) if they don't have it on hand. You can also find suppliers online. Keep either one in a jar with a tight lid, and it will never go bad. I bought a pound of guar about 15 years ago, and it's still going strong!

Low-Carbohydrate Bake Mix

There are several brands of low-carbohydrate bake mix on the market. These are generally a combination of some form of powdery protein and fiber, such as soy, whey, and sometimes oat, plus baking powder, and sometimes salt. These mixes are the low-carb world's equivalent of Bisquick, although they do not have shortening added. You will need to add butter, oil, or some other form of fat when using them to make pancakes, waffles, biscuits, and such. I mostly use low-carb bake mix in lesser quantities, for "flouring" chicken before baking or frying or replacing flour as a "binder" in a casserole. If you can't find low-carbohydrate bake mix locally, there are many Web sites that sell it.

Oat Flour

A handful of recipes in this book call for oat flour. Because of its high fiber content, oat flour has a lower usable carb count than most other flours. Even so, it must be used in very small quantities. Oat flour is available at natural food stores. In a pinch, you can grind up oatmeal in your blender or food processor.

Psyllium Husks

This is another fiber product. It's the same form of fiber that is used in Metamucil and similar products. Because psyllium has little flavor of its own, it makes a useful high-fiber "filler" in some low-carb bread recipes. Look for plain psyllium husks at your natural food store. Mine carries them in bulk, quite cheaply, but if yours doesn't, look for them among the laxatives and "colon health" products. (A brand called "Colon Cleanse" is widely available.)

Pumpkin Seed Meal

A few recipes in this book call for pumpkin seed meal—I started experimenting with it after getting a fair amount of e-mail from folks who couldn't make my baked goods because of an allergy to nuts, and I've found it works quite well. (If you're allergic to nuts and want to make any of my recipes that call for almond meal, I'd try substituting pumpkin seed or sunflower seed meal.)

It's very easy to make pumpkin seed meal. Just buy raw shelled pumpkin seeds at your natural food store or at any market that caters to a Mexican-American population—sometimes they'll be labeled "pepitas." Then put the pumpkin seeds in your food processor and grind them with the S-blade until they reach a cornmeal consistency. That's all. (Do not try this with the salted pumpkin seeds in the shell that are sold as snacks! You'll get salty food with a texture like wood pulp.)

By the way, when I first published my recipe for Zucchini Bread, which calls for pumpkin seed meal, a few *Lowcarbezine!* readers wrote to tell me that their bread was tasty, but that it had come out green. I assume this is because of the green color of the seeds. I haven't had this problem, but it's harmless.

Rice Protein Powder

For savory recipes such as main dishes, you need a protein powder that isn't sweet and preferably one that has no flavor at all. There are a number of these on the market, and some are blander than others. I tried several kinds, and I've found that rice protein powder is the one I like best. I buy Nutribiotics brand, which has 1 gram of carbohydrates per tablespoon, but any unflavored rice protein powder with a similar carb count should work fine. For that matter, I see no reason not to experiment with other unflavored protein powders, if you like.

Rolled Oats

Also known as old-fashioned oatmeal, rolled oats are oat grains that have been squashed flat. These are available in every grocery store in the Western Hemisphere. Do not substitute instant or quick-cooking oatmeal.

Soy Powder, Soy Flour, and Soy Protein Isolate

Some of my recipes call for soy *powder*. None call for soy *flour*. If you use soy flour in a recipe that calls for soy powder, you won't get the results I got. You also won't get the right results with *soy protein powder*, also known as *soy protein isolate*. What is the difference? Soy protein isolate is a protein that has been extracted from soybeans and concentrated into a protein powder. Soy flour is made from raw soybeans that have simply been ground up into flour, and it has a strong bean flavor. Soy powder, also known as *soy milk powder*, is made from whole soybeans, like soy flour, but the beans are cooked before they're ground up. For some reason I don't pretend to understand, this gets rid of the strong flavor and makes soy powder taste quite mild. If your local natural food store doesn't stock soy powder, they can no doubt order it for you; I recommend Fearn brand.

You should be aware that despite the tremendous marketing buildup soy has enjoyed for the past several years, there are some problems emerging. Soy is well known to interfere with thyroid function, which is the last thing you need if you're trying to lose weight. It also can interfere with mineral absorption. It is also less certain, but still possible, that regular consumption of soy causes brain deterioration and genital defects in boy babies born to mothers with soy-heavy diets. For these reasons, although I do not shun soy entirely, I use other options when possible.

Vital Wheat Gluten

Gluten is a grain protein. It's the gluten in flour that makes bread dough stretchy so that it will trap the gas released by the yeast, letting your bread rise. We are not, of course, going to use regular, all-purpose flour, with its high carbohydrate content. Fortunately, it is possible to buy concentrated wheat gluten. This high-protein, low-starch flour is absolutely essential to making low-carbohydrate yeast breads.

Buying vital wheat gluten can be a problem, however, because the nomenclature is not standardized. Some packagers call this "vital wheat gluten" or "pure gluten flour," whereas others simply call it "wheat gluten." Still others call it "high-gluten flour." This is a real poser, since the same name is frequently used for regular flour that has had extra gluten added to it; that product is something you definitely do not want.

To make sure you're getting the right product, you'll simply have to read the label. The product you want, regardless of what the packager calls it, will have between 75 and 80 percent protein or about 24 grams in ¼ cup (30 g). It will also have a very low carbohydrate count, somewhere in the neighborhood of 6 grams of carbohydrates in that same ¼ cup (30 g). If your natural food store has a bulk bin labeled "high-gluten flour" or "gluten flour" but there's no nutrition label attached, ask to see the bulk food manager and request the information off of the sack the flour came in. If the label on the bin says "vital wheat gluten" or "pure gluten flour," you can probably trust it.

At this writing, the most widely distributed brand of vital wheat gluten in the United States is Bob's Red Mill. More and more grocery stores are beginning to carry this line of products. If your grocery store doesn't yet, you might request that they start.

Wheat Germ

The germ is the part of the wheat kernel that would have become the plant if the grain had sprouted. It is the most nutritious, highest-protein part of the wheat kernel, and it is much lower in carbohydrates than the starchy part that becomes white flour. A few recipes in this book call for raw wheat germ, which is available at natural food stores. Raw wheat germ should be refrigerated because it goes rancid pretty easily. If your natural food store doesn't keep the raw wheat germ in the cooler, I'd look for another natural food store.

If you can't get raw wheat germ, toasted wheat germ, such as Kretchmer's, is a usable second-best. It's widely available in grocery stores.

Wheat Protein Isolate

A few of these recipes, particularly some of the baked goods, call for wheat protein isolate. This is just what it sounds like—it's a protein powder made from wheat. It has a high gluten content but also contains other proteins found in wheat. Wheat protein isolate has very little flavor and very little carbohydrate—just 1.5 grams per cup.

Wheat protein isolate is not widely distributed yet, but it is available through a few online sources. In particular, www.locarber.com and www.carbsmart.com both carry it.

Whey Protein Powder

Whey is the liquid part of milk. If you've ever seen yogurt that has separated, the clearish liquid on top is the whey. Whey protein is of extremely good quality, and the protein powder made from it is tops in both flavor and nutritional value. For any sweet recipe, the vanilla-flavored whey protein powder is best, and it's readily available in natural food stores. Keep in mind that protein powders vary in their carbohydrate counts, so look for the one with the fewest carbohydrates. Also beware of sugar-sweetened protein powders, which can be higher in carbs. The one I use is sweetened with stevia and has a little less than 1 gram of carbohydrates per tablespoon.

Natural whey protein powder is just like vanilla-flavored whey protein powder, except that it has not been flavored or sweetened. Its flavor is bland, so it is used in recipes where a sweet flavor is not desirable. Natural whey protein powder is called for in some of the recipes that other folks have donated to my books; I generally use rice protein powder when a bland protein powder is called for.

Ketatoes

Ketatoes is a low-carb version of instant mashed potatoes. It actually contains some dehydrated potato, diluted with a lot of fiber. You simply mix the powder with equal amounts of water. Personally, I find Ketatoes made according to package directions unappealing—they smell good, but the texture is off. However, used in small quantities, Ketatoes mix allows us to give a convincingly potatoey flavor to a variety of dishes. I've used Ketatoes mix in a number of the recipes in this book. Be aware that Ketatoes come in a variety of flavors, but all my recipes call for Ketatoes Classic—that is, plain potato flavor.

If you can't buy Ketatoes in your hometown, there are about a billion online merchants who would be only too happy to ship them to you.

Liquids

Beer

A few recipes in this book call for beer. The lowest carbohydrate beers currently on the market are Michelob Ultra, at 2.8 grams per bottle, and Miller Lite and Milwaukee's Best Light, both 3.5 grams per can. These are what I recommend you use. These are also what I recommend you drink if you are a beer fan.

Broths

Canned or boxed chicken and beef broths are very handy items to keep around, and it's certainly quicker to make dinner with these than it would be if you had to make your own from scratch. However, the quality of most of the canned broth you'll find at your local grocery store is appallingly bad. The chicken broth has all sorts of chemicals in it and often sugar, as well. The "beef" broth is worse, frequently containing no beef whatsoever. I refuse to use these products, and you should too.

However, there are a few canned and boxed broths worth buying. Many grocery stores now carry a brand called Kitchen Basics, which contains no chemicals at all. It's packaged in 1-quart (960-ml) boxes, much like soy milk, and it's available in both chicken and beef. Natural food stores also have good quality canned and boxed broths. Both Shelton and Health Valley brands are widely distributed in the United States.

Decent packaged broth won't cost you a whole lot more than the stuff that is made of salt and chemicals. If you watch for sales, you can often get it as cheaply as the bad stuff; stock up on it then. (When my natural food store runs a sale of good broth for 89 cents a can, I buy piles of the stuff!)

One last note: You will also find canned vegetable broth, particularly at natural food stores. This is tasty, but it runs much higher in carbohydrates than the chicken and beef broths. I'd avoid it.

Carb Countdown Dairy Beverage

A very useful addition to low-carb cuisine is this carbohydrate-reduced milk product, available in full-fat, 1%, and skim, not to mention an exceedingly yummy chocolate variety. To me, Carb Countdown tastes just like milk, and I've used it pretty extensively in these recipes.

I checked with the manufacturer, and Carb Countdown is nationally distributed, so you should be able to find it near you. However, if you cannot, try substituting half-and-half or equal parts of heavy cream and water. For that matter, if you're on the South Beach Diet, low-fat milk is allowed; feel free to use it in place of Carb Countdown wherever I've specified it.

Vinegar

Various recipes in this book call for wine vinegar, cider vinegar, sherry vinegar, rice vinegar, tarragon vinegar, white vinegar, balsamic vinegar, and even raspberry vinegar, for which you'll find a recipe. If you've always thought that vinegar was just vinegar, think again! Each of these vinegars has a distinct flavor all its own, and if you substitute one for the other, you'll change the whole character of the recipe. Add just one splash of cider vinegar to the Asian Chicken Salad (page 159), and you've traded your Chinese accent for an American twang. Vinegar is such a great way to give bright flavors to foods while adding very few carbs that I keep all of these varieties on hand. This is easy to do, because vinegar keeps for a very long time.

As with everything else, read the labels on your vinegar. I've seen cider vinegar that has 0 grams of carbohydrates per ounce and I've seen cider vinegar that has 4 grams of carbohydrates per ounce—a huge difference. Beware, also, of apple cider–*flavored* vinegar, which is white vinegar with artificial flavors added. I bought

this once by mistake. (You'd think someone who constantly reminds others to read labels would be beyond such errors, wouldn't you?)

Wine

There are several recipes in this cookbook calling for either dry red or dry white wine. I find the inexpensive box wines, which come in a mylar bag inside a cardboard box, very convenient to keep on hand for cooking. The simple reason for this is that they don't go bad because the contents are never exposed to air. These are not fabulous vintage wines, but they're fine for our modest purposes, and they certainly are handy. I generally have both Burgundy and Chablis wine-in-a-box on hand. Be wary of any wine with "added flavors." Too often, one of those flavors will be sugar. Buy wine with a recognizable name, such as Burgundy, Rhine, Chablis, Cabernet, and the like, rather than stuff like "Chillable Red," and you'll get better results.

Low-Carb Tortillas

These are becoming easier and easier to find. I can get them at every grocery store in town. If you can't buy them at a local store, you can order them online. They keep pretty well. I've had them hang around for 3 or 4 weeks in a sealed bag without getting moldy or stale, so you might want to order more than one package at a time.

I use La Tortilla Factory brand because they've got the lowest usable carb count of any I've found, just 3 grams. They're mostly made of fiber!

Beware: I have recently seen "low-carb" tortillas with deceptive packaging. The listed serving size turned out to equal only half of one tortilla. That's not a serving, as far as I'm concerned!

Nuts, Seeds, and Nut Butters

Nuts and Seeds

Low in carbohydrates and high in healthy fats, protein, and minerals, nuts and seeds are great foods for us. Not only are they delicious for snacking or for adding crunch to salads and stir-fries, but when ground, they can replace some of the flour in low-carb baked goods. In particular, you'll find quite a few recipes in this book calling for ground almonds, ground hazelnuts, and ground sunflower seeds. Since these ingredients can be pricey, you'll want to shop around. In particular, natural food stores often carry nuts and seeds in bulk at better prices than you'll find at the grocery store. I have also found that specialty ethnic groceries often have good prices on nuts. I get my best deal on almonds at my wonderful Middle Eastern grocery, Sahara Mart.

By the way, along with pumpkin and sun-flower seeds, you can buy sesame seeds in bulk at natural food stores for a fraction of what they'll cost you in a little shaker jar at the grocery store. Buy them "unhulled" and you'll get both more fiber and more calcium. You can also get unsweet-ened coconut flakes at natural food stores.

Flaxseed

Flaxseed comes from the same plant that gives us the fabric linen, and it is turning out to be one of the most nutritious seeds there is. Along with good-quality protein, flaxseeds have tons of soluble, cholesterol-reducing fiber and are a rich source of eicosapentaenoic acid (EPA), the same fats that make fish so heart-healthy.

Most of the recipes in this book that use flaxseed call for it to be ground up into a coarse meal. You can buy pre-ground flaxseed meal (Bob's Red Mill sells it, among others), but I much prefer to grind my own. The simple reason for this is that the fats in flaxseeds are very stable so long as the seeds are whole, but they go rancid pretty quickly after the seed coat is broken.

Grinding flaxseed is very easy if you have a food processor. Simply put the seeds in your ood processor with the S-blade in place, turn on the machine, and forget about it for about 5 minutes. (Yes, it takes that long!) I have heard from a few people that a far better tool is an electric coffee grinder, though you'll want to use one you don't use for coffee or clean it meticu-lously of coffee residue before using it. You can then add your flaxseed meal to whatever it is you're cooking.

If you don't have a food processor or a coffee grinder, you'll just have to buy flaxseed meal pre-ground. If you do, keep it in an airtight container, refrigerate or freeze it, and use it up as quickly as you can.

Nut Butters

The only peanut butter called for in this cookbook is "natural" peanut butter, the kind made from ground, roasted peanuts, peanut oil, and salt—nothing else. Most big grocery stores now carry natural peanut butter; it's the stuff with the layer of oil on top. The oil in standard peanut butter has been hydrogenated to keep it from separating out (that's what gives big name-brand peanut butters that extremely smooth, plastic consistency) and it's hard to think of anything worse for you than hydrogenated vegetable oil—except for sugar, of course, which is also added to standard peanut butter. Stick to the natural stuff.

Natural food stores carry not only natural peanut butter but also almond butter, sunflower butter, and sesame butter, generally called "tahini." All of these are useful for low-carbers. Keep all natural nut butters in the refrigerator unless you're going to eat them up within a week or two.

Seasonings

Bouillon or Broth Concentrates

Bouillon or broth concentrate comes in cubes, crystals, or liquids. It is generally full of salt and chemicals, and it doesn't taste notably like the animal it supposedly came from. It definitely does not make a suitable substitute for good-quality broth if you're making a pot of soup. However, these products can be useful for adding a little kick of flavor here and there, more as seasonings than as soups, and for this, I keep them on hand. I use a paste bouillon concentrate product called Better Than Bouillon, which comes in both chicken and beef flavors; I do find it preferable to the other kinds. But, use what you have on hand; it should be okay. If you can get the British product Bovril, it might even be better!

Chili Garlic Paste

This is a traditional Asian ingredient, consisting mostly, as the name strongly implies, of hot chilies and garlic. If, like me, you're a chili-head, you'll find endless ways to used the stuff once you have it on hand. Chili garlic paste comes in jars and keeps for months in the refrigerator. It's worth seeking out at Asian markets or in the international foods aisle of big grocery stores.

Chipotle Peppers Canned in Adobo Sauce

Chipotle peppers are smoked jalapeños. They're very different from regular jalapeños, and they're quite delicious. Look for them, canned in adobo sauce, in the Mexican foods section of big grocery stores. Because you're unlikely to use the whole can at once, you'll be happy to know that you can store your chipotles in the freezer, where they'll keep for months. I just float my can in a bowl of hot tap water for 5 minutes until it's thawed enough to peel off one or two peppers, then I put it right back in the freezer.

Diet-Rite Tangerine Soda

Just a few recipes in this book call for Diet-Rite tangerine soda. I've specified Diet-Rite brand because it's sweetened with sucralose (Splenda) rather than with aspartame. This is important because aspartame loses its sweetness when heated for any length of time while sucralose does not. Diet-Rite is nationally distributed, I understand, so you should be able to find it. If you can find another brand of tangerine- or orange-flavored diet soda that is sweetened with sucralose instead of aspartame, feel free to substitute it (and let me know!). However, do not substitute aspartame-sweetened soda. Your recipe won't come out right.

Fish Sauce or Nuoc Mam or Nam Pla

This is a salty, fermented seasoning widely used in Southeast Asian cooking. It's available in Asian grocery stores and in the Asian food section of big grocery stores. Grab it when you find it; it keeps nicely without refrigeration. Fish sauce is used in a few (really great) recipes in this book, and it adds an authentic flavor. In a pinch, you can substitute soy sauce, although you'll lose some of your Southeast Asian accent.

Fruit$_2$O

Say "fruit two-oh," as in H$_2$O with fruit flavor added. Fruit$_2$O is a new, nationally distributed beverage line consisting of water with natural fruit flavors and a touch of Splenda. It's a wonderful, refreshing thing to drink. More important for our purposes here, however,

is the fact that it lets us add fruit flavors to recipes without adding carbohydrates or calories. You'll find a few recipes calling for peach-flavored, lemon-flavored, and orange-flavored Fruit$_2$O in this book. Look for Fruit$_2$O in the water aisle of your grocery store.

Garlic

Garlic is a borderline vegetable. It's fairly high in carbohydrates, but it's very, very good for you. Surely you've heard all about garlic's nutritional prowess by now. Garlic also, of course, is an essential flavoring ingredient in many recipes. However, remember that there is an estimated 1 gram of carbohydrates per clove, so go easy. A "clove," by the way, is one of those little individual bits you get in a whole garlic bulb. If you read "clove" and use a whole bulb (also called a "head") of garlic, you'll get lots more carbs—and a lot stronger garlic flavor—than you expected.

I only use fresh garlic, except for in the occasional recipe that calls for a sprinkle-on seasoning blend. Nothing else tastes like the real thing. To my taste buds, even the jarred, chopped garlic in oil doesn't taste like fresh garlic. And we won't even talk about garlic powder. You may use jarred garlic if you like; ½ teaspoon should equal about 1 clove of fresh garlic. If you choose to use powdered garlic, well, I can't stop you, but I'm afraid I can't promise the recipes will taste the same either. Figure that ¼ teaspoon of garlic powder is roughly equivalent to 1 clove of fresh garlic.

By the way, the easiest way to crush a clove or two of garlic is to put the flat side of a big knife on top of it and smash it with your fist. Pick out the papery skin, which will now be easy, chop your garlic a bit more, and toss it into your dish. Keep in mind that the distinctive garlic aroma and flavor only develops after the cell walls are broken (that's why a pile of fresh garlic bulbs in the grocery store doesn't reek), so the more finely you crush or mince your garlic, the more flavor it will release.

Fresh Ginger

Many recipes in this book call for fresh ginger, sometimes called gingerroot. Fresh ginger is an essential ingredient in Asian cooking, and dried, powdered ginger is not a substitute. Fortunately, fresh ginger freezes beautifully; just drop your whole gingerroot (called a "hand" of ginger) into a resealable plastic freezer bag and toss it in the freezer. When the time comes to use it, pull it out, peel enough of the end for your immediate purposes, and grate it. (It will grate just fine while still frozen.) Throw the remaining root back in the bag and toss it back in the freezer.

Ground fresh ginger in oil is available in jars at some very comprehensive grocery stores. I like freshly grated ginger better, but this jarred ginger will also work in these recipes.

Low-Sugar Preserves

In particular, I find low-sugar apricot preserves to be a wonderfully versatile ingredient. I buy Smucker's brand and like it very much. This is lower in sugar by far than the "all fruit" preserves, which replace sugar with concentrated fruit juice. Folks, sugar from fruit juice is still sugar. I also have been known to use low-sugar orange marmalade and low-sugar raspberry preserves.

Vege-Sal

If you've read my newsletter, *Lowcarbezine!*, you know that I'm a big fan of Vege-Sal. What is Vege-Sal? It's a salt that's been seasoned, but don't think "seasoned salt." Vege-Sal is much milder than traditional seasoned salt. It's simply salt that's been blended with some dried, powdered vegetables. The flavor is quite subtle, but I think it improves all sorts of things. I've given you the choice between using regular salt or Vege-Sal in a wide variety of recipes. Don't worry, they'll come out fine with plain old salt, but I do think Vege-Sal adds a little something extra. Vege-Sal is also excellent sprinkled over chops and steaks in place of regular salt. Vege-Sal is made by Modern Products and is widely available in natural food stores.

Sweeteners

Blackstrap Molasses

What the heck is molasses doing in a low-carb cookbook? It's practically all carbohydrates, after all. Well, yes, but I've found that combining Splenda (see page 28) with a very small amount of molasses gives a good brown-sugar flavor to all sorts of recipes. Always use the darkest molasses you can find; the darker it is, the stronger the flavor and the lower the carb count. That's why I specify blackstrap—the darkest, strongest molasses there is. It's nice to know that blackstrap is also where all the minerals they take out of sugar end up, so it may be full of carbs, but at least it's not a nutritional wasteland. Still, I only use small amounts.

Most natural food stores carry blackstrap molasses, but if you can't find it, always buy the darkest molasses available, keeping in mind that most grocery store brands come in both light and dark varieties.

Why not use some of the artificial brown sugar–flavored sweeteners out there? Because I've tried them, and I haven't tasted even one I would be willing to buy again. Ick.

Polyols

Polyols, also known as sugar alcohols, are widely used in sugar-free candies and cookies. There are a variety of polyols, and their names all end with "tol": sorbitol, maltitol, mannitol, lactitol, xylitol, and the like. (Okay, there's one exception: isomalt. I don't know what happened there.) Polyols are, indeed, carbohydrates, but they are carbohydrates that are made up of molecules that are too big for the human gut to digest or absorb easily. As a result, polyols don't create much rise in blood sugar, nor much of an insulin release.

This does not, however, mean that polyols are completely unabsorbed. I have seen charts of the relative absorption rates of the various polyols, and I am here to tell you that you do, indeed, absorb carbohydrates from these sweeteners, in varying degrees. Sadly, the highest absorption rate seems to be for maltitol, which is the most widely used of the polyols. You absorb about 2.5 calories for every gram of maltitol you eat. Since you would absorb 4 calories for a gram of sugar, simple arithmetic tells us that you're absorbing more than half of the carbohydrate in the maltitol you eat.

Why do manufacturers use polyols instead of sucralose (Splenda)? Polyols are used in commercial sugar-free sweets because, unlike Splenda and other artificial sweeteners, they will give all of the textures that can be achieved with sugar. Polyols can be used to make crunchy toffee, chewy jelly beans, slick hard candies, moist brownies, and creamy chocolate, just as sugar can.

However, there are one or two problems with polyols. First of all, there is some feeling that different people have differing abilities to digest and absorb these very long-chain carbohydrates, which means that for some people, they may cause more of a derangement of blood sugar than for others. Once again, my only advice is to pay attention to your body.

The other problem with polyols is one that is inherent in all indigestible, unabsorbable carbohydrates: they can cause gas and diarrhea. Unabsorbed carbs ferment in your gut, you see, with intestinal gas as a result; it's the exact same thing that happens when people eat beans. I find that even half of a low-carb chocolate bar is enough to cause me social embarrassment several hours later. And I know of a case where eating a dozen and a half sugar-free taffies before bed caused the hapless consumer forty-five minutes of serious gut-cramping intestinal distress at four in the morning.

Don't think, by the way, that you can get around these effects of polyol consumption by taking enzymes that help you digest complex carbohydrates, such as Beano. It will work, but it will work by making the carbohydrates digestible and absorbable—meaning that any low-carb advantage is gone. I've known folks who have gained weight this way.

What we have here, then, is a sweetener that enforces moderation. Personally, I think this is a wonderful thing!

Polyols have become available for the home cook. I have started to use them in my recipes, because they do, indeed, offer a textural advantage. In particular, my cookie recipes were often too crumbly and sometimes too dry. Polyols solve this problem.

However, I have become increasingly wary of using polyols in any great quantity, because I am convinced we absorb more carbohydrate from them than the food processors want to let on. So here's what I do: When I feel that adding polyol sweetener to a recipe will improve the texture, I use just enough of the sweetener to get the effect I want, and then I add Splenda to bring the recipe up to the level of sweetness I'm looking for. This

has worked very well for me. It also makes the resulting food easier on both your gut and your blood sugar than it would be if I'd used all polyol.

I use erythritol whenever possible, in preference to maltitol, isomalt, or any of the other granular polyols. Why? Because erythritol has the lowest digestion and absorption rate of all the polyols—you get only 0.3 calories per gram of erythritol, which tells us that we're absorbing very little indeed. Erythritol also seems to be easier on the gut than the other polyols.

There are, however, recipes where I use other polyols. I use sugar-free dark chocolate not infrequently (and if you haven't tried the sugar-free chocolate yet, you're missing something!). I also use sugar-free pancake syrup and the new sugar-free imitation honey. Obviously, with these products, I'm stuck with whichever polyol the manufacturer used.

I also have found one application in which I can get only maltitol to work: Chocolate sauce. I have tried repeatedly to make a decent no-sugar-added chocolate sauce with erythritol, and it simply isn't happening. The stuff starts out looking all right, but as soon as it cools, it turns grainy on me. Maltitol makes a perfectly textured chocolate sauce. So for that purpose alone, I keep a little maltitol in my pantry.

I confess, I am at a loss as to how to count the carbohydrate grams that polyols add to my recipes, since I can't know which of the polyol sweeteners you'll be using, and they do, indeed, have differing absorption rates. Therefore, I have left them out of the nutritional analyses in this cookbook, which puts me on the same footing as the food processors, I guess. I have mentioned this in the recipe analyses. Be aware that you're probably getting at least a few grams of extra carb per serving in these recipes.

Splenda

Splenda is the latest artificial sweetener to hit the market, and it blows all of the competition clear out of the water! Feed nondieting friends and family Splenda-sweetened desserts, and they will never know that you didn't use sugar. It tastes that good.

Splenda has some other advantages. The table sweetener has been bulked so that it measures just like sugar, spoon-for-spoon and cup-for-cup. This makes adapting recipes much easier. Also, Splenda stands up to heat, unlike aspartame, which means you can use it for baked goods and other things that are heated for a while.

Be aware that Splenda granular—the stuff that comes in bulk in a box or the new "Baker's Bag"—is different than the stuff that comes in the little packets. The stuff in the packets is considerably sweeter—one packet equals 2 teaspoons granular. Whenever the ingredients list says only "Splenda," it means Splenda granular, the stuff you buy in bulk.

However, Splenda is not completely carb-free. Because of the maltodextrin used to bulk it, Splenda has about 0.5 gram of carbohydrates per teaspoon, or about $\frac{1}{8}$ of the carbohydrates of sugar. So count half a gram per teaspoon, 1½ grams per tablespoon (1.5 g), and 24 grams per cup (25 g). At this writing, McNeil, the company that makes Splenda, has no plans to release liquid Splenda in the United States, but I am hoping that they will change their minds. The liquid, available in some foreign countries, is carb-free. So while it will take a little more finesse to figure out quantities, it will also allow me to slash the carb counts of all sorts of recipes still further! Stay tuned.

Stevia/FOS Blend

Stevia is short for *Stevia rebaudiana*, a South American shrub with very sweet leaves. Stevia extract, a white powder from stevia leaves, is growing in popularity with people who don't care to eat sugar but who are nervous about artificial sweeteners.

However, stevia extract has a couple of faults: First, it's so extremely sweet that it's hard to know just how much to use in any given recipe. Second, it often has a bitter taste as well as a sweet one. This is why some smart food packagers have started blending stevia with fructooligosaccharide, also known as FOS. FOS is a sugar, but it's a sugar with a molecule so large that humans can neither digest nor absorb it, so it doesn't raise blood sugar or cause an insulin release. FOS has a nice, mild sweetness to it; indeed, it's only half as sweet as table sugar. This makes it the perfect partner for the too-sweet stevia.

This stevia/FOS blend is called for in just a few recipes in this book. It is available in many natural food stores, both in packets and in shaker jars. The brand I use is called SteviaPlus, and it's from a company called Sweet Leaf, but any stevia/FOS blend should do for the recipes that call for it.

My favorite use for this stevia/FOS blend, by the way, is to sweeten my yogurt. I think it tastes quite good, and FOS actually helps the good bacteria take hold in your gut, improving your health.

Sugar-Free Imitation Honey

This is one of those "I knew low carb had really hit the mainstream when . . ." products. I knew we were mainstream when my grocery store started carrying sugar-free imitation honey! This is a polyol syrup with flavoring added to make it taste like honey, and the two I've tried, one by Honey Tree and the other by Steele's, are not bad imitations.

Sugar-free imitation honey is becoming more and more available, and a useful little product it is—in baked goods it adds some extra moisture, while in things like barbecue sauces it adds the familiar syrupy quality. I can get sugar-free imitation honey here in Bloomington at my local Marsh grocery store, and I've heard that Wal-Mart now carries a brand. For that matter, many of the low-carb online retailers carry Steele's brand of imitation honey. In short, it shouldn't be too hard to get your hands on some.

Remember that sugar-free imitation honey is pretty much pure polyol. Slather it on your low-carb pancakes or biscuits with too free a hand, and you'll pay the price in gastric distress.

Sugar-Free Pancake Syrup

This is actually easy to find; all my local grocery stores carry it—indeed, they have more than one brand. It's usually with the regular pancake syrup, but it may be lurking with the diabetic or diet foods. It's just like regular pancake syrup, only it's made from polyols instead of sugar. I use it in small quantities in a few recipes to get a maple flavor.

Vegetables

Avocados

Several recipes in this book call for avocados. Be aware that the little, black, rough-skinned California avocados are lower in carbohydrate (and higher in healthy monounsaturated fat) than the big green Florida avocados. All nutritional analyses were done assuming you used California avocados.

Carrots

Because carrots have a higher glycemic index than many vegetables, a lot of low-carbers have started avoiding them with great zeal. But while carrots do have a fairly high blood sugar impact, you'd have to eat pounds of them to get the quantity that is used to test with. So don't freak when you see a carrot used here and there in these recipes, okay? I've kept the quantities small, just enough to add flavor, color, and a few vitamins. There's certainly not enough to torpedo your diet.

Frozen Vegetables

You'll notice that many of these recipes call for frozen vegetables, particularly broccoli, green beans, and cauliflower. I use these because I find them very convenient, and I think that the quality is quite good. If you like, you may certainly substitute fresh vegetables in any recipe. You will need to adjust the cooking time, and if the recipe calls for the vegetable to be used thawed but not cooked, you'll need to "blanch" your vegetables by boiling them for just three to five minutes.

It's important to know that frozen vegetables are not immortal, no matter how good your freezer is. Don't buy more than you can use up in four to six weeks, even if they're on sale. You'll end up throwing them away.

Onions

Onions are borderline vegetables. They're certainly higher in carbohydrates than, say, lettuce or cucumbers. However, they're loaded with valuable phytochemicals, so they're very healthful, and of course they add an unmatched flavor to all sorts of foods. Therefore I use onions a lot, but I try to use the smallest quantity that will give the desired flavor. Indeed, one of the most common things I do to cut carb counts on "borrowed" recipes is to cut back on the amount of onion used. If you have serious diabetes, you'll want to watch your quantities of onions pretty carefully, and maybe even cut back further on the amounts I've given.

Different types of onions are good for different things. There are mild onions, which are best used raw, and there are stronger onions, which are what you want if you're going to be cooking them. My favorite mild onions are sweet red onions; these are widely available, and you'll see I've used them quite a lot in the recipes here. However, if you prefer, you can substitute Vidalia or Bermuda onions anywhere I've specified sweet red onions. Scallions, also known as green onions, also are mild and are best eaten raw or quickly cooked in stir-fries. To me, scallions have their own flavor, and I generally don't substitute for them, but your kitchen won't blow up or anything if you use another sort of sweet onion in their place.

When a recipe simply says "onion," what I'm talking about is good old yellow globe onions, the ones you can buy 3 to 5 pounds at a time in net sacks. You'll be doing yourself a favor if you pick a sack with smallish onions in it so that when a recipe calls for just a ¼ or ½ cup (40 or 80 g) of chopped onion, you won't be left with half an onion. For the record, when I say "small onion," I mean one about 1½ inches (3.8 cm) in diameter, or about ¼ to ⅓ cup (40 to 50 g) when chopped. A medium onion would be about 2 inches (5 cm) in diameter and would yield between ½ and ¾ cup (80 and

120 g) when chopped. A large onion would be 2½ to 3 inches (6.3 to 7.5 cm) across and would yield about 1 cup (160 g) when chopped. Personally, I'm not so obsessive about exact carb counts that I bother to measure every scrap of onion I put in a dish; I think in terms of small, medium, and large onions, instead. If you prefer to be more exact, that's up to you.

Tomatoes and Tomato Products

Tomatoes are another borderline vegetable, but like onions, they are so nutritious, so flavorful, and so versatile that I'm reluctant to leave them out of low-carb cuisine entirely. After all, lycopene, the pigment that makes tomatoes red, has been shown to be a potent cancer-fighter, and who wants to miss out on something like that?

You'll notice that I call for canned tomatoes in a fair number of recipes, even in some where fresh tomatoes might do. This is because fresh tomatoes aren't very good for much of the year, whereas canned tomatoes are all canned at the height of ripeness. I'd rather have a good canned tomato in my sauce or soup than a mediocre fresh one. Since canned tomatoes are generally used with all the liquid that's in the can, the nutritional content doesn't suffer the way it does with most canned vegetables.

I also use plain canned tomato sauce, canned pizza sauce, canned pasta sauce, and jarred salsa. When choosing these products, you need to be aware that tomatoes, for some reason, inspire food packers to flights of sugar-fancy. They add sugar, corn syrup, and other carb-laden sweeteners to all sorts of tomato products, so it is very important that you *read the labels* on all tomato-based products to find the ones with no added sugar. And keep on reading them, even after you know what's in them. The good, cheap brand of salsa I used for quite a while showed up one day with "New, Improved!" on the label. Can you guess how they improved it? Right—they added sugar. So I found a new brand.

Here is a small note on ketchup: Commercially-made low-carb ketchup is now available and is often lower carb than my version. All recipes containing ketchup in this book are based on the nutritional analysis of my ketchup recipe.

Yeast

All of the bread recipes in this book were developed using plain old active dry yeast, not "bread machine yeast" and certainly not "rapid rise" yeast. Indeed, one of my testers had some spectacular failures using rapid rise yeast in her bread machine with one of my recipes, but the recipe worked brilliantly for another tester who used regular yeast.

The best place to buy yeast is at a good natural food store, where yeast is generally available in bulk for a tiny fraction of what it would cost you in little packets at the grocery store. Yeast should be stored in a cooler at the natural food store and the refrigerator at home.

One last note: Don't buy more yeast than you're likely to use up in four to six weeks. It will eventually die on you, and you'll end up with dough that won't rise. When you're using expensive ingredients, like we do, this is almost more than a body can bear.

Yogurt and Buttermilk

Yogurt and buttermilk both fall into the category of "cultured milks"—milk that has deliberately had a particular bacteria added to it and then been kept warm until the bacteria grows. These bacteria give yogurt and buttermilk their characteristic thick textures and tangy flavors.

If you look at the label of either of these cultured milk products, you'll see that the nutrition label claims 12 grams of carbohydrates per cup (and by the way, 8 grams of protein). This is the same carbohydrate count as the milk these products are made from. For this reason, many low-carbers avoid yogurt and buttermilk.

However, in *GO-Diet*, Dr. Goldberg and Dr. O'Mara explain that in actuality, most of the lactose (milk sugar) in the milk is converted into lactic acid by the bacteria. This is what gives these foods their sour taste. According to the doctors, the labels say "12 grams carbohydrate" largely because carbohydrate count is determined by "difference." What this means is that the calorie count is determined first. Then the protein and fat fractions are measured, and the number of calories they contribute is calculated. Any calories left over are assumed to come from carbohydrate.

However, Goldberg and O'Mara say that this is inaccurate in the cases of yogurt and buttermilk, and they say we should count just 4 grams of carbohydrates per cup for these cultured milks. Accordingly, I have added them back to my diet, and I have had no trouble with them, meaning no weight gain and no triggering of "blood sugar hunger." I really enjoy yogurt as a snack! Based on this, the carb counts in this book are calculated using that 4-grams-of-carbohydrates-per-cup figure.

Keep in mind that these numbers *only* apply to *plain* yogurt. The sweetened kind is always higher in carbohydrate. If you like fruit-flavored yogurt, flavor it yourself. You'll find a recipe for making your own plain yogurt, easy as pie, in Chapter 4, but any store-bought plain yogurt is fine.

2

Beverages

Florida Sunshine Smoothie

Mixed citrus flavors really sing together to make this smoothie a dose of morning sunshine in a glass.

1 cup (245 g) plain non-fat yogurt

½ cup (120 ml) Carb Countdown dairy beverage

¼ teaspoon pink grapefruit sugar-free drink mix powder

⅛ teaspoon orange sugar-free drink mix powder

⅛ teaspoon sugar-free lemonade mix

Combine all of the ingredients in your blender and blend until smooth and well combined.

Yield: 1 serving

Each with 19 g protein, 5 g carbohydrate, 0 g dietary fiber, 5 g usable carbs.

Honeydew Lime Cooler

1 cup (245 g) plain non-fat yogurt

½ cup (120 ml) Carb Countdown dairy beverage

½ cup (90 g) honeydew melon chunks or balls, frozen

¼ teaspoon lemon-lime sugar-free drink mix powder

Guar or xanthan

Combine all of the ingredients in your blender and blend until smooth and well combined.

Yield: 1 serving

Each with 19 g protein, 15 g carbohydrate, 1 g dietary fiber, 14 g usable carbs

Peach-Orange Pleasure

1 cup (245 g) plain non-fat yogurt

½ cup (120 ml) Carb Countdown dairy beverage

½ cup (125 g) sliced peaches, frozen

½ teaspoon orange sugar-free drink mix powder

½ teaspoon guar or xanthan

Combine all of the ingredients in your blender and blend until smooth and well combined.

Yield: 1 serving

Each with 20 g protein, 15 g carbohydrate, 2 g dietary fiber, 13 g usable carbs.

Apple Pie Smoothie

This smoothie is cinnamon-apple spicy, and the vanilla protein powder adds that à la mode note!

1 cup (245 g) plain non-fat yogurt

½ cup (120 ml) Carb Countdown dairy beverage

2 tablespoons (16 g) vanilla whey protein
   powder
2 tablespoons (28 ml) green apple sugar-free
   syrup
¼ teaspoon ground cinnamon
1 pinch ground cloves

Combine all of the ingredients in your blender and blend until smooth and well combined.

Yield: 1 serving

Each with 41 g protein, 8 g carbohydrate, 1 g dietary fiber, 7 g usable carbs.

Cantaloupe-Watermelon Smash

If you'd like to make this even more mixed-melon-y, use half cantaloupe and half honeydew, but the color won't be as pretty.

1 cup (245 g) plain non-fat yogurt
½ cup (120 ml) Carb Countdown dairy beverage
½ cup (90 g) cantaloupe chunks or balls, frozen
2 tablespoons (28 ml) watermelon sugar-free
   syrup
Guar or xanthan

Combine all of the ingredients in your blender and blend until smooth and well combined.

Yield: 1 serving

Each with 20 g protein, 12 g carbohydrate, 1 g dietary fiber, 11 g usable carbs.

Cherry Vanilla Sundae in a Glass

Do you love cherry-vanilla ice cream? Try this smoothie!

½ cup (70 g) no-sugar-added vanilla ice cream
1½ cups (355 ml) Carb Countdown dairy
   beverage
¼ cup (30 g) canned sour cherries in water,
   drained
2 tablespoons (16 g) vanilla whey protein
   powder
1 tablespoon (15 ml) cherry sugar-free syrup
½ teaspoon vanilla extract
Guar or xanthan

Combine all of the ingredients in your blender and blend until smooth and well combined.

Yield: 1 serving

Each with 40 g protein, 13 g carbohydrate, 1 g dietary fiber, 12 g usable carbs. *The carb count does not include the polyols in the sugar-free ice cream or syrup.

Razzleberry Smoothie

1 cup (245 g) plain non-fat yogurt
½ cup (120 ml) Carb Countdown dairy beverage
⅓ cup (85 g) raspberries, frozen
2 tablespoons (30 ml) strawberry sugar-free
   syrup

(continued on page 36)

Combine all of the ingredients in your blender and blend until smooth and well combined.

Yield: 1 serving

Each with 19 g protein, 10 g carbohydrate, 3 g dietary fiber, 7 g usable carbs. Carb count does not include polyol in syrup.

Strawberry-Kiwi Sparkler

You got your kiwi-strawberry soda, you got your strawberries, you got your kiwi. What could be easier? Fortunately, the combination of colors doesn't turn this smoothie brown. I was a little worried about that.

1 cup (245 g) plain non-fat yogurt
½ cup (120 ml) kiwi-strawberry Diet Rite soda
½ kiwi fruit, peeled (I didn't bother to freeze mine.)
5 medium strawberries, frozen

Combine all of the ingredients in your blender and blend until smooth and well combined.

Yield: 1 serving

Each with 14 g protein, 14 g carbohydrate, 3 g dietary fiber, 11 g usable carbs.

Blueberry Pancakes in a Glass

I figured if blueberries are good in pancakes, with syrup and all, why not try the same flavors in a smoothie?

1 cup (245 g) plain non-fat yogurt
½ cup (120 ml) Carb Countdown dairy beverage
½ cup (75 g) blueberries, frozen
2 tablespoons (30 ml) sugar-free pancake syrup
¼ teaspoon ground cinnamon

Combine all of the ingredients in your blender and blend until smooth and well combined.

Yield: 1 serving

Each with 19 g protein, 16 g carbohydrate, 2 g dietary fiber, 14 g usable carbs.* The carb count does not include the polyols in the sugar-free pancake syrup.

The King's Smoothie

Reportedly, Elvis's favorite food was fried peanut-butter-and-banana sandwiches on white bread. If he'd drunk these instead, he would have been healthier!

1½ cups (355 ml) Carb Countdown dairy beverage
3 tablespoons (50 g) natural peanut butter

2 tablespoons (16 g) vanilla whey protein
  powder
2 tablespoons (30 ml) banana sugar-free syrup
Guar or xanthan

Combine all of the ingredients in your blender and blend until smooth and well combined.

Yield: 1 serving

Each with 49 g protein, 17 g carbohydrate, 4 g dietary fiber, 13 g usable carbs.

Hazelnut-Amaretto Frozen Latte

This is nutty-good. Atkins makes hazelnut syrup, and DaVinci makes amaretto syrup.

½ cup (70 g) no-sugar-added vanilla ice cream
1 cup (240 ml) Carb Countdown dairy beverage
1 tablespoon (8 g) vanilla whey protein powder
1½ teaspoons instant coffee granules
1 tablespoon (15 ml) hazelnut sugar-free syrup
1 tablespoon (15 ml) amaretto sugar-free syrup
Guar or xanthan

Combine all of the ingredients in your blender and blend until smooth and well combined.

Yield: 1 serving

Each with 23 g protein, 5 g carbohydrate, trace dietary fiber, 5 g usable carbs. Carb count does not include polyol in syrups.

Almond Joy in a Glass

Make this without the almond extract if you like for a Mounds smoothie.

1½ cups (360 ml) chocolate-flavored Carb
  Countdown dairy beverage
2 tablespoons (16 g) chocolate whey protein
  powder
2 tablespoons (10 g) unsweetened cocoa
  powder
¼ teaspoon almond extract
¼ teaspoon coconut extract

Combine all of the ingredients in your blender and blend until smooth and well combined.

Yield: 1 serving

Each with 24 g protein, 8 g carbohydrate, 4 g dietary fiber, 4 g usable carbs.

Death by Chocolate

I put every chocolate ingredient I had on hand in this. Not surprisingly, it was great!

½ cup (70 g) no-sugar-added chocolate ice cream
1½ cups (360 ml) chocolate-flavored Carb
  Countdown dairy beverage
2 tablespoons (16 g) chocolate whey protein
  powder

(continued on page 38)

**2 tablespoons (30 ml) chocolate sugar-free
syrup**

**2 tablespoons (10 g) unsweetened cocoa
powder**

Combine all of the ingredients in your blender and
blend until smooth and well combined.

Yield: 1 serving

Each with 24 g protein, 8 g carbohydrate, 4 g dietary
fiber, 4 g usable carbs. Carb count does not include
polyol in syrup.

Root Beer Float

My sister keeps IBC Sugar-Free Root Beer and
Dreyer's Vanilla No-Sugar-Added Ice Cream in the
house for this purpose and this purpose alone.

**1 small scoop vanilla no-sugar-added ice cream
or 1 serving Atkins Endulge Super Premium
Ice Cream, vanilla flavor**

**1 can or bottle (12 ounces, or 360 ml) sugar-
free root beer, well chilled**

Put the ice cream in a large glass or mug and
pour the root beer over it. Serve with straws and
a long-handled spoon.

Yield: 1 serving

The carb count will depend on your brand of no-sugar-
added ice cream.

Chocolate Float

If you can get chocolate-flavored diet soda in your
region, this is a nice variant of the Root Beer Float.

**1 small scoop vanilla no-sugar-added ice cream
or 1 serving Atkins Endulge Super Premium
Ice Cream, vanilla flavor**

**1 can (12 ounces, or 360 ml) sugar-free
chocolate-fudge flavored soda, well chilled**

Put the ice cream in a large glass or mug and
pour the soda over it. Serve with a straw and a
long-handled spoon.

Yield: 1 serving

The carb count will depend on your brand of no-sugar-
added ice cream.

Canfield's makes diet chocolate-fudge flavored
soda. If you can't find it in a local grocery store,
there are several websites that sell it. Be aware,
however, that this is one of those love-it-or-hate-it
products. Faygo also makes a chocolate soda.

Dreamsicle Float

If you were a fan of Dreamsicles as a kid, you'll
love this float!

**1 small scoop no-sugar-added vanilla ice cream
or 1 serving Atkins Endulge Super Premium
Ice Cream, vanilla flavor**

**1 can (12 ounces, or 360 ml) sugar-free orange
soda, well chilled**

Put the ice cream in a large glass or mug and pour the soda over it. Serve with a straw and a long-handled spoon.

Yield: 1 serving

The carb count will depend on your brand of no-sugar-added ice cream.

Farmer's Soda

This is simpler than a float and a bit lower carb.

¼ cup (60 ml) heavy cream
1 can (12 ounces, or 360 ml) sugar-free soda, flavor of your choice, well chilled

Simply pour the cream into the bottom of a large glass and pour the soda over it.

Yield: 1 serving

3 grams of carbohydrates, no fiber, and no protein.

Cyndy Riser's Spiced Tea

This is a low-carb version of an old favorite.

1 package sugar-free Tang (makes 6 quarts [5.7 L])
²/₃ cup (80 g) instant tea mix
2 packages sugar-free lemonade (each makes 2 quarts [1.9 L])
1 tablespoon (6.3 g) ground cloves

1 tablespoon (6.9 g) ground cinnamon
2 cups (50 g) Splenda

Mix all ingredients. Store it in an airtight container. Add 1 heaping teaspoon to 1 cup (240 ml) hot water.

Yield: 40 servings

Each with trace protein; 1 g carbohydrate; trace dietary fiber; 1 g usable carb.

Spices can be adjusted to taste. Cindy likes a little more cinnamon and cloves than indicated. However, my family likes it just the way it is.

Sweet Tea

Sweet tea—iced tea with plenty of sugar in it—is the default summer beverage in the South. Here are the proportions for making a big pitcher of this classic, without the sugar.

6 cups (1.5 L) water
4 family-sized tea bags
1 cup (25 g) Splenda
Water to fill

Bring the 6 cups (1.5 L) of water to a boil in a saucepan and then add the tea bags. Let it simmer for just a minute and then remove from heat and let it sit for about 10 minutes. Remove the tea bags, squeezing them out in the process.

Add the Splenda and stir briefly to dissolve. Now pour this concentrate into a 1-gallon (3.8-L) pitcher and fill with water. Serve over ice!

(continued on page 40)

Yield: Makes 16 servings of 8 ounces (240 ml) each

3 grams of carbohydrate, a trace of fiber, a trace of protein.

Do you want to make this virtually zero carb? Order some Zero Carb Syrup Base Concentrate—a concentrated liquid form of Splenda—from www.locarber.com. If you want a version with no artificial sweeteners, you can try using stevia; I know people who like stevia even better than sugar or Splenda in iced tea. I favor a blend of stevia extract and FOS (a naturally occurring long-chain sugar too big to be digested by the human gut) called Stevia Plus—look for it at natural food stores. The label says 2 tablespoons equals 1 cup of sugar in sweetness, but I'd taste as you go.

Eggiweggnog

This is for those of you who are able to consume raw eggs. My husband would gladly have this for breakfast every day!

3 eggs
½ cup (120 ml) heavy cream
½ cup (120 ml) half-and-half
2 tablespoons (3 g) Splenda
1 teaspoon vanilla extract
Pinch of salt
Pinch of nutmeg

Put the eggs, heavy cream, half-and-half, Splenda, vanilla, and salt in a blender and run it for 30 seconds or so. Pour into glasses, sprinkle a little nutmeg on top, and drink up.

Yield: 2 servings

Each with 9 grams of carbohydrates, no fiber, and 11 grams of protein.

Cooked Eggnog

This is for you folks who cannot consume a raw egg—and it's mighty tasty, too. It just takes more work.

2 cups (475 ml) half-and-half
1 cup (240 ml) heavy cream
¼ cup (6 g) Splenda
1 teaspoon vanilla extract
¼ teaspoon salt
6 eggs
1 cup (240 ml) water
Pinch of nutmeg

In a big glass measuring cup, combine the half-and-half and cream. Microwave it at 70 percent power for 3 to 4 minutes or until it's very warm through but not boiling. (This is simply a time-saver and is not essential; if you prefer, you can simply heat the half-and-half and cream over a low flame in the saucepan you'll use to finish the recipe.)

After microwaving, pour the half-and-half mixture into a heavy-bottomed saucepan and whisk in the Splenda, vanilla, salt, and eggs. Turn the burner to lowest heat (if you have a heat diffuser or a double boiler, this would be a good time to use it) and stand there and stir your eggnog constantly until it's thick enough to coat a metal spoon with a thin film. This will, I'm sorry to say, take at least 5 minutes and maybe as many as 20.

Stir in the water and chill. Sprinkle a little nutmeg on each serving and feel free to spike this, if you like!

Yield: About 6 servings of 1 cup (240 ml)

Each with 5 grams of carbohydrates, a trace of fiber, and 9 grams of protein.

Chai

My darling friend Nicole is a devotee of this spiced Indian tea. She suggested I come up with a low-carb version, and here it is. Make up a batch, and your whole house will smell wonderful.

1 tablespoon (6 g) fennel seed or anise seed
6 green cardamom pods
12 whole cloves
1 cinnamon stick
¼ inch (6 mm) of fresh ginger root, thinly sliced
¼ teaspoon whole black peppercorns
2 bay leaves
7 cups (1.7 L) water
2 tablespoons (13.5 g) loose Darjeeling tea
⅓ cup (8 g) Splenda
⅛ tablespoon blackstrap molasses
½ cup (120 ml) heavy cream mixed with
½ cup (120 ml) water, or 1 cup (240 ml)
half-and-half

Combine the fennel, cardamom, cloves, cinnamon, ginger, peppercorns, bay leaf, and water. Bring this to a simmer, and let it simmer for 5 minutes.

Add the tea, turn off the heat, cover, and let the mixture steep for 10 minutes.

Strain and stir in the Splenda, molasses, and cream. You can refrigerate this for a day or two and reheat it in the microwave whenever you want a cup.

Yield: 8 servings of 1 cup (240 ml) each.

Made with heavy cream, each serving will have about 7 grams of carbohydrates, no fiber (you've strained it out), and 2 grams of protein. Made with half-and-half, it'll have 8 grams of carbs, no fiber, and 2 grams of protein.

Cocoa

The lowest carbohydrate hot chocolate mix on the market is Swiss Miss Diet, but this is much better.

1 cup (240 ml) heavy cream
1 cup (240 ml) water
2 tablespoons (11 g) unsweetened cocoa
powder
1½ or 2 tablespoons (2 or 3 g) Splenda
2 tablespoons (16 g) vanilla whey protein
powder
Tiny pinch of salt

Over the lowest possible heat (it doesn't hurt to use a heat diffuser or a double-boiler) combine the cream and water. When they're starting to get warm, add the cocoa, Splenda, protein powder, and salt; whisk until well combined. Bring just barely to a simmer and then pour into cups.

Yield: 2 servings

Each with 10 grams of carbohydrates and 2 grams of fiber, for a total of 8 grams of usable carbs and 15 grams of protein.

(continued on page 42)

The amount of protein in this cocoa means that a cup of this doesn't make a bad breakfast. And for grownups, this is very nice with a shot of Mockahlua or Mochahlua (page 46) in it—but not in the morning!

Hot Cinnamon Mocha

Assemble this in your slow cooker before going skating, caroling, or to a football game and have a winter party waiting when you get home!

½ gallon (1.9 L) chocolate-flavored Carb
   Countdown dairy beverage
2 cinnamon sticks
3 tablespoons (9 g) instant coffee granules
1½ teaspoons vanilla extract

Combine everything in your slow cooker and give it a stir. Cover the slow cooker, set it to high, and let it cook for 3 hours. Turn the slow cooker to low and serve from the slow cooker.

If it's a grown-up party, put a bottle of Mockahlua (page 46) on the side for spiking!

Yield: 10 servings

Each with 10 g protein, 5 g carbohydrate, 2 g dietary fiber, 3 g usable carbs.

Creamy Vanilla Coffee

Reader Honey Ashton sends this sweet little treat and says it's also good iced.

1 hot cup (240 ml) decaffeinated coffee
2 tablespoons (56 g) low-carb vanilla shake
   meal-replacement powder
1 to 2 teaspoons sugar-free vanilla coffee-
   flavoring syrup
Cinnamon (optional)

Combine the coffee, vanilla shake powder, and coffee-flavoring syrup. Garnish with cinnamon (if using).

Yield: 1 serving

No more than 2 grams of carbohydrates, no fiber, and no protein. Carb count does not include polyol in syrup.

Irish Coffee

If you're having this after dinner, you may want to use decaf instead of regular coffee.

2 ounces (60 ml) Irish whisky
6 ounces (170 ml) hot coffee
1 to 2 teaspoons Splenda
1 tablespoon Whipped Topping (page 552)

Put the whisky into a stemmed Irish coffee glass or a mug. Fill with coffee. Stir in Splenda and top with whipped cream.

Yield: 1 serving

2 grams of carbohydrates, no fiber, and only a trace of protein.

Café Chantilly

This is a classic!

1 tablespoon (15 ml) cognac
4 ounces (120 ml) brewed coffee
Unsweetened whipped cream (Whip chilled
heavy cream by itself with an electric mixer.)

Just stir the cognac into the coffee, top with a dollop of whipped cream, and serve.

Yield: 1 serving, with just 1 gram of carbohydrates, no fiber, and no protein.

Each serving has only 65 calories!

Mexican Coffee

Traditionally this is made with pilloncillo sugar—Mexican brown sugar—and milk, but that's too many carbs for us. Here's the reduced-carb version.

6 ounces (170 ml) brewed coffee
2 to 3 tablespoons (30 to 45 ml) heavy cream
2 teaspoons Splenda
2 drops blackstrap molasses*
Tiny pinch of ground cinnamon
Tiny pinch of ground cloves

Pour the coffee and stir in the cream, Splenda, and molasses. Sprinkle the spices over the top and serve.

Yield: 1 serving

3 grams of carbohydrates, the merest trace of fiber, and 1 gram of protein.

*It helps to keep your blackstrap molasses in a squeeze bottle. I buy mine in bulk from my natural food store and keep it in one of those "honey bears."

Café Vienna

This is either coffee for chocolate lovers or chocolate for coffee lovers.

6 ounces (170 ml) brewed coffee
2 tablespoons (30 ml) sugar-free chocolate
coffee flavoring syrup
2 tablespoons (30 ml) heavy cream
Tiny pinch of ground cinnamon

Pour the coffee, stir in the chocolate syrup and heavy cream, dust the cinnamon over the top, and serve.

Yield: 1 serving

Assuming you use Atkins or Da Vinci coffee flavoring syrup (which are made with Splenda instead of polyols), this will have 2 grams of carbohydrates, a trace of fiber, and 1 gram of protein.

(continued on page 44)

If you'd like to spiff this up for company, use whipped cream (see Whipped Topping on page 552) instead of the plain heavy cream.

Chocolate Orange Coffee

I came up with this one morning when my husband was out of cream for his coffee—it kept me from having to run out to the store before breakfast, and he loved it!

6 ounces (170 ml) brewed coffee
1 tablespoon (15 ml) sugar-free chocolate coffee flavoring syrup
1 or 2 drops orange extract

Pour the coffee and stir in the syrup and the extract. That's all!

Yield: 1 serving

Again assuming you use Atkins or Da Vinci brand syrup, you'll have just 1 gram of carbohydrates here, no fiber, and no protein.

Café Incontro

This is for adults only, of course!

6 ounces (170 ml) brewed coffee
1 scant shot (about 1 ounce, 28 ml) dark rum
2 teaspoons sugar-free chocolate coffee flavoring syrup
Splenda to taste, if desired

Pour the coffee, add the rum, syrup, and Splenda, and serve. That's all!

Yield: 1 serving

Just 1 gram of carbohydrates (again, we're talking the Atkins or Da Vinci syrup), no fiber, and no protein. Add 0.5 grams of carbohydrates for each teaspoon of Splenda you add.

Kay's Hot Rum Toddy

This a delicious winter libation is for adults only! The rum is carb-free, but it will slow down your metabolism, so go easy.

2¼ cups (56 g) Splenda
2 teaspoons blackstrap molasses
1 teaspoon ground nutmeg
1 teaspoon ground cinnamon
1 teaspoon ground cloves
1 teaspoon ground cardamom
1 bottle (750 ml) top-quality dark rum

Put the Splenda, molasses, nutmeg, cinnamon, cloves, and cardamom in a food processor with the S-blade in place. Process until it's smooth and creamy, scraping down the sides of the processor once or twice to make sure everything combines evenly.

Scoop this "batter" mixture into a snap-top container and keep it in the fridge. (The batter will keep well, and that means you can make only a serving or two at a time, if you like.)

To serve the toddy, warm a coffee mug by filling it with boiling water and pouring it out. Then fill it again, halfway, with more boiling water. Add 1 to 2 tablespoons of the batter and stir until it dissolves into the water (a small whisk works well for this). Add two shots of dark rum, stir, and sip.

Yield: About 12 servings.

Each 2 tablespoon serving of batter will have 5 grams of carbohydrates, a trace of fiber, and a trace of protein.

Kay says that one theory of hot-toddy making is that it is impossible to use too much batter and you should keep stirring more in until you are bored with stirring. Another theory of hot toddy making is that it is impossible to use too much rum, and that you should keep stirring in more until your friends panic. Use your best judgment.

Laure's Homemade LC "Bailey's Mae"

This is named in honor of Laure's chocolate lab! Barbo Gold, our tester, had a really good time testing this recipe and says it's tops.

2 cups (480 ml) any booze (rum, vodka, bourbon, Southern Comfort, or brandy)
14 ounces (415 ml) heavy cream
1 cup (240 ml) half-and-half
2 tablespoons (15 ml) no-sugar chocolate syrup (Laure uses Walden Farms brand)
2 teaspoons instant coffee granules
1 teaspoon vanilla

½ cup (12 g) Splenda
½ teaspoon almond extract

Combine all in a blender. Put in a tall jar. Store in fridge. Stir before serving. YUM!

Yield: 10 servings, ½ cup (120 ml) each

Each with 2 g protein; 2 g carbs; no fiber; 2 g usable carbs. Carb count does not include polyol in syrup.

Dana Massey's Low-Carb Irish Cream Liqueur

Our tester, Barbo Gold, loved this. (Come to think of it, how come Barbo gets all the really fun recipes?)

1¼ cups (300 ml) heavy whipping cream
3 egg yolks
¼ cup (6 g) Splenda
¼ cup (60 g) erythritol (can be replaced with another ¼ cup [6 g] Splenda)
1 tablespoon (8 g) DiabetiSweet

Whisk all ingredients together in the order given in a saucepan over low heat. Stir constantly until thickened and be careful not to overcook. Cool completely and set aside.

3 eggs (or equivalent egg substitute, if you prefer not to use raw egg)

(continued on page 46)

2 tablespoons (30 ml) sugar-free chocolate syrup (like Hershey's syrup; Walden Farms makes one and so does Sorbee)

2 tablespoons (30 ml) vanilla extract

1 tablespoon (3 g) instant coffee powder (not granular)

1/3 cup (80 ml) water

1 1/3 cups (320 ml) Irish Whiskey

In a blender, blend eggs, chocolate syrup, vanilla, coffee powder, and water until well mixed. Stir in whipping cream mixture and whiskey (don't blend). Pour into container with a tight-fitting lid. Refrigerate up to 3 weeks. Enjoy!

Yield: About 20 1½-ounce (40 ml) "shots"

Each with 2 g protein; 1 g carbohydrate; 0 g dietary fiber; 1 g usable carb. Carb count does not include the polyol in the syrup.

Dana's note: Feel free to use a combined 5 tablespoons of any polyol sweetener in place of the erythritol and DiabetiSweet.

Mockahlua

My sister, a longtime Kahlua fan, says this is addictive. And my husband demanded to know, "How did you do that?" You can make this with decaf if caffeine bothers you. This recipe makes quite a lot, but don't worry about that; 100-proof vodka's a darned good preservative. Your Mockahlua will keep indefinitely.

2½ cups (570 ml) water

3 cups (75 g) Splenda

3 tablespoons (9 g) instant coffee granules

1 teaspoon vanilla

1 bottle (750 ml) 100-proof vodka (Use the cheap stuff.)

In a large pitcher or measuring cup, combine the water, Splenda, coffee crystals, and vanilla. Stir until the coffee and Splenda are completely dissolved.

Pour the mixture through a funnel into a 1.5- or 2-liter bottle. (A clean 1.5-liter wine bottle works fine, so long as you've saved the cork.) Pour in the vodka. Cork and shake well.

Yield: 32 servings of 1½ ounces (42 ml)—a standard "shot."

Each will have 2 grams of carbohydrates, no fiber, and the merest trace of protein.

Variation: Mochahlua. Try this one if you like a little chocolate with your coffee. Just cut the water back to 1½ cups (360 ml) and substitute a 12-ounce (355 ml) bottle of sugar-free chocolate coffee flavoring syrup for the Splenda and vanilla. This has only a trace of carbohydrates per shot, because the liquid Splenda used to sweeten the chocolate coffee flavoring syrup doesn't have the maltodextrin used to bulk the granular Splenda.

Variation: Mockahlua and Cream. This makes a nice "little something" to serve at the end of a dinner party, in lieu of a heavier dessert. For each serving you'll need a shot of Mockahlua (or Mochahlua) and 2 shots of heavy cream. Simply mix and sip! Each serving has 4 grams of carbohydrates, no fiber, and 2 grams of protein.

Black Russian

1 shot (1½ ounces, or 42 ml) vodka
½ shot (¾ ounce, or 20 ml) Mockahlua

Just pour both liquors over ice in a rocks glass. That's it!

Yield: 1 serving

2 grams of carbohydrate, no fiber, no protein.

White Russian

1 shot (1½ ounces, or 42 ml) vodka
½ shot (¾ ounce, or 20 ml) Mockahlua
1 shot (1½ ounces, or 42 ml) heavy cream

Combine and pour over ice if desired.

Yield: 1 serving

3 grams of carbohydrate, 0 grams fiber, 1 gram protein.

Frozen White Russian

This is seriously decadent and not as low carb as some of our other beverages—I'd recommend stopping at one! Still, this makes a great dessert for an adults-only cookout.

1 shot (1½ ounces, or 42 ml) Mockahlua
1 shot (1½ ounces, or 42 ml) vodka
½ cup (65 g) sugar-free vanilla ice cream

Put everything in a blender and run the blender until well combined. Pour into a smallish glass—a rocks glass or a wineglass will work nicely.

Yield: 1 serving

The carb count on this will depend on the brand of sugar-free vanilla ice cream you use. If you use one of the lowest-carb—Atkins Endulge or Breyer's Carb Smart—your drink will have 6 grams of carbohydrate, 0 grams fiber, 3 grams protein. And it will be unbelievably, decadently delicious.

Gin Rickey

This old-fashioned cocktail is one of my new favorites!

1 tablespoon lime juice
1 shot (1½ ounces, or 42 ml) gin
Club soda to fill

Put the lime juice and gin in the bottom of a tall glass. Fill with ice and then add club soda to the top.

Yield: 1 serving

1 gram of carbohydrate, a trace of fiber, and a trace of protein.

Daiquiri

Forget all those strawberry daiquiris and banana daiquiris—this is the original, and it's remarkably refreshing.

(continued on page 48)

1 shot (1½ ounces, or 42 ml) lime juice

2 shots (3 ounces, or 85 ml) white rum

1 tablespoon (1.5 g) Splenda

You can make this two ways: on the rocks or frozen. For a daiquiri on the rocks, simply mix all the ingredients well and pour over ice. For a frozen daiquiri, plunk all the ingredients plus 3 to 4 ice cubes in your blender and blend until the ice is pulverized.

Yield: 1 serving

4 grams of carbohydrate, no fiber, no protein (hah!).

Dana Massey's Low-Carb Strawberry Daiquiris

This is a sweet indulgence, so have fun!

3 to 4 cups (330 to 440 g) fresh or frozen unsweetened strawberries, thawed if using frozen

½ to ¾ cup (120 to 180 ml) light rum

¼ cup (60 ml) lime juice (Don't use Rose's bottled lime juice—it has sugar added.)

¼ to ⅓ cup (6 to 8 g) Splenda (you may use a different sugar substitute; adjust measurements accordingly)

Crushed ice

Place strawberries, rum, lime juice, and sugar substitute in a blender. Blend until smooth. Add ice; continue to blend until well combined.

Yield: 4 to 6 servings

Assuming 4, each will have 1 g protein; 11 g carbohydrate; 3 g dietary fiber; 8 g usable carbs.

To make Low-Carb Strawberry Margaritas, replace the rum with tequila.

Dana Massey's note: We use erythritol in this recipe.

Dana Carpender's note: I'd probably use Splenda, myself.

Margarita Fizz

1 shot (1½ ounces, or 42 ml) tequila

1 shot (1½ ounces, or 42 ml) lime juice

1½ teaspoons Splenda

8 ounces (240 ml) unsweetened orange-flavored sparkling water

Put the tequila, lime juice, and Splenda in the bottom of a tall glass and stir. Fill with ice and pour in orange-flavored sparkling water to fill.

Yield: 1 serving

4 grams of carbohydrate, a trace of fiber, and a trace of protein.

Seabreeze Sunrise

If you like fruity drinks, try this!

1 shot (1½ ounces, or 42 ml) tequila

1 shot (1½ ounces, or 42 ml) low-sugar cranberry juice cocktail (Ocean Spray makes one.)

8 ounces (240 ml) pink grapefruit–flavored Crystal Light (or any no-sugar grapefruit-flavored drink mix), prepared

Combine the tequila and cranberry juice cocktail in a tall glass, fill with ice, and pour in the grapefruit-flavored drink.

Yield: 1 serving

3 grams of carbohydrate, 0 grams fiber, and 0 grams protein.

Hard Lemonade

Commercially made hard lemonade is actually a malt beverage—in the same class as beer. That makes it high carb right there, plus it has sugar. But how hard can it be to make your own?

1 shot (1½ ounces, or 42 ml) vodka
Sugar-free lemonade (Both Country Time and Wyler's make a sugar-free lemonade mix.)

Just fill a tall glass with ice, pour in the vodka, and fill with sugar-free lemonade. Garnish with a lemon slice, if you like!

Yield: 1 serving

1 gram carbohydrate, 0 grams fiber, and 0 grams protein.

Mojito

I'm tragically unhip. I discovered the Mojito while writing this book and fell in love with it—only to learn it had been the hot drink for at least a year!

If you haven't tried this classic Cuban drink, you must. (Don't have fresh mint? There's nothing easier to grow—indeed, plant mint and it will threaten to take over your yard!)

1 shot (1½ ounces, or 42 ml) white rum
1 tablespoon (15 ml) lime juice
1 sprig fresh mint
1 teaspoon Splenda
Club soda to fill

Combine the rum, lime juice, mint, and Splenda in the bottom of a tall glass. Using the back of a spoon, press the mint well to release the flavor and stir everything together. Now fill the glass with ice, then with club soda.

Yield: 1 serving

2 grams carbohydrate, a trace of fiber, and a trace of protein.

Wine Spritzer

This is a great drink if you want something mild that you can sip on for a while without getting incapacitated. (A good thing to bear in mind if you have to play around with the grill rack and manipulate hot coals!)

3 ounces (90 ml) dry red wine
Unsweetened berry-flavored sparkling water

Pour the wine over ice in a tall glass and pour in berry-flavored sparkling water to fill.

(continued on page 50)

Yield: 1 serving

1 gram carbohydrate, 0 grams fiber, a trace of protein.

Wine Cooler

You have a lot of leeway here! Basically, you're combining wine and diet soda. Experiment to find your favorite combinations.

3 to 5 ounces (90 to 150 ml) dry wine—red or white, whichever you prefer
Diet soda—consider trying lemon-lime, red raspberry, tangerine or orange, or grapefruit (Fresca)

Pour the wine over ice in a tall glass and fill with the soda of your choice.

Yield: 1 serving

Assuming you use 3 ounces (90 ml) of wine, this will have about 1 gram of carbohydrate, 0 grams fiber, and a trace of protein.

Salty Dog

This old summer favorite is usually made with grapefruit juice—at 22 grams of carbohydrate per cup. We'd better use the pink grapefruit–flavored Crystal Light!

Coarse salt
1 shot (1½ ounces, or 42 ml) gin
Crystal Light pink grapefruit–flavored sugar-free drink mix (or any no-sugar grapefruit-flavored drink mix), prepared

Rim a tall glass with salt. Fill it with ice and add the gin and Crystal Light grapefruit-flavored drink.

Yield: 1 serving

1 gram carbohydrate, 0 grams fiber, 0 grams protein.

Dark and Stormy

A classic Dark and Stormy is made with ginger beer, not ginger ale, but there is no such thing as low-carb ginger beer, at least that I know of. So, I tried it with diet ginger ale and got a very tasty drink!

1 shot (1½ ounces, or 42 ml) dark rum
1 shot (1½ ounces, or 42 ml) lime juice
Vernor's Diet Ginger Ale (I like to use Vernor's because it's particularly crisp, but if you can't find it, use any diet ginger ale you can get.)

Put the rum and lime juice in a tall glass, add ice, and fill with ginger ale.

Yield: 1 serving

3 grams of carbohydrate, a trace of fiber, and a trace of protein.

Shandy

This is a classic British summer cooler. If you make two, you'll use up all the beer and all the ginger ale!

6 ounces (180 ml) chilled light beer
6 ounces (180 ml) chilled diet ginger ale

Simply combine the two in a tall beer glass.

Yield: 1 serving

Using the lowest-carb light beer, this will have less than 2 grams of carbohydrate per serving, with no fiber, and a trace of protein.

Cuba Libre

I bet most of you thought of this on your own, but here's for those of you who didn't.

1 shot (1½ ounces, or 42 ml) white rum
Diet cola
Wedge of lime

Put the shot of rum in a tall glass, fill with ice, and pour diet cola to the top. Squeeze in a wedge of lime.

Yield: 1 serving

2 grams of carbohydrate, a trace of fiber, and a trace of protein.

Sangria

This is a refreshing summer favorite!

1½-liter bottle of dry red wine—burgundy, merlot, or the like (You can use the cheap stuff!)
²/₃ cup (16 g) Splenda
½ teaspoon orange extract

½ teaspoon lemon extract
1 orange
1 lemon
1 lime
Orange- or lemon-flavored unsweetened sparkling water

Pour the wine into a nonreactive bowl. Stir in the Splenda and the extracts.

Now, you have to decide if you're going to serve your sangria from a punch bowl or put it into a clean old jug. Me, I put it in an old 1-gallon (3.8 L) vinegar jug, but I was taking my sangria camping.

If you're going to put your sangria in a punch bowl, simply scrub your fruit and slice it as thin as humanly possible. Put it in the punch bowl with the wine/Splenda mixture and let the whole thing macerate for an hour or so before serving.

If you're using a jug, you'll need to cut your fruit into small chunks that will fit through the neck. Force the fruit into the jug and then pour the wine/Splenda mixture over it. Again, let it macerate for at least an hour.

When the time comes to serve your sangria, fill a tall glass with ice, pour in 4 ounces (120 ml) of the wine mixture, and fill to the top with lemon- or orange-flavored sparkling water.

Yield: 12 servings

Each with 6 grams of carbohydrate (assuming you actually eat all the fruit, which you won't—I'm figuring it's really between 4 and 5 grams), a trace of fiber, and a trace of protein.

3

Appetizers and Snacks

Wicked Wings

Once you try these, you'll understand the name—they're "wicked good"! These are a bit messy and time-consuming to make, but they're worth every minute. They'll impress the heck out of your friends too, and you'll wish you'd made more of them. They also taste great the next day.

4 pounds (1.8 kg) chicken wings
1 cup (100 g) grated Parmesan cheese
2 tablespoons (2.6 g) dried parsley
1 tablespoon (5.4 g) dried oregano
2 teaspoons paprika
1 teaspoon salt
½ teaspoon pepper
½ cup butter

Preheat the oven to 350°F (180°C, or gas mark 4). Line a shallow baking pan with foil. (Do not omit this step, or you'll still be scrubbing the pan a week later.)

Cut the wings into "drummettes," saving the pointy tips. (Not sure what to do with those wing tips? Freeze them for soup—they make great broth.)

Combine the Parmesan cheese and the parsley, oregano, paprika, salt, and pepper in a bowl.

Melt the butter in a shallow bowl or pan.

Dip each drumstick in butter, roll in the cheese and seasoning mixture, and arrange in the foil-lined pan.

Bake for 1 hour—and then kick yourself for not having made a double recipe!

Yield: About 50 pieces

Each with only a trace of carbohydrates, a trace of fiber, and 4 grams of protein.

Chinese Peanut Wings

If you love Chinese barbecued spareribs, try making these.

¼ cup (60 ml) soy sauce
3 tablespoons (4.5 g) Splenda
3 tablespoons (48 g) natural peanut butter
2 tablespoons (30 ml) dry sherry
1 tablespoon (15 ml) oil
1 tablespoon (15 ml) apple cider vinegar
2 teaspoons Chinese Five Spice powder
¼ teaspoon red pepper flakes (or more, if you want them hotter)
1 clove garlic, crushed
12 chicken wings or 24 drumettes

Preheat the oven to 325°F (170°C, or gas mark 3).

Put the soy sauce, Splenda, peanut butter, sherry, oil, vinegar, spice powder, pepper flakes, and garlic in a blender or food processor and blend well.

If you have whole chicken wings and want to cut them into "drummettes," do it now. (This is a matter of preference and is not essential.)

Arrange the wings in a large baking pan, pour the blended sauce over them, and then turn them over to coat on all sides. Let them sit for at least half an hour (an hour is even better).

Bake the wings for an hour, turning every 20 minutes during baking.

When the wings are done, put them on a serving platter and scrape the sauce from the pan back into the blender or food processor.

(continued on page 54)

Blend again for just a moment to make it smooth and serve with the wings.

Yield: 24 pieces

Each with 1 gram of carbohydrates, a trace of fiber, and 5 grams of protein.

Chili Lime Wings

1 tablespoon (7 g) paprika
1 teaspoon chili powder
1 teaspoon dried oregano, crumbled
¼ teaspoon salt
¼ teaspoon pepper
½ teaspoon garlic powder
1½ pounds (680 g) chicken wings
3 tablespoons (45 ml) olive oil
1 lime, cut in wedges

Preheat oven to 375°F (190°C, or gas mark 5).

In a small bowl, combine the paprika and the next 5 ingredients (through garlic powder).

If you like individual "drummettes," cut your wings up (or you can buy them that way!). Arrange them in a pan and brush them with the olive oil. Now sprinkle the paprika mixture evenly over your wings.

Roast for at least 45 minutes, and an hour isn't likely to hurt. You want them crispy! If you have a rotisserie with a basket, that's a great way to cook these as well.

Serve hot, with wedges of lime to squeeze over the wings.

Yield: About 14 pieces

Each with 5 g protein; 1 g carbohydrate; trace dietary fiber; 1 g usable carb.

Chinese Sticky Wings

Mmmmm—everyone loves Chinese chicken wings.

3 pounds (1.4 kg) chicken wings
¼ cup (60 ml) dry sherry
¼ cup (60 ml) soy sauce
¼ cup (60 ml) sugar-free imitation honey
1 tablespoon (6 g) grated ginger root
1 clove garlic
½ teaspoon chili garlic paste

Cut your wings into "drummettes" if they are whole. Put your wings in a big resealable plastic bag.

Mix together everything else, reserving some marinade for basting, and pour the rest into the bag. Seal the bag, pressing out the air as you go. Turn the bag a few times to coat the wings and throw it in the fridge for a few hours (a whole day is brilliant).

Preheat oven to 375°F (190°C, or gas mark 5). Pull out the bag, pour off the marinade, and arrange the wings in a shallow baking pan. Give them a good hour in the oven, basting every 15 minutes with the reserved marinade. Use a clean utensil each time you baste.

Serve with plenty of napkins!

Yield: About 28 pieces

Each with 5 g protein; trace carbohydrate; trace dietary fiber; 0 usable carb. Carb count does not include polyols in the sugar-free imitation honey.

Lemon Soy Chicken Wings

These are Chinese-y too, just in a different sort of a way.

8 whole chicken wings
3 cloves garlic
1 tablespoon (6 g) grated ginger root
2 tablespoons (30 ml) lemon juice
3 tablespoons (45 ml) soy sauce
1 tablespoon (15 ml) sugar-free imitation honey
1 tablespoon (1.5 g) Splenda
½ teaspoon chili powder

If you like your wings cut into "drummettes," do that first. This keeps being repeated. Put wings in a resealable plastic bag.

Combine everything else. Reserve some liquid for basting and pour the rest over the wings. Seal the bag, pressing out the air as you go, and turn it a few times to coat. Let wings marinate for at least an hour, and all day won't hurt a bit.

Preheat oven to 375°F (190°C, or gas mark 5). While the oven's heating, drain the marinade off of the wings. Arrange wings in a shallow baking pan and roast for 1 hour, basting two or three times with the reserved marinade and using a clean utensil each time.

Yield: 16 pieces

Each with 5 g protein; 1 g carbohydrate; trace dietary fiber; 1 g usable carb. Carb count does not include polyol in sugar-free honey.

Lemon-Mustard Chicken Wings

10 chicken wings
3 tablespoons (45 ml) brown mustard
2 tablespoons (3 g) Splenda
2 tablespoons (30 ml) lemon juice
½ teaspoon chili paste
¼ teaspoon salt or Vege-Sal

Preheat your oven to 400°F (200°C, or gas mark 6). Cut wings into drummettes. Arrange the wings in a baking pan.

Mix together everything else. Brush half of the mixture over the wings and bake for 20 to 25 minutes. Turn the wings, brush with the rest of the mustard mixture using a clean utensil, and bake for another 20 to 25 minutes. Serve.

Yield: 20 pieces

Each with 5 g protein; trace carbohydrate; trace dietary fiber; no usable carb.

Stuffed Eggs

Don't save these recipes for parties: If you're a low-carb eater, a refrigerator full of stuffed eggs is a beautiful thing. Here are six varieties. Feel free to double or triple any of these recipes—you know they'll disappear.

Southwestern Stuffed Eggs

These spicy eggs were a huge hit at the party I took them to!

6 hard-boiled eggs
2 tablespoons (28 g) mayonnaise
1 tablespoon (15 g) plain yogurt
1 tablespoon (10 g) minced onion
¾ teaspoon chili powder
1 tablespoon (15 ml) cider vinegar
⅛ teaspoon garlic, finely minced

Peel the eggs and slice the eggs in half. Carefully remove the yolks to a mixing bowl and arrange the whites on a platter.

Mash the yolks well with a fork and then mash in the mayonnaise and yogurt. When the mixture is smooth, stir in the remaining ingredients.

Spoon the mixture back into the hollows in the egg whites. You may sprinkle a tiny bit of chili powder or paprika on top to make them look festive.

Yield: 12 pieces

Each with 3 g protein; 1 g carbohydrate; trace dietary fiber; 1 g usable carb.

Onion Eggs

6 hard-boiled eggs
5 tablespoons (70 g) mayonnaise
1 teaspoon spicy brown or Dijon mustard
2½ teaspoons very finely minced sweet
    red onion

5 drops hot pepper sauce
¼ teaspoon salt or Vege-Sal

Peel the eggs and slice the eggs in half.

Carefully remove the yolks into a mixing bowl and arrange the whites on a platter.

Mash the yolks with a fork. Stir in the mayonnaise, mustard, onion, hot pepper sauce, and salt and mix until creamy.

Spoon the mixture back into the hollows in the egg whites.

Yield: 12 halves

Each with a trace of carbohydrates, a trace of fiber, and 3 grams of protein.

Fish Eggs

That's eggs with fish, not eggs from fish. If you thought stuffed eggs couldn't go to an upscale party, these will change your mind.

6 hard-boiled eggs
2 tablespoons (28 g) mayonnaise
2 tablespoons (30 g) sour cream
¼ cup (50 g) moist smoked salmon,
    mashed fine
1 tablespoon (15 g) jarred, grated horseradish
2 teaspoons finely minced sweet red onion
⅛ teaspoon salt

Peel the eggs and slice the eggs in half.

Carefully remove the yolks into a mixing bowl and arrange the whites on a platter.

Mash the yolks with a fork. Stir in the mayonnaise, sour cream, salmon, horseradish, onion, and salt and mix until creamy.

Spoon the mixture back into the hollows in the egg whites.

Yield: 12 halves

Each with a trace of carbohydrates, a trace of fiber, and 3 grams of protein.

Stilton Eggs

This is for all you blue cheese fans! If you don't have Stilton—the particularly strong English blue cheese—on hand, go ahead and use whatever blue cheese you've got.

6 hard-boiled eggs
2 tablespoons (28 g) mayonnaise
2 tablespoons (30 g) plain yogurt
2 ounces (60 g) Stilton cheese, crumbled pretty fine
3 scallions, minced
¼ teaspoon salt or Vege-Sal

Peel the eggs and slice the eggs in half.

Carefully remove the yolks into a mixing bowl and arrange the whites on a platter.

With a fork, mash the yolks well. Stir in the mayonnaise and yogurt. When the yolks are smooth and creamy, mash in the Stilton, leaving some small lumps and then stir in the scallions and the salt.

Spoon the yolk mixture back into the hollows in the egg whites.

Yield: 12 pieces

Each with 3 g protein; 1 g carbohydrate; trace dietary fiber; 1 g usable carb.

Hammond Eggs

Deviled ham gives these eggs a country sort of kick.

6 hard-boiled eggs
1 can (2¼ ounces, or 62 g) of deviled ham
4 teaspoons spicy brown mustard
3 tablespoons (42 g) mayonnaise
¼ teaspoon salt
Paprika

Peel the eggs and slice the eggs in half.

Carefully remove the yolks into a mixing bowl and arrange the whites on a platter.

Mash the yolks with a fork. Stir in the ham, mustard, mayonnaise, and salt and mix until creamy.

Spoon the mixture back into the hollows in the egg whites. Sprinkle with a little paprika for color.

Yield: Makes 12 halves

Each with 1 gram of carbohydrates, a trace of fiber, and 4 grams of protein.

Cajun Eggs

6 hard-boiled eggs
⅓ cup (75 g) mayonnaise
2 teaspoons horseradish mustard
1 teaspoon Cajun Seasoning (page 484)

Peel the eggs and slice the eggs in half.

Carefully remove the yolks into a mixing bowl and arrange the whites on a platter.

Mash the yolks with a fork. Stir in the mayonnaise and mustard and mix until creamy.

(continued on page 58)

Add the Cajun seasoning and blend well.

Spoon the mixture back into the hollows in the egg whites.

Yield: 12 halves

Each with 1 gram of carbohydrates, a trace of fiber, and 3 grams of protein.

Artichoke Parmesan Dip

Serve this party favorite with pepper strips, cucumber rounds, celery sticks, or low-carb fiber crackers.

1 can (13½ ounces, or 380 g) artichoke hearts
1 cup (225 g) mayonnaise
1 cup (100 g) grated Parmesan cheese
1 clove garlic, crushed, or 1 teaspoon of jarred, chopped garlic
Paprika

Preheat the oven to 325°F (170°C, or gas mark 3).

Drain and chop the artichoke hearts.

Mix the artichoke hearts with the mayonnaise, cheese, and garlic, combining well.

Put the mixture in a small, oven-proof casserole dish, sprinkle a little paprika on top, and bake for 45 minutes.

Yield: 4 servings

Each with 3 grams of carbohydrates and 1 gram of fiber, for a total of 2 grams of usable carbs and 10 grams of protein. Analysis does not include dippers.

Spinach Artichoke Dip

This is a great, equally yummy version of the previous recipe, but keep in mind that it does make twice as much dip.

1 can (13½ ounces, or 380 g) artichoke hearts
1 package frozen chopped spinach (10 ounces, or 280 g), thawed
2 cups (450 g) mayonnaise
2 cups (200 g) grated Parmesan cheese
2 cloves garlic, crushed, or 2 teaspoons jarred, chopped garlic
Paprika

Preheat the oven to 325°F (170°C, or gas mark 3).

Drain and chop the artichoke hearts.

Combine the spinach, mayonnaise, cheese, and garlic in a large casserole dish (a 6-cup [1.4-L] dish is about right). Sprinkle with paprika.

Bake for 50 to 60 minutes.

Yield: 8 servings

Each with 4 grams of carbohydrates and 2 grams of fiber, for a total of 2 grams of usable carbs and 10 grams of protein.

Curried Chicken Dip

Not only will this mildly spicy dip please your friends and family, but carried in a snap-top container with a bag of cut-up veggies, it would make a great lunch.

1 can (5 ounces, or 140 g) chunk chicken, drained

3 ounces (85 g) light cream cheese

1 tablespoon (14 g) mayonnaise

2 tablespoons (20 g) minced red onion

¾ teaspoon curry powder

1 teaspoon brown mustard

¼ teaspoon hot pepper sauce, or to taste

2 tablespoons (10 g) minced fresh parsley

This is pretty darned easy—just assemble everything in your food processor with the S-blade in place and pulse until it's smooth. Put your dip in a pretty bowl and surround it with cucumber slices, celery sticks, and/or pepper strips.

Yield: 6 servings

Each with 7 g protein; 2 g carbohydrate; trace dietary fiber; 2 g usable carbs. Carb count does not include vegetable dippers.

Guacamole

This is a very simple guacamole recipe, without sour cream or mayonnaise, that lets the taste of the avocados shine through.

4 ripe black avocados

2 tablespoons (20 g) minced sweet red onion

3 tablespoons (45 ml) lime juice

3 cloves garlic, crushed

¼ teaspoon hot pepper sauce

Salt or Vege-Sal to taste

Halve the avocados and scoop the flesh into a mixing bowl. Mash coarsely with a fork.

Mix in the onion, lime juice, garlic, hot pepper sauce, and salt, stirring to blend well and mashing to the desired consistency.

Yield: 6 generous servings

Each with 11 grams of carbohydrates and 3 grams of fiber, for a total of 8 grams of usable carbs and 3 grams of protein.

This recipe contains lots of healthy fats and almost three times the potassium found in a banana.

Dill Dip

This easy dip tastes wonderful with all sorts of raw vegetables; try serving it with celery, peppers, cucumber, broccoli, or whatever else you have on hand.

1 pint (460 g) sour cream

¼ small onion

1 heaping tablespoon (3 g) dry dill weed

½ teaspoon salt or Vege-Sal

Put the sour cream, onion, dill weed, and salt in a food processor and process until the onion disappears. (If you don't have a food processor, mince the onion very fine and just stir everything together.)

You can serve this right away, but it tastes even better if you let it chill for a few hours.

Yield: 1 pint

(continued on page 60)

25 grams of carbohydrates and 1 gram of fiber, for a total of 24 grams of usable carbs and 16 grams of protein in the batch. (This is easily enough for 10 to 12 people, so no one's going to get more than a few grams of carbs.) Analysis does not include vegetable dippers.

Hot Crab Dip

Here's hot crab, hot cheese, and garlic—what's not to like?

1 cup (225 g) mayonnaise
8 ounces (225 g) shredded cheddar cheese
4 scallions, minced
6 ounces (170 g) canned crabmeat, drained
1 clove garlic, crushed
3 ounces (85 g) cream cheese, softened,
     cut into chunks

Combine everything in your slow cooker and stir together. Cover the slow cooker, set it to low, and let it cook for 1 hour. Remove the lid and stir to blend in the now-melted cream cheese. Re-cover and cook for another hour.

Serve with celery, pepper, and cucumber dippers.

Yield: 8 servings

Each with 13 g protein, 1 g carbohydrate, trace dietary fiber, 1 g usable carbs. Analysis does not include vegetable dippers.

Clam Dip

With some celery sticks and pepper strips for scooping, this would make a good lunch. Of course, you can also serve it at parties with celery, green pepper, cucumber rounds, or fiber crackers for you and crackers or chips for the non-low-carbers.

2 packages (8 ounces, or 225 g each) cream
     cheese, softened
½ cup (115 g) mayonnaise
2 to 3 teaspoons Worcestershire sauce
1 tablespoon (15 ml) Dijon mustard
8 to 10 scallions, including the crisp part of
     the green shoot, minced
2 cans (6½ ounces, or 185 g each) minced
     clams, drained
Salt or Vege-Sal
Pepper

Combine all the ingredients well. A food processor or blender works well for this, or if you prefer to leave chunks of clam, you could use an electric mixer. Chill and serve.

Yield: 12 servings

Each with just under 4 grams of carbohydrates, a trace of fiber, and 10 grams of protein. Analysis does not include vegetable dippers or crackers.

Bacon-Cheese Dip

Bacon and cheese together—It just makes you glad to be a low-carber, doesn't it?

16 ounces (455 g) light or regular cream cheese, softened
2 cups (225 g) shredded cheddar cheese
2 cups (230 g) shredded Monterey Jack cheese
½ cup (120 ml) Carb Countdown dairy beverage
½ cup (120 ml) heavy cream
2 tablespoons (30 ml) brown mustard
1 tablespoon (10 g) minced onion
2 teaspoons Worcestershire sauce
½ teaspoon salt or Vege-Sal
¼ teaspoon cayenne
1 pound (455 g) bacon, cooked, drained, and crumbled

Cut the cream cheese in cubes and put them in your slow cooker. Add the cheddar cheese, Monterey Jack cheese, Carb Countdown, cream, mustard, onion, Worcestershire sauce, salt, and cayenne. Stir to distribute the ingredients evenly. Cover the slow cooker, set it to low, and let it cook for 1 hour, stirring from time to time. When the cheese has melted, stir in the bacon.

Serve with cut-up vegetables, fiber crackers, or other low-carb dippers.

Yield: 12 servings

Each with 25 g protein, 2 g carbohydrate, trace dietary fiber, 2 g usable carbs. Carb count does not include vegetable dippers or crackers.

Avocado Cheese Dip

This dip has been known to make my mom a very popular person at parties. Dip with pork rinds, vegetables, or purchased protein chips. It can also be served over steak, and it makes perhaps the most elegant omelets on the face of the earth.

2 packages (8 ounces, or 225 g each) cream cheese, softened
1½ cups (180 g) shredded white Cheddar or Monterey jack cheese
1 ripe black avocado, peeled and seeded
1 small onion
1 clove garlic, crushed
1 can (3 to 4 ounces, or 85 to 115 g) green chilies, drained, or jalapeños, if you like it hot

Combine all the ingredients in a food processor and process until very smooth.

Scrape into a pretty serving bowl and place the avocado seed in the middle. For some reason, placing the seed in the middle helps keep the dip from turning brown as quickly while it sits out. But if you're making this a few hours ahead of time, cover it with plastic wrap, making sure the wrap is actually touching the surface of the dip. Don't make this more than a few hours before you plan to serve it.

Yield: About 5 cups (1.1 L), plenty for a good-size party

(continued on page 62)

The batch contains 45 grams of carbohydrates and 9 grams of fiber, for a total of 36 grams of usable carbs and a whopping 83 grams of protein. Analysis is for dip only.

Smoked Gouda Veggie Dip

This dip is great with celery, peppers, or any favorite raw veggie. Combine your ingredients with a mixer, not a food processor, so you have actual little bits of Gouda in the dip.

1 package (8 ounces, or 225 g) cream cheese, softened
2/3 cup (150 g) mayonnaise
1 cup (150 g) shredded smoked Gouda
6 scallions, including the crisp part of the green shoot, sliced
2 tablespoons (12.5 g) grated Parmesan cheese
1/2 teaspoon pepper

Beat the cream cheese and mayonnaise together until creamy, scraping the sides of the bowl often.

Add the Gouda, scallions, Parmesan, and pepper and beat until well blended.

Chill and serve with raw vegetables.

Yield: At least 8 servings

Each with 2 grams of carbohydrates, a trace of fiber, and 7 grams of protein. Analysis does not include vegetable dippers.

Dukkah

My friend Lou Anne brought this Turkish "dry dip" along on a campout, and I've been nagging her for the recipe ever since. Although Dukkah is traditionally eaten with bread, it also adds an exotic, fascinating flavor to simple raw vegetables.

1/3 cup (50 g) almonds or hazelnuts
1/4 cup (30 g) white sesame seeds
1/4 cup (20 g) coriander seeds
1/4 cup (24 g) cumin seeds
Salt and pepper to taste

In a dry saucepan, toast the nuts, sesame seeds, coriander seeds, and cumin seeds over high heat for 1 minute, stirring constantly.

Use a food processor, coffee grinder, or mortar and pestle to crush the toasted mixture and then season it with salt and pepper. (Don't over-grind; you want a consistency similar to coarse-ground cornmeal.)

Put your Dukkah in a bowl next to a bowl of olive oil and set out cut-up raw vegetables. Dip the vegetables first into the oil, then into the Dukkah, and eat.

Yield: Just over a cup, or about 10 servings

Each with 4 grams of carbohydrates and 1 gram of fiber, for a total of 3 grams of usable carbs and 2 grams of protein. (Analysis does not include vegetables.)

Country-Style Paté

This is really good. Plus, as paté goes, it's easy to make.

6 slices bacon
2 tablespoons (28 g) butter
1 cup (70 g) sliced mushrooms
½ cup (80 g) chopped onion
1 cup (225 g) chicken livers
½ teaspoon Worcestershire sauce
2 tablespoons (28 g) mayonnaise
Scant ½ teaspoon salt or Vege-Sal
¼ teaspoon pepper

In a heavy skillet over medium heat, fry the bacon until it just starts to get crisp. Remove the bacon and then drain and reserve the grease.

Turn the heat down to low and melt the butter and a little bacon grease in the skillet. Sauté the mushrooms and onion in the skillet until they're quite limp (about 15 minutes).

While they're sautéing, fill a medium saucepan with water and bring it to a boil.

Put the chicken livers in the water (make sure you keep stirring those sautéing vegetables) and bring the water back to a boil. Cover the pan, turn off the heat, and let it sit for 15 minutes.

Drain the chicken livers. Put them in a food processor with the S-blade in place and pulse two or three times to grind the chicken livers. Crumble and add the bacon and the mushroom and onion mixture. Pulse to combine. Add the Worcestershire sauce, mayonnaise, salt, and pepper, and pulse again until well combined. Serve with celery sticks, pepper strips, or low-carb crackers.

Yield: 12 servings

Each with 2 grams of carbohydrates, a trace of fiber, and 5 grams of protein. Analysis does not include vegetable dippers or crackers.

Tuna Paté

If you throw in some veggies for dipping, this versatile dish makes a great snack, first course at a dinner party, or even a fine brown bag lunch.

2 tablespoons (28 g) butter
2 cloves garlic, crushed
½ medium onion, chopped
1 can (4 ounces, or 115 g) mushrooms, drained
½ teaspoon orange extract
1 tablespoon (1.5 g) Splenda
1 package (8 ounces, or 225 g) cream cheese, softened
1 can (6 ounces, 170 g) tuna, drained
2 tablespoons (7.6 g) fresh parsley
Grated rind of half an orange
¼ teaspoon salt
¼ teaspoon pepper

In a small, heavy skillet over medium heat, melt the butter and sauté the garlic, onion, and mushrooms until the onion is limp. Add the orange extract and Splenda and stir well. Cool.

Place the cream cheese, tuna, parsley, orange rind, salt, and pepper in a food processor with the S-blade in place. Pulse to blend. Add the sautéed mixture and pulse until smooth and well blended.

Spoon into a serving bowl and chill. Serve with celery sticks, pepper strips, cucumber rounds, and crackers (for the carb-eaters).

(continued on page 64)

Each with 3 grams of carbohydrates and 1 gram of fiber, for a total of 2 grams of usable carbs and 11 grams of protein. Analysis does not include vegetable dippers or crackers.

Tuna Puffs

1 egg
2 tablespoons (20 g) pumpkin seed meal or almond meal
2 tablespoons (20 g) rice protein powder
1 tablespoon (14 g) butter, melted
2 tablespoons (30 ml) half-and-half
1½ teaspoons lemon juice
½ teaspoon chili garlic paste
6 ounces (170 g) canned tuna, drained
4 scallions, sliced thin
Salt and pepper to taste
Easy Orange Salsa (page 496)

Preheat oven to 375°F (190°C, or gas mark 5) and spray a mini-muffin pan with nonstick cooking spray.

In a mixing bowl, beat the egg for a minute or so. Now stir in the pumpkin seed meal, rice protein powder, melted butter, half-and-half, lemon juice, and chili garlic paste.

Add the tuna, breaking it up well as you stir it in. Stir in the scallions and add salt and pepper to taste.

Spoon into prepared mini-muffin cups and bake for 12 to 15 minutes.

When Tuna Puffs are done, place on a platter surrounding a bowl of Easy Orange Salsa.

Yield: 24 puffs

Each with 3 g protein; 1 g carbohydrate; trace dietary fiber; 1 g usable carb. Analysis includes the Easy Orange Salsa.

Marinated Mushrooms

The quality of the vinaigrette dressing makes all the difference here, so use the best you can make or buy.

8 ounces (225 g) small, fresh mushrooms
1½ cups (360 ml) vinaigrette dressing (home-made or store-bought)

Thoroughly wipe the mushrooms clean with a soft cloth.

Place them in a saucepan, cover them with the dressing, and simmer over medium-low heat for 15 minutes.

Chill and drain the mushrooms, saving the dressing to store any leftover mushrooms in. (You can even simmer another batch of mushrooms in it when the first batch is gone.) Arrange the mushrooms on lettuce with toothpicks for spearing.

Yield: Depending on the size of your mushrooms, this will make about 12 to 15 servings

Each with about 1 gram of carbohydrates and not enough fiber or protein to talk about.

Garlic Cheese Stuffed Mushrooms

These are the easiest stuffed mushrooms you'll ever make and really yummy, too.

6 small portobello mushrooms, totaling 6 ounces (170 g)

1 package (6 ounces, or 170 g) garlic and herb spreadable cheese (such as Boursin or Alouette)

2 tablespoons (10 g) crushed pork rinds

Preheat oven to 350°F (180°C, or gas mark 4).

Wipe the mushrooms clean and remove the stems (save them to slice and sauté to serve over steaks or in omelets). Divide the cheese between the mushroom caps. Sprinkle each one with a teaspoon of pork rind crumbs.

Arrange your mushrooms in a shallow baking pan. Add just enough water to cover the bottom of the pan. Bake for 30 minutes and serve hot. These are good with the Mustard-Horseradish Dipping Sauce (page 477), but they're just fine as is.

Yield: 6 servings

Each with 1 g protein; 1 g carbohydrate; trace dietary fiber, 1 g usable carb.

Spinach Stuffed Mushrooms

People scarf these right down!

1½ pounds (680 g) mushrooms, wiped clean

2 tablespoons (28 g) butter

½ cup (80 g) chopped onion

4 cloves garlic, crushed

10 ounces (280 g) frozen chopped spinach, thawed

4 ounces (115 g) cream cheese

¼ teaspoon pepper

½ teaspoon salt or Vege-Sal

1½ teaspoons Worcestershire sauce

¼ cup (25 g) Parmesan cheese, plus a little extra for sprinkling

Preheat oven to 350°F (180°C, or gas mark 4).

Wipe the mushrooms clean and remove the stems. Set the caps aside and chop the stems fairly fine.

In a large, heavy skillet, over medium-low heat, melt the butter. Add the chopped stems and the onion. Sauté these until the mushroom bits are changing color and the onion is soft and translucent. Add the garlic, stir it up, and sauté for another couple of minutes.

While that's happening, dump your thawed spinach into a strainer and press all the water out of it that you can. Now stir it into the mushroom-onion mixture. Next, stir in the cream cheese. When it's melted, add the pepper, salt, Worcestershire sauce, and Parmesan.

(continued on page 66)

Stuff the spinach/mushroom mixture into the mushroom caps. Arrange the stuffed caps in a baking pan as you stuff them.

When they're all stuffed, sprinkle a little Parmesan cheese over them to make them look nice. Add enough water to just barely cover the bottom of the pan. Bake for 30 minutes. Serve warm.

Yield: About 40 pieces

Each with 1 g protein; 1 g carbohydrate; trace dietary fiber; 1 g usable carb.

Two-Cheese Tuna-Stuffed Mushrooms

Of all the stuffed mushrooms I've cooked or sampled, these are my absolute favorites.

½ pound (225 g) fresh mushrooms
1 can (6 ounces, or 170 g) tuna
½ cup (60 g) shredded smoked Gouda
2 tablespoons (12.5 g) grated Parmesan cheese
3 tablespoons (42 g) mayonnaise
1 scallion, finely minced

Preheat the oven to 350°F (180°C, or gas mark 4).

Wipe the mushrooms clean with a damp cloth and remove their stems.

Combine the tuna, Gouda, Parmesan, mayonnaise, and minced scallion and mix well.

Spoon the mixture into the mushroom caps and arrange them in a shallow roasting pan. Add just enough water to cover the bottom of the pan. Bake for 15 minutes and serve hot.

Yield: About 15 servings

Each with 1 gram of carbohydrates, a trace of fiber, and 4 grams of protein.

Turkey-Parmesan Stuffed Mushrooms

1 pound (445 g) ground turkey
¾ cup grated (75 g) Parmesan cheese
½ cup (115 g) mayonnaise
1 teaspoon dried oregano
1 teaspoon dried basil
2 cloves garlic, crushed
1 teaspoon salt or Vege-Sal
¼ teaspoon pepper
1½ pounds (670 g) mushrooms

Preheat the oven to 350°F (180°C, or gas mark 4).

Combine the turkey, Parmesan, mayonnaise, oregano, basil, garlic, salt, and pepper, mixing well.

Wipe the mushrooms clean with a damp cloth and remove their stems.

Spoon the mixture into the mushroom caps and place them in a shallow roasting pan. Add just enough water to cover the bottom of the pan. Bake for 20 minutes and serve hot.

Yield: About 45 mushrooms

Each with 1 gram of carbohydrates, a trace of fiber, and 3 grams of protein.

Soy and Ginger Pecans

I gave away tins of these for Christmas one year and got rave reviews.

2 cups (200 g) shelled pecans
4 tablespoons (56 g) butter, melted
3 tablespoons (45 ml) soy sauce
1 teaspoon ground ginger

Preheat the oven to 300°F (150°C, or gas mark 2).
    Spread the pecans in a shallow roasting pan. Stir in the butter, coating all the nuts.
    Roast for 15 minutes and then remove from the oven and stir in the soy sauce. Sprinkle the ginger evenly over the nuts and stir that in as well.
    Roast for another 10 minutes.

Yield: 8 servings

Each with 6 grams of carbohydrates and 2 grams of fiber, for a total of 4 grams of usable carbs and 3 grams of protein.

Worcestershire Nuts

I like to use this combination of nuts, but feel free to use just one or the other or to experiment with your own proportions.

1 cup (150 g) shelled walnuts
1 cup (100 g) shelled pecans
4 tablespoons (56 g) butter, melted
3 tablespoons (45 ml) Worcestershire sauce

Preheat the oven to 300°F (150°C, or gas mark 2).
    Spread the nuts in a shallow baking pan and stir in the butter, coating all the nuts.
    Roast for 15 minutes and then remove from the oven and stir in the Worcestershire sauce.
    Roast for another 10 minutes.

Yield: 8 servings

Each with 6 grams of carbohydrates and 2 grams of fiber, for a total of 4 grams of usable carbs and 3 grams of protein.

Smoked Almonds

These are crunchy with a nice kick!

1 pound (455 g) almonds
3 tablespoons (42 g) butter
2 teaspoons Classic Barbecue Rub (page 486, or use purchased rub)
2 teaspoons salt
2 teaspoons liquid smoke

Preheat the oven to 300°F (150°C, or gas mark 2).
    Lay a big flat roasting pan over a burner and melt the butter in it.
    Stir in the seasonings, making sure they're blended into the butter.
    Now add the almonds and stir until they're well-coated. Roast for 30 to 40 minutes. Store in an airtight container.

Yield: 12 servings

Each with 8 g protein; 8 g carbohydrate; 4 g dietary fiber; 4 grams usable carbs.

Blue Cheese Dressing Walnuts

I originally wanted to make these with powdered blue cheese dressing mix, only to find that there is no such thing, at least not in my grocery stores. So I tried using liquid dressing instead. It didn't end up tasting a lot like blue cheese, but it did end up tasting really good.

4 cups (400 g) walnuts
½ cup (120 ml) blue cheese salad dressing
1 teaspoon garlic salt

Combine the walnuts and dressing in your slow cooker. Stir until the nuts are evenly coated with the dressing. Cover the slow cooker, set it to low, and let it cook for 3 hours, stirring once halfway through.

Stir in the garlic salt just before serving.

Yield: 16 servings

Each with 8 g protein, 4 g carbohydrate, 2 g dietary fiber, 2 g usable carbs.

Maple-Glazed Walnuts

3 cups (300 g) walnuts
1½ teaspoons ground cinnamon
1 tablespoon (14 g) butter, melted
¼ teaspoon salt
2 teaspoons vanilla extract
⅓ cup (78 ml) sugar-free pancake syrup
⅓ cup (8 g) Splenda, divided

Put the walnuts in your slow cooker.

In a bowl, mix together the cinnamon, butter, salt, vanilla extract, pancake syrup, and ¼ cup (6 g) of the Splenda. Pour the mixture over the nuts and stir to coat. Cover the slow cooker, set it to low, and let it cook for 2 to 3 hours, stirring every hour or so.

Then uncover the slow cooker and cook, stirring every 20 minutes, until the nuts are almost dry. Stir in the remaining Splenda, cook for another 20 minutes, and then remove from the slow cooker and cool. Store in an airtight container.

Yield: 9 servings

Each with 10 g protein, 6 g carbohydrate, 2 g dietary fiber, 4 g usable carbs. Analysis does not include polyol in sugar-free syrup.

Dana's Snack Mix

You can buy shelled sunflower seeds and pumpkin seeds in bulk at most natural food stores, and you should be able to get raw cashew pieces there, too. For variety, try adding 2½ cups (75 g) of low-carb garlic croutons along with the seeds and nuts.

6 tablespoons (84 g) butter
3 tablespoons (45 ml) Worcestershire sauce
1½ teaspoons garlic powder
2½ teaspoons seasoned salt
1 teaspoon onion powder
2½ cups (560 g) raw, shelled sunflower seeds
2½ cups (560 g) raw, shelled pumpkin seeds
1 cup (150 g) almonds
1 cup (100 g) pecans

1 cup (150 g) walnuts

1 cup (150 g) raw cashew pieces

Preheat the oven to 250°F (120°C, or gas mark ½).

In a small pan, melt the butter and stir in the Worcestershire sauce, garlic powder, seasoned salt, and onion powder.

In a large bowl, combine the seeds and nuts. Pour the melted butter mixture over them and mix very well.

Put the mixture in large roasting pan and bake for 2 hours, stirring occasionally.

Allow the mixture to cool; store in an airtight container.

Yield: 18 servings

Each with 14 grams of carbohydrates and 5 grams of fiber, for a total of 9 grams of usable carbs and 13 grams of protein.

Ranch Mix

2 cups (450 g) raw, shelled pumpkin seeds

2 cups (450 g) raw, shelled sunflower seeds

2 cups (290 g) dry-roasted peanuts

1 cup (150 g) raw almonds

1 cup (150 g) raw cashew pieces

2 tablespoons (30 ml) canola oil

1 packet dry ranch salad dressing mix

1 teaspoon lemon pepper

1 teaspoon dried dill

½ teaspoon garlic powder

Preheat the oven to 350°F (180°C, or gas mark 4).

In large mixing bowl, combine the pumpkin seeds, sunflower seeds, peanuts, almonds, and cashews. Add the canola oil and stir to coat. Add the dressing mix, lemon pepper, dill, and garlic powder and stir until well distributed.

Put the seasoned nuts in shallow roasting pan and roast for 45 to 60 minutes, stirring occasionally, until the almonds are crisp through.

Yield: 16 servings

Each with 15 grams of carbohydrates and 5 grams of fiber, for a total of 10 grams of usable carbs and 16 grams of protein.

Pepitas Calientes

Hot and sweet and crunchy—these Mexican-style pumpkin seeds will be the hit of any gathering you serve them at. Feel free to double or triple this!

1 cup (225 g) raw, shelled pumpkin seeds

2 teaspoons garlic powder

¼ teaspoon salt

2 teaspoons chili garlic paste

1 teaspoon Splenda

1 teaspoon lime juice

Heat a medium-size heavy skillet over medium-high heat. Add the pumpkin seeds and dry-fry them for a few minutes, stirring constantly. After a little while, you'll see them swell a bit and become a bit plumper. This means they're just about done.

(continued on page 70)

Stir in the garlic powder, salt, chili garlic paste, Splenda, and lime juice, making sure all the seeds are well coated. Continue to stir over heat until they dry and then serve hot.

Yield: 4 servings of ¼ cup (60 g) each

Each with 3 g protein; 10 g carbohydrate; 2 g dietary fiber; 8 g usable carbs.

Asian Punks

Pumpkin seeds are terrific for you—they're a great source of both magnesium and zinc. And they taste great, too.

2 cups (450 g) raw, shelled pumpkin seeds
2 tablespoons (30 ml) soy sauce
½ teaspoon powdered ginger
2 teaspoons Splenda

Preheat the oven to 350°F (180°C, or gas mark 4).

In a mixing bowl, combine the pumpkin seeds, soy sauce, ginger, and Splenda, mixing well.

Spread the pumpkin seeds in a shallow roasting pan and roast for about 45 minutes or until the seeds are dry, stirring two or three times during roasting.

Yield: 4 servings

Each with 13 grams of carbohydrates and 3 grams of fiber, for a total of 10 grams of usable carbs and 17 grams of protein. (These are also a terrific source of minerals.)

Indian Punks

You can actually buy curry-flavored pumpkin seeds, but these are better tasting and better for you.

4 tablespoons (56 g) butter
2½ tablespoons (15 g) curry powder
2 cloves garlic, crushed
2 cups (450 g) raw, shelled pumpkin seeds
Salt

Preheat the oven to 300°F (150°C, or gas mark 2).

Melt the butter in a small skillet over medium heat. Add the curry and garlic and stir for 2 to 3 minutes.

In a mixing bowl, add the seasoned butter to the pumpkin seeds and stir until well coated.

Spread the pumpkin seeds in a shallow roasting pan and roast for 30 minutes. Sprinkle lightly with salt.

Yield: 4 servings

Each with 15 grams of carbohydrates and 4 grams of fiber, for a total of 11 grams of usable carbs and 18 grams of protein.

In addition to all the minerals found in the pumpkin seeds, you get the turmeric in the curry powder, which is believed to help prevent cancer.

Punks on the Range

This snack is spicy-chili-crunchy. If you miss barbecue-flavored potato chips, try snacking on these.

2 cups (450 g) raw, shelled pumpkin seeds
1 tablespoon (15 ml) canola oil
1 tablespoon (7.8 g) chili powder
1 teaspoon salt

Preheat the oven to 350°F (180°C, or gas mark 4).

In a mixing bowl, combine the pumpkin seeds and canola oil, stirring until well coated. Add the chili powder and salt and stir again.

Spread the seeds in a shallow roasting pan and roast for about 30 minutes.

Yield: 4 servings

Each with 13 grams of carbohydrates and 3 grams of fiber, for a total of 10 grams of usable carbs and 17 grams of protein.

Barbecued Peanuts

1 tablespoon (15 ml) liquid smoke flavoring
1 teaspoon Worcestershire sauce
Dash of hot pepper sauce
½ cup (120 ml) water
1½ cups (220 g) dry-roasted peanuts
3 tablespoons (42 g) butter
Garlic salt

Preheat the oven to 250°F (120°C, or gas mark ½).

In a saucepan, combine the liquid smoke, Worcestershire sauce, hot pepper sauce, and water.

Bring to a simmer.

Turn off the heat and stir in the peanuts. Let the peanuts sit in the liquid for 30 minutes, stirring occasionally.

Drain off the liquid and spread the peanuts in a shallow roasting pan. Bake for at least 1 hour or until good and dry. (Stir occasionally to help speed up the process.)

When the peanuts are thoroughly dry, melt the butter and stir it into the peanuts to coat. Sprinkle lightly with garlic salt.

Yield: 3 servings

Each with 16 grams of carbohydrates and 6 grams of fiber, for a total of 10 grams of usable carbs and 17 grams of protein.

Brie and Walnut Quesadillas

⅓ cup (40 g) chopped walnuts
8 ounces (225 g) Brie
6 low-carb tortillas

Preheat your oven to 350°F (180°C, or gas mark 4). Spread your walnuts in a shallow roasting pan. Put them in the oven and let them roast for 8 to 10 minutes—set the oven timer!

(continued on page 72)

While that's happening, cut your Brie into quarters and thinly slice off the rind. Now, slice the Brie. If it's too soft for that, cut it into little cubes.

Lay a tortilla in a big, heavy skillet over medium-low heat. Cover it with slices or small hunks of Brie and let it heat until the cheese begins to melt and the walnuts are done. Scatter 1/3 of the walnuts over the cheese and top the whole thing with another tortilla. Turn your quesadilla over and continue to cook until the cheese i s good and melty. Transfer to a plate and cover with a lid to keep warm while you make two more!

Cut into wedges and serve.

Yield: 6 servings

Each with 15 g protein; 12 g carbohydrate; 8 g dietary fiber; 4 g usable carbs.

Warm Brie with Sticky Nuts

This is an unusual and delectable party offering. It is also very rich; if you're planning on serving dinner as well, consider sharing this six ways! I think this would also make an elegant dessert.

8-ounce (225 g) wheel of Brie (Don't buy a slice from a bigger wheel.)
1/3 cup (40 g) chopped pecans
3 tablespoons (45 g) butter
1 tablespoon (15 g) polyol
1 teaspoon sugar-free imitation honey
1 tablespoon (1.5 g) Splenda
1/4 teaspoon blackstrap molasses
1 pinch salt

Preheat oven to 350°F (180°C, or gas mark 4). Unwrap cheese and place it in a shallow baking dish. Put it the oven and set your timer for 10 minutes.

Meanwhile, in a saucepan, start sautéing the chopped pecans in the butter—give them about 5 minutes over medium-low heat. Then stir in the polyol, imitation honey, Splenda, and molasses and keep stirring for 3 or 4 minutes. When the cheese is just about ready, stir in the salt.

Fetch the Brie out of the oven and place it on a serving plate. Scoop the nuts—they'll now be sticky and clumping a bit—out of the butter and spread them evenly across the top of the cheese.

Serve by cutting into 4 wedges and eat with a fork.

Yield: 4 servings

Each with 13 g protein; 2 g carbohydrate; 1 g dietary fiber; 1 g usable carb. Carb count does not include polyols.

Cheese-Pecan Nibbles

These are quite simple to make and sure to delight your guests. Feel free to use either the regular or the light garlic and herb cheese—they have about the same carb count.

2 cups (300 g) pecan halves
4 ounces (115 g) garlic and herb spreadable cheese (such as Boursin or Alouette)

You can make this with canned, roasted, and salted pecans, or if you prefer, you can roast your own. If you choose the latter, preheat your oven to 350°F (180°C, or gas mark 4). Spread 2 cups (300 g) of unbroken pecan halves in a shallow baking pan. Stir in 1 teaspoon oil to coat—it will take a fair amount of stirring to get that little oil to coat this many nuts, so keep stirring! Sprinkle with salt and roast for 8 to 10 minutes. Remove from oven and let them cool before the next step.

Spread a dollop—between ¼ and ½ teaspoon— of garlic and herb spreadable cheese on the flat side of a pecan half, and then press the flat side of another pecan half against it to make a pecan-and-cheese sandwich! Place on a serving plate and continue with the rest of the cheese and the rest of the pecans.

Yield: Enough for about 6 people

Each of person will get 4 g protein; 7 g carbohydrate; 3 g dietary fiber; 4 g usable carbs.

Fried Cheese

This is the sort of decadence I would never have considered in my low-fat days. If you miss cheese-flavored snacks, you've got to try this.

2 or 3 tablespoons (30 or 45 ml) olive or canola oil

½ to ¾ cup (60 to 90 g) shredded Cheddar, Monterey Jack, or jalepeño Jack cheese

Spray a small, heavy bottomed, nonstick skillet with nonstick cooking spray and place over medium-high heat.

Add the oil and then the cheese. The cheese will melt and bubble and spread to fill the bottom of the skillet.

Let the cheese fry until it's crisp and brown around the edges. Use a spatula to lift up an edge and check whether the cheese is brown all over the bottom; if it isn't, let it go another minute or so.

When the fried cheese is good and brown, carefully flip it and fry the other side until it is brown.

Remove the cheese from the skillet, drain, and lie it flat to cool. Break into pieces and eat.

Yield: 2 servings

Each with 1 gram of carbohydrates, no fiber, and 11 grams of protein.

Variation: Cheesy Bowls and Taco Shells—For a tasty, cheesy, tortilla-like bowl, follow the directions for Fried Cheese until both sides are cooked. Remove and drain the cheese but drape it over the bottom of a bowl to cool. When it cools and hardens, you'll have a cheesy, edible bowl to eat a taco salad out of.

You can also make a taco shell by folding the cheese disc in half and propping it partway open. Be careful when handling it; hot cheese can burn you pretty seriously.

Saganaki

If you've never tried the Greek cheese Kasseri, you're in for a treat. This dish is fantastically delicious, and it has a dramatic, fiery presentation to boot.

¼ **pound (115 g) Kasseri, in a slab ½ inch**
     (1.3 cm) thick
1 **egg, beaten**
2 **to 3 tablespoons (16 to 24 g) rice protein**
     powder, (10 to 15 g) soy powder, or (14 to
     21 g) low-carb bake mix
Olive oil
1 **shot (1½ ounces, or 42 ml) brandy**
¼ **lemon**

Dip the slab of cheese in the beaten egg, then in the protein powder, coating it all over.

Heat ¼ inch (65 cm) of olive oil in a heavy skillet over medium heat. When the oil is hot, add the cheese.

Fry until golden and crisp on both sides, turning only once. Remove from the pan and put on a fire-proof plate.

Pour the brandy evenly over the hot cheese, strike a match, and light the brandy on fire. It is traditional to shout "Opa!" at this moment.

Squeeze the lemon over the flaming cheese, putting out the fire. Divide in half and scarf it down!

Yield: 2 servings

Each with 3 grams of carbohydrates, a trace of fiber, and 17 grams of protein.

Southwestern Saganaki

This is a yummy twist on the traditional Saganaki and a perfect starter for a fiery Mexican dinner for two.

¼ **pound (115 g) pepper Jack cheese, in a slab**
     ½ inch (1.3 cm) thick
1 **egg, beaten**
2 **to 3 tablespoons (16 to 24 g) rice protein**
     powder, (10 to 15 g) soy powder, or
     (14 to 21 g) low-carb bake mix
Olive oil
1 **shot (1½ ounces, or 42 ml) tequila**
¼ **lime**

Dip the slab of cheese in the beaten egg, then in the protein powder, coating it all over.

Heat ¼ inch (65 cm) of olive oil in a heavy skillet over medium heat. When the oil is hot, add the cheese.

Fry until golden and crisp on both sides, turning only once. Remove from the pan and put on a fire-proof plate.

Pour the tequila evenly over the hot cheese, strike a match, and light the tequila on fire.

Squeeze the lime over the flaming cheese, putting out the fire.

Yield: 2 servings

Each with 3 grams of carbohydrates, a trace of fiber, and 17 grams of protein.

Cheese Cookies

This recipe requires a food processor, so if you only have a tiny one, cut the recipe in half. Despite the name, these are not sweet; they're more like cheese crackers.

½ pound (225 g) processed American loaf cheese, like Velveeta (Store brand works fine.)
½ pound (225 g) sharp cheddar cheese
¼ pound (115 g) butter
1 cup (80 g) soy powder
About 6 dozen pecan or walnut halves (optional)

Preheat the oven to 400°F (200°C, or gas mark 6).

Cut the loaf cheese, cheddar, and butter into chunks.

Put the cheese chunks, butter, and soy powder in the food processor and pulse until the dough is well combined.

Coat a cookie sheet with nonstick cooking spray. Drop spoonfuls of dough onto the cookie sheet and press half a pecan or walnut in the top of each one (if using).

Bake for 8 to 10 minutes or until the cookies are just getting brown around the edges.

Yield: This will depend on how big you make your cookies. I make mine small and get 6 dozen.

Each with 1 gram of carbohydrates, a trace of fiber, and 2 grams of protein.

Antipasto

This easy dish makes a nice light summer supper. Use some or all of the ingredients listed here, adjusting quantities as necessary.

Wedges of cantaloupe
Salami
Boiled ham
Pepperoncini (mildly hot salad peppers, available in jars near the pickles and olives)
Halved or quartered hard-boiled eggs
Marinated mushrooms
Black and green olives (Get the good ones.)
Strips of canned pimento
Solid-pack white tuna, drizzled with olive oil
Sardines
Marinated artichoke hearts (available in cans)

Simply arrange some or all of these things decoratively on a platter, put out a stack of small plates and some forks, and dinner is served.

Yield: Varies with your taste and needs, but here are the basic nutritional breakdowns for the items on your antipasto platter:

Cantaloupe, ⅛ of a small melon: 4.5 grams of carbohydrates and 0.5 grams of fiber, for a total of 4 grams of usable carbs and 0.5 grams of protein

Salami, 1 average slice: 0.5 grams of carbohydrates, a trace of fiber, and 3 grams of protein

Boiled ham, 1 average slice: a trace of carbohydrates, no fiber, and 3.5 grams of protein

Pepperoncini, 1 average piece: 0.5 grams of carbohydrates, a trace of fiber, and no protein

(continued on page 76)

Hard-boiled eggs, ½: 0.3 grams of carbohydrates, no fiber, and 3 grams of protein

Marinated mushrooms, 1 average piece: 1 gram of carbohydrates, a trace of fiber, and no protein

Black olives, 1 large: 0.5 grams of carbohydrates, a trace of fiber, and no protein

Green olives, 1 large: a trace of carbohydrates, a trace of fiber, and no protein

Pimento, 1 slice: a trace of carbohydrates, a trace of fiber, and no protein

Tuna, 3 ounces: no carbohydrates, no fiber, and 22 grams of protein

Sardines, 2 average: no carbohydrates, no fiber, and 5 grams of protein (not to mention 91 milligrams of calcium)

Artichoke hearts, 2 quarters: 2 grams of carbohydrates, 1 gram of fiber, and no protein

Pickled Shrimp

This recipe will feed a crowd, so make it when you have plenty of people to share with.

6 cups (1.4 L) water
¼ cup (60 ml) dry sherry
½ teaspoon peppercorns
1 bay leaf
6 teaspoons (36 g) salt, divided
3 pounds (1.4 kg) raw shrimp, shelled and deveined

1 cup (240 ml) oil
²/₃ cup (160 ml) lemon juice
½ cup (120 ml) white vinegar
3 tablespoons (20 g) mixed pickling spice
2 teaspoons Splenda
2 sprigs fresh dill, coarsely chopped

In a large saucepan over high heat, bring the water, sherry, peppercorns, bay leaf, and 2 teaspoons (12 g) of salt to a boil.

Add the shrimp and bring back to a boil. Cook 1 minute longer and drain.

In a large bowl, combine the oil, lemon juice, vinegar, pickling spice, Splenda, dill, and the remaining 4 teaspoons (24 g) of salt. Add the shrimp and toss with this pickling mixture.

Cover the bowl and chill it and the platter you will serve the shrimp on in the refrigerator overnight.

To serve, drain off and discard the marinade and arrange the shrimp on the platter. Garnish with additional dill, if desired.

Yield: This is enough for a party of a few dozen people, but the carb count will differ according to how big your shrimp are, of course! Figure 24 servings.

Each with less than 1 gram of carbohydrates, a trace of fiber, and 12 grams of protein.

If it's going to be a long party, it's a good idea to set the platter or bowl on a bed of crushed ice in another container to keep the shrimp cold.

Easy Party Shrimp

How easy is this? Yet your guests will devour it. If you can't find the crab boil spices in the spice aisle at your grocery store, ask the fish guys. They should know where it is.

1 envelope (3 ounces, or 85 g) crab boil spices
12 ounces (360 ml) light beer
1 tablespoon (18 g) salt or Vege-Sal
4 pounds (2 kg) easy-peel shrimp or frozen shrimp, unthawed

Drop the crab boil spice net bag in your slow cooker and pour in the beer. Add the salt or Vege-Sal and stir. Add the shrimp. Add just enough water to bring the liquid level up to the top of the shrimp. Cover the slow cooker, set it to high, and let it cook for 1 to 2 hours or until the shrimp are pink through. Set the pot to low.

Serve the shrimp straight from the slow cooker with low-carb cocktail sauce, lemon butter, or mustard and mayo stirred together, for dipping. Or heck, serve all three. This is enough shrimp for a good-sized party, at least 15 or 20 people, if you're serving it as an appetizer/party snack.

Yield: 20 servings

Each with 18 g protein, 1 g carbohydrate, 0 g dietary fiber, 1 g usable carbs. (Analysis does not include any dipping sauces.)

Crab and Bacon Bundles

This quick, hot appetizer will impress your guests.

1 can (6 ounces, or 170 g) crab, drained
1 scallion, finely minced
½ pound (225 g) bacon
Duck Sauce (page 465)

Preheat the broiler.

Flake the crab, removing any bits of shell or cartilage. Stir in the minced scallion and set aside.

Cut all your bacon strips in half crosswise to make two shorter strips. Place a rounded ½ teaspoon or so of the crab mixture on the end of a bacon strip and roll the strip up around it, stretching the bacon slightly as you go. Pierce the bundle with a toothpick to hold. Repeat until all the crab and bacon strips are used up.

Broil about 8 inches (20 cm) from heat, turning once or twice, until the bacon is crisp—no more than 10 minutes. Serve with Duck Sauce for dipping.

Yield: About 2 dozen servings

Each with only a trace of carbohydrates, a trace of fiber, and 4 grams of protein. (Analysis does not include Duck Sauce.)

Cocktail Ham Tartlets

These hot appetizers are a throwback to the 1960s, but they're darned tasty.

Pie Crust (page 520)
2 cans deviled ham, one the 4.25-ounce (120 g) size, the other the 2.25-ounce (60 g) size
¾ cup (180 g) Simple No-Sugar Pickle Relish (page 497)
2 teaspoons spicy brown mustard

Make your pie crust first, but don't pat it into a pie pan. Instead, you're going to use two 12-cup muffin tins. Spray them with nonstick cooking spray, nip off 1-inch (2.5-cm) balls of dough with your fingers, and press each one evenly over the bottom of a muffin cup.

Now, preheat your oven to 375°F (190°C, or gas mark 5). Mix together all the remaining ingredients and spoon about a teaspoon of the mixture into each muffin cup, spreading it with the back of the spoon.

Bake your Cocktail Ham Tartlets for about 20 minutes and then let them cool just a bit before using the rounded tip of a butter knife to loosen each one and lift it out to a serving plate. Serve warm.

Yield: 24 servings

Each with 6 g protein; 2 g carbohydrate; trace dietary fiber; 2 g usable carbs.

Cranberry Barbecue Meatballs

Boring old ground turkey does a Cinderella turn and comes to the party in this dish!

2 pounds (1 kg) ground turkey
2 eggs
4 scallions, minced
2 tablespoons (28 ml) soy sauce
¼ teaspoon orange extract
½ teaspoon pepper
1 teaspoon Splenda
¼ cup (60 ml) oil
1 cup (240 ml) low-carb barbecue sauce (your choice from the Sauces and Seasonings chapter, or purchased)
1 cup (110 g) cranberries (These are strictly seasonal, but they freeze well.)
¼ cup (6 g) Splenda

In a big mixing bowl, combine the turkey, eggs, and scallions.

In another bowl, mix together the soy sauce, orange extract, pepper, and 1 teaspoon Splenda and pour into the bowl with the turkey. Now use clean hands to smoosh it all together until it's very well blended. Make 1-inch (2.5-cm) meatballs from the mixture.

Heat half the oil in a big, heavy skillet over medium heat. Brown the meatballs in a few batches, adding the rest of the oil as needed. Transfer the browned meatballs to your slow cooker.

In a blender or food processor with an S-blade, combine the barbecue sauce, cranberries, and ¼ cup (6 g) Splenda. Run it until the berries are puréed. Pour this mixture over the meatballs.

Cover the slow cooker, set to low, and let it cook for 5 to 6 hours. Serve hot from the slow cooker with toothpicks for spearing!

Yield: 48 meatballs

Each with 4 g protein, 1 g carbohydrate, trace dietary fiber, 1 g usable carbs.

Colombo Meatballs with Jerk Sauce

Colombo is the Caribbean version of curry, and jerk is the notoriously fiery barbecue marinade from Jamaica. The heat of this recipe is best controlled by choosing your hot sauce wisely. If you use Tabasco or Louisiana hot sauce, they'll be spicy. If you use Jamaican Scotch Bonnet sauce or habanero sauce, they'll take the top of your head right off!

FOR MEATBALLS:
1 pound (455 g) ground lamb
1 egg
¼ cup (40 g) minced onion
¼ teaspoon ground coriander
¼ teaspoon ground turmeric
⅛ teaspoon anise seed, ground
1 clove garlic, minced
¼ teaspoon dry mustard
2 teaspoons lemon juice
½ teaspoon Splenda
½ teaspoon salt
2 tablespoons (30 ml) olive oil
1 bay leaf

FOR SAUCE:
¼ cup (40 grams) minced onion
1 teaspoon ground allspice
1 tablespoon (6 g) grated ginger root
1 tablespoon (15 ml) soy sauce
¼ teaspoon dried thyme
¼ teaspoon ground cinnamon
1 tablespoon (1.5 g) Splenda
2 cloves garlic, crushed
¼ cup (60 ml) low-carb ketchup
1 tablespoon (15 ml) lemon juice
1 tablespoon (15 ml) lime juice
1½ teaspoons hot pepper sauce

To make the meatballs: In a big mixing bowl, add the lamb, egg, minced onion, coriander, turmeric, anise seed, minced garlic, dry mustard, lemon juice, Splenda, and salt. Using clean hands, moosh it all together till it's well blended. Then make 1-inch (2.5-cm) meatballs, pressing them together firmly.

Heat the oil in a big, heavy skillet over medium heat and brown the meatballs in two batches. Drop the bay leaf in the bottom of the slow cooker and then put the meatballs on top of it.

To make the sauce: Mix together the minced onion, allspice, ginger, soy sauce, thyme, cinnamon, Splenda, crushed garlic, ketchup, lemon juice, lime juice, and hot pepper sauce. Pour this sauce evenly over the meatballs. Cover the slow cooker, set it to low, and let it cook for 3 hours. Serve hot from the slow cooker. Remove the bay leaf before serving.

Yield: 35 servings

Each with 2 g protein, 1 g carbohydrate, trace dietary fiber, 1 g usable carbs.

Zippy Cocktail Dogs

Here's an easy way to jazz up little cocktail wieners.

¼ cup (60 ml) Dana's No-Sugar Ketchup (page 463) or purchased low-carb ketchup
¼ cup (6 g) Splenda
½ teaspoon blackstrap molasses
1 teaspoon Worcestershire sauce
¼ cup (60 ml) bourbon
½ pound (225 g) cocktail-size hot dogs

In a large bowl, stir together the ketchup, Splenda, molasses, Worcestershire sauce, and bourbon.

Put the hot dogs in the slow cooker and pour the sauce over them. Cover the slow cooker, set it to low, and let it cook for 2 hours. Then uncover and cook for 1 more hour. Serve with toothpicks for spearing.

Yield: 6 servings

Each with 5 g protein, 4 g carbohydrate, trace dietary fiber, 4 g usable carbs.

If you can't get cocktail-size hot dogs, use regular hot dogs cut in chunks. They're not as cute, but they should taste the same!

Orange Smokies

Put these out at your next Super Bowl party and watch people eat!

1 pound (455 g) small smoked sausage links
¼ cup (60 ml) Dana's No-Sugar Ketchup (page 463) or purchased low-carb ketchup
¼ cup (60 ml) lemon juice
2 tablespoons (3 g) Splenda
¼ teaspoon orange extract
¼ teaspoon guar or xanthan (optional)

Put the sausage in your slow cooker.

In a small bowl, stir together the ketchup, lemon juice, Splenda, and orange extract. Thicken the mixture just a little, if you think it needs it, with guar or xanthan. Pour the sauce over the sausage. Cover the slow cooker, set it to low, and let it cook for 3 hours. Keep the sausages hot in the slow cooker to serve.

Yield: 8 servings

Each with 8 g protein, 1 g carbohydrate, trace dietary fiber, 1 g usable carbs.

4

Eggs and Dairy

Dana's Easy Omelet Method

If I had to choose just one skill to teach to every new low-carber, it would be how to make an omelet. They're fast, they're easy, and they make a wide variety of simple ingredients seem like a meal!

First, have your filling ready. If you're using vegetables, you'll want to sauté them first. If you're using cheese, have it grated or sliced and ready to go. If you're making an omelet to use up leftovers—a great idea, by the way—warm them through in the microwave and have them standing by.

Spray your omelet pan well with cooking spray if it doesn't have a good nonstick surface and put it over medium-high heat. While the skillet's heating, grab your eggs—2 is the perfect number for this size pan, but 1 or 3 will work—and a bowl, crack the eggs, and beat them with a fork. Don't add any water or milk or anything while mixing.

The pan is hot enough when a drop of water thrown in sizzles right away. Add a tablespoon of oil or butter, spread it around to cover the bottom, and then pour in the eggs all at once. They should sizzle and immediately start to set. When the bottom layer of egg is set around the edges—this should happen quite quickly—lift the edge using a spatula and tip the pan to let the raw egg flow underneath. Do this all around the edges until there's not enough raw egg to run.

Now, turn your burner to the lowest heat if you have a gas stove. If you have an electric stove, you'll have to have a "warm" burner standing by; electric elements don't cool off fast enough for this job. Put your filling on one half of the omelet, cover it, and let it sit over very low heat for a minute or two, no more. Peek and see if the raw, shiny egg is gone from the top surface (although you can serve it that way if you like— that's how the French prefer their omelets) and the cheese, if you've used it, is melted. If not, re-cover the pan and let it go another minute or two.

When your omelet is done, slip a spatula under the half without the filling and fold it over; then lift the whole thing onto a plate. Or you can get fancy and tip the pan, letting the filling side of the omelet slide onto the plate, folding the top over as you go, but this takes some practice.

This makes a single-serving omelet. I think it's a lot easier to make several individual omelets than to make one big one, and omelets are so fast to make that it's not that big a deal. Anyway, that way you can customize your omelets to each individual's taste. If you're making more than 2 or 3 omelets, just keep them warm in your oven, set to its very lowest heat.

Now here are some ideas for what to put in your omelets!

Macro Cheese Omelet

This is my husband's favorite! With all that cheese, this is mighty filling.

1 tablespoon (14 g) butter
2 eggs, beaten
1 to 2 ounces (28 to 55 g) cheddar, sliced or shredded
1 to 2 ounces (28 to 55 g) Monterey Jack, sliced or shredded
1 slice processed Swiss

Make your omelet according to Dana's Easy Omelet Method (page 82), placing the cheese over half of your omelet when you're ready to add the filling. Cover, turn the heat to low, and cook until the cheese is melted (3 to 4 minutes). Follow the directions to finish making the omelet.

Yield: 1 serving

3 grams of carbohydrates, no fiber, and 46 grams of protein.

Apple, Bacon, and Blue Cheese Omelet

These are three of my favorite things—wrapped in eggs, another of my favorite things!

3 slices bacon
¼ Granny Smith or other crisp, tart apple, thinly sliced
2 teaspoons butter, divided
2 eggs, beaten
1 ounce (30 g) crumbled blue cheese

Start the bacon cooking in the microwave—if you don't own a microwave bacon rack, a glass pie plate will work just fine. (In my microwave, 3 to 4 minutes on high is about right, but microwave power varies.)

While the bacon's cooking, melt 1 teaspoon of butter in your omelet pan over medium-high heat. Add the apples and fry for 2 to 3 minutes per side or until they're slightly golden. Remove the apple slices and keep them on hand.

Melt the remaining butter in the skillet, spread it about, and make your omelet according to Dana's Easy Omelet Method (page 82), using nonstick cooking spray if necessary. Arrange the fried apples on half the omelet, top with the blue cheese, cover the pan, and turn the heat to low.

Go check on that bacon! If it needs another minute, do that now, while the cheese is melting. Then drain it and crumble it over the now-melted blue cheese. Fold and serve.

Yield: 1 serving

6 grams of carbohydrates and 1 gram of fiber, for a total of 5 grams of usable carbs and 23 grams of protein.

Mexican Omelet

This will open your eyes in the morning! It's one of my favorites—I enjoy breathing fire.

1 tablespoon (14 g) butter
2 eggs, beaten
2 ounces (55 g) jalapeño Jack cheese, shredded or sliced
2 tablespoons (32 g) salsa
Hot pepper sauce (optional)

Make your omelet according to Dana's Easy Omelet Method (page 82), placing the cheese over half of your omelet when you're ready to add the filling. Cover, turn the heat to low, and cook until the cheese is melted (3 to 4 minutes). Follow the directions to finish making the omelet. Top with salsa and hot sauce (if using).

Yield: 1 serving

5 grams of carbohydrates and 1 gram of fiber, for a total of 4 grams of usable carbs and 25 grams of protein.

Taco Omelet

This is a great way to use up leftover taco filling.

1 tablespoon (14 g) butter
2 eggs, beaten
¼ cup (50 g) beef, turkey, or chicken taco filling, warmed.
2 tablespoons (15 g) shredded Cheddar cheese
2 tablespoons (32 g) salsa
1 tablespoon (15 g) sour cream

Make your omelet according to Dana's Easy Omelet Method (page 82), placing the taco filling and cheese over half of your omelet when you're ready to add the filling. Cover, turn the heat to low, and cook until the cheese is melted (3 to 4 minutes). Follow the directions to finish making the omelet. Top with salsa and sour cream.

Yield: 1 serving

3 grams of carbohydrates and 1 gram of fiber, for a total of 2 grams of usable carbs and 24 grams of protein. (Analysis does not include garnishes.)

You can, if you like, jazz up this omelet with a little diced onion, olives, or whatever else you like on a taco.

Fajita Omelet

Again, this is a great way to use up leftovers!

1 tablespoon (15 ml) olive oil
2 eggs
Leftover steak or chicken fajita, warmed
1 tablespoon (15 g) sour cream

Make your omelet according to Dana's Easy Omelet Method (page 82), placing the fajita filling over half of your omelet when you're ready to add the filling. Cover, turn the heat to low, and cook for 2 to 3 minutes. Follow the directions to finish making the omelet and top with the sour cream.

Yield: 1 serving

The carb count for this omelet will depend on your recipe for fajitas. The eggs and sour cream will add only 2 grams of carbs, no fiber, and 11 grams of protein.

Kasseri Tapenade Omelet

This omelet is loaded with cool Greek flavors! Look for jars of tapenade, an olive relish, in big grocery stores. Kasseri is a Greek cheese; all my local grocery stores carry it, so I'm guessing yours do too.

2 to 3 teaspoons olive oil
2 eggs, beaten
1 ounce (30 g) kasseri cheese, sliced or shredded
1½ tablespoons (23 ml) tapenade

Make your omelet according to Dana's Easy Omelet Method (page 82). Cover half the omelet with the cheese and then top with the tapenade when you're ready to add the filling. Cover, turn the heat to low, and let it cook for a couple of minutes until the cheese is melted. Fold and serve.

Yield: 1 serving

4 grams of carbohydrates, no fiber, and 18 grams of protein.

Club Omelet

One of the few high-carb meals I miss is the turkey club sandwich—so here's the omelet equivalent!

2 slices bacon, cooked and drained
2 ounces (55 g) turkey breast slices
½ small tomato, sliced
1 scallion, sliced
2 eggs
1 tablespoon (15 g) mayonnaise

Have your bacon cooked and drained—I like to microwave mine and crumble it up. Cut the turkey into small squares and have the tomato and scallion sliced and at hand.

Beat the eggs, and make your omelet according to Dana's Easy Omelet Method (page 82), adding just the bacon and turkey while it's still cooking. Once it's cooked to your liking, sprinkle the tomato and scallion over the meat, spread the mayo on the other side, fold, and serve.

Yield: 1 serving

Each with 29 g protein; 5 g carbohydrate; 1 g dietary fiber; 4 g usable carbs.

Tuna Melt Omelet

It's worth making extra tuna salad just to make this omelet. This is a great lunch.

1 tablespoon (14 g) butter
2 eggs, beaten
1 ounce (28 g) Swiss cheese or processed Swiss-style singles
½ cup (100 g) leftover tuna salad, warmed to room temperature

(continued on page 86)

Make your omelet according to Dana's Easy Omelet Method (page 82), placing the Swiss cheese over half of your omelet when you're ready to add the filling. Spread the tuna salad over the cheese, cover, turn the heat to low, and cook until hot all the way through (3 to 4 minutes). Follow the directions to finish making the omelet.

Yield: 1 serving

The carb count of this omelet will depend on your recipe for tuna salad. The eggs and cheese will add only 2 grams of carbohydrates, no fiber, and 19 grams of protein.

Denver Omelet

1 tablespoon (14 g) butter
2 eggs
1 ounce (28 g) cheddar cheese, shredded
   or sliced
¼ cup (40 g) diced cooked ham
¼ green pepper, cut in small strips and
   sautéed
¼ small onion, sliced and sautéed

Make your omelet according to Dana's Easy Omelet Method (page 82), placing the cheese and the sautéed ham and vegetables over half of your omelet when you're ready to add the filling. Cover, turn the heat to low, and cook until the cheese is melted (3 to 4 minutes). Follow the directions to finish making the omelet.

Yield: 1 serving

7 grams of carbohydrates and 1 gram of fiber, for a total of 6 grams of usable carbs (and you can cut that by using seriously low-carb ham) and 25 grams of protein.

Artichoke Parmesan Omelet

This is a terrific combination.

1 tablespoon (14 g) butter
2 eggs, beaten
1 to 2 tablespoons (14 to 28 g) mayonnaise
1 canned artichoke heart, sliced
2 tablespoons (12.5 g) grated Parmesan
   cheese

Make your omelet according to Dana's Easy Omelet Method (page 82), spreading mayonnaise over one half of your omelet and topping it with the artichoke heart and Parmesan when you're ready to add the filling. Cover, turn the heat to low, and cook until the cheese is melted (3 to 4 minutes). Follow the directions to finish making the omelet.

Yield: 1 serving

11 grams of carbohydrates and 5 grams of fiber, for a total of 6 grams of usable carbs and 18 grams of protein.

Roman Mushroom Omelet

Believe it or not, this is classical Italian food, with no pasta in sight.

2 cups (200 g) sliced mushrooms
¼ small onion, sliced thin
1 stalk celery, diced fine
2 tablespoons (30 ml) olive oil
1 clove garlic
½ teaspoon chicken bouillon granules
½ teaspoon Splenda
Salt and pepper
4 eggs
½ cup (80 g) shredded Romano cheese, divided

In your big skillet, start sautéing the mushrooms, onion, and celery in the olive oil. When the mushrooms have changed color and the onion is translucent, add the garlic, chicken bouillon granules, and Splenda, stirring until the bouillon dissolves. Let cook for another minute or so. Add salt and pepper to the mushroom mixture to taste and remove from skillet.

Now, in your omelet pan, make 2 omelets, one after the other, according to Dana's Easy Omelet Method (page 82), using the mushrooms as filling and ¼ cup (40 g) of shredded Romano cheese per omelet on top. Cover and cook until the cheese melts, fold, and serve. (You can keep the first omelet warm long enough to make the second omelet by simply covering the plate with a spare pot lid. For that matter, you can halve this recipe to make one omelet!)

Yield: 2 omelets

Each with 22 g protein; 8 g carbohydrate; 1 g dietary fiber; 7 g usable carbs.

Curried Cheese and Olive Omelets

This was originally a spread for English muffins and the like, but it makes a wicked omelet. I know that this combination of ingredients sounds a little odd, but the flavor is magical.

1 cup (120 g) shredded cheddar cheese
5 or 6 scallions, finely sliced, including the crisp part of the green
1 can (4.25 ounces, or 120 g) chopped ripe olives, drained
3 tablespoons (42 g) mayonnaise
½ teaspoon curry powder
6 eggs, beaten

Simply plunk the cheese, scallions, olives, mayonnaise, and curry powder in a mixing bowl and combine well. Now, make 3 omelets according to Dana's Easy Omelet Method (page 82), using the cheese-and-olive mixture as the filling. If there's only one of you, however, just use 2 eggs to make 1 omelet. The cheese mixture will keep well for a couple of days in a closed container in the refrigerator, letting you make fabulous omelets very quickly for a few days running.

Yield: 3 servings

Each with 6 grams of carbohydrates and 3 grams of fiber, for a total of 3 grams of usable carbs and 21 grams of protein. (As a bonus, you get 372 milligrams of calcium!)

"My Day to Crab" Omelet

My grandmother never got to go crabbing when the family was at the shore because she was too busy keeping house. Finally she declared, "It's my day to crab!" If it's your day to crab, this omelet will cheer you up.

¼ **cup (35 g) canned crabmeat, flaked and picked over for shells and cartilage**
2 **scallions, sliced, including the crisp part of the green**
1 **tablespoon (14 g) butter**
2 **eggs, beaten**
1 **to 2 tablespoons (14 to 28 g) mayonnaise**

Mix the crab meat with the scallions and have the mixture standing by. Make your omelet according to Dana's Easy Omelet Method (page 82), spreading mayonnaise over half the omelet and topping it with the crab and scallion mixture when you're ready to add the filling. Cover, turn the heat to low, and cook until the cheese is melted (3 to 4 minutes). Follow the directions to finish making the omelet.

Yield: 1 serving

3 grams of carbohydrates and 1 gram of fiber, for a total of 2 grams of usable carbs and 19 grams of protein.

Leftover Lamblet

I adore roast lamb, and the leftovers are way too good to waste! This is very hearty and would make a great quick supper.

¼ **pound (115 g) leftover roast lamb, cut into small chunks**
½ **small onion**
2 **tablespoons (12.5 g) grated Parmesan cheese**
3 **tablespoons (42 g) mayonnaise**
½ **teaspoon prepared horseradish**
1 **tablespoon (14 g) butter**
2 **eggs, beaten**

In a food processor with the S-blade in place, grind the lamb and the onion together. When you have a pretty uniform consistency, add the Parmesan, mayonnaise, and horseradish and pulse until everything is combined. Place in a microwave-safe bowl and microwave on 50 percent power for just 1 minute or so to warm through.

Make your omelet according to Dana's Easy Omelet Method (page 82), placing the lamb mixture evenly over half of your omelet when you're ready to add the filling. Cover, turn the heat to low, and cook until the eggs are set (60 to 90 seconds). Follow the directions to finish making the omelet.

Yield: 1 serving

6 grams of carbohydrates and 1 gram of fiber, for a total of 5 grams of usable carbs and 38 grams of protein.

Sloppy Tom Omelet

I like this omelet as a quick lunch. Indeed, I've been known to make Sloppy Toms just to have them on hand for this purpose. If you have a favorite low-carb Sloppy Joe recipe, feel free to use it instead.

2 eggs
¼ cup (50 g) Sloppy Toms (page 354)
1 ounce (30 g) cheddar cheese or Monterey Jack, sliced or shredded

If your Sloppy Toms are left over, straight out of the fridge, warm them a bit in the microwave before you start cooking the eggs. Then make your omelet according to Dana's Easy Omelet Method (page 82), adding the cheese first, then the Sloppy Toms on top of the cheese. Cover, turn heat to low and finish cooking, and then fold and serve.

Yield: 1 serving

Each with 27 g protein; 7 g carbohydrate; 1 g dietary fiber; 6 g usable carbs.

Pizza Omelet

Remember that the pizza sauce is where the carbs are in this omelet, so govern yourself accordingly.

1 tablespoon (15 ml) olive oil
2 eggs, beaten
2 ounces (55 g) mozzarella cheese
2 tablespoons (30 ml) jarred no-sugar-added pizza sauce, warmed
1 teaspoon grated Parmesan cheese

Make your omelet according to Dana's Easy Omelet Method (page 82), placing the mozzarella over half of your omelet when you're ready to add the filling. Cover, turn the heat to low, and cook until the cheese is melted (2 to 3 minutes). Follow the directions to finish making the omelet and top with the pizza sauce and Parmesan.

Yield: 1 serving

6 grams of carbohydrates (and you can lower that if you use the lowest-carb pizza sauce), no fiber, and 24 grams of protein.

California Omelet

I've had breakfast down near the waterfront in San Diego. This is what it tastes like.

1 tablespoon (15 ml) olive oil
2 eggs, beaten
2 ounces (55 g) Monterey Jack cheese, shredded
3 or 4 slices ripe black avocado
¼ cup (4 g) alfalfa sprouts

Make your omelet according to Dana's Easy Omelet Method (page 82), placing the Monterey Jack over half of your omelet when you're ready to add the filling. Cover, turn the heat to low, and cook until the cheese is melted (2 to 3 minutes). Arrange the avocado and sprouts over the cheese and follow the directions to finish making the omelet.

Yield: 1 serving

4 grams of carbohydrates and 1 gram of fiber, for a total of 3 grams of usable carbs and 26 grams of protein (and as much potassium as a banana!).

Guacomelet

Should you happen to have leftover guacamole—an unlikely circumstance, I'll admit—this is a fine thing to do with it.

1 tablespoon (15 ml) oil
2 eggs, beaten
2 ounces (55 g) Monterey Jack cheese, sliced or shredded
¼ cup (59 g) guacamole

Make your omelet according to Dana's Easy Omelet Method (page 82), placing the cheese over half of your omelet when you're ready to add the filling. Spread the guacamole over the cheese, cover, turn the heat to low, and cook until the cheese is melted (3 to 4 minutes). Follow the directions to finish making the omelet.

Yield: 1 serving

6 grams of carbohydrates and 1 gram of fiber, for a total of 5 grams of usable carbs and 26 grams of protein (and a whopping 487 milligrams of potassium!).

Avocado Cheese Dip Omelet

This is perhaps the most decadently delicious omelet I know how to make, and it's certainly a good enough reason to hide some of the Avocado Cheese Dip at your next party.

1 tablespoon (15 ml) olive oil
2 eggs, beaten
⅓ cup (80 g) Avocado Cheese Dip (page 61)

Make your omelet according to Dana's Easy Omelet Method (page 82), placing the Avocado Cheese Dip over half of your omelet when you're ready to add the filling. Cover, turn the heat to low, and cook until hot all the way through (3 to 4 minutes). Follow the directions to finish making the omelet.

Yield: 1 serving

6 grams of carbohydrates and 1 gram of fiber, for a total of 5 grams of usable carbs and 19 grams of protein.

"Clean the Fridge" Omelet

The name is not a joke—I made this omelet up out of whatever I found kicking around in the refrigerator, needing to be used up before it went bad. The results were definitely good enough to make it again.

½ red bell pepper, cut into thin strips
¼ medium onion, thinly sliced
3 tablespoons (45 ml) olive oil
2 eggs, beaten
1 ounce (30 g) jalapeño jack, shredded or sliced
½ black avocado, sliced

In your skillet over medium-high heat, sauté the pepper and onion in the oil until the onion is translucent and the pepper is going limp. Remove from the pan and keep on hand. If your pan isn't nonstick, give it a shot of nonstick cooking spray before putting it back on the heat and increasing the heat a touch to high.

Make your omelet according to Dana's Easy Omelet Method (page 82). Put the cheese on half the omelet and top with the avocado and then the pepper and onion. Cover, turn the heat to low, and let it cook until the cheese is melted. Fold and serve.

Yield: 1 serving

14 grams of carbohydrates and 6 grams of fiber, for a total of 8 grams of usable carbs and 21 grams of protein. (This also contains a whopping 821 milligrams of potassium!)

New York Sunday Brunch Omelet

My husband was absolutely blown away by this. It's unbelievably filling, by the way.

1 tablespoon (14 g) butter
2 eggs, beaten
2 ounces (55 g) cream cheese, thinly sliced
¼ cup (50 g) flaked smoked salmon
2 scallions, sliced

Make your omelet according to Dana's Easy Omelet Method (page 82), placing the cream cheese over half of your omelet when you're ready to add the filling. (Don't try to spread the cream cheese—it won't work!) Top with the salmon, cover, turn the heat to low, and cook until hot all the way through (2 to 3 minutes). Scatter the scallions over salmon and follow the directions to finish making the omelet.

Yield: 1 serving

5 grams of carbohydrates and 1 gram of fiber, for a total of 4 grams of usable carbs and 22 grams of protein.

Ropa Vieja Omelet

Here's another way to use your Ropa Vieja (page 380)

⅓ cup (70 g) Ropa Vieja
1 ounce (30 g) Monterey Jack cheese
¼ black avocado, sliced
2 eggs

Warm your Ropa Vieja in the microwave, slice or shred your cheese, and slice your avocado; have everything standing by!

Now heat your omelet pan and add a little oil. Beat up your eggs, and when the skillet's hot, pour them in and make your omelet according to Dana's Easy Omelet Method (page 82). When it's time to add the filling, put the cheese in first, then the Ropa Vieja, and then the avocado. Cover, turn heat to low, and finish cooking. Fold and serve.

Yield: 1 serving

Each with 29 g protein; 5 g carbohydrate; 2 g dietary fiber; 3 g usable carbs.

Omelet Cordon Bleu

Canned asparagus is fine for this, but you may cook some up if you prefer or use leftover asparagus, should you have any.

1 tablespoon (14 g) butter
2 eggs
¼ cup (30 g) shredded Gruyère cheese
1 ounce (28 g) boiled or baked deli ham
   (or sliced leftover ham)
3 asparagus spears, cooked

Make your omelet according to Dana's Easy Omelet Method (page 82), placing the Gruyère, ham, and asparagus over half of your omelet when you're ready to add the filling. Cover, turn the heat to low, and cook until the cheese is melted (2 to 3 minutes). Follow the directions to finish making the omelet.

Yield: 1 serving

3 grams of carbohydrates and 1 gram of fiber, for a total of 2 grams of usable carbs and 25 grams of protein.

Braunschweiger Omelet

Hey, don't look like that! Some of us love liverwurst!

1 tablespoon (14 g) butter
2 eggs, beaten
2 ounces (55 g) braunschweiger (liverwurst),
   mashed a bit with a fork

2 or 3 slices ripe tomato

Make your omelet according to Dana's Easy Omelet Method (page 82), spooning the mashed braunschweiger over half of your omelet and topping with the tomato slices when you're ready to add the filling. Cover, turn the heat to low, and cook until heated through (2 to 3 minutes). Follow the directions to finish making the omelet.

Yield: 1 serving

4 grams of carbohydrates, a trace of fiber, and 19 grams of protein.

Chili Omelet

You can use either beef chili or turkey chili. It doesn't matter—they both make a great omelet.

1 tablespoon (15 ml) olive oil
2 eggs, beaten
½ cup (100 g) all-meat chili, warmed
2 tablespoons (8 g) shredded cheddar cheese
1 tablespoon (15 g) sour cream

Make your omelet according to Dana's Easy Omelet Method (page 82), placing the chili over half of your omelet when you're ready to add the filling. Top with the cheddar, cover, turn the heat to low, and cook until the cheese is melted (2 to 3 minutes). Follow the directions to finish making the omelet and top with the sour cream.

Yield: 1 serving

About 6 grams of carbohydrates (depending on your chili recipe), no fiber, and 33 grams of protein.

Blintzlets

This falls somewhere between a blintz and an omelet—hence the name. These are not dirt-low in carbs, but they're really yummy. They can be a special breakfast—you'll want to add a little more protein on the side, maybe some ham—or even a light dessert.

1 cup (225 g) 4% or 2% cottage cheese
2 tablespoons (30 g) sour cream
½ teaspoon vanilla extract
1 tablespoon (1.5 g) Splenda
4 eggs
¼ cup (30 g) vanilla whey protein powder
6 tablespoons (90 ml) low-sugar strawberry
    preserves

Put the cottage cheese, sour cream, vanilla, and Splenda in your food processor with the S-blade in place. Process until smooth.

Put the eggs and the protein powder in a blender and whirl for 20 seconds or so.

Heat an 8- or 9-inch (20- or 25-cm) nonstick skillet over medium-high heat. Make sure it's hot before you cook! Even though it's nonstick, spray it with nonstick cooking spray. Now, pour in a small puddle of the egg mixture and swirl the pan to coat the whole bottom—the idea is to use just enough of the egg mixture to cover the bottom of the skillet with a thin but solid layer. Cook until the top of the egg is set—this takes only a minute or so—and then turn briefly. The protein powder makes this mixture very fragile, so be careful.

Lay the thin, eggy pancake on a plate, spread 1 tablespoon of the preserves on one half, and spoon 3 tablespoons of the cottage cheese mixture over it. Fold and serve. Repeat with remaining ingredients.

Yield: Makes 6

Each with 9 grams of carbohydrates and 11 grams of protein. You can cut the carb count of each serving 3 grams by using just ½ tablespoon of preserves in each one. Or you could thaw ½ cup (150 g) of frozen unsweetened strawberries, mash them with a tablespoon or two of Splenda, and use them in place of the preserves. This would save 5 grams of carbs per serving.

Frittatas

The frittata is the Italian version of the omelet, and it involves no folding! If you're still intimidated by omelets, try a frittata.

Confetti Frittata

¼ pound (115 g) bulk pork sausage
¼ cup (38 g) diced green pepper
¼ cup (38 g) diced sweet red pepper
¼ cup (40 g) diced sweet red onion
¼ cup (25 g) grated Parmesan cheese
1 teaspoon salt-free seasoning, such as
    original flavor Mrs. Dash
8 eggs, beaten

Preheat the broiler.

In a large, oven-proof skillet, start browning and crumbling the sausage over medium heat. As some fat starts to cook out of it, add the green peppers, red peppers, and onion to the skillet. Cook the sausage and veggies until

(continued on page 94)

there's no pink left in the sausage. Spread the sausage and veggie mixture into an even layer in the bottom of the skillet.

In a medium bowl, beat the Parmesan cheese and seasoning into the eggs and pour the mixture over the sausage and veggies in the skillet.

Turn the heat to low and cover the skillet. (If your skillet doesn't have a cover, use foil.) Let the frittata cook until the eggs are mostly set. This may take up to 25 to 30 minutes, but the size of your skillet will affect the speed of cooking, so check periodically.

When all but the very top of the frittata is set, slide it under the broiler for about 5 minutes or until the top is golden. Cut into wedges and serve.

Yield: 4 servings

Each with 4 grams of carbohydrates and 1 gram of fiber, for a total of 3 grams of usable carbohydrates and 17 grams of protein.

Artichoke Mushroom Frittata

3 tablespoons (42 g) butter

1 cup (300 g) canned, quartered artichoke hearts, drained

4 ounces (115 g) fresh mushrooms, sliced

½ small onion, sliced

8 eggs, beaten

6 ounces (170 g) shredded Gruyère cheese

Preheat the broiler.

In a heavy skillet, melt the butter and sauté the artichoke hearts, mushrooms, and onion over medium-low heat until the mushrooms are limp.

Spread the vegetables evenly over the bottom of the skillet and pour the eggs over them.

Turn the heat to low and cover the skillet. (If your skillet doesn't have a cover, use foil.) Let the frittata cook until mostly set (7 to 10 minutes).

Top with the Gruyère and slide the skillet under the broiler, about 4 inches (10 cm) from the heat. Broil for 2 to 3 minutes or until the eggs are set on top and the cheese is lightly golden. Cut into wedges and serve.

Yield: 4 servings

Each with 7 grams of carbohydrates and 3 grams of fiber, for a total of 4 grams of usable carbs and 26 grams of protein.

Artichoke and Friends Frittata

3 tablespoons (45 ml) olive oil

¼ pound (115 g) zucchini (about 1 really little zucchini), diced small

3 tablespoons (30 g) chopped onion

1 clove garlic, crushed

½ small green pepper, diced

½ small red pepper, diced

1 cup (300 g) canned artichoke hearts, drained and chopped

1 cup (110 g) ¼-inch (6-mm) ham cubes

¼ cup (15 g) chopped fresh parsley

10 eggs

1 tablespoon (5 g) oregano

⅓ cup (33.3 g) grated Parmesan cheese

Preheat the broiler.

For this you need an oven-safe skillet—a big cast-iron skillet works great. Spray the skillet with nonstick cooking spray and put it over medium-high heat. Add the olive oil and start sautéing the zucchini, onion, garlic, and peppers. When the vegetables are starting to soften, stir in the artichoke hearts, ham cubes, and fresh parsley. Let the whole thing continue cooking while you prepare the eggs.

Scramble up the eggs with the oregano and Parmesan.

Arrange everything in the skillet in an even layer and pour in the eggs. Cover the pan, turn the heat to low, and let the whole thing cook for 15 to 20 minutes or until all but the top is set.

Run the skillet under the broiler for 3 or 4 minutes until it starts to brown a little. Then cut frittata in wedges to serve.

Yield: 4 to 5 servings

Assuming 5 servings, each will have 20 g protein; 8 g carbohydrate; 1 g dietary fiber; 7 g usable carbs.

Chorizo Frittata

This recipe is very South of the Border. If you like chorizo (Mexican sausage), you might cook some up, drain it well, and keep it in a container in the freezer so you can whip up one of these omelets on short notice.

1 tablespoon (15 ml) oil

½ green pepper, diced

1 small onion, sliced

⅔ cup (75 g) cooked, crumbled, drained chorizo

⅔ cup (173 g) salsa

8 eggs, beaten

6 ounces (170 g) shredded cheddar or Monterey Jack

Preheat the broiler.

In a large, heavy skillet over medium heat, heat the oil and sauté the green pepper and onion for a few minutes until tender-crisp. Add the chorizo and the salsa, stir well, and heat through.

Spread the mixture into an even layer on the bottom of the skillet and pour in the eggs.

Turn the heat to low and cover the skillet. (If your skillet doesn't have a cover, use foil.) Let the frittata cook until the eggs are mostly set (7 to 10 minutes).

Top with the shredded cheese and slide the skillet under the broiler, about 4 inches (10 cm) from the heat. Broil for 2 to 3 minutes or until the eggs are set and the cheese is melted. Cut into wedges and serve.

Yield: 4 servings

Each with 8 grams of carbohydrates and 1 gram of fiber, for a total of 7 grams of usable carbs and 32 grams of protein.

UnPotato Tortilla

Don't think Mexican flatbread, think eggs. In Spain, a "tortilla" is much like an Italian frittata—a substantial egg dish, cooked in a skillet and served in wedges. This one is my version of a traditional dish served in tapas bars all over Spain. As bar food goes, it's a heckuva step up from beer nuts and stale popcorn!

¼ **head cauliflower**
1 **medium turnip**
1 **medium onion, sliced thin**
3 **tablespoons (45 ml) olive oil, divided**
6 **eggs**
Salt and pepper

Thinly slice your cauliflower—include the stem—and peel and thinly slice your turnip. Put them in a microwaveable casserole dish with a lid, add a couple of tablespoons of water, and microwave on high for 6 to 7 minutes.

In the meanwhile, start the onion sautéing in 2 tablespoons (30 ml) of the olive oil in an 8- to 9-inch (20- to 23-cm) skillet—a nonstick skillet is ideal, but it's not essential. If your skillet isn't nonstick, give it a good squirt of nonstick cooking spray first. Use medium heat.

When your microwave goes beep, pull out the veggies, drain them, and throw them in the skillet with the onion. Continue sautéing everything, adding a bit more oil if things start to stick, until the veggies are getting golden around the edges—about 10 to 15 minutes. Turn the heat to low and spread the vegetables in an even layer on the bottom of the skillet.

Mix up the eggs with a little salt and pepper and pour over the vegetables. Cook on low for 5 to 7 minutes, lifting the edges frequently to let uncooked egg run underneath. When it's all set except for the top, slide the skillet under a low broiler for 4 to 5 minutes or until the top of your tortilla is golden. (If your skillet doesn't have a flameproof handle, wrap it in foil first.) Cut in wedges to serve. A sprinkling of chopped parsley is nice gainish.

Yield: 6 servings

Each with 6 g protein; 4 g carbohydrate; 1 g dietary fiber; 3 g usable carbs.

Scrambles

When both omelets and frittatas are too much trouble, just make a scramble. The ways of varying scrambled eggs are endless, so you could have them several times a week and never get bored. These have been analyzed assuming a three-egg serving, but if you want a lighter meal, leave out one egg and subtract 0.5 gram of carbohydrates and 6 grams of protein from my analysis.

Country Scramble

This fast-and-filling family-pleaser is a great way to use up leftover ham.

1 **tablespoon (14 g) butter**
¼ **cup (40 g) diced cooked ham**
¼ **cup (38 g) diced green pepper**
2 **tablespoons (20 g) diced onion**
3 **eggs, beaten**
Salt and pepper

Melt the butter in a skillet over medium heat. Add the ham, green pepper, and onion and sauté for a few minutes until the onion is softened.

Pour in the eggs and scramble until the eggs are set. Add salt and pepper to taste and serve.

Yield: 2 servings

Each with 7 grams of carbohydrates and 1 gram of fiber, for a total of 6 grams of usable carbs and 23 grams of protein.

Don't look at the number of servings and assume you can't feed a hungry family with a scramble—these recipes are a snap to double, as long as you have a skillet large enough to scramble in.

Huevos Con El Sabor de Chiles Rellenos

Chiles Rellenos—green chilies stuffed with cheese, dipped in batter, and then fried—are irresistible, and very time-consuming to make. However, since the traditional batter is egg-rich, it occurred to me to incorporate the chilies and the cheese into a scramble. It's delicious! If you haven't tried canned green chilies, you should know that they're only slightly spicy—this recipe won't leave you gasping and reaching for a glass of water.

6 eggs
¼ cup (30 g) canned diced green chilies
1 tablespoon (14 g) butter or oil
4 ounces (115 g) Monterey Jack cheese, cut into small chunks

Beat the eggs with the chilies. Spray a large, heavy skillet with nonstick cooking spray and put it over medium-high heat. When the skillet is hot, add the butter or oil, and move it around to coat the bottom of the skillet.

Pour in the beaten eggs with chilies and scramble them until they're about half-set. Add the chunks of Monterey Jack, continue scrambling until set, and then serve.

Yield: 2 or 3 servings

Assuming 2 servings, each will have 4 grams of carbohydrates, a trace of fiber, and 31 grams of protein.

Inauthentic Machaca Eggs

True Machaca is made with beef that you've salted and dried, then rehydrated in boiling water, and pounded into shreds. It's very tasty, but I don't know a lot of people who want to do that much work. The beef shreds from the Ropa Vieja work beautifully in this scramble!

2 tablespoons (30 ml) olive oil
1 cup (200 g) Ropa Vieja (page 380)
½ green bell pepper, diced
½ onion, chopped
1 clove garlic, crushed
1 cup (240 g) canned tomatoes with green chilies, drained
5 eggs
¼ cup (16 g) chopped fresh cilantro

(continued on page 98)

Heat the olive oil in a large, heavy skillet and add the Ropa Vieja, diced pepper, onion, and garlic. Sauté them together, stirring often, until the onion and pepper are becoming a little soft. In the meanwhile, measure your tomatoes and beat your eggs.

Okay, your onion is translucent, and your pepper's starting to soften. Add the tomato, stir it up, and then pour in the beaten eggs. Scramble until the eggs are set. Divide evenly between two plates, top each serving with half the cilantro, and serve.

Feel free to add some chopped jalapeños or more green chilies to this, if you'd like it spicy. Or you could use a pasilla or Anaheim chili in place of the green pepper.

Yield: 2 to 3 servings

Assuming 2 servings, each will have 30 g protein; 12 g carbohydrate; 2 g dietary fiber; 10 g usable carbs.

Curry Scramble

I'm in love with curry. With a green salad, this makes a great light supper whether you're a devoted curry lover or not.

1 tablespoon butter
¼ teaspoon curry powder
½ clove garlic, crushed
3 eggs
1 tablespoon (15 ml) heavy cream
3 slices bacon, cooked until crisp

Melt the butter in a heavy skillet and sauté the curry powder and garlic over medium-low heat for a minute or two.

Beat the eggs and cream together, pour into the skillet, and scramble until the eggs are set. Crumble bacon over the top.

Yield: 1 serving

3 grams of carbohydrates, a trace of fiber, and 23 grams of protein.

Smoked Salmon and Goat Cheese Scramble

This sounds fancy, I know, but it takes almost no time and is very impressive. It's terrific to make for a special brunch or a late-night supper. A simple green salad with a classic vinaigrette dressing would be perfect with this.

4 eggs
½ cup (120 ml) heavy cream
1 teaspoon dried dill weed
4 scallions
¼ pound (115 g) chevre (goat cheese)
¼ pound (115 g) moist smoked salmon
1 to 2 tablespoons (14 to 28 g) butter

Whisk the eggs together with the cream and dill weed. Slice the scallions thin, including the crisp part of the green. Cut the chevre—it will have a texture similar to cream cheese—into little hunks. Coarsely crumble the smoked salmon.

In a big (preferably nonstick) skillet, melt the butter over medium-high heat. (If your skillet doesn't have a nonstick surface, give it a shot of nonstick cooking spray before adding the butter.) When the butter's melted, add the scallions first and sauté them for just a minute. Add the egg mixture and cook, stirring frequently, until the eggs are halfway set—about 1 minute to 90 seconds. Add the chevre and smoked salmon, continue cooking and stirring until the eggs are set, and serve.

Yield: 3 servings

Each with 5 grams of carbohydrates and 1 gram of fiber, for a total of 4 grams of usable carbs and 27 grams of protein.

Springtime Scramble

4 stalks asparagus
8 fresh snow pea pods
1 scallion
3 eggs
1 teaspoon olive oil

Snap the bottoms off your asparagus where they break naturally and then cut the stalks into ½-inch (1.25-cm) pieces on the diagonal. Pinch the ends off the snow peas and pull off the strings. Then cut them into ½-inch (1.25-cm) pieces, too. Put the two in a microwaveable bowl, add a couple of teaspoons of water, cover, and microwave on high for just 3 minutes. Uncover as soon as the microwave beeps! While this is happening, slice your scallion, including the crisp part of the green, and whisk your eggs.

Okay, pull your asparagus and snow peas out of the microwave. Spray a medium skillet with nonstick cooking spray and place over medium heat. Add the olive oil and let it start heating. Drain the asparagus and snow peas and throw them in the skillet, along with the scallion. Now pour in the eggs and scramble until set. That's it!

Yield: 1 serving

Each with 19 g protein; 8 g carbohydrate; 2 g dietary fiber; 6 g usable carbs.

Piperade

Say "peep-er-ahd." This Basque peasant dish has so many vegetables in it that it's a whole meal in itself.

2 tablespoons bacon grease
¼ cup diced onion
½ cup diced green pepper
⅓ cup diced tomato (very ripe fresh or canned)
3 eggs, beaten
Salt and pepper

Heat the bacon grease in a heavy skillet over lowest heat. Add the onion and sauté for 5 to 7 minutes or until the onion is soft.

Add the pepper and the tomato. Stir, cover, and cook at lowest heat for 15 minutes, stirring once or twice. (You want the vegetables to be quite soft.)

(continued on page 100)

Pour in the eggs and scramble slowly until the eggs are just set. Add salt and pepper to taste and serve.

Yield: 1 serving

13 grams of carbohydrates and 3 grams of fiber, for a total of 10 grams of usable carbs and 18 grams of protein.

Variation: Hearty Piperade—Make just as you would regular Piperade, but add ¼ cup (40 g) diced ham for each serving. (This is a great time to use up any leftovers you've been saving.) Sauté the ham with the vegetables and then add the eggs and scramble as usual.

Yield: 1 serving

14 grams of carbohydrates and 3 grams of fiber, for a total of 11 grams of usable carbs and 24 grams of protein.

Moroccan Scramble

With all these vegetables, this is a meal in itself. It's exotic and fabulous.

1 tablespoon (15 ml) olive oil
¼ cup (30 g) chopped onion
½ teaspoon minced garlic or 1 clove garlic, crushed
1 tablespoon (15 ml) tapenade
¼ cup (60 g) canned diced tomatoes
3 eggs
½ teaspoon ground cumin

2 tablespoons (8 g) chopped fresh cilantro
Salt and pepper

In a skillet, heat the olive oil over high heat and start sautéing the onion and garlic. When the onion is translucent, add the tapenade and tomatoes and stir. Now, whisk the eggs with the cumin and pour into the vegetable mixture. Scramble until mostly set and then add the cilantro and scramble until done. Add salt and pepper to taste and serve.

Yield: 1 serving

11 grams of carbohydrates and 1 gram of fiber, for a total of 10 grams of usable carbs and 18 grams of protein.

Italian Scramble

This is a good quick supper. Serve it with a green salad and some garlic bread for the kids.

2 tablespoons (30 ml) olive oil
¼ cup (40 g) diced green pepper
¼ cup (40 g) chopped onion
1 clove garlic, crushed
3 eggs
1 tablespoon (6.3 g) grated Parmesan cheese

Heat the olive oil in a heavy skillet over medium heat and sauté the pepper, onion, and garlic for 5 to 7 minutes or until the onion is translucent.

Beat the eggs with the Parmesan and pour into the skillet. Scramble until the eggs are set and serve.

8 grams of carbohydrates and 1 gram of fiber, for a total of 7 grams of usable carbs and 17 grams of protein.

Parmesan Rosemary Eggs

This is so simple and so wonderful. If you like Italian food, you have to try this. It's also easy to double or triple.

3 eggs
2 tablespoons (30 ml) heavy cream
¼ cup (25 g) grated Parmesan cheese
½ teaspoon ground rosemary*
½ teaspoon minced garlic
½ tablespoon butter

Whisk together the eggs, cream, cheese, rosemary, and garlic. Put a medium-size skillet over medium-high heat (if it isn't nonstick, give it a shot of nonstick cooking spray first). When the pan is hot, add the butter, give the egg mixture one last stir to make sure the cheese hasn't settled to the bottom, and then pour the egg mixture into the skillet. Scramble until the eggs are set and serve.

Yield: 1 serving

3 grams of carbohydrates, a trace of fiber, and 25 grams of protein.

*You can use whole, dried rosemary, but you'll have little needles in your food. If you do use whole rosemary, increase the amount to 1 teaspoon.

Greek Scramble

2 tablespoons (30 ml) olive oil
1 tablespoon (10 g) minced onion
6 good, strong, black Greek olives, chopped
3 eggs, beaten
¼ cup (38 g) crumbled feta cheese

Heat the oil in heavy skillet over medium heat. Sauté the onion for a minute or two and then add the olives and sauté for a minute more.

Pour in the eggs and add the feta. Scramble until set and serve.

Yield: 1 serving

6 grams of carbohydrates, a trace of fiber, and 22 grams of protein.

French Country Scramble

This is for anyone who doesn't think that eggs can be elegant.

4 ounces (115 g) sliced mushrooms
3 scallions, coarsely sliced
1 tablespoon (14 g) butter

(continued on page 102)

2 canned artichoke hearts, chopped
6 eggs
½ cup (120 g) shredded Gruyère

If you haven't purchased your mushrooms already sliced, slice them up while you slice the scallions. In a large, heavy skillet over medium-high heat, sauté the mushrooms and scallions in the butter. When the mushrooms have turned darker, add the artichoke hearts (I just slice mine right into the skillet) and stir the whole thing up. Then beat the eggs, add them to the skillet, and scramble the whole thing. When the eggs are about half-set, add the cheese and scramble until done. Serve.

Yield: 2 or 3 servings

Assuming 3 servings, each will have 10 grams of carbohydrates and 4 grams of fiber, for a total of 6 grams of usable carbs and 19 grams of protein. Note: Keep in mind that much of the carbohydrate in artichokes is in the form of inulin, about the lowest-impact carbohydrate yet discovered, so the blood sugar impact is less than the numbers would imply—which is pretty low to begin with.

Hangtown Fry

This is a very famous dish originating, I believe, in the Gold Rush days of California.

8 large oysters
2 tablespoons (16 g) low-carb bake mix or rice protein powder
4 tablespoons (55 g) butter
4 eggs

2 tablespoons (30 ml) cream
2 tablespoons (12.5 g) grated Parmesan cheese
2 tablespoons (7.6 g) chopped fresh parsley

Coat the oysters with the bake mix or protein powder, either by putting the bake mix or protein powder in a shallow dish and rolling the oysters in it or by shaking them in a small brown paper bag with the mix in it.

Melt the butter over medium heat in a large, heavy skillet. Add the oysters and fry until golden all over, about 5 to 7 minutes.

While the oysters are frying, beat the eggs and the cream together. When the oysters are golden, pour the beaten eggs into the skillet and scramble until set. Divide between 2 serving plates, sprinkle a tablespoon of Parmesan and a tablespoon of parsley over each portion, and serve.

Yield: 2 servings

Each with 5 grams of carbohydrates and 1 gram of fiber, for a total of 4 grams of usable carbs and 21 grams of protein.

Hot Dog Scramble

Okay, it's not haute cuisine, but I'll bet your kids will eat it without complaining.

1 tablespoon (14 g) butter
1 hot dog, sliced into rounds
½ small onion, chopped
3 eggs, beaten
¼ cup (30 g) shredded cheddar cheese

Melt the butter in a heavy skillet over medium heat. Add the hot dog slices and onion and sauté until the onion is limp and the hot dog slices are starting to brown.

Add the eggs and scramble until half-set. Add the cheese and continue to scramble until the eggs are set and the cheese is melted. Serve.

Yield: 1 serving

8 grams of carbohydrates and 1 gram of fiber, for a total of 7 grams of usable carbs and 31 grams of protein.

Chipotle Eggs

Smoky and complex in flavor, chipotle peppers—smoked jalapeños—are very special, and they make these eggs very special, too. Personally, I think a side of avocado slices with a little lime or lemon juice would be nice with this.

½ cup (80 g) finely chopped onion
½ teaspoon minced garlic or 1 clove garlic, crushed
1 tablespoon (15 ml) oil
2 small chipotle peppers canned in adobo sauce, finely minced—about 2 teaspoons
6 eggs
½ cup (50 g) shredded Monterey Jack cheese

Spray a large, heavy skillet with nonstick cooking spray, place it over medium-high heat, and start sautéing the onion and garlic in the oil. When the onion is translucent, add the chopped chipotles, stir them in, and let the whole thing cook for another minute. (This is a good time to break and scramble the eggs.)

Pour the eggs into the skillet and scramble until nearly set. Scatter the cheese evenly over the top, turn the heat to low, cover the skillet, and let it keep cooking until the cheese is melted—just a minute or two. Serve.

Yield: 2 or 3 servings.

(continued on page 104)

Assuming 2 servings, each will have 5 grams of carbohydrates and 1 gram of fiber, for a total of 4 grams of usable carbs and 24 grams of protein. This also contains 285 milligrams of calcium and 248 milligrams of potassium. (They'll be more potassium if you have those avocado slices!)

Fried Eggs

Are you tired of all that scrambling? These next few recipes are, in one form or another, good old fried eggs.

Fried Eggs Not Over Really Easy

If you're like me, you like your eggs over-easy so that the whites are entirely set and the yolks are still soft—but you find it maddeningly difficult to flip a fried egg without breaking the yolk. Here's the solution!

3 eggs
½ tablespoon butter or oil
1 teaspoon water

Spray your skillet with nonstick cooking spray and place it over medium-high heat. When the skillet is hot, add the butter and coat the bottom of the pan with it. Crack your eggs into the skillet—careful not to break the yolks!—and immediately cover them.

Wait about 2 minutes and check your eggs. They should be well set on the bottom but still a bit slimy on top. Add a teaspoon of water for each serving (you can approximate this; the quantity isn't vital), turn the heat to low, and

cover the pan again.

Check after a minute; the steam will have cooked the tops of the eggs. If there's still a bit of uncooked white, give it another 30 seconds to 1 minute. Lift out and serve.

Yield: 1 serving

About 1.5 grams of carbohydrates, no fiber, and 16 grams of protein.

For the easiest eggs, use a skillet that fits the number of eggs you're frying. A 7-inch (18-cm) skillet is just right for a single serving, but if you're doing two servings, use a big skillet.

Huevos Rancheros

1 tablespoon (14 g) butter or oil
2 eggs
3 tablespoons (49 ml) salsa (hot or mild, as you prefer)
2 ounces (55 g) Monterey Jack cheese, shredded

Spray a heavy skillet with nonstick cooking spray and set it over medium heat. Add the butter or oil and crack the eggs into the skillet. Turn down the heat and cover. Let the eggs fry for 4 to 5 minutes.

While the eggs are frying, warm the salsa in a saucepan or in the microwave.

When your fried eggs are set on the bottom but still a little underdone on top, scatter the cheese evenly over the fried eggs, add a teaspoon or two of water to the skillet, and cover it again. In a minute or two, the tops of the eggs should be set (but the yolks still soft) and the cheese melted.

Transfer the eggs to a plate with a spatula, top with warmed salsa, and serve.

Yield: 1 serving

4 grams of carbohydrates and 1 gram of fiber, for a total of 3 grams of usable carbohydrates and 25 grams of protein.

Asparagi All'Uovo

This Italian dish turns a couple of eggs into a light supper. This looks like a lot of instructions, but none of the steps takes much time.

1 pound (455 g) asparagus
½ teaspoon minced garlic or 1 clove garlic, crushed
¼ cup (60 ml) olive oil
½ cup (50 g) grated Parmesan cheese
8 eggs

Preheat the broiler.

Snap the bottoms off the asparagus where they break naturally. Put the asparagus in a microwaveable casserole dish or a glass pie plate. Add a couple of tablespoons of water and cover. (Use plastic wrap or a plate to cover a pie plate.) Microwave on high for 3 to 4 minutes.

While the asparagus is cooking, stir the garlic into the olive oil.

When the asparagus is done, drain it. If you have 4 single-serving oven-proof dishes long enough to hold asparagus, they're ideal for this recipe—divide the asparagus between the 4 dishes. If not, you'll need to use a rectangular glass baking dish. Arrange the asparagus in 4 groups in the baking dish.

Whether you're using the individual dishes or the single baking dish, drizzle each serving of asparagus with the garlic and olive oil. Sprinkle lightly with salt and pepper and divide the cheese between the 4 servings. Put the asparagus under the broiler, about 4 inches (10 cm) from low heat. Let it broil for 4 to 5 minutes.

While the asparagus is broiling, fry the eggs to your liking. Either use your biggest skillet to do them all at once or divide them between two skillets.

When the Parmesan is lightly golden, take the asparagus out of the broiler. If you've cooked it in one baking dish, use a big spatula to carefully transfer each serving of asparagus to a plate. Top each serving of asparagus with 2 fried eggs and serve.

Yield: 4 servings

Each with 4 grams of carbohydrates and 1 gram of fiber, for a total of 3 grams of usable carbs and 16 grams of protein. If you'd like 22 grams of protein, add a third egg to each serving.

Rodeo Eggs

This was originally a sandwich recipe, but it works just as well without the bread.

4 slices bacon, chopped into 1-inch (2.5-cm) pieces
4 thin slices onion
4 eggs
4 thin slices cheddar cheese

(continued on page 106)

Begin frying the bacon in a heavy skillet over medium heat. When some fat has cooked out of it, push it aside and put the onion slices in, too. Fry the onion on each side, turning carefully to keep the slices together, until it starts to look translucent. Remove the onion from the skillet and set aside.

Continue frying the bacon until it's crisp. Pour off most of the grease and distribute the bacon bits evenly over the bottom of the skillet. Break in the eggs and fry for a minute or two until the bottoms are set but the tops are still soft. (If you like your yolks hard, break them with a fork; if you like them soft, leave them unbroken.)

Place a slice of onion over each yolk and then cover the onion with a slice of cheese. Add a teaspoon of water to the skillet, cover, and cook for 2 to 3 minutes or until the cheese is thoroughly melted.

Cut into four separate eggs with the edge of a spatula and serve.

Yield: This serves 2 if they're good and hungry or 4 if they're only a bit peckish or if they're kids.

In 2 servings, each will have 4 grams of carbohydrates, a trace of fiber, and 27 grams of protein.

Gruyère Eggs

1 tablespoon (14 g) butter
2 eggs
¼ cup (30 g) shredded Gruyère cheese
1 scallion, sliced

Spray a heavy skillet with nonstick cooking spray and melt the butter in it over medium-high heat. Crack the eggs into the skillet and fry them until the bottoms are done but the tops are still a little soft.

Scatter the Gruyère over the eggs. Add a couple of teaspoons of water to the skillet, cover, and let cook another couple of minutes until the cheese is melted and the whites are set.

Move the eggs to a serving plate, scatter the sliced scallion on top, and serve.

Yield: 1 serving

2 grams of carbohydrates, a trace of fiber, and 19 grams of protein.

Chili Egg Puff

Serve this versatile dish for brunch or supper. And don't be afraid of those chilies: The mild ones aren't hot, they're just very flavorful. (And if you like hot foods, feel free to use hotter chilies.)

5 eggs
3 tablespoons (15 g) soy powder or (24 g) rice protein powder
½ teaspoon salt or Vege-Sal
½ teaspoon baking powder
1 cup (225 g) small-curd cottage cheese
8 ounces (225 g) Monterey Jack cheese, grated
3 tablespoons (42 g) butter, melted
1 can (4 ounces, or 115 g) diced green chilies, drained

Preheat the oven to 350°F (180°C, or gas mark 4). Spray a 6-cup (1.4-L) casserole dish with nonstick cooking spray or butter it generously.

Break the eggs into a bowl and beat them with a whisk. Whisk in the soy powder, salt, and baking powder, mixing very well.

Beat in the cottage cheese, Monterey Jack, melted butter, and chilies. Pour the whole thing into the prepared casserole dish, put it in the oven, and bake for about 35 minutes. (It's okay if it's a little runny in the very center when you spoon into it; that part acts as a sauce for the rest.)

Yield: 4 servings

Each with 7 grams of carbohydrates and 1 gram of fiber, for a total of 6 grams of usable carbohydrates and 30 grams of protein.

Don't know how big your casserole dish is? Fill it with water using a measuring cup. You want one that just holds 6 cups (1.4 L) of water, although just a tad bigger or smaller won't matter.

Swiss Puff

This is a great comfort-food-type supper.

4 eggs
1 batch Ultimate Fauxtatoes (page 209)
¾ teaspoon salt or Vege-Sal
½ teaspoon pepper
1 tablespoon (15 g) butter
2 cups (240 g) shredded Swiss cheese
4 scallions, sliced, including the crisp part of the green shoot
2 tablespoons (7.6 g) chopped parsley
4 drops hot pepper sauce

Preheat oven to 375°F (190°C, or gas mark 5).

Separate your eggs. (Since whites with even a tiny speck of yolk in them will stubbornly refuse to whip up, do yourself a favor and separate each egg into a small cup or bowl.) Dump the yolks into the Fauxtatoes and beat them in; add the salt, pepper, and butter. Dump your (presumably yolkless) egg whites into a deep mixing bowl and set aside.

Stir the shredded Swiss cheese into the Fauxtatoes and then stir in the scallions, parsley, and hot pepper sauce.

Now, using an electric mixer, beat the whites until they stand in soft peaks. Fold gently into the Fauxtatoes. Spoon the whole thing into a 6-cup (1.4-L) casserole dish you've sprayed with nonstick cooking spray. Bake for 40 to 45 minutes.

Yield: 4 to 5 servings

Assuming 4 servings, each will have 32 g protein; 18 g carbohydrate; 8 g dietary fiber; 10 g usable carbs.

Ham and Cheese Puff

This dish reheats particularly well, making it the perfect leftover meal.

¼ pound (115 g) ham
¼ pound (115 g) cheddar cheese
1 green pepper
1 can (4 ounces, or 115 g) mushrooms, well drained
5 eggs

(continued on page 108)

3 tablespoons (15 g) soy powder or (24 g) unflavored protein powder
½ teaspoon baking powder
½ teaspoon salt or Vege-Sal
1 cup (225 g) small-curd cottage cheese
2 tablespoons (30 g) grated horseradish

Preheat the oven to 350°F (180°C, or gas mark 4). Spray a 6-cup (1.4-L) casserole dish with nonstick cooking spray or butter it generously.

Use a food processor with the S-blade in place to grind the ham, cheddar, green pepper, and mushrooms together until finely chopped (no chunks of pepper or ham should be bigger than a ½-inch [1.3-cm] cube).

In a large bowl, beat the eggs well. Add the soy or protein powder, baking powder, and salt and beat well again.

Beat in the cottage cheese and horseradish and then add the chopped ham mixture.

Pour the egg mixture into the prepared casserole dish. Bake for about 40 minutes or until it is puffy and set but still jiggles a bit in the middle when you shake it.

Yield: 4 servings

Each with 10 grams of carbohydrates and 2 grams of fiber, for a total of 8 grams of usable carbohydrates and 29 grams of protein.

The carb analysis of your recipe may vary from mine, depending on the ham, cheddar, and cottage cheese you use. As always, you can trim this carb count by using the lowest-carbohydrate ingredients you can find. And watch out when you buy your horseradish: I had to read a lot of labels to find one that didn't add sugar.

Turkey Club Puff

Disguise your Friday-after-Thanksgiving leftovers in this delicious puff.

5 eggs
¼ cup (20 g) soy powder or (32 g) unflavored protein powder
½ teaspoon salt
½ teaspoon baking powder
1 cup (225 g) cottage cheese
½ pound (225 g) Swiss cheese, cubed
¼ cup (120 ml) melted butter
¾ cup (130 g) cubed cooked turkey
6 slices bacon, cooked until crisp

Preheat the oven to 350°F (180°C, or gas mark 4). Spray a 6-cup (1.4-L) casserole dish with nonstick cooking spray or butter generously.

Break the eggs into a bowl and beat them with a whisk. Whisk in the soy powder, salt, and baking powder, mixing very well.

Beat in the cottage cheese, Swiss cheese, melted butter, cubed turkey, and crumbled bacon. Pour the whole thing into the prepared casserole dish. Bake for 35 to 40 minutes or until set.

Yield: 5 servings

Each with 5 grams of carbohydrates, a trace of fiber, and 33 grams of protein.

Sausage, Egg, and Cheese Bake

1 pound (455 g) pork sausage (hot or mild, as you prefer)
½ cup (75 g) diced green pepper
½ cup (80 g) diced onion
8 eggs
¼ teaspoon pepper
1 cup (120 g) shredded cheddar cheese
1 cup (110 g) shredded Swiss cheese

Preheat the oven to 350°F (180°C, or gas mark 4).

In a large, heavy, oven-proof skillet, start browning and crumbling the sausage over medium heat.

When some grease has cooked out of the sausage, add the green pepper and the onion and continue cooking, stirring frequently, until the sausage is no longer pink.

In a large bowl, beat the eggs and pepper together and stir in the cheddar and Swiss cheeses.

Spread the sausage and vegetables evenly on the bottom of the skillet and pour the egg and cheese mixture over it. Bake for 25 to 30 minutes or until mostly firm but still just a little soft in the center.

Yield: 6 servings

Each with 4 grams of carbohydrates, a trace of fiber, and 26 grams of protein.

Quiche Lorraine

Quiche has somehow acquired a reputation for being foofy, girly food—but it's entirely made of stuff men love! So tell your husband this is "Bacon, Egg, and Cheese Pie" and watch him it down.

1 Pie Crust, unbaked (page 520)
8 ounces (225 g) Gruyère cheese
12 slices bacon
5 eggs
½ cup (120 ml) Carb Countdown dairy beverage
½ cup (120 ml) heavy cream, or you can use 1 cup (240 ml) half-and-half in place of the Carb Countdown and the cream
1 pinch ground nutmeg
1 tablespoon (15 ml) dry vermouth
½ teaspoon salt or Vege-Sal
¼ teaspoon pepper

Have your crust ready in the pan and standing by. Preheat oven to 350°F (180°C, or gas mark 4).

Shred your cheese and cook and drain your bacon—I microwave my bacon, and I find that 1 minute per slice on high is about right, but your microwave may be a little different.

First put the cheese in the pie shell, covering the bottom evenly. Crumble the bacon evenly over the cheese.

Now whisk together the eggs, Carb Countdown dairy beverage, cream, nutmeg, vermouth, salt, and pepper. Pour this over the cheese and bacon. Bake for 45 minutes and then cool. It's actually traditional to serve Quiche Lorraine at room temperature, but you certainly may warm it if you like.

(continued on page 110)

Yield: 8 servings

Each with 32 g protein; 4 g carbohydrate; 1 g dietary fiber; 3 g usable carbs.

Spinach Mushroom Quiche

1 Almond-Parmesan Crust, prebaked (page 136)

8 ounces (225 g) sliced mushrooms

½ cup (80 g) chopped onion

2 tablespoons (30 g) butter

10 ounces (280 g) frozen chopped spinach, thawed

3 eggs

¾ cup (175 ml) heavy cream

¾ cup (175 ml) Carb Countdown dairy beverage

2 tablespoons (30 ml) dry vermouth

½ teaspoon salt

¼ teaspoon pepper

1½ cups (180 g) shredded Monterey Jack cheese

Have your crust ready first. Preheat oven to 325°F (170°C, or gas mark 3).

In a large, heavy skillet over medium-high heat, sauté the mushrooms and onion in the butter until the onion is translucent and the mushrooms are limp. Transfer the mixture into a large mixing bowl, preferably one with a pouring lip.

Dump your thawed spinach into a strainer and using clean hands, squeeze all the moisture out of it you can. Add it to the mushroom mixture.

Now add the eggs, cream, and Carb Countdown dairy beverage. Whisk the whole thing up until well combined. Whisk in the vermouth, salt, and pepper.

Cover the bottom of the Almond-Parmesan Crust with the Monterey Jack and put it in the oven for a couple of minutes until the cheese just starts to melt. Take it out of the oven and pour in the egg-vegetable mixture—your quiche will be very full! Very carefully place it back in the oven. It's a good idea to place a flat pan under it, on the floor of the oven, to catch any drips.

Bake for 50 to 60 minutes or until just set in the center. Let cool. Quiche is traditionally served at room temperature, but if you like it warm, it's better to make this ahead, let it cool, chill it, and then cut slices and warm them for a minute or two on 70 percent power in your microwave, rather than serving it right out of the oven.

Yield: 8 servings

Each with 17 g protein; 10 g carbohydrate; 4 g dietary fiber; 6 g usable carbs.

Broccoli-Bacon-Colby Quiche

This crustless quiche is wonderful, but feel free to make any quiche recipe you've got, minus the crust, in the same way. For this recipe, I use broccoli cuts that are bigger than chopped broccoli but smaller than florets, and I think they're ideal.

2 cups (500 g) frozen broccoli florets, thawed and coarsely chopped, or a bag of broccoli cuts
2 cups (225 g) shredded Colby cheese
6 slices cooked bacon
4 eggs
2 cups (475 ml) Carb Countdown dairy beverage
1 teaspoon salt or Vege-Sal
1 teaspoon dry mustard
2 teaspoons prepared horseradish
¼ teaspoon pepper

Spray a 1½-quart (1.4-L) glass casserole dish (make sure it fits inside your slow cooker) with nonstick cooking spray.

Put the broccoli in the bottom of the casserole dish. Spread the cheese evenly on top of the broccoli and crumble the bacon evenly over the cheese.

In a bowl, whisk together the eggs, Carb Countdown, salt or Vege-Sal, dry mustard, horseradish, and pepper and pour it over the broccoli in the casserole dish.

Place the casserole dish in your slow cooker and carefully pour water around the casserole dish to within 1 inch (2.5 cm) of the rim. Cover the slow cooker, set it to low, and let it cook for 4 hours.

Turn off the slow cooker, uncover it, and let the water cool until you can remove the casserole dish without risk of scalding your fingers. Serve hot or at room temperature.

Yield: 6 servings

Each with 20 g protein, 6 g carbohydrate, 2 g dietary fiber, 4 g usable carbs.

Eggs Fu Yong

This can be made on the stove top, is quick and cheap to make, uses up any sort of leftover meat, is high in protein and low in carbohydrates, needs no side dishes, is infinitely variable, and tastes good to boot! How much more can you ask from a recipe? Because this recipe can be varied so much, what I've given you is more a guideline than hard and fast rules.

4 eggs
2 teaspoons dry sherry
1 tablespoon (15 ml) soy sauce
Peanut oil, or other bland oil for frying
½ teaspoon grated ginger
2 to 3 ounces (50 to 90 g) leftover cooked meat, cut into small strips,* or canned chunk turkey, chicken, or ham, or canned shrimp or crabmeat
1 cup (75 g) Napa cabbage or green cabbage, finely shredded, or bagged coleslaw mix, or 1 cup (50 g) bean sprouts, or some combination of the two
¼ cup (30 g) mushrooms, canned or fresh, finely chopped
¼ cup (40 g) onion or scallions, finely minced
¼ cup (30 g) bamboo shoots, cut into matchstick strips

Beat the eggs with the sherry and the soy sauce. Set aside. In a large skillet, heat a few tablespoons of oil over high heat. Add the ginger, then the meat and remaining ingredients. Stir-fry until the onion is translucent and the cabbage or bean

(continued on page 112)

sprouts are tender-crisp. Stir the meat and vegetables into the seasoned eggs. Add another few tablespoons of oil to the skillet and heat.

Ladle about ½ cup (120 ml) of the egg mixture at a time into the skillet and fry on both sides until the egg is set.

You can cook this in a wok if you want to be authentic, but I actually find that a skillet is a lot easier for this recipe.

Yield: 2 servings

The carb count will vary a little, but each serving will have close to 6 grams of carbohydrates and 2 grams of fiber, for a total of 4 grams of usable carbs and 26 grams of protein.

* Use ham, pork, turkey, chicken, or shrimp—whatever you've got. If they're little bitty shrimp, leave 'em whole. If they're great big shrimp, chop them coarsely.

Vedgeree

Kedgeree is a traditional dish made with rice, flaked smoked mackerel or halibut, and hard-boiled eggs. I wanted to decarb it, but smoked mackerel and halibut are hard to come by, and I refuse to include impossible-to-find ingredients. Then I found a recipe for "Vedgeree," a vegetarian take-off, so I decarbed it, and it was yummy. This recipe will make a satisfying one-dish meal out of a couple of hard-boiled eggs. You do keep hard-boiled eggs in the fridge, don't you?

¼ **head cauliflower**
½ **cup (75 g) frozen cross-cut green beans**
¼ **cup (30 g) chopped onion**
1 **cup (100 g) sliced mushrooms**
½ **tablespoon butter**
2 **hard-boiled eggs**
Salt and pepper

Run the cauliflower through the shredding blade of a food processor. Put the cauliflower in a microwaveable dish, put the frozen green beans on top, add a couple of tablespoons of water, cover, and microwave on high for 7 minutes.

While the cauliflower and beans are cooking, sauté the onion and mushrooms in the butter until the onions are limp and translucent and the mushrooms have turned dark. Peel the eggs, quarter them lengthwise, and set them aside.

When the cauliflower and beans are done, pull them out, drain them, and stir them into the mushrooms and onions. Add salt and pepper to taste. Place the hard-boiled egg quarters on top of the vegetables, turn the heat to low, cover the pan, and let the whole thing cook for just another minute or two to heat the eggs through. Serve.

Yield: 1 serving

14 grams of carbohydrates and 4 grams of fiber, for a total of 10 grams of usable carbs and 16 grams of protein.

Yogurt

When I tell people I make my own yogurt, they react as if I'd said I could transmute base metals into gold. But as you'll see, it's easy to make and considerably cheaper than buying the commercial stuff. "Officially," plain yogurt has 12 grams of carbohydrates per cup, but Dr. Goldberg and Dr. O'Mara point out in *The GO-Diet* that most of the lactose (milk sugar) is converted to lactic acid, leaving only about 4 grams per cup. So if you like yogurt, enjoy!

1 tablespoon (15 g) plain yogurt
1½ to 2 cups (180 to 240 g) instant dry milk, or a 1-quart (960-ml) envelope

Fill a clean, 1-quart (960-ml) snap-top container half full with water.

Put the plain yogurt in the water and stir. Add the powdered milk and whisk until the lumps are gone.

Fill the container to the top with water, whisk it one last time, and put the lid on.

Put your yogurt-to-be in a warm place. I use a bowl lined with an old electric heating pad set on low, but any warm spot will do, such as inside an old-fashioned gas oven with a pilot light, on the stove top directly over the pilot light, or even near a heat register in winter.

Let your yogurt sit for 12 hours or so. It should be thick and creamy by then, but if it's still a little thin, give it a few more hours. When it's ready, stick it in the refrigerator and use it just like store-bought plain yogurt. Or flavor it with vanilla or lemon extract and some Splenda or stevia/FOS blend. You can also stir in a spoonful of sugar-free preserves or mash a few berries with a fork and stir them in.

For your first batch, you'll use store-bought plain yogurt as a starter, but after that you can use a spoonful from the previous batch. Every so often it's a good idea to start over with fresh, store-bought yogurt.

Regarding those two different amounts of dry milk: Using the full 2 cups will give you richer, creamier yogurt with more protein and more calcium but with a couple extra grams of carbohydrates as well. It's up to you. If you'd like, you can add ¼ cup (60 ml) of heavy cream in place of ¼ cup (60 ml) of the water to make a higher-fat "whole milk" yogurt. You can also, if you prefer, make your yogurt from liquid milk, but it's a pain. You have to scald the milk first and then cool it again before adding the "starter" yogurt, which seems like a lot of bother to me.

One last useful tidbit: If you find you use a lot of buttermilk—for example, if you decide you really enjoy low-carb muffins and such—you can make your own buttermilk exactly the same way you'd make yogurt. Simply substitute a couple of tablespoons of commercial buttermilk for a "starter" instead of the yogurt.

5

Breads

White Bread

This bread has a firm, fine texture and a great flavor.

1 cup (240 ml) water
¼ cup (25 g) oat bran
2 tablespoons (22 g) psyllium husks
¾ cup (75 g) vital wheat gluten
½ cup (64 g) vanilla whey protein powder
⅓ cup (40 g) rice protein powder
1 teaspoon salt
1 tablespoon (15 ml) oil
1 tablespoon (1.5 g) Splenda
2 teaspoons yeast

Put the ingredients in your bread machine in the order given and run the machine. When finished, promptly remove the loaf from the machine and bread case to cool.

Yield: About 10 slices

Each with 5 grams of carbohydrates and 1 gram of fiber, for a total of 4 grams of usable carbs and 24 grams of protein.

"Whole Wheat" Bread

Slice this extra-thin so you can "afford" two slices, and it makes a great grilled cheese sandwich.

½ cup (120 ml) warm water
½ cup (120 ml) heavy cream
1 tablespoon (14 g) butter, softened
1 egg

1 teaspoon salt
¾ cup (75 g) vital wheat gluten
2 tablespoons (14 g) raw wheat germ
2 tablespoons (14 g) wheat bran
¼ cup (45 g) psyllium husks
½ cup (60 g) oat flour
½ cup (64 g) vanilla whey protein powder
2 teaspoons yeast

Put the ingredients in your bread machine in the order given and run the machine. When finished, promptly remove the loaf from the machine and bread case to cool.

Yield: About 10 slices

Each with 13 grams of carbohydrates and 7.5 grams of fiber, for a total of 5.5 grams of usable carbs and 19 grams of protein (more than two eggs!).

Seed Bread

This bread is nutty and filling! Make sure you chop your sunflower seeds, or they'll mostly sink to the bottom of your loaf.

½ cup (120 ml) warm water
½ cup (120 ml) heavy cream
1 tablespoon (15 ml) oil
1 egg
½ teaspoon salt
¾ cup (75 g) vital wheat gluten
½ cup (50 g) oat bran
⅓ cup (40 g) ground almonds
⅓ cup (40 g) sunflower seeds, coarsely chopped

(continued on page 116)

¼ cup (32 g) rice protein powder

2 tablespoons (14 g) ground flaxseed

½ teaspoon blackstrap molasses

1 teaspoon Splenda

2 teaspoons yeast

Put the ingredients in your bread machine in the order given and run the machine. When finished, promptly remove the loaf from the machine and bread case to cool.

Yield: About 10 slices

Each with 8 grams of carbohydrates and 2 grams of fiber, for a total of 6 grams of usable carbs and 21 grams of protein.

Mom's Oatmeal Molasses Bread

This is my de-carbed version of the bread that won my mom first prize at the county fair. This has the best texture of any low-carb bread I know!

¼ cup (20 g) rolled oats

2 tablespoons (14 g) raw wheat germ

⅔ cup (160 ml) boiling water

1 tablespoon (15 ml) blackstrap molasses

1 tablespoon (1.5 g) Splenda

1 tablespoon (14 g) butter, softened

1 teaspoon salt

½ cup (60 g) ground almonds

¾ cup (75 g) vital wheat gluten

¼ cup (32 g) vanilla whey protein powder

2 tablespoons (30 ml) water

2 teaspoons yeast

Put the rolled oats and wheat germ in the bread case of your bread machine. Pour the boiling water over them and let them sit for at least 15 minutes.

Add everything else in the order given and run the machine. When finished, promptly remove the loaf from the machine and bread case to cool.

Yield: 8 slices

Each with 5.5 grams of carbohydrates and 0.5 gram of fiber, for a total of 5 grams of usable carbs and 25 grams of protein.

Maple Oat Bread

Sugar-free pancake syrup gives this bread a very special flavor.

7 ounces (205 ml) water

2 teaspoons sugar-free pancake syrup

¾ cup (75 g) wheat gluten

½ cup (60 g) wheat protein isolate

¼ cup (20 g) rolled oats

2 tablespoons (14 g) wheat bran

¼ cup (25 g) wheat germ

2 tablespoons (14 g) ground flaxseed

1 tablespoon (8 g) oat flour

¼ teaspoon salt

1 tablespoon (14 g) butter, softened

2 teaspoons active baker's yeast (one packet)

Put the ingredients in your bread machine in the order given, unless the instructions with your unit call for something quite different—then do it according to instructions!

Run the bread machine through two knead-and-rise cycles. In my cheapie, low-tech, twelve-year-old bread machine, this means unplugging the machine when the first knead-and-rise cycle is through, plugging it back in, and hitting start again—but if your machine will automatically run two knead-and-rise cycles before baking, go with it. After the second rise, let the bread bake. Promptly remove the loaf from the bread case when done and cool before slicing and/or wrapping.

Yield: 12 slices

Each with 21 g protein; 5 g carbohydrate; 2 g dietary fiber; 3 g usable carbs. Carb count does not include the polyols in the sugar-free pancake syrup.

Sesame Seed Bread

I like to eat this toasted, along with a bowl of soup.

1 cup (240 ml) warm water
¼ cup (25 g) oat bran
¼ cup (25 g) wheat bran
¼ cup (30 g) sesame seeds
¼ cup (32 g) vanilla whey protein powder
1 cup (100 g) vital wheat gluten
1¼ teaspoons salt
1 tablespoon (15 ml) blackstrap molasses
2 teaspoons yeast

Put the ingredients in your bread machine in the order given and run the machine. When finished, promptly remove the loaf from the machine and bread case to cool.

Yield: 12 slices

Each with 6.5 grams of carbohydrates and 1.7 grams of fiber, for a total of 4.8 grams of usable carbs and 18 grams of protein.

Poppy Seed Bread

This bread has a firm, close-grained texture that lends itself to thin slicing. It also doesn't rise more than about 4 inches (10 cm), but I liked the flavor and texture so much, I thought I'd include it anyway. Don't eat poppy seeds if you're facing a drug test! You run the risk of testing positive for opiates.

⅔ cup (160 ml) water
⅔ cup (70 g) gluten
3 tablespoons (20 g) wheat bran
3 tablespoons (25 g) oat flour
⅔ cup (80 g) almond meal
⅓ cup (35 g) wheat protein isolate
2 tablespoons (18 g) poppy seeds
3 tablespoons (25 g) powdered milk
1 tablespoon (14 g) butter, softened
2 teaspoons active baker's yeast
½ teaspoon salt
1 tablespoon (1.5 g) Splenda

Put everything in a bread machine in the order specified in the instructions that come with your unit. Run the dough through two knead-and-rise cycles and then bake. When finished, promptly remove the loaf from the bread case and cool before slicing thin to serve.

Yield: About 12 slices

Each with 19 g protein; 6 g carbohydrate; 2 g dietary fiber; 4 g usable carbs.

Rye Bread

I love rye bread, and it's so nice to be able to have it again! Leave out the caraway if you don't like it, but to many of us, it's just not proper rye bread without it.

1 cup (240 ml) warm water
½ cup (50 g) wheat bran
½ cup (60 g) whole grain rye flour
¼ cup (32 g) rice protein powder
¾ cup (75 g) vital wheat gluten
1 teaspoon salt
1 tablespoon (15 ml) oil
1 tablespoon (6.3 g) caraway seeds
1½ teaspoons yeast

Put the ingredients in your bread machine in the order given and run the machine. When finished, promptly remove the loaf from the machine and bread case to cool.

Yield: 12 slices

Each with 6.8 grams of carbohydrates and 2 grams of fiber, for a total of 4.8 grams of usable carbs and 14 grams of protein.

Cinnamon Raisin Bread

This is so sweet and cinnamony! Have a slice of this toasted and slathered with butter for break-fast, and you'll never know you're on a low-carb diet!

¾ cup plus 2 tablespoons (190 ml) warm water
¼ cup (25 g) oat bran
½ cup (60 g) ground almonds
⅓ cup (40 g) vanilla whey protein powder
1½ teaspoons cinnamon
¾ cup plus 3 tablespoons (95 g) vital wheat gluten
¼ cup (6 g) Splenda
1 tablespoon (15 ml) oil
1 teaspoon salt
2 teaspoons yeast
2 tablespoons (18 g) raisins, each snipped in half

Put the ingredients in your bread machine in the order given and run the machine. When finished, promptly remove the loaf from the machine and bread case to cool.

Yield: 12 slices

Each with 6 grams of carbohydrates and 0.6 grams of fiber, for a total of 5.4 grams of usable carbs and 19 grams of protein.

The reason you cut the raisins in half is to let them distribute more evenly throughout the bread; even so, there aren't a lot of them, I'll admit. That's because the raisins are the highest-carb part of this bread. If you want, you can leave them whole so each one will be more noticeable.

Zucchini Bread

Many low carbers tell me they miss having "a little something" with a cup of coffee or tea for breakfast and express a profound weariness with eggs. Here's something for you! This Zucchini Bread is moist, sweet, cinnamon-y, and delicious—not to mention being low carb and having as much protein per slice as a couple of eggs!

½ cup (120 ml) canola oil
¼ cup (60 ml) sugar-free imitation honey
2 eggs
⅓ cup (80 g) plain yogurt
1 cup (125 g) pumpkin seed meal*
1 cup (125 g) vanilla whey protein powder
1½ teaspoons baking soda
½ teaspoon salt
1 teaspoon cinnamon
⅓ cup (18 g) Splenda granular
1 cup (125 g) chopped walnuts
1½ cups (180 g) shredded zucchini (about one 6-inch [15-cm] zucchini)

Preheat the oven to 350°F (180°C, or gas mark 4).

In a good-sized mixing bowl, combine the oil, imitation honey, eggs, and yogurt. Whisk these together. Now, in a second bowl, add the dry ingredients: the ground pumpkin seeds, vanilla whey protein powder, baking soda, salt, cinnamon, and Splenda. Stir them together, making sure any little lumps of baking soda get broken up. Now whisk the dry ingredients into the wet ingredients. Stir just until everything is well combined; There is no need for prolonged beating. Finally, stir in the walnuts and the shredded zucchini, mixing well.

Pour the mixture into a loaf pan you've sprayed well with nonstick cooking spray—my loaf pan is large, 5 × 9 inches (13 × 23 cm). Bake for about 50 minutes or until a toothpick inserted into the center comes out clean. Turn the bread out onto a wire rack for cooling.

Yield: About 16 slices

Each with 14 g protein; 5 g carbohydrate; 2 g dietary fiber—for a usable carb count of just 3 g a slice. Carb count does not include polyols in the sugar-free imitation honey.

*To make your own pumpkin seed meal, buy raw shelled pumpkin seeds, which are sometimes called pepitas (not the salted pumpkin seeds in the shell sold as snacks). Grind them in your food processer with the S-blade until they reach a cornmeal consistency.

Heart-y Bread

This is so named because both rice bran and flax are known to lower cholesterol. Want more good news? This bread tastes as good as it is good for you.

1 cup plus 2 tablespoons (270 ml) water
⅓ cup (30 g) rice bran
⅓ cup (20 g) flaxseed meal
1 cup (100 g) vital wheat gluten
⅓ cup (40 g) vanilla whey protein powder
2 teaspoons blackstrap molasses
1 teaspoon salt
1 tablespoon (15 ml) oil
2 teaspoons yeast

(continued on page 120)

Put the ingredients in your bread machine in the order given and run the machine. When finished, promptly remove the loaf from the machine and bread case to cool.

Yield: 11 slices

Each with 6.7 grams of carbohydrates and 2.6 grams of fiber, for a total of 4.1 grams of usable carbs and 19 grams of protein.

Dinner Rolls

These have a more elastic texture than carb-y dinner rolls; it comes from the high protein content. (They're so high in protein, you could have a leftover roll in the morning and call it breakfast.) But they come out wonderfully crusty and have a good yeasty flavor. We had them for a holiday meal, and everyone liked them, texture and all.

5½ ounces (155 ml) water
3 tablespoons (25 g) instant dry milk
¾ cup (75 g) wheat gluten
¾ cup (75 g) wheat protein isolate
½ cup (60 g) oat flour
2 tablespoons (28 g) butter
½ teaspoon salt
2 teaspoons active baker's yeast (one packet)

Put everything in your bread machine in the order specified with your unit. Put the dough through two knead-and-rise cycles. Remove from the machine.

Spray a 12-cup muffin tin with nonstick cooking spray.

Nip off bits of dough and roll them into balls about 1 inch (2.5 cm) in diameter. Place three dough balls in a cloverleaf configuration in each muffin tin.

The dough will be extremely elastic! Don't worry about trying to make each ball completely smooth.

Let rolls rise for 60 to 90 minutes in a warm place. Preheat oven to 350°F (180°C, or gas mark 4) and bake rolls for 10 to 15 minutes or until golden. Serve with plenty of butter!

Yield: 12 rolls

Each with 26 g protein; 8 g carbohydrate; 1 g dietary fiber; 7 g usable carbs. Analysis does not include butter.

Buttermilk Drop Biscuits

You wouldn't believe how much trouble I had coming up with a decent low-carb biscuit! Everything I made either ran all over the baking sheet or was unpleasantly heavy. And I couldn't get a dough that could be rolled out and cut without sticking! Finally, I hit on the idea of drop biscuits baked in a muffin tin, and sure enough, it worked out great.

1 cup (125 g) almond meal
½ cup (125 g) rice protein
¼ cup (25 g) gluten
2 tablespoons (28 g) butter
2 tablespoons (30 ml) coconut oil
½ teaspoon salt

2 teaspoons baking powder
½ teaspoon soda
¾ cup (180 ml) buttermilk

Preheat oven to 475°F (240°C, or gas mark 9)—the oven must be up to temperature before you add the buttermilk to the dry ingredients, so do this first!

Put everything but the buttermilk into your food processor with the S-blade in place. Pulse the food processor to cut in the butter—you want it evenly distributed in the dry ingredients. Dump this mixture, which should have a mealy texture, into a mixing bowl.

Spray a 12-cup muffin tin with nonstick cooking spray. Don't use paper muffin cups; you want the browning you'll get from direct contact with the hot metal.

Check to make sure your oven is up to temperature—if it isn't, have a quick cup of tea until it's hot. Now measure the buttermilk, pour it into your dry ingredients, and stir it in with a few swift strokes—don't overmix; you just want to make sure everything's evenly damp. This will make a soft dough. Spoon it into your prepared muffin tin, smoothing the tops with the back of the spoon. Put in the oven immediately and bake for 10 to 12 minutes or until golden on top. Serve hot with butter, and if you like, low-sugar preserves or sugar-free imitation honey.

Yield: 12 biscuits

Each with 14 g protein; 4 g carbohydrate; 1 g dietary fiber, 3 g usable carbs. Analysis does not incude toppings.

English Muffins

Yes, you can make your own low-carb English Muffins. The yogurt is what gives them that characteristic, mildly sour taste.

½ cup (120 ml) warm water
½ cup (115 g) yogurt
1 teaspoon salt
⅔ cup (70 g) vital wheat gluten
¼ cup (45 g) psyllium husks
2 tablespoons (14 g) raw wheat germ
¼ cup (25 g) wheat bran
½ cup (60 h) oat flour
½ cup (65 g) vanilla whey protein powder
1½ teaspoons yeast

Put the ingredients in your bread machine in the order given and run until the end of the "rise" cycle. Remove the dough from the machine.

Using just enough oat flour on your work surface to keep the dough from sticking, pat the dough out so it's ½ inch (1.3 cm) thick.

Using a tin can with both ends removed as a cutter (a tuna can works well), cut rounds from the dough. Cover them with a clean cloth, set them aside in a warm place, and let them rise for about 1 hour or until they've doubled in bulk.

Heat a heavy skillet or griddle over medium-low heat. Scatter the surface lightly with wheat germ to prevent sticking and place as many muffins in the skillet as will fit easily. Let the muffins cook for about 6 minutes per side or until they're browned. Eat these just like you would regular English muffins—split them, toast them, and butter them.

(continued on page 122)

Yield: About 6 muffins, or 12 servings

Each with 13 grams of carbohydrates and 6.5 grams of fiber, for a total of 6.5 grams of usable carbs and 14 grams of protein. Analysis does not include butter.

French Toast

Make this for breakfast some lazy weekend morning, and the family will think you're cheating on your diet!

4 eggs
½ cup (120 ml) heavy cream
½ cup (120 ml) water
1 teaspoon vanilla extract (optional)
6 slices low-carb bread of your choice (White, "whole wheat," cinnamon raisin, and oatmeal molasses are all good choices.)
Butter

Beat together the eggs, heavy cream, water, and vanilla extract (if using) and place the mixture in a shallow dish, such as a pie plate.

Soak the slices of bread in the mixture until they're well saturated; you'll have to do them one or two at a time. Let each slice soak for at least 5 minutes, turning once.

Fry each soaked piece of bread in plenty of butter over medium heat in a heavy skillet or griddle. Brown well on each side.

Serve with sugar-free syrup, cinnamon and Splenda, or sugar-free preserves, as you choose.

Yield: 6 servings

The carb count will vary with the type of bread you use, but the egg and cream add only 2 grams of carbs, no fiber, and 4 grams of protein per slice. Analysis does not include toppings.

Kim's Dutch Baby

A Dutch Baby is a big, puffy, eggy, baked pancake, and my sister Kim adores them, so I came up with this recipe for her. It's great for Sunday brunch.

2 tablespoons (28 g) butter
⅓ cup (37 g) low-carb bake mix
⅓ cup (40 g) rice protein powder
¼ cup (6 g) Splenda
½ teaspoon salt
½ teaspoon cinnamon
4 eggs
1 cup (240 ml) half-and-half
2 teaspoons canola or other vegetable oil
1 teaspoon vanilla extract

Preheat the oven to 425°F (220°C, or gas mark 7). It is essential that the oven be up to temperature before putting your Dutch Baby in, so don't combine the wet and dry ingredients until the oven is ready.

Spray a large, cast-iron skillet or a 10-inch (25-cm) pie pan with nonstick cooking spray and melt the butter in the bottom. Set aside.

In a bowl, combine the bake mix, protein powder, Splenda, salt, and cinnamon.

In a separate bowl, beat together the eggs, half-and-half, oil, and vanilla extract and whisk it vigorously for a couple of minutes. (Beating air into it will make the Dutch Baby puff more.)

Beat in the dry ingredients just until well mixed and then pour the batter into the prepared pan.

Bake for 20 minutes; reduce the temperature to 350°F (180°C, or gas mark 4), and bake for another 3 to 5 minutes.

Yield: 2 big servings or 4 small ones (if you serve 4, you'll want some sausage or something along with it, I think).

Depending on the brand of low-carb bake mix and protein powder you use, figure 20 to 25 grams of carbohydrates in the whole Dutch Baby and 3 to 4 grams of fiber. Two servings would each have about 10 grams of usable carbs and about 38 grams of protein.

Your Dutch Baby will come out gloriously puffed, but it will quickly sink in the middle. That's okay—it's supposed to. It will be crunchy around the

edges and soft in the middle. The traditional accompaniment for a Dutch Baby is a sprinkle of lemon juice and confectioner's sugar, but lemon and Splenda works great. You could also try cinnamon and Splenda, plain Splenda, some thawed frozen berries, or sugar-free jam or jelly. They're all Yummy!

"Whole Wheat" Buttermilk Pancakes

½ cup (60 g) almond meal
½ cup (65 g) vanilla whey protein powder
¼ cup (25 g) gluten

2 tablespoons (15 g) wheat germ
1 tablespoon (7 g) wheat bran
1 teaspoon baking powder
½ teaspoon baking soda
1 cup (240 ml) buttermilk
1 egg
2 tablespoons (28 g) butter, melted

In a mixing bowl, combine the almond meal and the next 6 ingredients (through baking soda). Stir together so everything is evenly distributed.

In a 2-cup (475 ml) glass measure, combine the buttermilk, egg, and melted butter; stir together.

Take a moment to set your big skillet or griddle over medium heat so it's ready when you are.

Now, pour the wet ingredients into the dry ingredients and stir together with a few swift strokes of your whisk.

When your skillet is hot enough that a single drop of water sizzles and dances around when dripped on the surface, you're ready to cook. If your skillet doesn't have a good nonstick surface, spray it with nonstick cooking spray. (Turn off the heat first or remove the skillet from the burner and turn away from the flame—that spray is flammable!) Now you're ready to fry your pancakes—I like to use 2 tablespoons (30 ml) of batter per pancake. Fry the first side until the bubbles around the edges leave little holes when they break and then flip and cook the other side. Repeat until all the batter is used up!

Serve with butter and your choice of low-sugar preserves, cinnamon and Splenda, or sugar-free syrup—and don't think you're limited to

(continued on page 124)

maple-flavored pancake syrup! Consider using your favorite sugar-free coffee-flavoring syrup.

Yield: 5 servings (about 15 pancakes total)

Each with 23 g protein; 7 g carbohydrate; 2 g dietary fiber; 5 g usable carbs. Analysis does not include toppings.

Perfect Protein Pancakes

These taste just like mom used to make—you'd never guess they were low carb.

2 eggs
½ cup (125 g) ricotta cheese
¼ cup (30 g) vanilla whey protein powder
½ teaspoon baking powder
⅛ teaspoon salt

Spray a heavy skillet or griddle with nonstick cooking spray and place it over medium heat.

In a mixing bowl, whisk together the eggs and ricotta until quite smooth. Whisk in the whey protein powder, baking powder, and salt, only mixing until well combined.

Drop batter onto the skillet or griddle by the tablespoonful. When the bubbles on the surface of the pancakes are breaking and staying broken, flip them and cook the other side.

Serve with butter and sugar-free syrup, sugar-free jelly, Splenda and cinnamon, or a few mashed berries sweetened with Splenda.

Yield: 14 "silver dollar" pancakes

Each with about 0.6 grams of carbohydrates, no fiber, and 2.5 grams of protein. Analysis does not include toppings.

I'd call five of these tiny pancakes a "serving," so double or triple your batches accordingly. Even better, make extras to freeze, and you can warm them up in the toaster oven for a healthy breakfast on a hurried morning.

Oat Bran Pancakes

I like these for their grainy-cinnamony flavor. I eat them with butter and a little cinnamon and Splenda.

½ cup (50 g) oat bran
1 cup (130 g) vanilla whey protein powder
1¼ cups (155 g) almond meal
¼ cup (6 g) Splenda
1 teaspoon baking powder
½ teaspoon baking soda
⅛ teaspoon salt
½ teaspoon cinnamon
2 cups (480 ml) buttermilk
2 eggs

In a medium-size mixing bowl, combine the oat bran and the next 7 ingredients (through cinnamon) and stir to distribute evenly. Measure the buttermilk in a glass measuring cup and break the eggs into it. Whisk the two together. Dump the buttermilk-and-egg mixture into the dry ingredients. Mix with a few quick strokes of the whisk, just enough to make sure all the dry ingredients are incorporated.

Heat a heavy skillet or griddle over a medium-high flame until a single drop of water skitters around when dripped on the surface. Using a pot holder, remove from the heat just long enough to spray with nonstick cooking spray and then return to the heat (the spray is flammable, so you don't want to be spraying it at a hot burner!).

Pour about 2 to 3 tablespoons (30 to 45 ml) of batter at a time onto the hot griddle. Cook until the bubbles around the edges start to break and leave little holes and then flip and cook the other side.

Serve with butter and your choice of sugar-free pancake syrup, sugar-free jelly or preserves, or cinnamon and Splenda.

Yield: 8 servings

Each with 32 g protein; 12 g carbohydrate; 3 g dietary fiber; 9 g usable carbs. Analysis does not include toppings.

Zucchini Pancakes

I know the name sounds strange, but if you like zucchini bread you should really try Vicki Cash's pancakes.

3 eggs (or 2 eggs and 2 egg whites)
2 tablespoons (30 ml) half-and-half
¼ cup (60 ml) canola oil
⅔ cup (75 g) low-carb bake mix
1 teaspoon cinnamon
½ teaspoon salt
½ teaspoon nutmeg
1 small zucchini, shredded (1 to 1½ cups [125 to 190 g])

Mix the eggs, half-and-half, canola oil, bake mix, cinnamon, salt, and nutmeg together until no longer lumpy. Mix in the zucchini and let the batter sit for 5 minutes.

While the batter sits, spray a nonstick griddle or skillet with canola cooking spray and place it over medium-high heat.

Pour the batter onto the griddle about ¼ cup (60 ml) at a time. Flip the pancakes when their edges are slightly brown and cook thoroughly on both sides. Serve with butter or puréed berries or peaches.

Yield: 3 servings

The carb count will vary with the brand of low-carb bake mix you use, but figure about 5 grams of usable carbs and about 20 grams of protein. Analysis does not include toppings.

Almond Pancake and Waffle Mix

This makes nice, tender pancakes and waffles that have a nutty taste and a texture similar to cornmeal pancakes and waffles.

2 cups (250 g) almond meal
½ cup (50 g) oat bran
½ cup (65 g) vanilla whey protein powder
½ cup (65 g) rice protein powder
2 tablespoons (14 g) wheat bran
2 tablespoons (14 g) raw wheat germ
2 tablespoons (14 g) vital wheat gluten
2½ teaspoons (12 g) baking powder
1½ teaspoons salt

(continued on page 126)

Assemble all the ingredients in a food processor with the S-blade in place. Run the processor for a minute or so, stopping once or twice to shake it so everything is well combined.

Store the mix in an airtight container in the refrigerator.

Yield: Makes about 4 servings of 1 cup (120 g)

Each with 33 grams of carbohydrates and 3 grams of fiber, for a total of 30 grams of usable carbs and 36 grams of protein.

Pancakes from Almond Mix

I like to eat these topped with sugar-free grape jelly, but you could also serve them with sugar-free syrup, sugar-free jam, thawed sugar-free frozen fruit, or Splenda and cinnamon.

2 cups (240 g) Almond Pancake and Waffle Mix (page 125)
2 eggs
1 cup (240 ml) water
1 tablespoon (15 ml) canola, peanut, or sunflower oil

Spray a skillet or griddle with nonstick cooking spray and set it over medium heat.

Mix all the ingredients with a whisk and drop the batter by the tablespoonful onto the griddle or skillet. Cook as you would regular pancakes, turning to brown lightly on each side. Stir the batter between batches to prevent it from settling.

Yield: About 16 pancakes

Each with 4 grams of carbohydrates, a trace of fiber, and 6 grams of protein.

For a little added flavor, melt a little butter on the griddle or skillet before you cook the batter.

Waffles from Almond Mix

These remind me a lot of cornmeal waffles, and they're really good with bacon on the side.

1 cup (120 g) Almond Pancake and Waffle Mix (page 125)
1 teaspoon Splenda
½ cup (120 ml) half-and-half
1 egg
¼ cup (60 ml) oil

Preheat a waffle iron.

In a mixing bowl, stir together the mix and Splenda.

In a separate bowl, stir together the half-and-half, egg, and oil and pour the mixture into the dry ingredients. Stir only until everything is wet, and there are no big lumps of dry mix.

Bake in the waffle iron according to the machine's directions. Serve with butter and sugar-free syrup, cinnamon and Splenda, sugar-free jam or jelly, or another low-carb topping of your choice.

Yield: In my waffle iron, this makes 6 servings.

Each with 5 grams of carbohydrates, a trace of fiber, and 6 grams of protein. Analysis does not include toppings.

Crunchy Protein Waffles

½ cup (50 g) raw wheat germ

1 cup (80 g) soy powder

½ cup (65 g) vanilla whey protein powder

½ teaspoon salt

1 tablespoon (6 g) Splenda

½ cup (60 g) sesame seeds

3 eggs

¾ cup (180 ml) heavy cream

½ cup (120 ml) water

4 to 6 tablespoons (60 to 90 ml) oil or
melted butter

Preheat a waffle iron.

Combine the wheat germ, soy powder, whey protein powder, salt, Splenda, and sesame seeds in a large bowl.

Separate the eggs, reserving the yolks. Whip the whites until they're stiff and set aside.

Whisk the cream, water, and oil together with the egg yolks and pour them into the dry ingredients. Mix well and gently fold in the egg whites.

Use a cup to pour the batter onto your waffle iron and bake until waffles are golden brown and crispy. Serve with butter and sugar-free syrup, sugar-free jam or jelly, cinnamon and Splenda, or—my favorite—thawed, frozen strawberries and whipped cream.

Yield: This depends on the size of your waffle iron; mine makes rectangular waffles, and I get about 10 servings.

Each with 8 grams of carbohydrates and 2 grams of fiber, for a total of 6 grams of usable carbs and 10 grams of protein. Analysis does not include toppings.

Gingerbread Waffles

Really make Sunday breakfast something special! Double or triple this recipe, and you'll have extra waffles to freeze and reheat on busy mornings. Tip—they'll be a lot crispier and tastier if you reheat them in the toaster than if you microwave them.

1 cup (125 g) almond meal

1 cup (120 g) vanilla whey protein powder

½ teaspoon salt

¼ cup (6 g) Splenda

1 tablespoon (14 g) baking powder

2 teaspoons ground ginger

1½ cups (360 ml) Carb Countdown dairy
beverage or ¾ cup (180 ml) heavy cream
and ¾ cup (180 ml) water

2 eggs

4 tablespoons (60 g) butter, melted

Preheat waffle iron.

Combine almond meal, protein powder, salt, Splenda, baking powder, and ginger. In a glass measuring cup, whisk together the Carb Countdown or cream and water and the eggs and then stir the butter into them. Pour this into the dry ingredients with a few quick strokes.

Ladle the batter into the waffle iron and bake until done—my waffle iron has a light that goes out when the waffle is ready, but follow the instructions for your unit.

Serve with whipped cream.

Yield: 6 servings

Each with 35 g protein; 9 g carbohydrate; 3 g dietary fiber, 6 g usable carbs. Analysis does not include whipped cream.

Exceedingly Crisp Waffles

You have to separate eggs and all, but these waffles are worth it!

½ cup (60 g) almond meal

⅓ cup (40 g) vanilla whey protein powder

¼ cup (30 g) oat flour

½ teaspoon baking powder

1 tablespoon (1.5 g) Splenda

¼ teaspoon baking soda

¾ cup (180 ml) buttermilk

¼ cup (60 ml) Carb Countdown dairy beverage or half-and-half

6 tablespoons (90 ml) canola oil

1 egg

In one mixing bowl, combine the almond meal, protein powder, oat flour, baking powder, Splenda, and baking soda. Stir the dry ingredients together.

Measure the buttermilk and Carb Countdown dairy beverage into a glass measuring cup. Add the canola oil.

Now's the time to plug in your waffle iron and get it heating; you want it to be ready as soon as your batter is!

Separate that egg, making sure you don't get even a tiny speck of yolk in the white. Add the yolk to the liquid ingredients. Put the white in a small, deep bowl and beat until stiff. Set aside.

Whisk all the liquid ingredients together and pour them into the dry ingredients. Mix everything quickly with a few quick strokes of your whisk. Mix only enough to be sure all the dry ingredients are moistened.

Add about ⅓ of the beaten egg white to the batter and fold in gently using a rubber scraper. Then fold in the rest of the egg white.

Bake immediately according to the directions that come with your waffle iron.

Serve with butter and sugar-free pancake syrup, cinnamon and Splenda, or low-sugar preserves.

Yield: How many waffles you get will depend on the size of your waffle iron; I got 6.

Each with 15 g protein; 9 g carbohydrate; 2 g dietary fiber, 7 g usable carbs. Analysis does not include toppings.

Buttermilk Bran Muffins

These muffins are tender, moist, sweet, and perfumed with cinnamon. And using the GO-Diet's figure of 4 grams of carbohydrates per cup of buttermilk, these are a bad deal, carbohydrates-wise.

⅔ cup wheat bran

¾ cup plus 2 tablespoons (105 g) vanilla whey protein powder

2 tablespoons (13 g) vital wheat gluten

¼ teaspoon salt

1 teaspoon baking soda

¼ cup (6 g) Splenda

½ teaspoon cinnamon

½ cup (60 g) chopped walnuts or pecans (optional)

1 cup (240 ml) buttermilk
1 egg
3 tablespoons (45 ml) oil
1 tablespoon (15 ml) blackstrap molasses

Preheat the oven to 350°F (180°C, or gas mark 4).

In a mixing bowl, combine the wheat bran, protein powder, wheat gluten, salt, baking soda, Splenda, cinnamon, and nuts and stir until well combined.

In a measuring cup, stir together the buttermilk, egg, oil, and molasses.

Spray 10 cups of a muffin tin well with nonstick cooking spray.

Give the wet ingredients one last stir and pour them into the dry ingredients. With a spoon, stir just long enough to moisten all the dry ingredients. Do not over-mix! The batter should look rough, and a few lumps are fine.

Spoon the batter into the prepared muffin cups, dividing the mixture evenly (the muffin cups should be about 2/3 full).

Bake for 20 to 25 minutes and then turn the muffins out of the muffin cups onto a wire rack to cool.

Yield: 10 muffins

Each with 13.5 carbohydrates and 6 grams of fiber, for a total of 7.5 grams of usable carbs and 9 grams of protein.

Sour Cream, Lemon, and Poppy Seed Muffins

1 cup (125 g) almond meal
1 cup (130 g) vanilla whey protein powder
1½ teaspoons baking powder
½ teaspoon salt
⅓ cup (8 g) Splenda
1 teaspoon baking soda
2 tablespoons (18 g) poppy seeds
1 cup (230 g) sour cream
2 eggs
2 tablespoons (30 ml) water
2 teaspoons lemon extract
Grated rind of 1 lemon

Preheat the oven to 400°F (200°C, or gas mark 6).

In a mixing bowl, combine the almond meal, protein powder, baking powder, salt, Splenda, baking soda, and poppy seeds and stir until well combined.

In a separate bowl, combine the sour cream, eggs, water, lemon extract, and lemon rind and whisk together well.

When your oven is up to temperature, spray 16 muffin cups well with nonstick cooking spray. (You can use paper liners, if you prefer.)

Pour the sour cream mixture into the dry ingredients and stir together with just a few strokes—just enough to make the mixture evenly moist. Do not over-mix.

Spoon the batter evenly into muffin cups and bake for 20 minutes.

(continued on page 130)

Yield: Makes 16 muffins

Each with 5.25 grams of carbohydrates and 1 gram of fiber, for a total of 4.25 grams of usable carbs and 7.75 grams of protein.

Cranberry Nut Muffins

I tried Cranberry Nut Bread, and it was a failure—all the cranberries rose, so the top of the bread was soggy. But muffins worked out fine!

½ cup (60 g) pecans

½ cup (50 g) cranberries

¾ cup plus 2 tablespoons (110 g) almond meal

¾ cup (90 g) vanilla whey protein powder

2 tablespoons (30 g) gluten

2 tablespoons (30 g) polyol

¼ cup (6 g) Splenda

2½ teaspoons baking powder

2 eggs

¾ cup (180 ml) Carb Countdown dairy beverage

3 tablespoons (42 g) butter, melted

¼ teaspoon orange extract

Preheat your oven to 400°F (200°C, or gas mark 6). Spray a 12-cup muffin tin with nonstick cooking spray or line it with paper muffin cups if you prefer.

Chop your pecans, then your cranberries—I do them by pulsing the S-blade of my food processor, and if you do them in this order, you won't have pecans sticking to the moisture left behind by the cranberries. Set aside.

In a mixing bowl, combine the almond meal and the next 5 ingredients (through baking powder). Stir together to make sure everything is distributed evenly.

Whisk together the eggs, Carb Countdown dairy beverage, melted butter, and orange extract.

Make sure your oven is up to temperature before you add the wet ingredients to the dry ingredients. When it is, pour the wet ingredients into the dry ingredients and stir the two together with a few swift strokes of your whisk or a spoon. Do not overmix! A few lumps are fine. Now add the pecans and cranberries and stir just enough to incorporate into the batter. Spoon the batter into the prepared muffin tin and bake for 20 minutes. Remove the muffins from the pan to a wire rack to cool.

Yield: 12 muffins

Each with 18 g protein; 5 g carbohydrate; 2 g dietary fiber; 3 g usable carb. Carb count does not include polyol sweetener.

Pumpkin Muffins

Just as with the Cranberry Nut Muffins, these muffins happened because I couldn't get pumpkin bread to work out!

⅓ cup (50 g) almond meal

¼ cup (25 g) gluten

¼ cup (30 g) vanilla whey protein powder

¼ teaspoon salt

¼ cup (6 g) Splenda

1 teaspoon baking powder

½ teaspoon ground cinnamon

½ teaspoon ground nutmeg

½ cup (120 g) canned pumpkin

1 egg

2 tablespoons (28 g) butter, melted

¼ teaspoon orange extract

⅓ cup (80 ml) Carb Countdown dairy beverage

½ cup (60 g) chopped pecans

Preheat oven to 400°F (200°C, or gas mark 6). Spray a 12-cup muffin tin with nonstick cooking spray, or if you prefer, line it with paper muffin cups.

In a mixing bowl, combine the almond meal and the next 7 ingredients (through nutmeg). Stir them together to evenly distribute ingredients.

In a separate bowl, combine the canned pumpkin, egg, melted butter, orange extract, and Carb Countdown dairy beverage and whisk together. Make sure your oven is up to temperature before you take the next step!

Pour the wet ingredients into the dry ingredients and with a few swift strokes, combine them. Stir just enough to make sure there are no big pockets of dry stuff; a few lumps are fine. Quickly stir in the pecans and spoon the batter into a prepared muffin tin. Bake for 20 minutes; remove the muffin's from the pan to a wire rack to cool.

Yield: 12 muffins

Each with 9 g protein; 3 g carbohydrate; 6 g usable carbs.

Granola

This isn't super-low in carbs, and it's really more for eating during maintenance than during weight loss. But it's far lower in carbs than standard granola, high in protein, very filling, and best of all, it tastes like real cereal!

2½ cups (200 g) rolled oats

¾ cup (170 g) sunflower seeds

¾ cup (90 g) sesame seeds

⅔ cup (70 g) wheat germ

¾ cup (50 g) flaked, unsweetened coconut

½ cup (60 g) chopped walnuts

½ cup (60 g) slivered almonds

½ cup (70 g) wheat bran

¼ cup (30 g) flaxseeds

1 teaspoon cinnamon

½ cup (12 g) Splenda

¾ cup (95 g) vanilla whey protein powder

¼ teaspoon blackstrap molasses

½ cup (120 ml) canola oil

Preheat the oven to 250°F (120°C, or gas mark ½).

In a large, shallow roasting pan, combine the rolled oats, sunflower seeds, sesame seeds, wheat germ, coconut, walnuts, almonds, bran, flaxseeds, cinnamon, Splenda, and protein powder, mixing them very well.

Stir the molasses into the canola oil; it won't really blend with it, but it will help the molasses get distributed evenly. Pour the mixture over the dry ingredients and stir until it's uniformly distributed.

Place in the oven and toast for an hour, stirring once or twice. Store in a tightly covered container. Serve topped with cream or half-and-half.

Yield: Makes about 16 servings of ½ cup

Each with 21.8 grams of carbohydrates and 6 grams of fiber, for a total of 15.8 grams of usable carbs and 11.6 grams of protein. Analysis does not include cream or half and half.

Hot Almond Cereal

Here's a recipe for all of you who miss hot cereal in the morning. It's loaded with fiber, and it's a great way to get the benefits of flax—not to mention that it's really, really tasty.

1 cup (170 g) flaxseeds
1 cup (125 g) ground almonds
½ cup (50 g) oat bran
1¼ cups (125 g) wheat bran
1 cup (130 g) vanilla whey protein powder

Preheat the oven to 300°F (150°C, or gas mark 2).

Grind your flaxseeds in a food processor with the S-blade in place. Flaxseeds take a while to grind up, so you may have to run the processor for several minutes. (You can buy flaxseed meal if you prefer, but flaxseed oil spoils pretty quickly after the seeds are ground, so I much prefer to grind my own.)

While the food processor is running, lightly toast your ground almonds by putting them in a shallow baking pan in the oven for 5 minutes or so.

When the flaxseeds are ground and the almonds are toasted, combine them with the oat bran, wheat bran, and protein powder and store in an airtight container.

To make a bowl of cereal, put ½ cup (60 g) of the mixture in a bowl and add ¾ cup (180 ml) of boiling water and a pinch of salt. Stir and let your cereal sit for a few minutes before eating.

Yield: About 9 servings

Each with about 16 grams of carbohydrates and 9 grams of fiber, for a total of 7 grams of usable carbs and 11 grams of protein.

Try this with a little Splenda and cream or even a little cinnamon. Personally, I like to add just a drop or two of blackstrap molasses to give it a brown-sugar flavor without many extra carbs.

Cinnamon Hot Cereal

This recipe is for those of you who used to eat your oatmeal with cinnamon and sugar. Add Splenda and cream to taste.

1 cup (110 g) ground flaxseeds
1 cup (125 g) ground almonds
½ cup (50 g) oat bran
1½ cups (150 g) wheat bran
½ cup (65 g) vanilla whey protein powder
2 teaspoons cinnamon

Combine all the ingredients well and store in an airtight container.

To make a bowl of cereal, put ½ cup (55 g) of the mixture in a bowl and add ¾ cup (180 ml) boiling water and a pinch of salt. Stir and let your cereal sit for a few minutes before eating.

Yield: About 5 servings

Each with 15 grams of carbohydrates and 9.5 grams of fiber, for a total of 5.5 grams of usable carbs and 11 grams of protein.

Graham Crackers

These are wonderful! Eat them as is, with some milk or reduced-carb dairy beverage, or spread them with a little cream cheese.

²/₃ cup (80 g) vanilla whey protein powder
²/₃ cup (80 g) almond meal
¹/₃ cup (35 g) oat bran
¹/₄ (25 g) wheat gluten
¹/₂ cup (50 g) wheat bran
¹/₂ cup (50 g) wheat germ
1 teaspoon baking powder
¹/₂ teaspoon baking soda
¹/₂ teaspoon salt
¹/₂ cup (120 ml) coconut oil
¹/₄ cup (50 g) granular polyol sweetener
¹/₄ cup (6 g) Splenda
1¹/₂ teaspoons blackstrap molasses
¹/₂ cup (120 ml) Carb Countdown dairy
    beverage

In a mixing bowl, combine the protein powder and the next 8 ingredients (through salt). Stir to evenly distribute the ingredients. Set aside.

Using an electric mixer, beat the coconut oil with the granular polyol sweetener, Splenda, and molasses until the mixture is fluffy. Now beat in the dry ingredients and the Carb Countdown gradually, alternating which you add.

When all the dry ingredients and milk are beaten in, scrape the dough into a ball and refrigerate overnight. (This does something magical to the texture. I don't understand it, myself.)

Okay, the next day you can pull your dough out of the fridge. Let it warm up for 15 or 20 minutes—while that's happening, you can preheat your oven to 350°F (180°C, or gas mark 4).

Divide the dough into two equal parts. Cover a cookie sheet with baking parchment or a Teflon pan liner and place one of the dough balls on it. Cover it with another sheet of baking parchment or another pan liner. Using a rolling pin, roll out the dough between the two layers of parchment or liner, just a little thinner than a commercial graham cracker. Peel off the top sheet and use a pizza cutter or a sharp, thin-bladed knife to score into squares. Prick each cracker 3 or 4 times with a fork.

Repeat this with the second dough ball and with a second set of parchment or pan liners (you can use the same top sheet for both).

Bake for about 15 to 20 minutes or until browned a bit around the edges. Let cool, rescore, and break apart. Store them in an airtight container.

Yield: 36 crackers

Each with 6 g protein; 3 g carbohydrate; 1 g dietary fiber, 2 g usable carbs. Carb count does not include polyol sweetener.

Sunflower Parmesan Crackers

These have a great, crunchy texture and a wonderful flavor.

1 cup (225 g) raw, shelled sunflower seeds
¹/₂ cup (50 g) grated Parmesan cheese
¹/₄ cup (60 ml) water

Preheat the oven to 325°F (170°C, or gas mark 3).

(continued on page 134)

Put the sunflower seeds and Parmesan in a food processor with the S-blade in place and process until the sunflower seeds are a fine meal almost the consistency of flour. Add the water and pulse the processor until the dough is well blended, soft, and sticky.

Cover a cookie sheet with a piece of baking parchment. Turn the dough out onto the parchment, tear off another sheet of parchment, and put it on top of the dough.

Through the top sheet of parchment, use your hands to press the dough into as thin and even a sheet as you can. Take the time to get the dough quite thin—the thinner, the better, so long as there are no holes in the dough. Peel off the top layer of parchment and use a thin, sharp, straight-bladed knife or a pizza cutter to score the dough into squares or diamonds.

Bake for about 30 minutes or until evenly browned. Peel the crackers off the parchment, break along the scored lines, and let them cool. Store them in a container with a tight lid.

Yield: How many carbs are these per cracker? It will vary with the size and thickness of your crackers. I get about 6 dozen.

Each with just a trace of carbohydrates, a trace of fiber, and 1 gram of protein. But you can eat the whole batch for just 13 grams of usable carbohydrates, so who's counting?

Sunflower Wheat Crackers

1 cup (225 g) sunflower seeds
½ cup (50 g) wheat germ
¼ cup (25 g) wheat bran
¼ cup (25 g) oat bran
½ teaspoon salt
1 tablespoon (1.5 g) Splenda
¼ cup (60 ml) canola oil
¼ cup (60 ml) water

In your food processor with the S-blade in place, grind the sunflower seeds until they're a fine meal. Add the wheat germ, wheat bran, oat bran, salt, and Splenda and pulse to mix. Now pour in the oil and pulse to mix that in. Finally, add the water and pulse to make an evenly blended dough.

Cover a cookie sheet with baking parchment or a Teflon pan liner. Turn the dough out onto this. Cover with another sheet of parchment or another pan liner. Now roll the dough out through the top sheet, making it as thin as you can without making holes in it. It's really worth the time to make this seriously thin.

Using a knife with a thin, straight, sharp blade or a pizza cutter, score the dough into squares or diamonds. I make mine about the size of Wheat Thins.

Bake for about 30 minutes or until evenly golden. Rescore to help you separate the crackers without breaking them. Store them in a tightly lidded container.

Yield: About 6 dozen small crackers

Each with 1 g protein; 1 g carbohydrate; trace dietary fiber; 1 g usable carb.

Sunflower Sesame Crackers

1 cup (225 g) raw, shelled sunflower seeds
½ cup (60 g) sesame seeds
½ teaspoon salt, plus additional for sprinkling
¼ cup (60 ml) water

Preheat the oven to 325°F (170°C, or gas mark 3).

In a food processor with the S-blade attached, grind the sunflower seeds to a fine meal.

Add the sesame seeds and salt and pulse the food processor just long enough to combine. (You want the sesame seeds to stay whole.) Add the water and pulse to make a dough.

Cover a cookie sheet with a piece of baking parchment. Turn the dough out onto the parchment, tear off another sheet of parchment, and put it on top of the dough.

Through the top sheet of parchment, use your hands to press the dough into as thin and even a sheet as you can. Take the time to get the dough quite thin—the thinner, the better, so long as there are no holes in the dough. Peel off the top layer of parchment and use a thin, sharp, straight-bladed knife or a pizza cutter to score the dough into squares or diamonds. If you like, you could sprinkle a little salt over the surface and gently press it into the dough before scoring the crackers.

Bake for about 30 minutes or until they're a light golden color. Peel the crackers off the parchment, break along the scored lines, and let them cool. Store them in a container with a tight lid.

Yield: About 6 dozen small crackers

Each with 1 gram of carbohydrates and about 0.5 gram of fiber, for a total of 0.5 gram of usable carbs and 1 gram of protein.

Sunflower Cheddar Crackers

Do you miss Cheese Nips? Try these.

1½ cups (340 g) raw, shelled sunflower seeds
1½ cups (180 g) grated cheddar cheese
½ teaspoon salt, plus additional for sprinkling
¼ cup (60 ml) water

Preheat the oven to 325°F (170°C, or gas mark 3).

In a food processor with the S-blade attached, grind the sunflower seeds to a fine meal.

Add the cheddar and salt and pulse the processor six to eight times to blend. Add the water and pulse until a dough ball forms.

Cover a cookie sheet with a piece of baking parchment. Turn the dough out onto the parchment, tear off another sheet of parchment, and put it on top of the dough.

Through the top sheet of parchment, use your hands to press the dough into as thin and even a sheet as you can. Take the time to get the dough quite thin—the thinner, the better, so long as there are no holes in the dough. Peel off the top layer of parchment. Sprinkle a little salt over the surface and gently press it in into place. Use a thin, sharp, straight-bladed knife or a pizza cutter to score the dough into squares or diamonds.

Bake for about 30 minutes. Peel the crackers off the parchment, break along the scored lines, and let them cool. Store them in a container with a tight lid.

Yield: About 6 dozen crackers

(continued on page 136)

Each with 1 gram of carbohydrates and 0.5 gram of fiber, for a total of 0.5 gram of usable carbs and 1 gram of protein.

Thanks to the cheese, these crackers come with a bonus: 21 milligrams of calcium!

Bran Crackers

Tired of paying through the nose for fiber crackers? These are similar to Fiber Rich or Bran-a-Crisp except that they're thinner, crispier, lower-carb—and a whole lot cheaper. Plus they're great with dips, patés, and tuna or egg salad.

1½ cups (150 g) wheat bran
½ cup (65 g) rice protein powder
1 teaspoon salt
1½ cups (360 ml) water

Preheat the oven to 350°F (180°C, or gas mark 4).

Combine the wheat bran, protein powder, and salt, stirring them together well. Stir in the water, making sure everything is wet, and let the mixture sit for about 5 minutes.

Cover a cookie sheet with baking parchment and turn the dough out onto the parchment (the dough will be very soft). Using the back of a spoon, pat and smooth this out into a thin, even, unbroken sheet.

Bake for 10 minutes and then use a pizza cutter or a knife with a thin, sharp blade to score the sheet of dough into crackers. Put the sheet back in the oven and bake for another 20 minutes.

Turn the oven to its lowest temperature and let the crackers sit in the warm oven for at least 3 hours until they're good and dry and crisp.

Break apart and store them in an airtight container.

Yield: 3 dozen crackers

Each with just over 2 grams of carbohydrates and 1 gram of fiber, for a total of about 1 gram of usable carbs and just a trace of protein.

Almond-Parmesan Crust

This is a good "crumb crust" for savory dishes, like quiche.

1⅓ cups (200 g) almonds
½ cup (50 g) grated Parmesan cheese
6 tablespoons (90 g) butter, melted
1 tablespoon (15 ml) water

Preheat oven to 350°F (180°C, or gas mark 4).

In your food processor with S-blade attached, grind the almonds until they're the texture of cornmeal. Add the Parmesan cheese and pulse to combine. Pour in the butter and the water and run the processor until a uniform dough is formed—you may need to stop the processor and run a butter knife around the bottom edge of the processor bowl halfway through.

Turn the mixture out into a 10-inch (25-cm) pie plate you've sprayed with nonstick cooking spray. Bake for about 10 to 12 minutes. Cool before filling.

Yield: 8 servings

Each with 7 g protein; 5 g carbohydrate; 3 g dietary fiber, 2 g usable carbs.

6

Salads

Greek Salad

This is a wonderful, filling, fresh-tasting salad we never get tired of.

1 large head romaine lettuce
1 cup (60 g) chopped fresh parsley
½ cucumber, sliced
1 green pepper, sliced
Greek Lemon Dressing (page 172)
¼ sweet red onion, thinly sliced into rings
12 to 15 Greek olives
2 ripe tomatoes, cut into wedges
4 to 6 ounces (115 to 170 g) feta cheese,
   crumbled
Anchovy fillets packed in olive oil (if desired)

Wash and dry your romaine and break or cut it into bite-sized pieces. Cut up and add the parsley, cucumber, and green pepper. (You can do this step ahead of time, if you like, which makes this salad very doable on a weeknight.)

Just before serving, pour on the Greek dressing and toss the salad like crazy.

Arrange the onions, olives, and tomatoes artistically on top and sprinkle the crumbled feta in the middle. You can also add the anchovies at this point, if you know that everybody likes them, but I prefer to make them available for those who like them to put on their individual serving.

Yield: 4 servings

Each with 16 grams of carbohydrates and 6 grams of fiber, for a total of 10 grams of usable carbs and 11 grams of protein.

Autumn Salad

The flavor contrasts in this salad are lovely, and I've kept the pear to a quantity that won't add too many carbs.

2 tablespoons (28 g) butter
½ cup (60 g) chopped walnuts
10 cups (200 g) loosely packed assorted greens
   (romaine, red leaf lettuce, and fresh spinach)
¼ sweet red onion, thinly sliced
¼ cup (60 ml) olive oil
2 teaspoons wine vinegar
2 teaspoons lemon juice
¼ teaspoon spicy brown or Dijon mustard
⅛ teaspoon salt
⅛ teaspoon pepper
½ ripe pear, chopped
⅓ cup (40 g) crumbled blue cheese

Melt the butter in a small, heavy skillet over medium heat. Add the walnuts and let them toast in the butter, stirring occasionally, for about 5 minutes.

While the walnuts are toasting—and make sure you keep an eye on them and don't burn them—wash and dry your greens and put them in salad bowl with the onion. Toss with the oil first. Then combine the vinegar, lemon juice, mustard, salt, and pepper and add that to the salad bowl. Toss until everything is well covered.

Top the salad with the pear, the warm toasted walnuts, and the crumbled blue cheese; serve.

Yield: 4 generous servings

Each with 13 grams of carbohydrates and 6 grams of fiber, for a total of 7 grams of usable carbs and 10 grams of protein.

Classic Spinach Salad

4 cups (80 g) fresh spinach

⅛ large, sweet red onion, thinly sliced

3 tablespoons (45 ml) oil

2 tablespoons (30 ml) apple cider vinegar

2 teaspoons tomato paste

1½ teaspoons Splenda

¼ small onion, grated

⅛ teaspoon dry mustard

Salt and pepper

2 slices bacon, cooked until crisp, and crumbled

1 hard-boiled egg, chopped

Wash the spinach very well and dry. Tear up the larger leaves. Combine with the onion in a salad bowl.

In a separate bowl, mix up the oil, vinegar, tomato paste, Splenda, onion, mustard, and salt and pepper to taste. Pour the mixture over the spinach and onion and toss.

Top the salad with the bacon and egg; serve.

Yield: 2 generous servings

Each with 7 grams of carbohydrates and 2 grams of fiber, for a total of 5 grams of usable carbs and 2 grams of protein.

Spinach-Strawberry Salad

This salad is simply extraordinary! For my money, this is the best salad in this book. If you don't try a single other salad recipe, try this one! It's beautiful, too, and very nutritious.

1 pound (455 g) bagged, prewashed baby spinach

1 batch Sweet Poppy Seed Vinaigrette (page 171)

1 cup (170 g) sliced strawberries

3 tablespoons (25 g) slivered almonds, toasted

½ cup (60 g) crumbled feta cheese

Put the baby spinach in a big salad bowl. Pour on the dressing and toss well. Top the with strawberries, almonds, and feta and serve.

Yield: 4 servings

Each with 8 g protein; 11 g carbohydrate; 5 g dietary fiber; 6 g usable carbs.

Summer Treat Spinach Salad

Worried about where you'll get your potassium now that you're not eating bananas? Each serving of this salad has more potassium than three bananas!

2 pounds (910 g) raw spinach

1 ripe black avocado

¼ cantaloupe

½ cup (15 g) alfalfa sprouts

2 scallions, sliced

French Vinaigrette Dressing (page 169)

Wash the spinach very well and dry. Tear up the larger leaves.

(continued on page 140)

Cut the avocado in half, remove the pit and the peel, and cut into chunks.

Peel and chunk the cantaloupe or use a melon baller.

Add the avocado and cantaloupe to the spinach, along with the alfalfa sprouts and scallions. Toss with the vinaigrette right before serving.

Yield: 6 servings

Each with 11 grams of carbohydrates and 5 grams of fiber, for a total of 6 grams of usable carbs and 5 grams of protein.

Dinner Salad Italiano

1 head romaine lettuce, washed, dried, and broken up
1 cup (70 g) sliced fresh mushrooms
½ cucumber, sliced
¼ sweet red onion, thinly sliced
½ pound (225 g) sliced salami, cut into strips
½ pound (225 g) sliced provolone, cut into strips
Italian or vinaigrette dressing (bottled, or page 169)
2 ripe tomatoes, cut into wedges

Make a big tossed salad from the lettuce, mushrooms, cucumber, onion, salami, and provolone. Toss with Italian or vinaigrette dressing and then add the sliced tomatoes and serve.

Yield: 3 servings

Each with 17 grams of carbohydrates and 6 grams of fiber, for a total of 11 grams of usable carbs and 36 grams of protein.

Orange, Avocado, and Bacon Salad

8 cups (160 g) mixed greens
Citrus Dressing (page 172)
½ navel orange
½ black avocado
6 slices bacon, cooked and drained
⅛ red onion

Put your greens in a big mixing bowl and pour the dressing over them. Toss well.

Peel your half-orange and separate the sections; halve each one again. Slice the avocado, crumble the bacon, and slice the red onion paper-thin. Now strew everything artfully over the greens and serve.

Yield: 4 servings

Each with 6 g protein; 9 g carbohydrate; 5 g dietary fiber; 4 g usable carbs.

Mixed Greens with Warm Brie Dressing

This elegant dinner party fare is a carbohydrate bargain with lots of flavor.

6 cups (120 g) torn romaine lettuce, washed
   and dried
6 cups (120 g) torn red leaf lettuce, washed
   and dried
2 cups (40 g) torn radicchio, washed and dried
1 cup (60 g) chopped fresh parsley
4 scallions, thinly sliced, including the crisp
   part of the green shoot
½ cup (120 ml) extra-virgin olive oil
½ small onion, minced
3 cloves garlic, crushed
6 ounces (170 g) Brie, rind removed, cut into
   small chunks
¼ cup (60 ml) sherry vinegar
1 tablespoon (15 ml) lemon juice
1½ teaspoons Dijon mustard

Put the lettuces, radicchio, parsley, and scallions
in a large salad bowl and keep cold.

Put the olive oil in a heavy-bottomed saucepan over medium-low heat. Add the onion and
garlic and let them cook for 2 to 3 minutes.

Melt in the Brie, one chunk at a time, continu-
ously stirring with a whisk. (It'll look dreadful at
first, but don't sweat it.)

When all the cheese is melted in, whisk in the
sherry vinegar, lemon juice, and Dijon mustard.
Let it cook for a few minutes, stirring all the while,
until your dressing is smooth and thick. Pour over
the salad and toss.

Yield: 6 servings

Each with 7 grams of carbohydrates and 3 of fiber,
for a total of 4 grams of usable carbs and 8 grams
of protein.

Chef's Salad

10 cups (200 g) romaine, iceberg, red leaf,
   or any other favorite lettuce
¼ pound (115 g) deli turkey breast
¼ pound (115 g) deli ham
¼ pound (115 g) deli roast beef
¼ pound (115 g) Swiss cheese
1 green pepper, cut into strips or rings
½ sweet red onion, cut into rings
4 hard-boiled eggs, halved or quartered
2 ripe tomatoes, cut vertically into 8 wedges
   each
Salad dressing

Make nice beds of the lettuce on 4 serving
plates.

Cut the turkey, ham, roast beef, and Swiss
cheese into strips. (It's nice, by the way, to get
fairly thickly sliced meat and cheese for this.)
Arrange all of this artistically on the beds of
lettuce and garnish with the pepper, onion,
eggs, and tomatoes. Let each diner add his or
her own dressing.

Yield: 4 servings

Each with 13 grams of carbohydrates and 4 grams
of fiber, for a total of 9 grams of usable carbs and
37 grams of protein. (Analysis does not include salad
dressing.)

This salad is infinitely variable, of course; if you don't
eat ham, hate roast beef, or love Swiss cheese, feel
free to play around with these instructions. I only put
down amounts so we could analyze the carb count
and give you a guide to work from.

Vietnamese Salad

This really exotic tossed salad from Southeast Asia makes a great first course!

4 cups (80 g) romaine lettuce, broken up
4 cups (80 g) torn butter lettuce
3 scallions, sliced, including the crisp part
    of the green shoot
1 ruby red grapefruit
1 tablespoon (1.5 g) Splenda
3 tablespoons (45 ml) fish sauce (nuoc mam
    or nam pla)
3 tablespoons (45 ml) lime juice
1½ teaspoons chili garlic paste
2 tablespoons (15 g) chopped peanuts
½ cup (32 g) chopped cilantro
½ cup (12.8 g) chopped fresh mint

Wash and dry your lettuce, combine it, and then divide it onto 4 salad plates.

Slice your scallions and scatter over the lettuce.

Halve your grapefruit and use a sharp, thin-bladed knife to cut around each section to loosen. Divide the grapefruit sections between the salads.

Mix together the Splenda, fish sauce, lime juice, and chili paste. Drizzle equal amounts of the dressing over each salad. Then top each portion with chopped peanuts, cilantro, and mint and serve.

Yield: 4 servings

Each with 4 g protein; 14 g carbohydrate; 4 g dietary fiber; 10 g usable carbs.

Our Favorite Salad

We've served this salad over and over, and we never tire of it. This dressing tastes a lot like Caesar, but it's less trouble, and there's no blender to wash afterwards.

1 clove garlic
½ cup (120 ml) extra-virgin olive oil
1 head romaine
½ cup (30 g) chopped fresh parsley
½ green pepper, diced
¼ cucumber, quartered and sliced
¼ sweet red onion
2 to 3 tablespoons (30 to 45 ml) lemon juice
2 to 3 teaspoons Worcestershire sauce
¼ cup (25 g) Parmesan cheese
1 medium ripe tomato, cut into thin wedges

Crush the clove of garlic in a small bowl, cover it with the olive oil, and set it aside.

Wash and dry your romaine, break it up into a bowl, and add the parsley, pepper, cucumber, and onion. Pour the garlic-flavored oil over the salad and toss until every leaf is covered.

Sprinkle on the lemon juice and toss again. Then sprinkle on the Worcestershire sauce and toss again. Finally, sprinkle on the Parmesan and toss one last time. Top with the tomatoes and serve.

Yield: 6 servings

Each with 7 grams of carbohydrates and 3 grams of fiber, for a total of 4 grams of usable carbs and 4 grams of protein.

Update Salad

This recipe went around in the 1960s, but it used curly endive instead of this mixture of bitter greens, and sugar in the dressing. I like to think I've brought it into the 21st century—hence the name.

FOR THE SALAD:
2 medium green peppers, cut in smallish strips
1 large bunch parsley, chopped
2/3 cup (13 g) torn radicchio
2/3 cup (13 g) chopped curly endive
2/3 cup (13 g) chopped frisée
3 tomatoes, each cut in 8 lengthwise wedges
1/8 of a large, sweet red onion, thinly sliced
2 tablespoons (18 g) chopped black olives

FOR THE DRESSING:
1/4 cup (60 ml) water
1/2 cup (120 ml) tarragon vinegar
1/2 teaspoon salt or Vege-Sal
1 1/2 tablespoons (23 ml) lemon juice
1 tablespoon (1.5 g) Splenda
1/8 teaspoon blackstrap molasses
6 tablespoons (90 g) sour cream

To make the salad: Put the peppers, parsley, radicchio, endive, frisée, tomatoes, onion, and olives in a big bowl and set aside.

To make the dressing: In a separate bowl, combine the water, vinegar, salt, lemon juice, Splenda, and molasses. Pour it all over the salad and toss.

Stick the whole thing in the refrigerator and let it sit there for a few hours, stirring it now and then if you think of it.

To serve, put a 1-tablespoon (15 g) dollop of sour cream on each serving.

Yield: 6 servings

Each with 9 grams of carbohydrates and 2 grams of fiber, for a total of 7 grams of usable carbs and 2 grams of protein.

Avocado-Walnut Salad

1/4 cup (30 g) chopped walnuts
8 cups (160 g) romaine lettuce, broken up
Cumin Vinaigrette (page 171)
1/2 black avocado, cut in 1/2-inch (1.3-cm) cubes
1 stalk celery, diced
1/3 medium cucumber, diced
1/4 small red onion, sliced paper-thin

Toast your walnuts—you can simply stir them in a hot skillet or toast them in a 300°F (150°C, or gas mark 2) oven while you're assembling the rest of the salad.

Toss the lettuce with the Cumin Vinaigrette. Top with everything else and serve.

Yield: About 4 to 5 servings

Assuming 5 servings, each will have 4 g protein; 8 g carbohydrate; 3 g dietary fiber; 5 g usable carbs.

Cauliflower Avocado Salad

4 cups (600 g) cauliflower
1 black avocado, peeled and diced
½ green bell pepper, diced
8 kalamata olives, pitted and chopped
4 scallions, thinly sliced, including the crisp part of the green shoot
Sun-Dried Tomato–Basil Vinaigrette (page 171)

Cut your cauliflower in roughly ½-inch (1.3-cm) chunks. Put it in a microwaveable bowl, add 1 tablespoon (15 ml) of water, and cover. Microwave on high for 7 minutes.

When the cauliflower is ready, drain it and dump it in a mixing bowl. Add everything else, including the Sun-Dried Tomato–Basil Vinaigrette, and toss. Serve warm on a bed of lettuce.

Yield: 6 servings

Each with 3 g protein; 11 g carbohydrate; 4 g dietary fiber; 7 g usable carbs.

Sour Cream and Cuke Salad

1 green pepper
2 cucumbers, scrubbed but not peeled
½ large, sweet red onion
½ head cauliflower
2 teaspoons salt or Vege-Sal
1 cup (230 g) sour cream

2 tablespoons (30 ml) vinegar (Apple cider vinegar is best, but wine vinegar will do.)
2 rounded teaspoons dried dill weed

Slice the pepper, cucumbers, onion, and cauliflower as thinly as you possibly can. The slicing blade on a food processor works nicely, and it saves you mucho time, but I've also done it with a good, sharp knife.

Toss the vegetables well with the salt and chill them in the refrigerator for an hour or two.

In a separate bowl, mix the sour cream, vinegar, and dill, combining well.

Remove the veggies from the fridge, drain off any water that has collected at the bottom of the bowl, and stir in the sour cream mixture.

Yield: 10 servings

Each with 4 grams of carbohydrates and 1 gram of fiber, for a total of 3 grams of usable carbs and 1 gram of protein.

You can eat this right away and it will be great, but it improves overnight.

Thai Cucumber Salad

This salad is sweet and hot and so good! This, by the way, is one of those magnificent recipes that is low-carb, low-fat, low-calorie, okay for vegetarians, and tastes great.

½ small red onion
1 small, fresh jalapeño, seeds removed

3 medium cucumbers
2 or 3 cloves fresh garlic, crushed
2 tablespoons (12 g) grated fresh ginger
½ cup (120 ml) rice vinegar
½ teaspoon salt
¼ teaspoon pepper
2 tablespoons (3 g) Splenda

Using a food processor with the S-blade in place, put the onion and jalapeño in the food processor and pulse until they are both finely chopped.

Remove the S-blade and put on the slicing disk. Quarter the cucumbers lengthwise and then run them through the processor. (If you're not using a food processor, you'll want to dice the onion and mince the jalapeño and then slice the cucumber as thin as you can.)

Put the onion, jalapeño, and cucumbers in a big bowl. In a separate bowl, thoroughly combine the garlic, ginger, vinegar, salt, pepper, and Splenda. Pour over the vegetables and mix well.

Chill for a few hours before serving for the best flavor.

Yield: 8 generous servings

Each with 6 grams of carbohydrates and 1 gram of fiber, for a total of 5 grams of usable carbs and 1 gram of protein.

Cauliflower-Olive Salad

This salad is unusual and unusually good.

½ head cauliflower, broken into small florets
½ cup (80 g) diced red onion
1 can (2¼ ounces, or 60 g) sliced ripe olives, drained
½ cup (30 g) chopped fresh parsley
¼ cup (60 ml) lemon juice
¼ cup (60 ml) olive oil
¼ cup (60 g) mayonnaise
½ teaspoon salt or Vege-Sal
About a dozen cherry tomatoes
Lettuce (optional)

Combine the cauliflower, onion, olives, and parsley in a bowl.

Combine the lemon juice, olive oil, mayonnaise, and salt in a separate bowl. Pour over the veggies and toss well.

Chill for at least an hour—a whole day wouldn't hurt a bit. When you're ready to serve the salad, cut the cherry tomatoes in half and add them to the salad. Serve on a bed of lettuce if you wish, but it's wonderful alone, too.

Yield: 4 servings

Each with 7 grams of carbohydrates and 2 grams of fiber, for a total of 5 grams of usable carbs and 1 gram of protein.

Ensalada de "Arroz"

½ head cauliflower, shredded
6 scallions, sliced, including the green
½ yellow pepper, diced
½ green pepper, diced
½ ripe tomato, diced
¼ cup (16 g) chopped fresh cilantro
¼ cup (60 ml) extra-virgin olive oil

(continued on page 146)

1 tablespoon (15 ml) red wine vinegar

1 tablespoon (15 ml) balsamic vinegar

1½ teaspoons Dijon mustard

Salt and pepper

Put the cauliflower in a microwaveable casserole dish with a lid, add a couple of tablespoons (30 to 45 ml) of water, cover, and microwave on high for 6 minutes.

When the microwave beeps, uncover the cauliflower immediately to stop the cooking. Drain it well and dump it into a large mixing bowl. Let it cool for 5 to 10 minutes (stir it once or twice during this time).

Stir the chopped vegetables into your "rice." Now, mix together everything else, pour over the salad, and toss well. Chill before serving.

Yield: 5 serving

Each with 1 g protein; 4 g carbohydrate; 1 g dietary fiber; 3 g usable carbs.

Broccoli Salad

½ cup (120 ml) olive oil

¼ cup (60 ml) vinegar

1 clove garlic, crushed

½ teaspoon Italian seasoning herb blend

½ teaspoon salt or Vege-Sal

⅛ teaspoon pepper

4 cups (1 kg) frozen broccoli "cuts"

Whisk the olive oil, vinegar, garlic, herbs, salt, and pepper together.

Don't even bother to thaw the broccoli—just put it in a bowl and pour the olive oil mixture on top of it. Mix well and let it sit for several hours in the fridge. Stir it now and then if you think of it and serve as-is or on greens.

Yield: 6 servings

Each with 7 grams of carbohydrates and 4 grams of fiber, for a total of 3 grams of usable carbs and 4 grams of protein.

Of course, if you prefer, you can use fresh broccoli to make this salad. You'll have to peel the stems, cut it up, and steam it for about 5 minutes first. And at that point, it will be very much like thawed frozen broccoli! Personally, I take the easy route.

Snow Pea Salad Wraps

This salad is unusual but very good.

2 cups (150 g) snow pea pods

4 medium celery stalks, diced fine

½ cup (80 g) minced red onion

½ cup (60 g) chopped peanuts

¼ cup (60 g) mayonnaise

¼ cup (60 g) plain nonfat yogurt

1 tablespoon (15 ml) lemon juice

⅛ teaspoon cayenne

8 slices bacon, cooked and drained

24 lettuce leaves

Pinch the ends off your snow peas and pull off any strings. Cut them into ½-inch (1.3-cm) pieces—measure them after cutting, not before.

Put the snow pea bits in a microwaveable bowl with just a teaspoon of water, cover, and microwave on high for just 1 minute. Uncover the bowl immediately!

Put your snow peas in a mixing bowl and add the celery, onion, and chopped peanuts. Mix together the mayonnaise, yogurt, lemon juice, and cayenne; pour over the veggies and toss. Crumble in the bacon and toss again.

Arrange four lettuce leaves on each plate—I like Boston lettuce for this. Spoon a mound of the snow pea salad next to the lettuce. To eat, spoon the snow pea mixture onto a lettuce leaf, wrap, and eat.

Yield: 6 servings

Each with 8 g protein; 8 g carbohydrate; 3 g dietary fiber; 5 g usable carbs.

Crunchy Snow Pea Salad

This salad is different and tasty! Do use snow peas instead of sugar snap peas—they're lower carb.

2 cups (150 g) snow peas
4 slices bacon
⅓ cup (50 g) roasted, salted cashews
1 cup (160 g) diced celery
1 cup (150 g) diced cauliflower (about ½-inch [1.3-cm] chunks)
½ cup (120 ml) ranch salad dressing
½ cup (120 g) plain yogurt
1 teaspoon spicy brown mustard

You'll want to pinch off the ends of your snow peas first and pull off any tough strings. Cut them into ½-inch (1.3-cm) pieces. Put your bits of snow peas in a microwavable bowl, add a tablespoon (15 ml) or so of water, and cover with a saucer or with plastic wrap. Microwave on high for just 1½ to 2 minutes and then remove from the microwave and uncover to stop the cooking.

Put the bacon on a microwave bacon rack or in a glass pie plate, microwave 4 minutes on high or until crisp, and then drain.

While the bacon's cooking, coarsely chop your cashews. Combine all the vegetables, including the snow peas, in a mixing bowl. Combine the ranch dressing, yogurt, and mustard; pour over the vegetables and toss. Crumble in the bacon, add the cashews, and toss again. Chill before serving.

Yield: 4 to 5 servings

Assuming 4, each will have 8 grams of carbohydrate and 2 grams of fiber, for a usable carb count of 6 grams; 5 grams of protein.

Parmesan Bean Salad

This salad is filling enough to make a nice light lunch.

1 pound (455 g) bag frozen, crosscut green beans
½ cup (80 g) minced red onion
¼ cup (60 ml) extra-virgin olive oil
5 tablespoons (75 ml) cider vinegar

(continued on page 148)

½ **teaspoon salt or Vege-Sal**
½ **teaspoon paprika**
¼ **teaspoon dried ginger**
¾ **cup (75 g) grated Parmesan cheese**

Steam or microwave the green beans until they're tender-crisp.

Let the beans cool a bit and then stir in the onion, oil, vinegar, salt, paprika, ginger, and Parmesan cheese. Chill well and serve.

Yield: 4 servings

Each with 12 grams of carbohydrates and 4 grams of fiber, for a total of 8 grams of usable carbs and 9 grams of protein.

Sauerkraut Salad

This salad has the advantage of using mostly stuff that keeps well—so you just might have the ingredients hanging around the house when you discover that the head of lettuce you bought last week has gone south.

2 **cups (280 g) sauerkraut, rinsed**
½ **green bell pepper**
1 **large rib celery**
¼ **medium red onion**
¼ **cup (6 g) Splenda**
2 **tablespoons (30 ml) cider vinegar**
2 **tablespoons (30 ml) oil**

Rinse your sauerkraut and put it in a bowl. Slice your pepper into matchstick strips and thinly slice your celery and onion; add all the vegetables to the sauerkraut. Now, add the Splenda, cider vinegar, and oil, toss, and stick the bowl in the

fridge. Let the whole thing marinate for a few hours before serving.

Yield: 4 to 5 servings

Assuming 5, each will have 7 grams of carbohydrate and 3 grams of fiber, for a usable carb count of 4 grams; 1 gram protein.

Low-Carb Rosy Radish Salad

This looks very pretty and tastes surprisingly mild.

1 **pound (455 g) bag frozen crosscut green beans**
4 **slices bacon, cooked until crisp, and crumbled**
1 **small onion, chopped**
1 **cup (100 g) sliced radishes**
3 **tablespoons (45 ml) cider vinegar**
1½ **tablespoons (2.3 g) Splenda**
¾ **teaspoon salt or Vege-Sal**
¼ **teaspoon pepper**

Steam or microwave the beans until they're tender-crisp.

Combine the beans, bacon, onion, and radishes in a mixing bowl. In a separate bowl, combine the vinegar, Splenda, salt, and pepper.

Pour the mixture over the salad, toss, and serve.

Yield: 5 servings

Each with 10 grams of carbohydrates and 3 grams of fiber, for a total of 7 grams of usable carbs and 4 grams of protein.

Nicer Niçoise

Salad niçoise is traditionally made with green beans and cold, boiled potatoes, but of course, we're not going to be eating those potatoes. I thought I'd try it with cauliflower, and sure enough, it worked great!

⅓ head cauliflower
1 pound (455 g) bag frozen, crosscut green beans, thawed but not cooked
1 clove garlic, crushed
¼ to ½ cup (15 to 30 g) fresh parsley, minced
¼ medium, red onion, diced
8 to 10 olives, sliced (I used stuffed olives, but use whatever you like best.)
½ to ¾ cup (120 to 180 ml) vinaigrette dressing (homemade or bottled)
Lettuce (to line plate)
3 cans (6 ounces, or 170 g each) tuna, drained
6 hard-boiled eggs, sliced
3 tomatoes, sliced

Slice your cauliflower quite thin. Put it in a micro-wave-safe bowl with about 1 tablespoon (15 ml) of water, cover, and cook it for 4 to 5 minutes (we're looking for it to be just tender).

Combine the green beans, garlic, parsley, onion, and olives in a good-size bowl. When the cauliflower is done, add that as well, and pour ½ cup (120 ml) of dressing over the whole thing. Stir well and stick it in the fridge. Let it marinate for several hours to a day, stirring now and then when you think of it.

When you're ready to eat the salad, put a few nice lettuce leaves on each plate and spoon a mound of the marinated mixture on top. Put the tuna on top and in the middle—use as much as you like—and surround it with slices of hard-boiled egg and tomato. Garnish it with more olives, drizzle more dressing on top, if you like, and serve.

Yield: 6 servings

Each with 12 grams of carbohydrates and 3 grams of fiber, for a total of 9 grams of usable carbs and 30 grams of protein.

UnPotato Salad

You are going to be so surprised; this is amazingly like potato salad.

1 large head of cauliflower, cut into small chunks
2 cups (240 g) diced celery
1 cup (160 g) diced red onion
2 cups (450 g) mayonnaise
¼ cup (60 ml) cider vinegar
2 teaspoons salt or Vege-Sal
2 teaspoons Splenda
½ teaspoon pepper
4 hard-boiled eggs, chopped

Put the cauliflower in a microwave-safe casserole dish, add just a tablespoon (15 ml) or so of water, and cover. Cook it on high for 7 minutes and let it sit, covered, for another 3 to 5 minutes. You want your cauliflower tender, but not mushy. (And you may steam it, if you prefer.)

Drain the cooked cauliflower and combine it with the celery and onions. (You'll need a big bowl.)

(continued on page 150)

In a separate bowl, combine the mayonnaise, vinegar, salt, Splenda, and pepper. Pour the mixture over the vegetables and mix well. Mix in the chopped eggs last and stir lightly to preserve some small hunks of yolk. Chill and serve.

Yield: 12 servings

Each with 3 grams of carbohydrates and 1 gram of fiber, for a total of 2 grams of usable carbs and 3 grams of protein.

Use the time while the cauliflower cooks to dice your celery and onions.

Southwestern UnPotato Salad

Of all the unpotato salads I've come up with, this one is my favorite!

½ **head cauliflower**
½ **cup (120 g) mayonnaise**
2 **tablespoons (30 ml) spicy mustard**
1 **tablespoon (15 ml) lime juice**
1 **small jalapeño**
½ **cup (30 g) chopped cilantro**
1 **clove garlic, crushed**
½ **cup (40 g) diced red onion**
1 **small tomato**

First, cut your cauliflower into ½-inch (1.3-cm) chunks—don't bother coring it first, just trim the bottom of the stem and cut up the core with the rest of it. Put your cauliflower chunks in a microwavable casserole dish with a lid, add a few tablespoons of water, and cook it on high for 7 minutes.

When your cauliflower is done, drain it and put it in a large mixing bowl. In a medium-size bowl, whisk together the mayo, mustard, and lime juice; then pour it over the cauliflower and mix well.

Cut the jalapeño in half, remove the seeds, and mince it fine. Add it to the salad along with the cilantro, garlic, and diced red onion (don't forget to wash your hands!); mix again.

Finally, cut the stem out of the tomato and cut the tomato into smallish dice. Then carefully stir it in. Chill the salad for a few hours before serving.

Yield: 6 servings

Each serving will have 3 grams of carbohydrate and 1 gram of fiber, for a usable carb count of 2 grams; 1 gram protein.

Curried Cauliflower Salad

I think this would be great with grilled or barbecued lamb, myself.

½ **head cauliflower**
5 **scallions**
4 **hard-boiled eggs**
½ **cup (120 g) mayonnaise**
1 **tablespoon (15 ml) spicy brown mustard**
1 **teaspoon curry powder**
1 **dash salt**
1 **dash pepper**

Chop your cauliflower, including the trimmed stem, into ½-inch (1.3-cm) bits. Put it in a microwavable casserole dish with a lid, add a couple of tablespoons of water, cover, and cook it on high for 7 minutes.

Meanwhile, slice your scallions, including the crisp part of the green, and chop up your hard-boiled eggs. Next, measure the mayonnaise, mustard, curry powder, salt, and pepper into a bowl and whisk them together.

Okay, the cauliflower is done now! Drain it, put it in a mixing bowl, and pour the dressing over it. Stir it up well so the cauliflower is coated with the dressing. When it's had a chance to cool a little, add the scallions and eggs and stir it up again. Refrigerate until a half hour before dinner. Remove from the fridge and let it warm up a little before serving—this is good at room temperature.

Yield: 4 to 5 servings

Assuming 4, each will have 3 grams of carbohydrate, with 1 gram of fiber, for a usable carb count of 2 grams; 8 grams protein.

Bacon, Tomato, and Cauliflower Salad

This recipe originally called for cooked rice, so I thought I'd try it with cauliflower "rice." I liked it so much, I made it again the very next day.

½ **head cauliflower**
½ **pound (225 g) bacon, cooked until crisp, and crumbled**

2 medium tomatoes, chopped
10 to 12 scallions, sliced, including all the crisp part of the green
½ **cup (115 g) mayonnaise**
Salt and pepper
Lettuce (optional)

Put the cauliflower through a food processor with the shredding disk. Steam or microwave it until it's tender-crisp (about 5 minutes on high in a microwave).

Combine the cooked cauliflower with the bacon, tomatoes, onions, and mayonnaise in a big bowl. Add salt and pepper to taste and mix.

This salad holds a molded shape really well, so pack it into a custard cup and unmold it on a plate lined with lettuce; it looks quite pretty served this way.

Yield: 5 servings

Each with 6 grams of carbohydrates and 2 grams of fiber, for a total of 4 grams of usable carbs and 15 grams of protein.

Cauliflower-Mozzarella Salad Basilico

Just like the Bacon, Tomato, and Cauliflower Salad, this originally called for rice, but it works great with cauliflower. Make your own pesto or use store-bought, whichever you prefer.

(continued on page 152)

½ head cauliflower, run through the shredding
blade of a food processor

15 cherry tomatoes, halved

15 strong black olives, pitted and coarsely
chopped

⅓ pound (150 g) mozzarella, cut in ½-inch
(1.3-cm) cubes

1 tablespoon (10 g) finely minced sweet
red onion

2 tablespoons (30 ml) olive oil

¼ cup homemade or purchased pesto

1 tablespoon (15 ml) wine vinegar

½ teaspoon salt

¼ teaspoon pepper

Cook the cauliflower "rice" until tender-crisp (about 5 minutes on high in a microwave). Let it cool.

When the "rice" is cool, add the tomatoes, olives, mozzarella, and onion and toss well.

Whisk together the olive oil, pesto, vinegar, salt, and pepper. Pour the mixture over the salad and toss.

Let the salad sit for at least a half an hour for the flavors to blend; overnight wouldn't hurt.

Yield: 5 servings

Each with 6 grams of carbohydrates and 1 gram of fiber, for a total of 5 grams of usable carbs and 9 grams of protein.

Mozzarella Salad

This is rich and filling. The texture is quite different depending on whether you use shredded or cubed cheese, but they're both good.

1½ cups (175 g) shredded or diced mozzarella

¼ cup (25 g) sliced scallions

½ cup (60 g) diced celery

¼ cup (60 g) mayonnaise

2 tablespoons (30 ml) wine vinegar

½ teaspoon oregano

½ teaspoon basil

Combine the mozzarella, scallions, and celery in a mixing bowl.

In a separate bowl, combine the mayonnaise, vinegar, oregano, and basil. Pour the mixture over the salad, stir to combine, and serve.

Yield: 2 servings

Each with 6 grams of carbohydrates and 2 grams of fiber, for a total of 4 grams of usable carbs and 20 grams of protein.

Avocado, Egg, and Blue Cheese Salad

This makes a very unusual egg salad! Avocados are not only delicious and low carb, but they're the best source of potassium on the planet!

1 stalk celery, diced

2 scallions, sliced, including the crisp part
of the green shoot

½ black avocado, diced

3 hard-boiled eggs, chopped

¼ cup (30 g) crumbled blue cheese

3 tablespoons (45 ml) vinaigrette dressing (I
like Paul Newman's Olive Oil and Vinegar.)

This is very simple. Just combine the vegetables, eggs, and cheese in a mixing bowl. Add the dressing and toss. Serve on a bed of lettuce.

Yield: 2 servings

Each with 14 g protein; 7 g carbohydrate; 2 g dietary fiber; 5 g usable carbs.

Egg Salad Francais

This recipe is completely different from any egg salad you've ever had and quite wonderful! It is actually a French tradition.

8 ounces (225 g) bagged European style salad*
2 scallions, sliced
1/3 cup (80 ml) bottled balsamic vinaigrette (I like Paul Newman's.)
Salt and pepper
1/4 cup (20 g) shredded Parmesan cheese**
1 tablespoon (15 ml) vinegar
4 very fresh eggs

First put 1 inch (2.5 cm) of water in a largish saucepan and put it over medium-high heat. Ignore that for a minute while you put the greens and scallions in a big salad bowl. Pour the vinaigrette over the whole thing, add salt and pepper as desired, and toss well. Set aside.

Spray a microwaveable plate with nonstick cooking spray and spread the Parmesan on it. Microwave on high for 1 minute.

While the cheese is cooking, let's get back to that water. It should be good and hot by now; turn it down to barely a simmer, add the vinegar, and poach the eggs in it. It helps to break each egg into a small cup or dish first to make sure that it's good and fresh and that the yolk doesn't break. (If it does, keep it for something else and use another egg for poaching.) Then slide each egg gently into the water and poach to the desired degree of doneness.

While the eggs are poaching, remove the Parmesan from the microwave—it will now be a crispy, lacy sheet. Break it up. Pile the salad on 2 serving plates and top each one with crispy Parmesan bits. Lift the now-poached eggs out of the pan with a slotted spoon, place 2 on each salad, and serve.

Yield: 2 servings

Each with 10 grams of carbohydrates and 4 grams of fiber, for a total of 6 grams of usable carbs and 20 grams of protein.

* The mixture should include some frisée, so read the label! If you can't find one with frisée, you can still make the salad, but it will be less authentic.

** It is very important to use good-quality shredded (not grated) Parmesan with no additives. Regular Parmesan in the round green shaker won't work; the cellulose in it messes it up for this.

Coleslaw

This is my standard coleslaw recipe, and it always draws compliments. The tiny bit of onion really sparks the flavor.

1 head green cabbage
1/4 sweet red onion
Coleslaw Dressing (page 176)

(continued on page 154)

Using a food processor's slicing blade or a sharp knife, reduce your cabbage to little bitty shreds and put those shreds in a great big bowl.

Mince the onion really fine and put that in the bowl, too.

Pour on the dressing and toss well.

Yield: 10 servings

Each with 1 gram of carbohydrates, a trace of fiber, and 1 gram of protein.

Did you just get invited to a picnic and are short on time for making something that'll feed a crowd? This recipe makes a veritable bucketful, and it's a wonderful side dish to almost any plain meat, including chops and chicken. If you like, you could even use bagged coleslaw from the grocery store and just add my dressing; I promise not to tell!

Coleslaw for Company

The colors in this slaw are so intense, it's almost too beautiful to eat.

1 head red cabbage
1 small carrot, shredded
¼ sweet red onion, finely minced
Coleslaw Dressing (page 176)

Using a food processor's slicing blade or a sharp knife, shred your cabbage and put it in a big bowl.

Add the carrot and onion and toss with the dressing. Admire and enjoy.

Yield: 10 servings

Each with 2 grams of carbohydrates, a trace of fiber, and 1 gram of protein.

Napa Mint Slaw

Napa's distinctive texture and mild flavor are quite different from the familiar green cabbage, and mint sets this recipe apart even more! As a result, this slaw appeals even to people who aren't big fans of standard coleslaw. If you decide you like fresh mint in cooking, consider growing some. It's a snap to grow—indeed, it's so invasive that once you plant it, you may have trouble growing anything else!

1½ pounds (680 g) Napa cabbage
½ cup (12.8 g) chopped fresh mint
3 scallions, sliced
Orange Bacon Dressing (page 173)
⅓ cup (40 g) chopped peanuts
5 slices bacon, cooked and drained

An average-sized head of Napa should be about 1½ pounds (680 g). Remove any bruised or wilted leaves and then lay the whole head on your cutting board and cut across it at ¼-inch (6 mm) intervals, all the way down to the bottom. Scoop your shredded Napa into a big bowl.

Add the chopped mint and sliced scallions to the cabbage.

Toss the salad with the dressing, add your peanuts and bacon to the slaw, toss again, and serve.

Yield: 5 servings

Each with 5 g protein; 4 g carbohydrate; 2 g dietary fiber; 2 g usable carbs.

Asian Ginger Slaw

Even my slaw-hating husband likes this! It's got a very different texture and flavor than your standard slaw.

4 cups (360 g) finely shredded napa cabbage
¼ cup (30 g) shredded carrot
2 scallions, thinly sliced
¼ cup (30 g) pale, inner celery stalk, thinly sliced
¼ cup (60 g) mayonnaise
1 teaspoon grated fresh ginger
2 tablespoons (30 ml) rice vinegar
1 teaspoon soy sauce
1 teaspoon Splenda

Combine the cabbage, carrot, scallions, and celery in a salad bowl.

In a separate bowl, combine the mayonnaise, ginger, vinegar, soy sauce, and Splenda. Beat together until smooth, pour over the vegetables, toss, and serve.

Yield: 8 servings

Each with 4 grams of carbohydrates and 1 gram of fiber, for a total of 3 grams of usable carbs and 1 gram of protein.

Spicy Peanut Slaw

I like peanuts in my coleslaw. Does it show? The chili garlic paste gives this a kick that sets it apart.

1 head cabbage, shredded, or 7 cups (525 g) bagged coleslaw mix
8 scallions sliced
1 cup (240 g) mayonnaise
1 tablespoon (1.5 g) Splenda

⅛ teaspoon blackstrap molasses
2 teaspoons chili garlic paste
½ cup (75 g) chopped dry-roasted peanuts

Put your cabbage in a big mixing bowl and add the scallions. Stir together the mayo, Splenda, molasses, and chili garlic paste; pour the dressing over the vegetables and toss. Add the peanuts and toss again.

Yield: 8 servings

Each serving will have 4 grams of carbohydrate and 1 gram of fiber, for a usable carb count of 3 grams; 3 grams protein.

Sesame-Almond Napa Slaw

I liked this slaw so much, I ate the whole danged batch right out of the mixing bowl! I suppose there are worse things I could binge on.

½ big head Napa cabbage—If they've got only smallish heads at the grocer, use the whole thing!
2 scallions
1 tablespoon (9 g) sesame seeds
¼ cup (30 g) slivered almonds
1 teaspoon butter
½ teaspoon chicken bouillon granules
2 tablespoons (30 ml) canola oil
2 tablespoons (30 ml) rice vinegar
1½ teaspoons soy sauce
1½ teaspoons sesame oil
1 tablespoon (1.5 g) Splenda

(continued on page 156)

Shred your Napa cabbage fine and slice your scallions; put them in a big mixing bowl.

In a medium skillet, over low heat, sauté the sesame seeds and almonds in the butter until the almonds are golden. Add to the cabbage.

Stir together everything else until the bouillon is dissolved; pour over the slaw and toss. You can eat this right away, but an hour's chilling is a fine idea. Toss again right before serving.

Yield: 5 servings, unless you're a cookbook author who waits to make dinner until 9 p.m., when she's starving.

Each with 2 g protein; 3 g carbohydrate; 1 g dietary fiber; 2 g usable carbs.

Lemon Slaw

The lemon flavor in this slaw makes it a natural with grilled fish, seafood, or poultry. And the combination of vegetables makes it appealingly colorful!

½ head cabbage, shredded, or 4 cups (300 g) bagged coleslaw mix
1 green pepper, cut in matchstick strips
½ cup (80 g) diced red onion
1 small carrot, shredded
¼ cup (15.2 g) chopped fresh parsley
½ cup (120 g) mayonnaise
½ cup (120 g) plain yogurt
¼ cup (60 ml) lemon juice
2 tablespoons (30 ml) olive oil
1 tablespoon (15 ml) white wine vinegar
½ teaspoon pepper
2 tablespoons (30 ml) Dijon mustard

1 tablespoon (1.5 g) Splenda
1 tablespoon (15 g) prepared horseradish
½ teaspoon celery seed

Combine the cabbage, pepper, onion, carrot, and parsley in a big mixing bowl. In a separate bowl, whisk together everything else, pour your dressing over the cabbage mixture, and toss well. Chill for at least a few hours before serving.

Yield: 6 servings

Each serving will have 7 grams of carbohydrate and 2 grams of fiber, for a usable carb count of 5 grams; 2 grams protein.

Confetti UnSlaw

This may be a raw cabbage salad, but it's not much like coleslaw. Plus, it's utterly gorgeous on the plate.

2 cups (180 g) shredded green cabbage
2 cups (180 g) shredded red cabbage
½ sweet red pepper, chopped
½ green pepper, chopped
4 scallions, sliced, including the crisp part of the green
⅓ cup (40 g) grated carrot
1 small celery rib, thinly sliced
2 tablespoons (7.6 g) minced fresh parsley
Creamy Garlic Dressing (page 175)

Just cut up and combine all these vegetables. Then toss with the Creamy Garlic Dressing.

Yield: 8 servings

Each with 6 grams of carbohydrates and 2 grams of fiber, for a total of 4 grams of usable carbs and 1 gram of protein.

Chicken Waldorf Salad

Measure your apple carefully since it's the main source of carbs here.

1½ cups (340 g) diced cooked chicken
½ cup (45 g) diced apple
2 big ribs celery, diced
½ cup (60 g) chopped walnuts
⅓ cup (75 g) mayonnaise

Combine all the ingredients, mix well, and serve.

Yield: 2 servings

Each with 9 grams of carbohydrates and 3 grams of fiber, for a total of 6 grams of usable carbs and 40 grams of protein.

Artichoke Chicken Salad

½ cup (150 g) canned artichoke hearts, sliced
2 cups (220 g) diced cooked chicken
⅓ cup (75 g) canned water chestnuts, diced or sliced
¼ cup (25 g) stuffed olives, sliced
1 tablespoon (15 ml) soy sauce

¼ cup (60 ml) Italian salad dressing, home-made or bottled
¾ cup (90 g) diced celery
1 tablespoon (15 g) butter
½ cup (60 g) pecans, chopped

Combine everything but the butter and pecans in a medium-size mixing bowl and toss well.

In a medium-size heavy skillet, over medium heat, melt the butter and add the pecans. Let them toast, stirring often, for 5 or 6 minutes. Add to the salad and toss.

Serve on a bed of lettuce, if you like.

Yield: 3 servings

Each with 31 g protein; 12 g carbohydrate; 3 g dietary fiber; 9 g usable carbs.

Cajun Chicken Salad

2 boneless, skinless chicken breasts
1 teaspoon Cajun Seasoning (store-bought, or page 484)
1 sweet red pepper, cut into small strips
1 green pepper, cut into small strips
¼ sweet red onion, thinly sliced
3 tablespoons (45 ml) tarragon vinegar
1 teaspoon spicy brown or Dijon mustard
1 clove garlic, crushed
⅓ cup (80 ml) olive oil
1 teaspoon dried tarragon
Salt and black pepper to taste

(continued on page 158)

Place a chicken breast in a large, heavy resealable plastic bag and pound with a meat tenderizer, hammer, or whatever you have available, until it's ¼-inch (6 mm) thick. Repeat with the second breast.

Sprinkle both sides of each pounded chicken breast with the Cajun seasoning. Grill or sauté until cooked through.

Cut both chicken breasts in strips about ¼-inch (6 mm) wide. Combine with the peppers and onion.

In a small bowl, combine the tarragon vinegar, mustard, garlic, oil, dried tarragon, and salt and pepper to taste; mix well. Pour over the chicken and vegetables and toss. Serve right away or let it sit for several hours for the flavors to blend.

Yield: 2 servings

Each with 11 grams of carbohydrates and 3 grams of fiber, for a total of 8 grams of usable carbs and 29 grams of protein.

Ginger-Almond Chicken Salad

1½ pounds (680 g) boneless, skinless chicken breast

¼ cup (60 ml) Teriyaki Sauce (page 465)

6 cups (120 g) iceberg lettuce, chopped

6 cups (120 g) red leaf lettuce, chopped

2 cups (150 g) shredded red cabbage

2 cups (150 g) shredded cabbage (Use bagged coleslaw mix, if you like.)

½ cup (60 g) shredded carrot

8 scallions, sliced, including the crisp part of the green shoot

1 tablespoon (15 g) butter

⅔ cup (80 g) slivered almonds

1 cup (240 ml) Ginger Salad Dressing (page 173)

Marinate the chicken breasts in the Teriyaki Sauce for at least 30 minutes, and all day won't hurt a bit.

When mealtime rolls around, plug in your electric tabletop grill to preheat. While that's happening, start assembling the lettuce, cabbage, carrot, and scallions in a big salad bowl.

Okay, the grill's hot. Throw your chicken breasts in and set a timer for 3 minutes.

Melt the butter in a medium skillet and start sautéing the almonds in it. You want them just barely golden.

While the chicken and almonds are cooking, pour the dressing over the vegetables and toss the salad.

The timer went off! Go baste the chicken on both sides with the Teriyaki Sauce it marinated in and close the grill again. Reset the timer for another 2 to 3 minutes. Stir the almonds while you're there!

Whew! Okay, the chicken is done, and the almonds are golden. First, take the almonds off the heat so they don't burn. Now remove your chicken from the grill to your cutting board.

Pile the salad on four serving plates. Slice the chicken breasts and divide between the four salads. Top each with almonds and serve.

Yield: 4 servings

Each with 48 g protein; 21 g carbohydrate; 8 g dietary fiber; 13 g usable carbs.

Dilled Chicken Salad

1½ cups (340 g) cooked chicken, diced
1 large rib celery, diced
½ green pepper, diced
¼ medium, sweet red onion, diced
3 tablespoons (42 g) mayonnaise
3 tablespoons (42 g) sour cream
1 teaspoon dried dill weed
Salt

Combine the chicken, celery, pepper, and onion in a bowl.

In a separate bowl, mix together the mayonnaise, sour cream, and dill. Pour the mixture over the chicken and veggies, toss, add salt to taste, and serve.

Yield: 2 servings

Each with 5 grams of carbohydrates and 1 gram of fiber, for a total of 4 grams of usable carbs and 24 grams of protein.

This is wonderful when made with leftover turkey, too.

Jerk Chicken Salad

1 cup (110 g) diced cooked chicken
4 scallions, sliced, including the crisp part of the green shoot
1 stalk celery, diced
2 tablespoons (30 g) mayonnaise
1 teaspoon spicy brown mustard
½ teaspoon sugar-free imitation honey

1 teaspoon lime juice
½ teaspoon jerk seasoning, purchased or homemade
¼ cup (50 g) diced peaches (I used frozen unsweetened peaches, but use fresh if you've got them.)

Put your chicken, scallions, and celery in a mixing bowl. Whisk together the mayo, mustard, sugar-free imitation honey, lime juice, and jerk seasoning; pour it over the chicken and toss.

Add the peach dice, toss again, and then serve on lettuce, if you like.

Yield: 2 servings

Each with 22 g protein; 6 g carbohydrate; 2 g dietary fiber; 4 g usable carbs. Analysis does not include polyol in sugar-free honey.

Asian Chicken Salad

This is an wonderful salad, different from any I've ever tried. Do use rice vinegar instead of another kind and napa cabbage instead of regular. They may seem like small distinctions, but they make all the difference.

2 tablespoons (30 ml) oil
½ cup (60 g) walnuts, chopped
4 boneless, skinless chicken breasts
3 cups (210 g) thinly sliced bok choy
3 cups (210 g) thinly sliced napa cabbage
¼ cup (30 g) grated carrots

(continued on page 160)

1 cucumber, thinly sliced

½ cup (50 g) sliced scallions

½ cup (30 g) chopped fresh cilantro

⅓ cup (80 ml) soy sauce

¼ cup (60 ml) rice vinegar

1 tablespoon (15 ml) lime juice

2 tablespoons (3 g) Splenda

3 cloves garlic, crushed

½ teaspoon red pepper flakes (or to taste)

Put the oil in a heavy skillet over medium heat and toast the walnuts, stirring for about 4 to 5 minutes or until they're brown and crisp. Set aside.

Grill your chicken breasts and slice them into strips. (I use my electric tabletop grill, but you can use whatever method you prefer.)

Combine the bok choy, cabbage, carrots, cucumber, scallions, and cilantro in a big bowl.

In a separate bowl, combine the soy sauce, rice vinegar, lime juice, Splenda, garlic, and red pepper flakes. Pour about two-thirds of this dressing over the salad and toss well, coating all the vegetables.

Heap the salad onto four serving plates, top each with a sliced chicken breast, and drizzle the rest of the dressing over them. Sprinkle with chopped walnuts and serve.

Yield: 4 generous servings

Each with 15 grams of carbohydrates and 4 grams of fiber, for a total of 11 grams of usable carbs and 36 grams of protein.

We generally only have 2 people to eat all this salad, so I set half of the vegetable mixture aside in a container in the refrigerator. Don't put

dressing on the half you plan to reserve, just put the dry, shredded vegetables in a container in the fridge, save half of your dressing to go with it, and reserve some of the walnuts, as well. This is wonderful to have on hand for a quick, gourmet lunch—just grill a chicken breast, toss the salad with the dressing, and presto, lunch is served.

Thai Cobb Salad

Hey, a classic salad deserves a variation!

12 ounces (340 g) boneless, skinless chicken breast

2 tablespoons (30 ml) Teriyaki Sauce (page 465)

6 cups (120 g) torn mixed greens (I used romaine, leaf lettuce, and iceberg.)

½ cup (30 g) chopped cilantro

½ cup (120 ml) Ginger Salad Dressing (page 173)

½ teaspoon red pepper flakes (optional)

½ black avocado

⅓ cup (40 g) shredded carrot

¼ cup (30 g) chopped peanuts

4 scallions, sliced, including the crisp part of the green shoot

1 cup (100 g) diced cucumber

Put the chicken in a resealable plastic bag with the Teriyaki Sauce. Seal the bag, pressing out the air as you go, and turn the bag a few times to coat. Let the chicken marinate for at least ½ hour, and longer would be nice.

When the time comes to actually make your salad, pull out your marinated chicken and pour off the marinade. Heat your electric tabletop grill.

While the grill is heating, put your greens in a big salad bowl with the cilantro, add the Ginger Salad Dressing and red pepper flakes, and toss well.

Okay, the grill is hot. Throw in the chicken and set a timer for 5 minutes.

While the chicken is cooking, slice your avocado.

Pile the dressed greens on two serving plates. Arrange the various ingredients in stripes or in spoke fashion, leaving room for the chicken.

When the timer beeps, pull out the chicken, throw it on your cutting board, and slice or cube it. Arrange it on the salads as well and serve.

Yield: 2 to 3 servings

Assuming 2, each will have 50 g protein; 25 g carbohydrate; 12 g dietary fiber; 13 g usable carbs.

Oriental Chicken, "Rice," and Walnut Salad Wrapped in Lettuce

½ **head cauliflower**

1 **tablespoon (15 g) butter**

½ **cup (60 g) walnuts, chopped**

4 **teaspoons soy sauce, divided**

2 **cups (220 g) diced cooked chicken**

2 **tablespoons (30 ml) rice vinegar**

2 **tablespoons (30 ml) oil**

3 **teaspoons grated ginger**

Salt

20 **lettuce leaves**

First, run your cauliflower through the shredding blade of your food processor. Put it in a microwaveable casserole dish with a lid, add a couple of tablespoons of water, cover, and cook it on high for 6 minutes. When the microwave beeps, uncover your cauliflower right away! You don't want white mush.

While that's happening, melt the butter in a medium skillet and add the walnuts. Stir over medium heat for a few minutes until they're getting crisp.

Stir in 2 teaspoons of the soy sauce and sauté for another minute to evaporate the soy sauce a bit. Remove from heat.

Put the diced chicken, walnuts, and cauli-rice in a big mixing bowl. In a separate bowl, stir together the rice vinegar, oil, grated ginger, and the remaining 2 teaspoons of soy sauce. Pour over the chicken and cauliflower and toss well. Add salt to taste.

Serve the salad mounded on 4 plates with lettuce leaves on the side. Wrap the salad up in the leaves to eat.

Yield: 4 servings

Each with 26 g protein; 5 g carbohydrate; 2 g dietary fiber; 3 g usable carbs.

Chicken Chili Cheese Salad

You got your chicken, you got your vegetables, and you got your cheese. Pretty nutritious, don't you think? All that and it tastes good, too. Feel

(continued on page 162)

free to make this with leftover turkey or ham, if you prefer. Or for that matter, make it with canned chunk chicken if you don't have any cold cooked chicken in the house.

½ **head cauliflower**
1 **cup (120 g) diced celery**
½ **red bell pepper, diced**
⅓ **cup (55 g) diced red onion**
¼ **cup (30 g) diced green chilies**
4 **ounces (115 g) Monterey Jack cheese, cut into ¼-inch (6-mm) cubes**
1½ **cups (340 g) diced cooked chicken**
⅓ **cup (80 g) mayonnaise**
½ **teaspoon ground cumin**
1 **teaspoon chili powder**
½ **teaspoon dried oregano**
1 **tablespoon (15 ml) white vinegar**
1½ **teaspoons lime juice**
2 **ounces (55 g) sliced black olives, drained**

First, chop your cauliflower into ½-inch (1.3-cm) chunks. Throw it in a microwaveable casserole dish with a lid, add a couple of tablespoons of water, cover, and cook it on high for 7 minutes.

While that's cooking, assemble the celery, pepper, onion, chilies, cheese, and chicken in a big mixing bowl.

As soon as the microwave beeps, pull out your cauliflower, uncover it, and drain it. Let it sit and cool for a few minutes, though—you don't want to melt your cheese. While you're waiting for the cauliflower to cool, combine the mayonnaise, cumin, chili powder, oregano, vinegar, and lime juice in a bowl. Stir everything together.

Okay, when the cauliflower has cooled a bit, dump it in with the chicken, cheese, and veggies

and stir everything to mix. Dump in the olives, pour on the mayonnaise mixture, and toss to coat. You can eat this right away, if you like, or chill it for a few hours. This is nice served on a bed of lettuce, but you could serve it stuffed into tomatoes, too.

Yield: 3 to 4 servings

Each with 24 g protein; 7 g carbohydrate; 2 g dietary fiber; 5 g usable carbs. Analysis is for salad only.

Tex-Mex Chicken Salad

½ **head cauliflower**
½ **red bell pepper, diced**
⅓ **cup (55 g) diced red onion**
¼ **cup (30 g) canned green chiles**
4 **ounces (115 g) Monterey Jack cheese, cut in ¼-inch (6 mm) cubes**
¼ **cup (25 g) sliced black olives**
1 **cup (225 g) diced cooked chicken**
⅓ **cup (80 g) mayonnaise**
½ **teaspoon ground cumin**
½ **teaspoon dried oregano**
1 **teaspoon chili powder**
1 **tablespoon (15 ml) white wine vinegar**
1½ **teaspoons lime juice**
⅓ **cup (21.3 g) chopped fresh cilantro**

Chop the cauliflower, including the stem, into ½-inch (1.3-cm) bits. Put them in a microwaveable casserole dish with a lid, add a couple of tablespoons of water, cover, and cook it on high for 7 minutes.

Assemble the red pepper and the next 5 ingredients (through chicken) in a big mixing bowl.

When the cauliflower comes out, uncover it and let it sit to cool for at least 5 minutes, and more won't hurt—you don't want it to melt your chunks of cheese. When the cauliflower has cooled a bit, drain it and add it to the chicken mixture.

Meanwhile, mix together the mayo, cumin, oregano, chili powder, white wine vinegar, and lime juice. Pour over the chicken-cauliflower mixture and toss well. Add the cilantro and toss again. Chill it if you have time, but it's pretty darned good even if it's still slightly warm!

Yield: 3 servings

Each with 25 g protein; 9 g carbohydrate; 3 g dietary fiber; 6 g usable carbs.

Taco Salad

This is a great summer supper. The wild card in this recipe is the ranch dressing—different brands vary tremendously in carb count. Choose a really, really low-carb one, and you'll drop the carb count below what's listed here.

8 cups (160 g) romaine or iceberg lettuce, washed, dried, and broken up

1 cup (150 g) diced green pepper

½ medium cucumber, sliced

1 medium tomato, sliced into thin wedges, or 15 cherry tomatoes, halved

½ cup (80 g) diced sweet red onion

½ ripe black avocado, peeled, seeded, and cut into small chunks

½ cup (32 g) cilantro, chopped (optional)

1 can (4 ounces, or 115 g) sliced black olives, drained (optional)

⅔ cup (173 g) salsa plus additional for topping

½ cup (120 ml) ranch dressing

1 batch Chicken or Beef Taco Filling*

1 cup (120 g) shredded Cheddar or Monterey Jack cheese

Sour cream

Put the lettuce, pepper, cucumber, tomato, onion, avocado, cilantro (if using), and olives (if using) in a large salad bowl.

Stir together the ⅔ cup (173 g) of salsa and the ranch dressing, pour it over the salad, and toss.

Divide the salad between the serving plates and top each one with the taco filling and shredded cheese. Put the salsa and sour cream on the table so that folks can add their own.

Yield: 6 servings

Each with 12 grams of carbohydrates and 4 grams of fiber, for a total of 8 grams of usable carbs and 22 grams of protein.

*To make chicken taco filling, combine 1 pound (455 g) boneless, skinless chicken breasts, 1 cup (240 ml) chicken broth, and 2 tablespoons Taco Seasoning (page 483) in a large, heavy-bottomed saucepan. Cover, put it over low heat, and simmer for 1½ hours. Tear chicken into shreds.

To make beef taco filling, crumble 1 pound (455 g) ground beef into a heavy skillet over medium-high heat and cook until brown. Drain and stir in 2 tablespoons Taco Seasoning (page 483) and ¼ cup (60 ml) water. Simmer for 5 minutes.

Souvlaki Salad

This skewered lamb is usually served as a sandwich in pita bread, but it makes a fabulous salad for a lot fewer carbs.

2 pounds (910 g) lean lamb, cut into 1-inch cubes

½ cup (120 ml) olive oil

1 cup (240 ml) dry red wine

1 teaspoon salt

¼ teaspoon pepper

1 teaspoon oregano

3 cloves garlic, crushed

1 head romaine lettuce

¼ sweet red onion, sliced paper-thin

24 cherry tomatoes, halved

⅔ cup (160 ml) Greek Lemon Dressing (page 172)

6 tablespoons (90 g) plain yogurt or sour cream (The yogurt is more authentic.)

Put the lamb cubes in a large resealable plastic bag.

Combine the oil, wine, salt, pepper, oregano, and garlic. Pour the mixture over the lamb cubes in the bag. Let this marinate for at least a few hours.

When you're ready to cook the lamb, pour off the marinade and thread the cubes onto skewers. You can grill these or broil them 8 inches (20 cm) or so from the broiler. Turn the kebabs while they're cooking and check for doneness by cutting into a chunk of meat after 10 minutes. They should be thoroughly cooked in 15 minutes. (If you don't have any skewers, you can always just lay the lamb cubes on the broiler pan. They're a lot easier to turn over if they're on skewers, however.)

While the meat is cooking, wash and dry your lettuce and arrange it on serving plates.

Push the cooked meat off the skewers and onto the prepared beds of lettuce. Scatter some red onion over each plate and arrange 8 cherry tomato halves on each. Drizzle each plate with a couple of tablespoons of dressing and top each with a tablespoon of yogurt.

Yield: 6 servings

Each with 11 grams of carbohydrates and 4 grams of fiber, for a total of 7 grams of usable carbs and 34 grams of protein.

Summer Tuna Salad

1 medium cucumber, cut into chunks

⅓ cup (50 g) sweet red onion, sliced

⅓ cup (20 g) chopped fresh parsley

½ large green pepper, cut into small strips

15 cherry tomatoes, quartered

1 can (6 ounces, or 170 g) tuna, drained

¼ cup (60 ml) extra-virgin olive oil

2 tablespoons (30 ml) wine vinegar

1 clove garlic, crushed

¼ teaspoon salt

⅛ teaspoon pepper

Put the cucumber, onion, parsley, pepper, tomatoes, and tuna in a salad bowl.

In a separate bowl, combine the oil, vinegar, garlic, salt, and pepper. Pour the mixture over the salad, toss, and serve.

Yield: 2 servings

Each with 16 grams of carbohydrates and 4 grams of fiber, for a total of 12 grams of usable carbs and 25 grams of protein.

Tuna Egg Waldorf

2 large ribs celery, diced
½ cup (80 g) diced red onion
½ cup (43 g) diced red apple
½ cup (60 g) chopped pecans
1 can (6 ounces, or 170 g) tuna, drained
3 hard-boiled eggs, chopped
¾ cup (175 g) mayonnaise
Salt
Lettuce

Put the celery, onion, apple, pecans, tuna, and hard-boiled eggs in a big bowl. Toss with the mayonnaise until it's all coated. Add salt to taste and serve on a lettuce-lined plate, if you like.

Yield: 3 servings

Each with 10 grams of carbohydrates and 3 grams of fiber, for a total of 7 grams of usable carbs and 23 grams of protein.

Thai-Style Crab Salad in Avocados

Short on time, I got my pal Julie McIntosh to try out this recipe for me. She loved it the way I'd conceived of it but suggested a little more cilantro, plus a little scallion, so that's what we did. Thanks, Julie!

1 ripe black avocado
3 tablespoons (45 ml) lime juice, divided
1 can (6 ounces, or 170 g) crabmeat, or
   6 ounces cooked lump crabmeat
1 teaspoon lemon juice
¼ cup (60 g) mayonnaise
2 tablespoons (8 g) chopped cilantro
1 scallion, thinly sliced
¼ teaspoon pepper, or to taste
Salt, if desired

Split the avocado in half, remove the seed, and sprinkle the cut surfaces with 1 tablespoon (15 ml) of the lime juice to prevent browning.

Combine the crabmeat, remaining 2 tablespoons (30 ml) lime juice, lemon juice, mayonnaise, cilantro, scallion, pepper, and salt in a mixing bowl and mix well. Stuff into the avocado halves, piling it high. Garnish with extra cilantro, if desired, and serve.

Yield: 2 servings

Each with 9 grams of carbohydrates and 5 grams of fiber, for a total of 4 grams of usable carbs and 20 grams of protein.

This salad also provides 932 milligrams of potassium and 110 milligrams of calcium.

Shrimp and Avocado Salad

Here's a cool summer night's dinner that will take all of 10 minutes to assemble, yet impress the heck out of any guests who might happen to have wandered in—or just the family.

2 pounds (910 g) shrimp, cooked and shelled
1 black avocado
10 scallions, sliced thin
⅔ cup (160 ml) bottled vinaigrette dressing (I like Paul Newman's Olive Oil and Vinegar.)
1 head romaine lettuce

This is very simple if you buy your shrimp already shelled and cooked. I like to use little bitty shrimp for this, but feel free to use middle-sized shrimp if that's what you have on hand. Put the shrimp in a big mixing bowl. Peel and seed your avocado and dice it, somewhere between ¼-inch (6 mm) and ½-inch (1.3 cm) big. Put that in the bowl, too. Slice your scallions, including the crisp part of the green, and throw them in the bowl as well.

Pour on the dressing and gently stir the whole thing up to coat all the ingredients. Let that sit for a few minutes while you break or cut up the lettuce. Arrange it in beds on 6 serving plates.

Now stir the shrimp salad one last time to get up any dressing that's settled to the bottom of the bowl and spoon it out onto the beds of lettuce. Serve immediately.

Yield: 6 servings

Each with 35 g protein; 8 g carbohydrate; 4 g dietary fiber; 4 g usable carbs.

Ham and Cheese Salad

When I tried this recipe, I didn't eat much else till it was gone!

½ head cauliflower
8 ounces (225 g) cooked ham, cut in ¼-inch (6 mm) cubes
8 ounces (225 g) Swiss cheese, cut in ¼-inch (6 mm) cubes
¼ cup (40 g) finely diced red onion
¾ cup (75 g) chopped dill pickle
¾ cup (60 g) snow pea pods, cut in ½-inch (1.3-cm) pieces
⅓ cup (80 g) mayonnaise
1 tablespoon (15 ml) brown mustard
1 tablespoon (15 ml) white wine vinegar
1 teaspoon dried tarragon

First chop your cauliflower into ½-inch (1.3-cm) chunks—include the stem. Put it in a microwave-able casserole dish with a lid, add a couple of tablespoons of water, and cover. Cook it on high for 7 minutes.

Use the time while your cauliflower is cooking to combine your ham, cheese, onion, and pickle in a big mixing bowl.

Then pinch the ends off of your snow pea pods and pull off any strings. Cut into ½-inch (1.3-cm) pieces and put those in a microwaveable bowl. Add a tablespoon (15 ml) of water and cover. When the cauliflower is done, pull it out of the microwave and uncover it immediately—both to stop the cooking and to let it cool. Put your snow peas in the microwave and cook them on high for just 1 minute. When they're done, uncover immediately, drain them, and add them to the mixing bowl.

While your cauliflower is cooling, combine the mayo, mustard, vinegar, and tarragon in a small bowl and stir together well.

When the cauliflower is cool enough to not melt the cheese, drain it and add it to the ham and cheese mixture. Add the dressing and toss to coat. This is good right away, but it's better if you let it sit in the fridge for at least a few hours to let the flavors blend.

Yield: 4 servings

Each with 28 g protein; 8 g carbohydrate; 1 g dietary fiber; 7 g usable carb.

Ham-Pecan Salad with Apricot Dressing

Always read the labels and buy the lowest-sugar ham you can find—they vary quite a lot in carbohydrate content. This recipe assumes ham with 1 gram of carbohydrate per 3-ounce (85 g) serving.

5 ounces (140 g) cooked ham, diced
1 stalk celery, diced
2 tablespoons (20 g) diced red onion
¼ cup (30 g) chopped pecans
2 tablespoons (30 g) mayonnaise
2 teaspoons low-sugar apricot preserves
1 teaspoon spicy brown or Dijon mustard
¼ teaspoon soy sauce

Mix together the ham, celery, onion, and pecans in a mixing bowl. Combine the mayonnaise, preserves, mustard, and soy sauce and pour this over the ham mixture. Mix well and serve. This is really nice on a bed of lettuce.

Yield: 1 serving

15 grams of carbohydrates and 4 grams of fiber, for a total of 11 grams of usable carbs and 29 grams of protein.

Artichoke Prosciutto Salad

This salad is rich and more filling than some others in this book. Serve it with a lighter grilled dish—maybe a seafood kebab or grilled chicken.

1 can (14 ounces, or 400 g) artichoke hearts, drained
2 ounces (55 g) prosciutto or good-quality deli ham, thinly sliced
½ cup (50 g) chopped kalamata olives
1 medium tomato
¼ cup (10 g) chopped fresh basil
3 tablespoons (45 ml) extra-virgin olive oil
1 tablespoon (15 ml) white wine vinegar
1 clove garlic
½ teaspoon Dijon mustard
1 teaspoon Splenda

Coarsely chop the artichoke hearts and throw them into a mixing bowl. Cut the prosciutto or ham into strips about 1 inch (2.5 cm) long and

(continued on page 168)

½ inch (6 mm) wide and throw that in, too. Chop the olives and add them; then dice the tomato and put that in. Finally, throw in the chopped fresh basil.

Mix together everything else and pour it over the vegetables. Stir. Let it marinate for several hours before serving.

Yield: 4 servings

Each serving will have 7 grams protein, 10 grams carbohydrate, and 1 gram fiber, for a usable carb count of 9 grams—but a lot of the fiber in artichokes is in the form of inulin, which has a very low glycemic index, so this is considerably easier on your blood sugar than that 9-gram figure would suggest.

Submarine Salad

Here's a salad with everything you'd find in a great submarine sandwich—except the bread! If your grocery store deli doesn't have some of these cold cuts, substitute your favorites. Except bologna. One slice of bologna, and you've lost your East Coast sub shop accent.

8 cups (160 g) shredded lettuce, loosely packed
1 ounce (30 g) prosciutto or boiled ham
1 ounce (30 g) capacolla
1 ounce (30 g) mortadella
1 ounce (30 g) Genoa salami
1 ounce (30 g) provolone cheese (smoked provolone if you can get it!)
1 ounce (30 g) mozzarella cheese
⅛ medium red onion, sliced paper-thin
3 tablespoons (21 g) roasted red pepper, diced
4 fresh basil leaves, minced
½ small tomato, sliced in thin wedges

2 tablespoons (30 ml) olive oil
½ clove garlic, crushed
1 tablespoon (15 ml) red wine vinegar
1 dash pepper
1 dash salt

Make a bed of lettuce on each of two serving plates.

Slice the meats and cheeses into strips. Arrange artistically on the beds of lettuce. Top that with the onion, diced red pepper, and chopped fresh basil. Add the tomato wedges, too. Now mix together the oil, garlic, vinegar, pepper, and salt. Drizzle it over the salads and then serve.

Yield: 2 servings

Each with 18 g protein; 13 g carbohydrate; 5 g dietary fiber; 8 g usable carbs.

Italian Roast Beef Salad

This makes a great meal, all from deli roast beef! Feel free to use leftover steak in this instead if you have that.

8 cups (160 g) bagged European or Italian blend greens
¼ cup (40 g) thinly sliced sweet red onion
¼ medium green pepper, sliced into small strips
3 tablespoons (45 ml) extra-virgin olive oil
½ teaspoon minced garlic or 1 clove garlic, crushed
1½ tablespoons (23 ml) balsamic vinegar
½ teaspoon spicy brown or Dijon mustard

¼ cup (30 g) crumbled Gorgonzola

4 ounces (115 g) sliced deli roast beef

2 tablespoons (18 g) toasted pine nuts

Place the greens, onion, and green pepper in a large salad bowl. Combine the oil and garlic, pour over the salad, and toss well. Stir together the balsamic vinegar and mustard and set them aside.

Crumble the Gorgonzola (if you didn't buy it precrumbled) and add it to the salad. Slice the roast beef into strips and throw it in there, too. Pour the balsamic vinegar mixture over the whole thing and toss very well. Pile onto 2 serving plates, top each with a tablespoon of pine nuts, and serve.

Yield: 2 servings

Each with 19 grams of carbohydrates and 9 grams of fiber, for a total of 10 grams of usable carbs and 27 grams of protein. You'll also get 1,153 milligrams of potassium and 247 milligrams of calcium, plus almost three times your daily requirements of vitamins C and A, and 100 percent of your daily requirement of folacin.

Gorgonzola is the Italian version of blue cheese. It is a bit milder and creamier than most blue cheeses. If you can't find it, substitute any blue cheese you like.

French Vinaigrette Dressing

No, this is not that sweet, tomatoey stuff that somehow has gotten the name "French dressing." No Frenchman would eat that stuff on a bet! This is a classic vinaigrette dressing.

½ teaspoon salt

¼ teaspoon pepper

¼ to ⅓ cup (60 to 80 ml) wine vinegar

½ teaspoon Dijon mustard

¾ cup (180 ml) extra-virgin olive oil

Put all the ingredients in a container with a tight lid and shake well. Shake again before pouring over salad and tossing.

Yield: 12 servings

Each with only a trace of carbohydrates, fiber, and protein.

The French Vinaigrette and Italian Vinaigrette Dressing recipes make approximately enough for two big, family-size salads, but feel free to double them and keep them in the fridge.

Italian Vinaigrette Dressing

Add a little zip to the French Vinaigrette, and you've got Italian Vinaigrette.

⅓ cup (80 ml) wine vinegar

2 cloves garlic, crushed

½ teaspoon oregano

¼ teaspoon basil

1 or 2 drops hot pepper sauce

⅔ cup (160 ml) extra-virgin olive oil

Put all the ingredients in a container with a tight-fitting lid and shake well.

Yield: 12 servings

(continued on page 170)

Each with 1 gram of carbohydrates, a trace of fiber, and a trace of protein.

Variation: Creamy Italian Dressing. This is a simple variation on the Italian Vinaigrette. Just add 2 tablespoons of mayonnaise to the Italian Vinaigrette Dressing and whisk until smooth.

Big Italian Restaurant Dressing

This is my clone of the dressing from a popular Italian restaurant chain—minus the sugar, of course.

½ cup (120 ml) white vinegar
⅓ cup (80 ml) water
⅓ cup (80 ml) olive oil
¼ cup (6 g) Splenda
2½ tablespoons (30 g) grated Romano cheese
2 tablespoons (30 ml) beaten egg
1¼ teaspoons salt
1 teaspoon lemon juice
1 clove garlic, crushed
1 tablespoon (3.8 g) minced parsley
1 pinch dried oregano
1 pinch red pepper flakes
½ teaspoon guar or xanthan

This one's really easy: Just assemble everything in your blender and run the sucker for 10 to 15 seconds. Keep in an airtight container in the fridge.

Yield: 1½ cups (360 ml), or 12 servings of 2 tablespoons (30 ml)

Each with 1 g protein; 1 g carbohydrate; trace dietary fiber, 1 g usable carb.

If you're uncomfortable using 2 tablespoons (30 ml) of raw egg, you can use egg substitute or pasteurized eggs instead.

Raspberry Vinaigrette Dressing

This dressing is so sweet and tangy. Raspberry vinaigrette is a favorite you'll get to enjoy more often once you're making your own low-carb variety.

¼ cup (60 ml) Raspberry Vinegar (see below)
¼ cup (60 ml) canola or other bland oil
3 tablespoons plus 1 teaspoon (45 g) mayonnaise
1 teaspoon spicy brown or Dijon mustard
Pinch salt and pepper

Blend all the ingredients and store in the refrigerator in a container with a tight-fitting lid.

Yield: 6 servings

Each with a trace of carbohydrates, fiber, and protein.

To make your own raspberry vinegar, combine ½ cup (120 ml) white vinegar, ¼ teaspoon raspberry cake flavoring (this is a highly concentrated oil in a teeny little bottle), and 3 tablespoons (4.5 g) Splenda and store in a container with a tight-fitting lid. This makes about ½ cup (120 ml), with 11.5 grams of carbohydrates in the whole batch or 1.5 grams of carbohydrates per tablespoon, with no fiber, and no protein.

Cumin Vinaigrette

This dressing is good with anything South-of-the-Border-ish or Middle Eastern, for that matter.

⅔ cup (160 ml) olive oil
⅓ cup (80 ml) lemon juice
2 teaspoons ground cumin
Salt and pepper to taste

Just whisk everything together and toss with your salad.

Yield: 1 cup (240 ml), or 8 servings of 2 tablespoons (30 g)

Each with trace protein; 1 g carbohydrate; trace dietary fiber; 1 g usable carb.

Sweet Poppy Seed Vinaigrette

½ cup (12 g) Splenda
¼ cup (60 ml) white wine vinegar
3 tablespoons (45 ml) olive oil
2 teaspoons minced red onion
1½ teaspoons poppy seeds
1 teaspoon paprika
¼ teaspoon salt

Measure everything into a bowl, whisk it together, and it's ready to go!

Yield: Makes roughly ½ cup (120 ml), or 4 servings of about 2 tablespoons (30 ml)

Each with trace protein; 2 g carbohydrate; trace dietary fiber; 2 g usable carbs.

Sun-Dried Tomato–Basil Vinaigrette

8 sun-dried tomato halves
2 tablespoons (30 ml) balsamic vinegar
2 tablespoons (30 ml) red wine vinegar
2 cloves garlic, crushed
½ teaspoon salt
½ cup (120 ml) extra-virgin olive oil
4 teaspoons dried basil, or 2 tablespoons (5.3 g) fresh, minced

Chop the sun-dried tomatoes quite fine. Now simply whisk everything together and toss with your salad.

Yield: Makes roughly ⅔ cup (160 ml), or about 5 servings of 2 tablespoons (30 ml)

Each with 1 g protein; 5 g carbohydrate; 1 g dietary fiber; 4 g usable carbs.

Balsamic-Parmesan Dressing

3 tablespoons (45 ml) balsamic vinegar
⅓ cup (80 ml) extra-virgin olive oil
1 tablespoon (14 g) mayonnaise
2 cloves garlic, crushed
1 teaspoon grated onion
¼ teaspoon salt or Vege-Sal
¼ teaspoon pepper
1 teaspoon spicy brown or Dijon mustard
1 tablespoon (6.3 g) grated Parmesan cheese

(continued on page 172)

Whisk all the ingredients together until smooth. Store in a container with a tight-fitting lid and shake or whisk again before tossing with salad.

Yield: 6 servings

Each with 1 gram of carbohydrates, a trace of fiber, and a trace of protein.

Citrus Dressing

2 tablespoons (30 ml) lemon juice
2 tablespoons (30 ml) lime juice
1 tablespoon (15 ml) white vinegar
2 tablespoons (30 ml) canola oil
¼ teaspoon orange extract
1 tablespoon (1.5 g) Splenda
1½ teaspoons sugar-free imitation honey

Simply combine everything in a bowl and whisk together. Alternately, assemble the ingredients in your blender and run it for a few seconds.

Yield: 4 to 5 servings

Assuming 4 servings, each will have trace protein; 2 g carbohydrate; trace dietary fiber; 2 g usable carbs. Analysis does not include polyol in imitation honey.

Greek Lemon Dressing

The use of lemon juice in place of vinegar in salad dressings is distinctively Greek.

¾ cup (180 ml) extra-virgin olive oil
¼ cup (60 ml) lemon juice
2 tablespoons (10.8 g) dried oregano, crushed
1 clove garlic, crushed
Salt and pepper

Put all the ingredients in a container with a tight-fitting lid and shake well.

Yield: 12 servings

Each with 1 gram of carbohydrates, a trace of fiber, and a trace of protein.

This is best made at least a few hours in advance, but don't try to double the recipe and keep it around. Lemon juice just doesn't hold its freshness the way vinegar does.

Soy and Sesame Dressing

2 tablespoons (30 ml) soy sauce
1½ tablespoons (25 ml) oil
1½ tablespoons (25 ml) rice vinegar
1 tablespoon (1.5 g) Splenda
1 clove garlic, crushed
½ teaspoon dark sesame oil
1½ teaspoons lemon juice
¼ teaspoon pepper

Simply whisk everything together or whirl in your blender.

Yield: ⅓ cup (80 ml), or 3 servings of 2 tablespoons (30 ml)

Each with 1 g protein; 2 g carbohydrate; trace dietary fiber; 2 g usable carbs.

Orange Bacon Dressing

3 tablespoons (45 ml) bacon grease
¼ cup (60 ml) white wine vinegar
1 tablespoon (15 ml) lemon juice
1½ tablespoons (2.25 g) Splenda
¼ teaspoon orange extract

Simply combine everything in a bowl and whisk together.

Yield: ½ cup (120 ml), or 4 servings of 2 tablespoons (30 ml)

Each with trace protein; 1 g carbohydrate; trace dietary fiber; 1 g usable carb.

Ginger Salad Dressing

¼ cup (40 g) minced onion
½ cup (120 ml) canola oil
⅓ cup (80 ml) rice vinegar
2 tablespoons (30 ml) water
2 tablespoons (20 g) grated ginger
2 tablespoons (20 g) diced celery
2 tablespoons (30 g) Dana's No-Sugar
    Ketchup (page 463)
4 teaspoons soy sauce
2 teaspoons Splenda

2 teaspoons lemon juice
½ teaspoon salt
¼ teaspoon pepper
1 clove garlic

Simply assemble everything in your blender and run for 10 to 15 seconds. Store in a snap-top container in the fridge.

Yield: 1½ cups (360 ml), or 12 servings of 2 tablespoons (30 ml)

Each with trace protein; 2 g carbohydrate; trace dietary fiber; 2 g usable carbs.

Tangy "Honey" Mustard Dressing

You know that honey, despite being "natural," is pure sugar, right? Make this instead.

¼ cup (60 ml) canola oil
2 tablespoons (30 ml) apple cider vinegar
2 tablespoons (30 ml) spicy brown or Dijon
    mustard
1 tablespoon plus 2 teaspoons (2.5 g) Splenda
⅛ teaspoon pepper
⅛ teaspoon salt

Combine all ingredients and store in a container with a tight-fitting lid.

Yield: 6 servings

Each with 1 gram of carbohydrates, a trace of fiber, and a trace of protein.

(continued on page 174)

This makes a little over ½ cup (120 ml), or just enough for one big salad, but feel free to double or even quadruple this recipe.

Catalina Dressing

Catalina dressing and its close relative, that red stuff that calls itself "French Dressing" (I'm betting it has nothing to do with French cuisine!), are some of the more sugary dressings on the market. I kept thinking I should come up with a low-carb version, but the truth is, I never liked the stuff. So when reader Emily Borman wrote me, asking me if I had a low-carb version, I jumped at the chance! I found a Catalina recipe, rewrote it with no-sugar ketchup and Splenda, and sent it to her. She promptly tried it, tweaked it with more ketchup and Splenda, and sent back the results. So here, thanks to Emily, is a Catalina dressing recipe for all you fans!

½ **cup plus 2 tablespoons (150 g) Dana's No-Sugar Ketchup (page 463)**
½ **cup plus 2 tablespoons (16 g) Splenda**
⅔ **cup (160 ml) canola or peanut oil**
⅔ **cup (160 ml) red wine vinegar**
2 cloves garlic, crushed
2 tablespoons (20 g) minced onion
Salt to taste

Simply assemble everything in a bowl or your blender and whisk or blend it together. Store in an airtight container in the fridge.

Yield: 1¾ cups (420 ml), or 14 servings of 2 tablespoons (30 ml)

Each with 1 g protein; 4 g carbohydrate; 1 g dietary fiber; 3 g usable carbs.

Blue Cheese Dressing

2 cups (450 g) mayonnaise
½ **cup (120 ml) buttermilk**
½ **cup (115 g) small-curd cottage cheese**
½ **teaspoon Worcestershire sauce**
1 clove garlic, crushed
1 teaspoon salt or Vege-Sal
3 ounces (85 g) crumbled blue cheese

Whisk together the mayonnaise, buttermilk, cottage cheese, Worcestershire, garlic, and salt, mixing well. Gently stir in the blue cheese to preserve some chunks. Store in a container with a tight-fitting lid.

Yield: Makes roughly 3 cups (720 ml)

A 2-tablespoon (30-ml) serving has 1 gram of carbohydrates, a trace of fiber, and 2 grams of protein.

Ranch Dressing

1 cup (225 g) mayonnaise
1 cup (240 ml) buttermilk
2 tablespoons (12 g) finely chopped scallions
¼ **teaspoon onion powder**
2 tablespoons (7.6 g) minced fresh parsley
1 clove garlic, crushed
¼ **teaspoon paprika**

⅛ teaspoon cayenne pepper or a few drops of hot pepper sauce
¼ teaspoon salt
¼ teaspoon black pepper

Combine all ingredients well and store in the refrigerator in a container with a tight-fitting lid.

Yield: Makes about 24 servings

Each with 1 gram of carbohydrates, a trace of fiber, and 1 gram of protein.

Parmesan Peppercorn Dressing

2 tablespoons (30 ml) olive oil
3 tablespoons (42 g) mayonnaise
2 tablespoons (30 ml) wine vinegar
3 tablespoons (18.8 g) grated Parmesan cheese
1 teaspoon freshly ground black pepper (Coarse-cracked pepper will do, if you don't have a pepper mill.)

Blend all the ingredients and store in the refrigerator in a container with a tight-fitting lid.

Yield: 6 servings

Each with 1 gram of carbohydrates, a trace of fiber, and 1 gram of protein.

Creamy Garlic Dressing

Look at all that garlic! If you plan to get kissed, make sure you share this salad with the object of your affections.

½ cup (115 g) mayonnaise
Pinch each of pepper and salt
8 cloves garlic, crushed
2 tablespoons (30 ml) olive oil
2 tablespoons (30 ml) wine vinegar

Combine all the ingredients well and store in the refrigerator in a container with a tight-fitting lid.

Yield: 6 servings

Each with 2 grams of carbohydrates, a trace of fiber, and a trace of protein.

This is only enough for one big salad, but I wouldn't double it; I'd make this one fresh so the garlic flavor will be better.

Caesar Dressing

If you cannot use raw eggs, you could use Egg Beaters or check your grocery store for pasteurized eggs. This is far better than any bottled Caesar dressing I've found, even if it's not quite as wonderful as what I had on my honeymoon in Mexico—although I suspect that the atmosphere had something to do with that.

(continued on page 176)

¼ cup (60 ml) lemon juice

¼ cup (60 ml) olive oil

1 teaspoon pepper

1½ teaspoons Worcestershire sauce

1 clove garlic, peeled and smashed

½ teaspoon salt or Vege-Sal

1 raw egg

½ cup (50 g) grated Parmesan

2 inches (5 cm) anchovy paste (You could use an anchovy fillet or two if you prefer, but anchovy paste is handier, and it keeps forever in the fridge.)

Put everything in a blender, run it for a minute, and toss with one really huge Caesar salad—dinner-party-sized—or a couple of smaller ones. Use it up pretty quickly and keep it refrigerated because of the raw egg.

Yield: 8 servings

Each with 1 gram of carbohydrates, a trace of fiber, and 3 grams of protein.

If you'd like this a little thicker, you could add ¼ teaspoon of guar or xanthan to the mix.

Coleslaw Dressing

Virtually all commercial coleslaw dressing is simply full of sugar, which is a shame, since cabbage is a very low-carb vegetable. I just love coleslaw, so I came up with a sugar-free dressing.

½ cup (115 g) mayonnaise

½ cup (115 g) sour cream

1 to 1½ tablespoons (15 to 23 ml) apple cider vinegar

1 to 1½ teaspoons prepared mustard

½ to 1 teaspoon salt or Vege-Sal

½ to 1 packet artificial sweetener, or 1 teaspoon of Splenda

Combine all the ingredients well and toss with coleslaw.

Yield: 12 servings

Each with 1 gram of carbohydrates, with a trace of fiber, and a trace of protein.

You may, of course, vary these proportions to taste. Also, a teaspoon or so of celery seed can be nice in this for a little variety. I use this much dressing for a whole head of cabbage. If you're used to commercial coleslaw, which tends to be simply swimming in dressing, you may want to double this or use this recipe for half a head.

7

Soups

California Soup

This makes a quick and elegant first course.

**1 large or 2 small, very ripe black avocados,
  pitted, peeled, and cut into chunks**
1 quart (960 ml) chicken broth, heated

Put the avocados in a blender with the broth,
purée until very smooth, and serve.

Yield: 6 servings (as a first course)

Each with 3 grams of carbohydrates and 1 gram of
fiber, for a total of 2 grams of usable carbs and
4 grams of protein.

If you like curry, you've got to try this: Melt a
tablespoon (14 g) or so of butter in a small
saucepan and add ½ teaspoon or so of curry
powder. Cook for just a minute and then add
the mixture to the blender with the broth and
avocados.

Corner-Filling Consommé

2 tablespoons (28 g) butter
4 ounces (115 g) sliced mushrooms
1 small onion, sliced paper-thin
1 quart (960 ml) beef broth
2 tablespoons (30 ml) dry sherry
¼ teaspoon pepper

Melt the butter in a skillet and sauté the mushrooms and onions in the butter until they're limp.
Add the beef broth, sherry, and pepper. Let it

simmer for 5 minutes or so, just to blend the
flavors a bit, and serve.

Yield: 6 appetizer-size servings

Each with 5 grams of carbohydrates and 1 gram
of fiber, for a total of 4 grams of usable carbs and
8 grams of protein.

Peanut Soup

If you miss split pea or bean soup, try this. Try it
even if you don't miss other soups—you may find
you have a new favorite.

3 tablespoons (42 g) butter
2 or 3 ribs celery, finely chopped
1 medium onion, finely chopped
2 quarts (1.9 L) chicken broth
½ teaspoon salt or Vege-Sal
**1¼ cups (325 g) natural peanut butter
  (I use smooth.)**
1 teaspoon guar gum (optional)
2 cups (420 ml) half-and-half or heavy cream
Salted peanuts, chopped

Melt the butter in a skillet and sauté the celery
and onion in the butter. Add the broth, salt, and
peanut butter, and stir. Cover and simmer on the
lowest temperature for at least 1 hour, stirring
now and then.

If you're using guar gum (it makes the soup
thicker without adding carbs; most peanut soup
is thickened with flour), scoop 1 cup (240 ml) of
the soup out of the pot about 15 minutes before
you want to serve it. Add the guar gum to this
cup, run the mixture through the blender for a
few seconds, and whisk it back into the soup.

Stir in the half-and-half and simmer for another 15 minutes. Garnish with the peanuts.

Yield: 5 servings

The carb count will depend on what brand of natural peanut butter you use (they have varying amounts of fiber) and whether you use half-and-half or heavy cream. Figure each serving has about 19 grams of carbohydrates and 3 grams of fiber, for a total of 16 grams of usable carbs and 29 grams of protein.

If your slow cooker will hold this quantity of ingredients (mine will), it's ideal for cooking this soup. Set it on High, cover it, and let it go for 2 to 3 hours.

Artichoke Soup

3 to 4 tablespoons (42 to 56 g) butter
1 small onion, finely chopped
2 stalks celery, finely chopped
1 clove garlic, crushed
1 can (14 ounces, or 400 g) quartered artichoke hearts, drained
4 cups (0.9 L) chicken broth, divided
½ teaspoon guar or xanthan
1 cup (240 ml) half-and-half
Juice of ½ lemon
Salt or Vege-Sal
Pepper

In a heavy skillet, melt the butter and sauté the onion, celery, and garlic over low to medium heat. Stir from time to time.

Drain the artichoke hearts and trim off any tough bits of leaf that got left on. Put the artichoke hearts in a food processor with the

S-blade in position. Add ½ cup (120 ml) of the chicken broth and the guar gum and process until the artichokes are a fine purée.

Scrape the artichoke mixture into a saucepan, add the remaining chicken broth, and set over medium-high heat to simmer.

When the onion and celery are soft, stir them into the artichoke mixture. When it comes to a simmer, whisk in the half-and-half. Bring it back to a simmer, squeeze in the lemon juice, and stir again. Add salt and pepper to taste. You can serve this immediately, hot, or in summer you can serve it chilled.

Yield: 6 servings

Each with 10 grams of carbohydrates and 3 grams of fiber, for a total of 7 grams of usable carbs and 4 grams of protein. (Note: Much of the carbohydrates in artichokes is inulin, which remains largely undigested, so this carb count is actually misleadingly high.)

Olive Soup

Olives are so good for you that you should be eating more of them! This makes a fine first course.

4 cups (0.9 L) chicken broth, divided
½ teaspoon guar or xanthan
1 cup (100 g) minced black olives (You can buy cans of minced black olives.)
1 cup (240 ml) heavy cream
¼ cup (60 ml) dry sherry
Salt or Vege-Sal
Pepper

(continued on page 180)

Put ½ cup (120 ml) of the chicken broth in the blender with the guar gum and blend for a few seconds. Pour into a saucepan and add the rest of the stock and the olives.

Heat until simmering and then whisk in the cream. Bring back to a simmer, stir in the sherry, and add salt and pepper to taste.

Yield: 6 servings

Each with 3 grams of carbohydrates and 1 gram of fiber, for a total of 2 grams of usable carbs and 2 grams of protein.

Eggdrop Soup

This soup is quick and easy, but it's filling and can practically save your life when you've got a cold. You don't have to use the guar, but it gives the broth the same rich quality that the cornstarch-thickened Chinese broths have.

1 quart (960 ml) chicken broth
¼ teaspoon guar (optional)
1 tablespoon (15 ml) soy sauce
1 tablespoon (15 ml) rice vinegar
½ teaspoon grated fresh ginger
1 scallion, sliced
2 eggs

Put 1 cup (240 ml) or so of the chicken broth in your blender, turn it on low, and add the guar (if using). Let it blend for a second and then put it in a large saucepan with the rest of the broth. (If you're not using the guar, just put all the broth directly in a saucepan.)

Add the soy sauce, rice vinegar, ginger, and scallion. Heat over medium-high heat and let it simmer for 5 minutes or so to let the flavors blend.

Beat your eggs in a glass measuring cup or small pitcher—something with a pouring lip. Use a fork to stir the surface of the soup in a slow circle and pour in about ¼ of the eggs, stirring as they cook and turn into shreds (which will happen almost instantaneously). Repeat three more times, using up all the egg and then serve!

Yield: 3 biggish servings, or 4 to 5 small ones (but this recipe is easy to double).

In 4 servings, each will have 2 grams of carbohydrates, a trace of fiber, and 8 grams of protein.

Stracciatella

This is the Italian take on eggdrop soup, and it's delightful.

1 quart (960 ml) chicken broth, divided
2 eggs
½ cup (50 g) grated Parmesan cheese
½ teaspoon lemon juice
Pinch of nutmeg
½ teaspoon dried marjoram

Put ¼ cup (60 ml) of the broth in a glass measuring cup or small pitcher. Pour the rest into a large saucepan over medium heat.

Add the eggs to the broth in the measuring cup and beat with a fork. Then add the Parmesan, lemon juice, and nutmeg and beat with a fork until well blended.

When the broth in the saucepan is simmering, stir it with a fork as you add small amounts of the egg and cheese mixture until it's all stirred in. (Don't expect this to form long shreds like Chinese eggdrop soup; because of the Parmesan, it makes small, fluffy particles instead.)

Add the marjoram, crushing it a bit between your fingers, and simmer the soup for another minute or so before serving.

Yield: 4 servings

Each with 2 grams of carbohydrates, a trace of fiber, and 12 grams of protein.

Sopa De Frijoles Negros

This is a really-truly bean soup! The high-carb but flavorful black beans are diluted with the low-carb black soybeans. Add plenty of seasonings, and you've got a great south-of-the-border soup.

2 cans (15 ounces, or 420 g) Eden brand black soybeans
1 can (15 ounces, or 420 g) black beans
1 can (14½ ounces, or 411 ml) chicken broth
1 tablespoon (15 ml) olive oil
½ cup (80 g) chopped onion
4 cloves garlic, crushed
1 cup (130 g) salsa
2 tablespoons (30 ml) lime juice
1 tablespoon (6.3 g) ground cumin
½ teaspoon red pepper flakes
½ teaspoon salt or Vege-Sal
½ cup (115 g) plain yogurt
¼ cup (16 g) chopped cilantro

Put half of the beans and half of the chicken broth in your blender or in your food processor with the S-blade in place. Run the machine until the beans are puréed. Dump the mixture into a bowl that holds at least 2 quarts (1.9 L) and purée the other half of the beans and the other half of the chicken broth. Add that to the first batch.

Heat the olive oil in a heavy-bottomed saucepan over medium-low heat and add the onion. Sauté until the onion starts turning translucent. Add the bean purée and the garlic. Now stir in the salsa, lime juice, cumin, red pepper flakes, and salt or Vege-Sal. Turn the heat up a bit until the soup is heated through and then turn it back down to the lowest setting and let your soup simmer for 30 to 45 minutes. Serve with a dollop of plain yogurt (or sour cream, if you prefer) and a sprinkling of chopped cilantro.

Yield: 6 servings

Each with 18 g protein, 25 g carbohydrate, 13 g dietary fiber, 13 g usable carbs. (This is obviously not an Induction dish, but for comparison, I analyzed a standard black bean soup recipe. It had 43 grams of carbohydrate and 10 grams of fiber per serving, for a usable carb count of 33 grams, or about two-and-a-half times as much. And it had less protein, too.)

Curried Pumpkin Soup

This is high enough in carbohydrate and low enough in protein that you should think of it as a first course, rather than a main course—and the yield for this recipe reflects that. But what a great starter for Thanksgiving dinner!

¼ cup (40 g) minced onion
1 clove garlic
1 tablespoon (14 g) butter
1 quart (960 ml) chicken broth
1½ cups (240 g) canned pumpkin
½ cup (120 ml) Carb Countdown dairy
   beverage
2 teaspoons curry powder
Salt and pepper to taste

In a large, heavy-bottomed saucepan, over medium-low heat, sauté the onion and garlic in the butter until just softened. Add the chicken broth and simmer for a half an hour.

Stir in the canned pumpkin, Carb Countdown dairy beverage, and curry powder. Bring back to a simmer and simmer gently for another 15 minutes. Add salt and pepper to taste and then serve.

Yield: 6 servings

Each with 5 g protein; 7 g carbohydrate; 2 g dietary fiber; 5 g usable carbs.

Sopa Aguacate

With a quesadilla on the side, this makes a nice light supper.

1 quart (960 ml) chicken broth
1 ripe black avocado
2 scallions
2 canned green chilies or 1 or 2 canned
   jalapeños, if you like it hot!
2 tablespoons (8 g) chopped cilantro
½ teaspoon salt or Vege-Sal

Start heating the broth—you can put it in a pan on the stove or you can put it in a large micro-waveable container in the microwave.

While the broth is heating, scoop the avocado out of its skin and into a food processor with the S-blade in place. Add the scallions, chilies, cilantro, and salt. Pulse to chop everything together—you can leave a few chunks of avocado or purée it smooth, whichever you prefer.

When the broth is hot, divide the avocado mixture between 4 smallish soup bowls. Ladle the hot broth over the avocado mixture and serve.

Yield: 4 servings

Each with 6 grams of carbohydrates and 3 grams of fiber, for a total of 3 grams of usable carbs and 6 grams of protein. Bonus: You'll get a whopping 572 mg potassium and only 125 calories!

Broccoli Blue Cheese Soup

I'd never had soup made with blue cheese before, but this is amazing. It certainly appealed to my blue-cheese-fan husband!

1 cup (160 g) chopped onion

2 tablespoons (28 g) butter

1 turnip, peeled and diced

1½ quarts (1.4 L) chicken broth

1 pound (455 g) frozen broccoli, thawed

1 cup (240 ml) Carb Countdown dairy beverage

¼ cup (60 ml) heavy cream

1 cup (120 g) crumbled blue cheese

In a large saucepan, sauté the onion in the butter over medium-low heat—you don't want it to brown.

When the onion's soft and translucent, add the turnip and the chicken broth to the pot. Bring the mixture to a simmer and let it simmer over medium-low heat for 20 to 30 minutes.

Add the thawed broccoli and let it simmer for another 20 minutes.

Scoop the vegetables out with a slotted spoon and place them in a blender. Add a ladleful of the broth and run the blender until the vegetables are finely puréed. Return the mixture to the pot.

Stir in the Carb Countdown, the heavy cream, and the blue cheese. Simmer for another 5 to 10 minutes, stirring occasionally, and serve.

Yield: 6 servings

Each with 14 g protein; 9 g carbohydrate; 3 g dietary fiber; 6 g usable carbs.

Swiss Cheese and Broccoli Soup

2 tablespoons (20 g) minced onion

1 tablespoon (14 g) butter

14 ounces (400 ml) chicken broth

10 ounces (280 g) frozen chopped broccoli, thawed

1 cup (240 ml) Carb Countdown dairy beverage

½ cup (120 ml) heavy cream

1½ cups (180 g) shredded Swiss cheese

Guar or xanthan

In a large, heavy-bottomed saucepan, sauté the onion in the butter until it's translucent. Add the chicken broth and the broccoli and simmer for 20 to 30 minutes until the broccoli is quite tender.

Stir in the Carb Countdown and cream. Bring it back up to a simmer. Now stir in the cheese, a little at a time, letting each batch melt before you add some more. When all the cheese is melted in, thicken a little with guar or xanthan, if you think it needs it, and serve.

Yield: 4 servings

Each with 20 g protein; 7 g carbohydrate; 2 g dietary fiber; 5 g usable carbs.

Tavern Soup

What's not to like about cheese soup with beer! Don't worry about the kids, the alcohol cooks off.

1½ **quarts (1.4 L) chicken broth**
¼ **cup (30 g) finely diced celery**
¼ **cup (30 g) finely diced green bell pepper**
¼ **cup (30 g) shredded carrot**
¼ **cup (15.2 g) chopped fresh parsley**
½ **teaspoon pepper**
1 **pound (455 g) sharp cheddar cheese, shredded**
12 **ounces (360 ml) light beer**
½ **teaspoon salt or Vege-Sal**
¼ **teaspoon hot pepper sauce**
Guar or xanthan

Combine the broth, celery, green pepper, carrot, parsley, and pepper in your slow cooker. Cover the slow cooker, set it to low, and let it cook for 6 to 8 hours (even a bit longer won't hurt).

When the time's up, either use a hand-held blender to purée the vegetables right there in the slow cooker or scoop them out with a slotted spoon, purée them in your blender, and return them to the slow cooker.

Now whisk in the cheese a little at a time until it's all melted in. Add the beer, salt or Vege-Sal, and hot pepper sauce and stir until the foaming stops. Use guar or xanthan to thicken your soup until it's about the texture of heavy cream. Re-cover the pot, turn it to high, and let it cook for another 20 minutes before serving.

Yield: 8 servings

Each with 18 g protein, 3 g carbohydrate, trace dietary fiber, 3 g usable carbs.

Cream of Mushroom Soup

If you've only ever thought of mushroom soup as gooey stuff that came in cans and was used in casseroles, you need to try this! It has a rich, earthy flavor. Even my mushroom-phobic husband liked it.

8 **ounces (225 g) mushrooms, sliced**
¼ **cup (25 g) chopped onion**
2 **tablespoons (28 g) butter**
1 **quart (960 ml) chicken broth**
½ **cup (120 ml) heavy cream**
½ **cup (120 g) light sour cream**
Guar or xanthan (optional)

In a big, heavy skillet, sauté the mushrooms and onion in the butter until the mushrooms soften and change color. Transfer them to your slow cooker. Add the broth. Cover the slow cooker, set it to low, and let it cook for 5 to 6 hours.

When the time's up, scoop out the vegetables with a slotted spoon and put them in your blender or food processor. Add enough broth to help them process easily and purée them finely. Pour the puréed vegetables back into the slow cooker, scraping out every last bit with a rubber scraper. Now stir in the heavy cream and sour cream and add salt and pepper to taste. Thicken the sauce a bit with guar or xanthan if you think it needs it. Serve immediately.

Yield: 5 servings

Each with 6 g protein, 5 g carbohydrate, 1 g dietary fiber, 4 usable carbs.

Cream of Cauliflower

You'll be surprised by how much this tastes like Cream of Potato!

3 tablespoons (42 g) butter
¾ cup (120 g) diced onion
¾ cup (90 g) diced celery
1 quart (960 ml) chicken broth
1 package (10 ounces, or 280 g) frozen cauliflower
½ teaspoon guar or xanthan (optional)
½ cup (120 ml) heavy cream
Salt and pepper

Melt the butter over low heat and sauté the onion and celery in it until they're limp. Combine this with the chicken broth and cauliflower in a large saucepan and simmer until the cauliflower is tender.

Use a slotted spoon to transfer the vegetables into a blender and then pour in as much of the broth as will fit. Add the guar or xanthan (if using) and purée the ingredients.

Pour the mixture back into the saucepan. Stir in the cream and add salt and pepper to taste.

Yield: 4 servings

Each with 9 grams of carbohydrates and 3 grams of fiber, for a total of 6 grams of usable carbs and 7 grams of protein.

Cheesy Cauliflower Soup

This was originally a potato-cheese soup, but it sure is good this way!

4 cups (600 g) cauliflower, diced small
1 tablespoon (10 g) finely chopped onion
2 tablespoons (20 g) finely chopped celery
1 tablespoon (7 g) grated carrot
3 cups (720 ml) chicken broth
1 teaspoon salt
2 teaspoons white vinegar
1½ cups (360 ml) Carb Countdown dairy beverage or half-and-half
1½ cups (180 g) shredded cheddar cheese
Guar or xanthan (optional)
2 slices bacon, cooked and drained
1 tablespoon (6 g) minced scallion

Put the cauliflower, onion, celery, and carrot in a large, heavy-bottomed saucepan. Add the chicken broth, salt, and vinegar; bring up to a simmer and let cook for 30 to 45 minutes.

Stir in the Carb Countdown or half-and-half and then whisk in the cheese a little at a time, giving each addition time to melt before adding more. Thicken it a little with guar or xanthan if you think it needs it.

Top each serving with a little crumbled bacon and minced scallions (though it's also wonderful without them!).

Yield: 5 servings

Each with 17 g protein; 7 g carbohydrate; 2 g dietary fiber; 5 g usable carbs.

Cauliflower, Cheese, and Spinach Soup

Maria's family gave this raves. It's easy, too!

6 cups (900 g) cauliflower florets, cut into
    ½-inch (1.3-cm) pieces
1 quart (960 ml) chicken broth
½ cup (80 g) minced red onion
5 ounces (140 g) bagged baby spinach leaves,
    pre-washed
¼ teaspoon cayenne
½ teaspoon salt or Vege-Sal
¼ teaspoon pepper
4 cloves garlic, crushed
3 cups (675 g) shredded smoked Gouda
    cheese
1 cup (240 ml) Carb Countdown dairy
    beverage
Guar or xanthan

In your slow cooker, combine the cauliflower, broth, onion, spinach, cayenne, salt or Vege-Sal, pepper, and garlic. Cover the slow cooker, set it to low, and let it cook for 6 hours or until the cauliflower is tender.

When the time's up, stir in the Gouda, a little at a time, and then the Carb Countdown. Re-cover the slow cooker and cook for another 15 minutes or until the cheese has thoroughly melted. Thicken soup a little with guar or xanthan.

Yield: 8 servings

Each with 17 g protein; 7 g carbohydrate, 2 g dietary fiber, 5 g usable carbs.

Cheesy Onion Soup

1 quart (960 ml) beef broth
1 medium onion
½ cup (120 ml) heavy cream
½ cup (120 ml) Carb Countdown dairy
    beverage
1½ cups (180 g) shredded sharp cheddar
    cheese
Guar or xanthan (optional)
Salt and pepper to taste

Pour the beef broth into a large saucepan and start it heating over a medium-high flame. Slice the onion paper-thin and add it to the broth. When the broth starts to boil, turn the heat to low and let the whole thing simmer for 1 hour. If you like, you can do this ahead of time; turn off the heat and let the whole thing cool, refrigerate it, and do the rest later. If you do this, bring the broth up to heat again before proceeding.

Gently stir in the cream and the Carb Countdown dairy beverage. Now stir in the cheese, a bit at a time, until it's all melted in. Thicken a little if you want with guar or xanthan but stir with a ladle or spoon instead of a whisk—you don't want to break up the strands of onion. Add salt and pepper to taste and serve.

Yield: 4 servings

Each with 24 g protein; 8 g carbohydrate; trace dietary fiber; 8 g usable carbs.

Cream of UnPotato Soup

I never cease to marvel at the versatility of cauliflower. This really does taste like potato soup.

1 quart (960 ml) chicken broth
½ head cauliflower, chunked
½ cup (50 g) chopped onion
½ cup (50 g) Ketatoes mix
½ cup (120 ml) heavy cream
½ cup (120 ml) Carb Countdown dairy beverage
Guar or xanthan (optional)
5 scallions, sliced

Put the broth, cauliflower, and onion in your slow cooker. Cover the slow cooker, set it to low, and let it cook for 4 to 5 hours.

I use a hand blender to purée my soup right in the slow cooker, but you may transfer the cauliflower and onion, along with 1 cup (240 ml) of broth, into your blender or food processor instead. Either way, purée until completely smooth and then blend in the Ketatoes. If you have removed the cauliflower from the slow cooker to purée, pour the purée back in and whisk it into the remaining broth.

Stir in the cream and Carb Countdown. Thicken it a bit further with guar or xanthan if you feel it needs it. Add salt and pepper to taste and stir in the sliced scallions. Serve hot right away or chill and serve as vichyssoise.

Yield: 6 servings

Each with 12 g protein, 13 g carbohydrate, 6 g dietary fiber, 7 g usable carbs.

German UnPotato Soup

This is worth the time you spend cutting things up! It's hearty and filling.

1 head cauliflower, chunked
2 stalks celery, sliced
1 medium onion, chopped
8 ounces (225 g) smoked sausage, sliced
1 tablespoon (15 ml) oil
4 cups (960 ml) beef broth, divided
2 tablespoons (30 ml) vinegar
1 tablespoon (1.5 g) Splenda
¼ teaspoon celery seed
½ teaspoon dry mustard
¼ teaspoon pepper
2 cups (240 g) bagged coleslaw mix

Place the cauliflower, celery, and onion in your slow cooker.

In a big, heavy skillet, brown the sausage a bit in the oil. Transfer the sausage to the slow cooker.

Pour 1 cup (240 ml) of the broth into the skillet and stir it around a bit to dissolve the flavorful bits. Pour it into the slow cooker.

In a bowl, combine the rest of the broth with the vinegar, Splenda, celery seed, dry mustard, and pepper. Pour over the vegetables and sausage. Cover the slow cooker, set it to low, and let it cook for 8 hours.

When the time's up, stir in the coleslaw mix and let it cook for another 20 to 30 minutes.

Yield: 4 servings

Each with 20 g protein, 17 g carbohydrate, 2 g dietary fiber, 15 g usable carbs.

Spring Chicken Soup

This soup is a great way to use up leftovers—just substitute 1 cup (110 g) of leftover chicken for the chicken breast called for in the ingredients list.

6 cups (1.4 L) chicken broth
1 can (6½ ounces, or 185 g) mushrooms
1 can (6½ ounces, or 185 g) cut asparagus
1 boneless, skinless chicken breast, diced into small cubes
¼ cup (60 ml) dry sherry
1 tablespoon (15 ml) soy sauce
Pepper
Sliced scallions

Combine the broth, mushrooms, asparagus, chicken, sherry, and soy sauce in a pot and heat. If you're using raw chicken, let it cook for 5 to 10 minutes (that's all it should take to cook small cubes of chicken through). Add pepper to taste and serve with a scattering of scallions on top.

Yield: 4 servings

Depending on the broth you use, this should have no more than about 17 grams of usable carbs in the whole pot, plus about 0.5 gram for the little bit of scallion you put on top of each bowl. Figure each serving has 6 grams of carbohydrates and 2 grams of fiber, for a total of 4 grams of usable carbs and 23 grams of protein.

If you're feeling ambitious, there's no reason you couldn't make this with fresh mushrooms and fresh asparagus; you'll just have to simmer it a little longer. As it is, though, this soup is practically instantaneous!

Chicken Minestrone

Here's a decarbed version of the Italian favorite. You'll never miss the pasta!

3 slices bacon, chopped
1 medium onion, chopped
2 medium turnips, cut into ½-inch (1.3-cm) cubes
1 medium carrot, thinly sliced
2 small zucchini, quartered and sliced
2 stalks celery, thinly sliced
3 tablespoons (45 ml) olive oil
1½ quarts (1.4 L) chicken broth
1½ pounds (700 g) skinless chicken thighs, boned and cubed
1 tablespoon (3.9 g) Italian seasoning
1 can (14½ ounces, or 410 g) diced tomatoes, undrained
1 can (15 ounces, or 425 g) black soybeans
Salt and pepper

Spray a big, heavy skillet with nonstick cooking spray and start the bacon frying over medium heat. As some grease cooks out of the bacon, add as many of the vegetables as will fit in the skillet and sauté them until they soften just a bit. Transfer the vegetables to your slow cooker and continue sautéing the rest of the vegetables, adding oil as needed, until all the vegetables are softened a bit and in the slow cooker.

Place the broth, chicken, Italian seasoning, tomatoes, soybeans, and salt and pepper to taste in the slow cooker. Cover the slow cooker, set it to low, and let it cook for 7 to 8 hours.

Yield: 6 servings

Each with 21 g protein, 18 g carbohydrate, 6 g dietary fiber, 12 g usable carbs.

Sopa Tlalpeno

This simple Mexican soup takes no more than 20 to 25 minutes to make!

1½ quarts (1.4 L) chicken broth
1 pound (455 g) boneless, skinless chicken breast
1 chipotle chile canned in adobo
1 black avocado
4 scallions, sliced
Salt and pepper
¾ cup (90 g) shredded Monterey Jack cheese

Pour the chicken broth into a large, heavy-bottomed saucepan, reserving ½ cup (120 ml), and place it over medium-high heat. While it's heating, cut your chicken breast in thin strips or small cubes and then add it to the broth. Let the whole thing simmer for 10 to 15 minutes or until the chicken is cooked through.

Put the reserved chicken broth in your blender with the chipotle and blend until the chipotle is puréed. Pour this mixture into the soup and stir.

Split the avocado in half, remove the seed, peel it, and cut it into ½-inch (1.3-cm) chunks. Add to the soup, along with the scallions, and salt and pepper to taste.

Ladle the soup into bowls and top each serving with shredded cheese.

Yield: 6 servings

Each with 26 g protein; 4 g carbohydrate; 2 g dietary fiber; 2 g usable carbs.

Spicy Chicken and Mushroom Soup

This is exotic and delicious.

3 tablespoons (42 g) butter
1 leek, thinly sliced (white part only)
8 ounces (225 g) sliced mushrooms
1 clove garlic, crushed
2 teaspoons Garam Masala
1 teaspoon pepper
¼ teaspoon cayenne
¼ teaspoon ground nutmeg
1 quart (960 ml) chicken broth
12 ounces (340 g) boneless, skinless chicken breasts, cut into thin strips
½ cup (120 ml) Carb Countdown dairy beverage
½ cup (120 ml) heavy cream
3 tablespoons (12 g) chopped fresh cilantro (optional)

(continued on page 190)

Melt the butter in a big, heavy skillet over medium heat and sauté the leek with the mushrooms until they both soften. Stir in the garlic, Garam Masala, pepper, cayenne, and nutmeg and sauté for another minute or two. Transfer to your slow cooker. Pour in the broth and add the chicken. Cover the slow cooker, set it to low, and let it cook for 6 to 7 hours.

When the time's up, use a slotted spoon to scoop roughly two-thirds of the solids into your blender or food processor. Add 1 cup (240 ml) or so of the broth and purée until smooth. Stir the purée back into the rest of the soup. (You may want to rinse the blender or food processor out with a little broth to get all of the purée.) Stir in the Carb Countdown and cream. Re-cover the pot and let it cook for another 30 minutes. Serve it with cilantro on top or not. It's nice either way.

Yield: 6 servings

Each with 18 g protein, 6 g carbohydrate, 1 g dietary fiber, 5 g usable carbs.

Mulligatawny

This is a curried soup that came out of the British Colonial times in India. It's also wonderful made with broth made from a turkey carcass, or for that matter, from the remains of a leg of lamb.

2 quarts (1.9 L) chicken broth
2 cups (220 g) or more diced cooked chicken
or diced boneless, skinless chicken breast
3 tablespoons (42 g) butter

1 clove garlic, crushed
1 medium onion, chopped
1 small carrot, shredded
2 ribs celery, diced
2 teaspoons to 1½ heaping tablespoons curry powder (I like it with lots of curry!)
1 bay leaf
½ tart apple, chopped fine
1 to 2 teaspoons salt or Vege-Sal
½ teaspoon pepper
½ teaspoon dried thyme
Zest of 1 fresh lemon, grated, or ½ to 1 teaspoon dehydrated lemon zest
1 cup (240 ml) heavy cream

Put the broth and diced chicken in a large stockpot and set the stockpot over low heat.

Melt the butter in a heavy skillet and add the garlic, onion, carrot, celery, and curry powder. Sauté until the vegetables are limp and add them to the stockpot.

Add the bay leaf, apple, salt, pepper, thyme, and lemon to the pot and simmer for 30 minutes. Just before serving, stir in the cream and remove the bay leaf.

Yield: 6 servings

Each with 8 grams of carbohydrates and 2 grams of fiber, for a total of 6 grams of usable carbs and 18 grams of protein.

Thai Chicken Soup

You can have this light but filling soup done in half an hour!

1 quart (960 ml) chicken broth

1 pound (455 g) boneless, skinless chicken breast

1 tablespoon (15 ml) lemon juice

1 tablespoon (15 ml) lime juice

2 tablespoons (12 g) grated fresh ginger

½ cup (120 ml) coconut milk

8 scallions

2 teaspoons chili garlic paste

1 teaspoon fish sauce (nuoc mam or nam pla)

3 tablespoons (12 g) chopped fresh cilantro

In a big, heavy saucepan, start heating the chicken broth while you cut the chicken breast into small cubes or thin strips. Throw your cut-up chicken into the pot, along with the lemon juice, lime juice, and ginger. Let the whole thing simmer for 20 minutes.

Stir in the coconut milk and scallions and let it cook another 10 minutes or so.

Stir in the chili garlic paste and fish sauce. Ladle into bowls, top each serving with chopped cilantro, and serve.

Yield: 3 to 4 servings

Assuming 4, each will have 32 g protein; 6 g carbohydrate; 2 g dietary fiber; 4 g usable carbs.

Sopa Azteca

That's soup made by Aztecs, not soup made from Aztecs!

3 quarts (2.8 L) chicken broth

2 cups (220 g) diced cooked chicken or boneless, skinless chicken breast

¼ cup (60 ml) olive oil

1 medium onion, chopped

4 or 5 cloves garlic, crushed

2 or 3 ribs celery, diced

1 green pepper, diced

1 small carrot, shredded

1 small zucchini, diced

2 tablespoons (10.8 g) dried oregano

2 tablespoons (9 g) dried basil

2 teaspoons pepper

2 cans (14½ ounces, or 410 g each) diced tomatoes, including juice

1 package (10 ounces, or 280 g) frozen chopped spinach

At least 8 ounces (225 g) Mexican Queso Quesadilla or Monterey Jack cheese, shredded

Chipotle peppers in adobo sauce (These come canned.)

5 ripe black avocados

Heat the broth and the chicken in a large pot over low heat.

Heat the olive oil in a skillet over medium heat and sauté the onion, garlic, celery, pepper, carrot, and zucchini together until they're limp. Stir the oregano, basil, and pepper into the vegetables and sauté for another minute and add them to the soup, along with the tomatoes and spinach. Let the whole thing simmer for 30 minutes to 1 hour to let the flavors blend.

When you're ready to serve the Sopa Azteca, put at least ¼ to ½ cup (30 to 60 g) of cheese (more won't hurt) in the bottom of each bowl and anywhere from 1 to 3 chipotles, depending on how spicy you like your food. (If you don't like spicy food at all, leave the chipotles out entirely.) Ladle the hot soup over the cheese and peppers.

(continued on page 192)

Use a spoon to scoop chunks of half of a ripe avocado onto the top of each bowl of soup.

Yield: 10 servings

Each serving of soup alone has 21 grams of carbohydrates and 6 grams of fiber, for a total of 15 grams of usable carbs and 25 grams of protein. One-half cup (60 g) of shredded cheese adds only a gram or so of carbohydrates and 14 grams of protein. Each chipotle pepper adds no more than 1 gram or so of carbs, and half an avocado has about 6 grams of carbohydrates and 2.5 grams of fiber, for a total of 3.5 grams of usable carbs per serving.

The totals on this soup may sound like a lot when you add them all up, but don't forget that this is a whole meal in a bowl: meat, vegetables, melted cheese, and lovely ripe avocado in each bite! You don't need to serve another thing with it, although you could serve tortillas or quesadillas for the carb-eaters in the crowd.

Instant Chicken Soup

Okay, so this isn't quite as instant as those little packets you mix with boiling water. But it's a lot tastier, a lot heartier, and a lot better for you.

¼ head cauliflower
1 quart (960 ml) or 2 cans (14.5 ounces, or 410 ml) chicken broth
10 to 12 ounces (280 to 340 g) boneless, skinless chicken breast
1 stalk celery
1 medium carrot
¼ medium onion
1 tablespoon (14 g) butter
1½ teaspoons poultry seasoning
Salt and pepper

Run the cauliflower through the shredding blade of your food processor. Put it in a microwaveable bowl, add a tablespoon of water, cover, and microwave on high for 5 minutes.

While that's cooking, pour the broth into a large saucepan over high heat. Dice the chicken breast into small bits—about ½-inch (1 cm) cubes—and add it to the pot.

Take the shredding disc out of the food processor and put the S-blade in place. Cut the celery, carrot, and onion into a few big chunks and place in the food processor bowl. Pulse until vegetables are chopped to a medium-fine consistency.

Melt the butter in a medium-size heavy skillet over medium-high heat and add the vegetables and the poultry seasoning. Sauté, stirring frequently.

When the microwave goes "ding," pull the cauliflower out of the microwave and add it to the soup. You can add the other veggies straight from the skillet or if you'd like them to be a little softer, put them in the bowl you cooked the cauliflower in, add 1 tablespoon (15 ml) of the broth from the soup, cover, and microwave for 3 to 4 minutes on high before adding them to the soup.

Either way, stir the vegetables into the soup, add salt and pepper to taste, and serve.

Yield: 3 or 4 servings

Assuming 3 servings, each will have 6 grams of carbohydrates and 1 gram of fiber, for a total of 5 grams of usable carbs and 28 grams of protein.

If you'd prefer, you can make this with egg threads instead of the cauliflower rice, and it will be higher in protein. Just beat a couple of eggs in a measuring cup and pour the beaten egg over the simmering soup, stirring slowly with a fork.

Chicken Soup with Wild Rice

Wild rice has more fiber and therefore fewer usable carbs than regular rice, either white or brown. And it adds a certain cachet to your soup!

2 quarts (1.9 L) chicken broth
2 carrots, thinly sliced
2 stalks celery, diced
½ cup (50 g) chopped onion
1 pound (455 g) boneless, skinless chicken breast, cut into ½-inch (1.3-cm) cubes
¼ cup (40 g) wild rice
1 teaspoon poultry seasoning

Simply combine everything in your slow cooker, cover, set it to low, and let it cook for 6 to 7 hours.

Yield: 6 servings

Each with 25 g protein, 10 g carbohydrate, 2 g dietary fiber, 8 g usable carbs.

Chunky Cream of Chicken and Portobello Soup

This soup is so elegant!

4 tablespoons (56 g) butter
1 cup (160 g) chopped onion
2 stalks celery, diced
1 large carrot, shredded
2 cups (200 g) portobello mushrooms, cut in matchstick strips
2 quarts (1.9 L) chicken broth
2 bay leaves
1 pound (455 g) boneless, skinless chicken breast
½ cup (120 ml) heavy cream
Salt and pepper
Guar or xanthan

Melt the butter in a large, heavy-bottomed saucepan and add the vegetables. Sauté until the onion is translucent and the mushrooms change color. Add the chicken broth and the bay leaves, bring to a simmer, and let cook on low for 30 minutes.

Scoop out about half of the broth and vegetables into your blender and purée. Return to the pan. Stir in the diced chicken breast and let simmer for another 20 minutes. Stir in the cream, add salt and pepper to taste, and thicken just a little with guar or xanthan. Remove the bay leaves and serve.

Yield: 6 servings

Each with 26 g protein; 11 g carbohydrate; 2 g dietary fiber; 9 g usable carbs.

Turkey Meatball Soup

This makes a light, quick, and tasty supper all by itself.

½ pound (225 g) ground turkey
1½ tablespoons (9 g) oat bran
2 tablespoons (7.6 g) minced fresh parsley
½ teaspoon salt or Vege-Sal
½ teaspoon poultry seasoning
⅛ teaspoon pepper
1 tablespoon (15 ml) olive oil
½ cup (60 g) grated carrot
2 cups (250 g) diced zucchini
1 tablespoon (10 g) minced onion
1 clove garlic, crushed
1 quart (960 ml) chicken broth
1 teaspoon dried oregano
2 eggs, beaten
¼ cup (25 g) grated Parmesan cheese

In a mixing bowl, combine the ground turkey with the oat bran, parsley, salt or Vege-Sal, poultry seasoning, and pepper. Mix well and form into balls the size of marbles or so. Set aside.

In a large, heavy-bottomed saucepan, heat the olive oil over medium-high heat. Add the carrot and let it sauté for 2 to 3 minutes. Then add the zucchini, onion, and garlic and sauté the vegetables for another 5 to 7 minutes.

Add the chicken broth and oregano and bring the soup to a simmer for 15 minutes. Drop the turkey meatballs into the soup one by one and let it simmer for another 10 to 15 minutes. (Taste the soup at this point and add more salt and pepper to taste, if desired.)

Just before you're ready to serve the soup, stir it slowly with a fork as you pour the beaten eggs in quite slowly. Simmer another minute and ladle into bowls. Top each serving with 1 tablespoon (6.3 g) of Parmesan and serve.

Yield: 4 servings

Each with 7 grams of carbohydrates and 2 grams of fiber, for a total of 5 grams usable carbs and 21 grams of protein.

Turkey Sausage Soup

This is a great, filling family soup for a cold night.

1½ pounds (700 g) bulk turkey sausage
1 can (14½ ounces, or 410 g) diced tomatoes
1 can (8 ounces, or 225 g) sliced mushrooms
1 turnip, diced
1 cup (150 g) cauliflower, diced
½ cup (50 g) chopped onion
1 cup (120 g) chopped green bell pepper
1 quart (960 ml) chicken broth
2 teaspoons chicken bouillon concentrate
1 teaspoon dried basil
2 teaspoons prepared horseradish
1 cup (240 ml) heavy cream

In a large, heavy skillet, brown and crumble the sausage. Pour off the fat and put the sausage in your slow cooker. Add the tomatoes, mushrooms, turnip, cauliflower, onion, and green pepper.

In a bowl, stir the broth and bouillon together. Stir in the basil and horseradish. Pour the mixture into the slow cooker. Cover the slow cooker, set it to low, and let it cook for 7 to 8 hours.

When the time's up, stir in the cream and let it cook for another 10 to 15 minutes.

Yield: 6 servings

Each with 17 g protein, 12 g carbohydrate, 2 g dietary fiber, 10 g usable carbs.

Tuscan Soup

This Italian-style soup somehow manages to be delicate and substantial at the same time. It is really addictive.

16 ounces (455 g) hot Italian sausage links
2 quarts (1.9 L) chicken broth
1 cup (240 ml) heavy cream
½ head cauliflower, sliced ¼-inch (6 mm) thick
6 cups (120 g) chopped kale
½ teaspoon red pepper flakes
2 cloves garlic, crushed

First, sauté the sausage until it's done. Remove from your skillet and let it cool a little. Meanwhile, start heating the chicken broth and cream in a big, heavy-bottomed saucepan over medium heat. Add the cauliflower and the kale to the soup.

Okay, your sausage is cool enough to handle! Slice it on the diagonal, about ½ inch (1.3 cm) thick. I like to cut each slice in half, too, to make more bites of sausage, but that's not essential. Put the sliced sausage in the soup.

Stir in the red pepper flakes and the garlic. Turn the burner to lowest heat and let the whole thing simmer for an hour, stirring now and then.

Yield: 6 servings

Each with 20 g protein; 10 g carbohydrate; 2 g dietary fiber; 8 g usable carbs.

Portuguese Soup

If this were really authentic, it would have potatoes in it. But this decarbed version is delicious, and it's a full meal in a bowl. Read the labels on the smoked sausage carefully—they range from 1 gram of carb per serving up to 5.

⅓ cup (80 ml) olive oil, divided
¾ cup (120 g) chopped onion
3 cloves garlic, crushed
2 cups (300 g) diced turnip
2 cups (300 g) diced cauliflower
1 pound (455 g) kale
1½ pounds (680 g) smoked sausage
1 can (14½ ounces, or 410 g) diced tomatoes
2 quarts (1.9 L) chicken broth, divided
¼ teaspoon hot pepper sauce
Salt and pepper

Put ¼ cup (60 ml) of the olive oil in a large soup pot and sauté the onion, garlic, turnip, and cauliflower over medium heat.

While that's cooking, chop the kale into bite-sized pieces and add it to the pot as well. (You may need to cram it in at first, but don't

(continued on page 196)

worry—it cooks down quite a bit.) Let the vegetables sauté for another 10 minutes or so, stirring to turn the whole thing over every once in a while.

Slice the smoked sausage lengthwise into quarters, then crosswise into ½-inch (1.3-cm) pieces. Heat the remaining oil in a heavy skillet over medium heat and brown the smoked sausage a little.

Add the browned sausage, tomatoes, and 7½ cups (1.8 L) of the chicken broth to the pot. Use the last ½ cup (120 ml) of broth to rinse the tasty browned bits out of the frying pan and add that too. Bring to a simmer and cook until the vegetables are soft (30 to 45 minutes). Stir in the hot pepper sauce, add salt and pepper to taste, and serve.

Yield: 10 servings

Each with 13 grams of carbohydrates and 2 grams of fiber, for a total of 11 grams of usable carbs and 23 grams of protein.

Bollito Misto

All this Italian soup-stew needs with it is a green salad and maybe some crusty bread for the carb-eaters.

1 large onion, sliced
2 carrots, cut ½ inch (1.3 cm) thick
3 stalks celery, cut ½ inch (1.3 cm) thick
2 pounds (1 kg) beef round, cubed
½ teaspoon salt
½ teaspoon pepper

2 tablespoons (7.6 g) chopped fresh parsley
1 bay leaf
3 teaspoons chicken bouillon concentrate
1 quart (960 ml) chicken broth
2 pounds (910 g) boneless, skinless chicken thighs, cubed
1 pound (455 g) Italian sausage links
½ cup (115 g) purchased pesto sauce

Put the onion, carrots, and celery in your slow cooker. Season the beef with the salt and pepper and place them on top. Add the parsley and bay leaf. Stir the bouillon into the chicken broth and pour it into the slow cooker. Cover the slow cooker, set it to low, and let it cook for 5 to 6 hours.

Add the chicken, turn the heat up to high, and let the whole thing cook another hour.

While it's cooking, pour yourself a glass of Chianti and put out some vegetables and dip for the kids. In a big, heavy skillet, place the sausages, cover with water, slap a lid on, and simmer for 20 minutes over medium heat. Remove the skillet from the heat and leave the sausages in the water, keeping the lid on.

When the slow cooker's time is up, drain the sausage and cut it into 1-inch (2.5-cm) chunks. Stir the sausage into the soup in the slow cooker. Remove the bay leaf and ladle the soup into soup bowls. Top each serving with 1 tablespoon (14.4 g) of pesto.

Yield: 8 servings

Each with 44 g protein, 6 g carbohydrate, 1 g dietary fiber, 5 g usable carbs.

Chicken and Andouille Gumbo

This chunky, vegetable-rich soup is spicy and filling! I've replaced the traditional gumbo *file* (powdered sassafras leaves) thickener with guar or xanthan, because I figure you'll have one of these in the house anyway.

2 tablespoons (28 g) butter

2 cloves garlic, crushed

¾ cup (120 g) chopped onion

½ cup (60 g) diced celery

10 ounces (280 g) frozen sliced okra, thawed

1 pound (455 g) boneless, skinless chicken breast, cut in ½-inch (1.3-cm) cubes

1 quart (960 ml) chicken broth

1 can (14½ ounces, or 410 g) diced tomatoes

1 tablespoon (3.8 g) chopped fresh parsley

1 teaspoon dried thyme

1 bay leaf

½ teaspoon cayenne

¼ teaspoon pepper

1 pound (455 g) andouille sausage links

2 tablespoons (30 ml) Worcestershire sauce

1 tablespoon (15 ml) lemon juice

Hot pepper sauce to taste

Guar or xanthan

Melt the butter in a big soup pot over medium-low heat and add the garlic, onion, and celery. Sauté them together for 5 minutes or so until the onion is just starting to soften.

Add the thawed sliced okra and the cubes of chicken and continue to sauté until the chicken is white all over. Add the chicken broth, the can of diced tomatoes, parsley, thyme, bay leaf, cayenne, and pepper, bring the whole thing up to a simmer, turn the heat down, and simmer for an hour.

When the hour's up, put the andouille links in a skillet over medium-high heat. Brown them all over—prick the casings all over with a fork as you do this. When the sausages are browned, remove them from the skillet to your cutting board and slice ½ inch (1.3 cm) thick. You can leave the slices round or cut each round in half, which is what I do—it depends on how big a bite of sausage you want! Add the sausage slices to the pot. Ladle a little of the broth into the skillet, stir it around to dissolve the nice brown crusty stuff, and pour it back into the pot.

Add the Worcestershire sauce and lemon juice to the soup and stir it up. Let the whole thing simmer for another 15 minutes or so. Now check—is the level of heat right? Or do you want it hotter? If so, stir in a little hot pepper sauce. Thicken the broth just a tad with guar or xanthan, remove bay leaf, and serve.

Now, you get to decide how you want to serve your gumbo. You can serve it as is, of course, and it will be nice as can be. But the traditional way to serve gumbo is ladled over rice, and you certainly may serve yours over cauli-rice. And here in my hometown of Bloomington, Indiana, there is a popular restaurant that serves its "gumbo of the day" Hoosier-style—over mashed potatoes. So you could have your gumbo over a scoop of Ultimate Fauxtatoes (page 209)!

Yield: 6 servings

Each with 31 g protein; 13 g carbohydrate; 2 g dietary fiber; 11 g usable carbs. Analysis does not include any cauli-rice or fauxtatoes you may serve with your gumbo.

UnPotato and Sausage Soup

Talk about comfort food! This is creamy and filling, with a good, rich potato flavor. Just the thing for a stormy winter night.

1 pound (455 g) Polish sausage
2 tablespoons (28 g) butter
¾ cup (120 g) chopped onion
4 cups (600 g) cauliflower, diced
½ cup (60 g) shredded carrot
1 small green pepper, diced
3 cups (720 ml) water, divided
1 teaspoon salt or Vege-Sal
½ teaspoon pepper
3 cups (720 ml) Carb Countdown dairy beverage
½ cup (25 g) Ketatoes mix
Guar or xanthan (optional)

Slice your sausage into rounds. Melt 1 tablespoon (14 g) of the butter in a big skillet over medium heat and start frying the sausage slices in it—you're just browning them a little. You can skip this step if you're in a hurry, but I think it adds a bit of flavor.

In a big, heavy-bottomed saucepan, melt the rest of the butter and start sautéing the onion over medium-low heat.

When the onions are turning golden, throw in the cauliflower, carrot, and green pepper. Pour in 2 cups (480 ml) of the water. When the sausage slices are browned on both sides, add them to the pot. Pour the remaining 1 cup (240 ml) of water into the skillet and scrape the bottom with a spatula to get all the good brown flavor stuck to the skillet. Pour this into the saucepan, too. Add the salt and pepper. Bring everything to a simmer and let it cook for 30 minutes.

When the cauliflower is soft, stir in the Carb Countdown dairy beverage and then whisk in the Ketatoes mix. Thicken your soup a little more with guar or xanthan, if you like, and bring it back to a simmer. Serve.

Yield: 6 servings

Each with 25 g protein; 19 g carbohydrate; 8 g dietary fiber; 11 g usable carbs.

Italian Sausage Soup

It would take some serious multi-tasking, but this soup can be ready in 15 minutes.

1½ quarts (1.4 L) chicken broth
1-pound (455-g) bag frozen Italian vegetable blend
1 pound (455 g) Italian sausage, mild or hot, as you prefer
½ medium onion, chopped
1 teaspoon minced garlic or 2 cloves garlic, crushed
2 teaspoons Italian seasoning
3 eggs
5 tablespoons (31.3 g) grated or shredded Parmesan cheese

First, put the broth in a large saucepan, cover it, and place it over high heat. Next, put the Italian vegetable blend in a microwaveable casserole dish, add a couple of tablespoons (30 ml) of water, cover, and microwave on high for 12 minutes.

Okay, that stuff is under control. Now, in a heavy-bottomed soup pot, start browning the Italian sausage over medium-high heat. If the sausage is in links, slit the skins and squeeze it out, so you can crumble it; bulk sausage you can just plunk into the pot. As a bit of grease starts to cook out of the sausage, add the onion and the garlic (you can chop the onion while the sausage is browning) and let them sauté together.

When the sausage is cooked through, add the chicken broth, which should be hot by now. Stir and add the Italian seasoning. Let the mixture simmer while you crack the eggs into a glass measuring cup and beat them with a fork. Pour the eggs in, a little bit at a time—pour, then stir, pour some more, and then stir some more. This will make lovely egg shreds in your soup.

The vegetables should be done by now, so pull them out of the microwave, drain, and dump them into the soup. Stir, let the whole thing simmer for just another minute, and serve with 1 tablespoon (6.3 g) of Parmesan cheese on each serving.

Yield: 5 servings

Each with 11 grams of carbohydrates and 2 grams of fiber, for a total of 9 grams of usable carbs and 26 grams of protein.

Hot-and-Sour Soup

Really authentic Hot-and-Sour Soup uses Chinese mushrooms, but this is mighty good with any variety—especially when you have a cold!

2 quarts (1.9 L) chicken broth

1 piece of fresh ginger about the size of a walnut, peeled and thinly sliced

½ pound (225 g) lean pork (I use boneless loin.)

3 tablespoons (45 ml) soy sauce

1 to 1½ teaspoons pepper

½ cup (120 ml) white vinegar

2 cans (6½ ounces, or 170 g each) mushrooms

1 cake (about 10 ounces, or 280 g) firm tofu

1 can (8 ounces, or 225 g) bamboo shoots

5 eggs

Put the broth in a soup pot and set it over medium heat. Add the ginger to the broth and let it simmer for a few minutes.

While the broth simmers, slice the pork into small cubes or strips. (I like strips.) Stir the pork, soy sauce, pepper, vinegar, and mushrooms (you don't need to drain them) into the broth. Let it simmer for 10 minutes or so until the pork is cooked through.

Cut the tofu into small cubes. If you like, you can also cut the canned bamboo shoots into thinner strips. (I like them better that way, but sometimes I don't feel like doing the extra work.) Stir the tofu and bamboo shoots into the soup and let it simmer another few minutes. Taste the soup; it won't be very hot—spicy-hot, that is, not temperature-hot—so if you like it hotter, add more pepper and some hot pepper sauce. If you like, you can also add a little extra vinegar.

Beat the eggs in a bowl and then pour them in a thin stream over the surface of the soup. Stir them in, and you'll get a billion little shreds of cooked egg in your soup. Who needs noodles?

(continued on page 200)

Yield: 6 servings

Each with 10 grams of carbohydrates and 2 grams of fiber, for a total of 8 grams of usable carbs and 25 grams of protein.

This is good served with a few finely sliced scallions on top (include some of the green part) and a few drops of toasted sesame oil. Since I like my soup hotter than my husband does, I use hot toasted sesame oil rather than putting hot sauce in the whole batch.

Stir-Fry Soup

The name says it all—a traditional stir-fry turned into a hearty soup. This works equally well with chicken or pork, so take your pick or use whatever is cluttering up the freezer.

2 quarts (1.9 L) chicken broth
1 pound (455 g) boneless pork loin or bone-
less, skinless chicken breast
1 medium onion
3 tablespoons (45 ml) oil
1-pound (455-g) bag frozen stir-fry vegetables,
thawed
1½ tablespoons (23 ml) soy sauce
1½ tablespoons (23 ml) dry sherry
1½ tablespoons (12 g) grated ginger
1½ teaspoons minced garlic
1½ teaspoons toasted sesame oil

Pour the chicken broth into a large microwave-able bowl or pitcher. Put it in the microwave and heat it for 10 minutes on high.

Slice the pork or chicken as thin as possible. (This is easier if the meat is partly frozen.) Thinly slice the onion as well. Heat the oil in the bottom of a large soup pot and add the meat, onion, and stir-fry vegetables. Stir-fry everything over highest heat while the broth is warming in the microwave.

By the time the microwave goes "ding," the pork or chicken should not be pink any more. Pour in the broth, add the soy sauce, sherry, ginger, garlic, and sesame oil, cover, and let the whole thing simmer for 4 to 5 minutes before serving.

Yield: 6 servings

Each with 9 grams of carbohydrates and 2 grams of fiber, for a total of 7 grams of usable carbs and 19 grams of protein.

Chinese Soup with Bok Choy and Mushrooms

1 quart (960 ml) chicken broth
2 tablespoons (16 g) grated ginger
2 teaspoons soy sauce
1 cup (100 g) sliced mushrooms
8 ounces (225 g) boneless pork loin, cut in
thin ½-inch (1.3-cm) strips
1½ cups (115 g) bok choy, sliced thin, leaves
and stems both
1 egg

In a large saucepan over medium-high heat, combine the chicken broth, ginger, and soy sauce. Let them simmer together for 5 minutes.

Now add the mushrooms and pork. Let the soup simmer for another 15 minutes.

Stir in the bok choy and let the soup simmer for another 5 to 10 minutes.

Beat the egg. Now pour it in a thin stream over the surface of the simmering soup, let it sit for 10 seconds, and then stir with the tines of a fork. Serve.

Yield: 4 servings

Each with 17 g protein; 3 g carbohydrate; 1 g dietary fiber; 2 g usable carbs.

Easy Tomato-Beef Soup

1¼ to 1½ pounds (570 to 680 g) ground beef
2 cans (14½ ounces, or 410 g each) beef broth
1 can (14½ ounces, or 410 g) diced tomatoes

In a skillet, brown the ground beef. Pour off the grease and add the broth and tomatoes. Heat through and serve.

Yield: 4 servings

Each with 9 grams of carbohydrates, a trace of fiber, and 19 grams of protein.

Mexican Cabbage Soup

This is great on a nasty, cold, rainy night! This is not hot, despite the chilies in the canned toma-toes—feel free to pass the hot sauce at the table if you want to spice it up. With all these vegetables, this is a complete meal, but if the family insists, you could add some corn tortillas for them.

1 quart (960 ml) beef broth
1 can (14 ounces, or 400 g) diced tomatoes with green chilies
1 pound (455 g) ground round or other very lean ground beef
1 tablespoon (15 ml) oil
½ cup (80 g) chopped onion
1 teaspoon minced garlic or 2 cloves garlic, crushed
1 teaspoon ground cumin
2 teaspoons oregano
2 cups (150 g) bagged coleslaw mix

In a large, microwaveable container combine the beef broth and canned tomatoes. Microwave on high for 8 to 10 minutes.

Meanwhile, in a large soup pot or heavy-bottomed saucepan, start browning and crumbling the beef in the oil. When the beef is about half browned, add the onion and garlic. Continue cooking until the beef is entirely browned. Add the cumin and oregano and then add the heated beef broth and tomatoes. Stir in the coleslaw mix and bring the whole thing to a simmer. Cook for another minute or so and serve.

Yield: 4 servings

Each with 9 grams of carbohydrates and 2 grams of fiber, for a total of 7 grams of usable carbs and 24 grams of protein.

Jamaican Pepperpot Soup

This soup is unbelievably hearty, almost like a stew, and very tasty!

½ pound (225 g) bacon, diced
2 pounds (910 g) boneless beef round or chuck, cut into 1-inch (2.5-cm) cubes
1 large onion, chopped
4 cups (960 ml) water
1 cup (240 ml) canned beef broth
2 packages (10 ounces, or 280 g each) frozen chopped spinach
½ teaspoon dried thyme
1 green pepper, diced
1 can (14½ ounces, or 410 g) sliced tomatoes
1 bay leaf
2 teaspoons salt
½ teaspoon pepper
1 teaspoon hot pepper sauce (or to taste)
1 package (10 ounces, or 280 g) frozen sliced okra, thawed
3 tablespoons (42 g) butter
½ cup (120 ml) heavy cream
Paprika

Place the bacon, beef cubes, onion, water, and beef broth in a large, heavy soup pot. Bring to a boil, turn the heat to low, and let the mixture simmer for 1 hour.

Add the spinach, thyme, green pepper, tomatoes, bay leaf, salt, pepper, and hot pepper sauce. Let it simmer for another 30 minutes.

Sauté the okra in the butter over the lowest heat for about 5 minutes, add it to the soup, and simmer just 10 minutes more.

Just before serving, remove the bay leaf, stir in the cream, and sprinkle just a touch of paprika on each serving.

Yield: 6 servings

Each with 16 grams of carbohydrates and 5 grams of fiber, for a total of 11 grams of usable carbs and 49 grams of protein.

Mexican Beef and Bean Soup

You know the family will love this!

12 ounces (340 g) ground round
1 medium onion, chopped
2 cloves garlic, crushed
1 medium green bell pepper, diced
1 quart (960 ml) beef broth
1 teaspoon beef bouillon concentrate
1 can (14½ ounces, or 410 g) tomatoes with green chiles
1 can (15 ounces, or 425 grams) black soybeans
2 teaspoons ground coriander
1 teaspoon ground cumin
¼ cup (16 g) chopped cilantro
6 tablespoons (70 g) sour cream

In a big, heavy skillet, brown and crumble the ground beef. Drain it well and transfer it to your slow cooker.

Add the onion, garlic, bell pepper, broth, bouillon, tomatoes, soybeans, coriander, and cumin and stir. Cover the slow cooker, set it to low, and let it cook for 7 to 8 hours.

Top each bowlful with cilantro and sour cream.

Yield: 6 servings

Each with 25 g protein, 14 g carbohydrate, 5 g dietary fiber, 9 g usable carbs.

Oyster Stew

This is a classic recipe that simply started out fast, easy, and low-carb. My husband prefers me to cut really big oysters into quarters. Since you can do this as the cream and half-and-half are heating, it doesn't add any time to the recipe—indeed, since the pieces of oyster cook faster than whole ones, it cuts the cooking time a bit.

5 tablespoons (70 g) butter
1 cup (240 ml) half-and-half
1½ cups (360 ml) heavy cream
½ cup (120 ml) water
1½ pints (700 g) oysters
Salt and pepper
⅛ teaspoon cayenne

Put the butter, half-and-half, heavy cream, and water in a heavy-bottomed saucepan over medium heat. As it comes to a simmer, add the oysters and stir. Simmer until the oysters are cooked, about 5 minutes. Add salt and pepper to taste, add the cayenne, and then serve.

Yield: 4 servings

Each with 8 grams of carbohydrates, no fiber, and 11 grams of protein. Despite the modest protein count, this is filling because it is so rich.

If you'd like to speed this recipe up, you can combine everything but the oysters in a large microwaveable container and cook it for 5 minutes on high, but it's not essential.

Italian Tuna Soup

Okay, it's not authentically Italian, but it's a lot like minestrone. It's easy, too.

1 quart (960 ml) chicken broth
1 can (14½ ounces, or 410 g) diced tomatoes
1 can (14½ ounces, or 410 g) Italian green beans or 1 package (10 ounces, or 280 g) frozen Italian green beans
½ cup (125 g) frozen broccoli cuts
½ cup (115 g) frozen cauliflower cuts
1 cup (115 g) thinly sliced zucchini, frozen or fresh
3 tablespoons (45 ml) tomato paste
1 teaspoon Italian seasoning
2 cans (6 ounces [170 g] each) tuna
Hot pepper sauce

Combine the broth, tomatoes, green beans, broccoli, cauliflower, zucchini, tomato paste, seasoning, and tuna. Add a few drops of hot pepper sauce (more if you like it hotter, less if you just want a little zip) and simmer until the vegetables are tender.

Yield: 5 servings

Each with 14 grams of carbohydrates and 3 grams of fiber, for a total of 11 grams of usable carbs and 23 grams of protein.

(continued on page 204)

Check the frozen foods section of your super-market for mixed bags of broccoli and cauliflower and substitute 1 cup (235 g) of the mix for the separate cauliflower and broccoli. That way, you'll only have one partially eaten bag of veggies in the freezer to use up, rather than two.

Cream of Salmon Soup

One person who sampled this soup pronounced it the best soup they'd ever had. And it's so easy!

1½ tablespoons (21 g) butter
¼ cup (40 g) finely minced onion
¼ cup (30 g) finely minced celery
2 cups (480 ml) heavy cream
1 can (14 ounces, or 400 g) salmon, drained
½ teaspoon dried thyme

In a heavy saucepan, melt the butter over medium-low heat and add the onion and celery. Sauté the vegetables for a few minutes until the onion starts turning translucent.

Meanwhile, pour the cream into a glass 2-cup (480 ml) measure or any other microwavable container big enough for it and from which you can pour. Place it in the microwave and heat it at 50 percent power for 3 to 4 minutes. (This just cuts the time needed to heat the cream through—you can skip this step and simply heat the soup on the stovetop a little longer, if you like.)

Pour the cream into the saucepan and add the salmon and thyme. Break up the salmon as you stir the soup—I found my whisk to be ideal for breaking the salmon into fine pieces. Heat until simmering and serve.

Yield: 4 servings

Each with 5 grams of carbohydrates, a trace of fiber, and 23 grams of protein.

Manhattan Clam Chowder

4 slices bacon, diced
1 large onion, chopped
2 ribs celery, diced
1 green pepper, chopped
2½ cups (375 g) diced white turnip
1 grated carrot
1 can (14½ ounces, or 410 g) diced tomatoes
3 cups (710 ml) water
1 teaspoon dried thyme
4 cans (6½ ounces, or 185 g each) minced
    clams, including liquid
Hot pepper sauce
1 teaspoon salt or Vege-Sal
1 teaspoon pepper

In a large, heavy bottomed soup pot, start the bacon cooking. As the fat cooks out of it, add the onion, celery, and green pepper and sauté them in the bacon fat for 4 to 5 minutes.

Add the turnip, carrot, tomatoes, water, and thyme and let the whole thing simmer for 30 minutes to 1 hour.

Add the clams, including the liquid, a dash of hot pepper sauce, the salt or Vege-Sal, and pepper. Simmer for another 15 minutes and serve.

Yield: 10 servings

Each with 11 grams of carbohydrates and 1 gram of fiber, for a total of 10 grams of usable carbs and 21 grams of protein.

Seafood Chowder

My sister Kim, who tested this for me, said that you don't have to stick to shrimp. You could use crab, chunks of lobster tail, or even a cut-up firm-fleshed fish fillet. Don't use fake seafood— "delicacies" and such. It has a lot of added carbs.

1½ cups (225 g) shredded cauliflower
⅓ cup (40 g) shredded carrots
1 teaspoon dried thyme
1 clove garlic
1 tablespoon (10 g) finely minced green bell pepper
⅛ teaspoon cayenne
¼ teaspoon pepper
3 cups (710 ml) chicken broth
1 cup (240 ml) Carb Countdown dairy beverage
¼ cup (60 ml) heavy cream
8 ounces (225 g) shrimp, shells removed
1 tablespoon (5 g) Ketatoes mix
¼ cup (25 g) scallions, thinly sliced
Guar or xanthan

Combine the cauliflower, carrots, thyme, garlic, green pepper, cayenne, pepper, and broth in your slow cooker. Cover the slow cooker, set it to low, and let it cook for 4 hours.

Turn the slow cooker to high and stir in the Carb Countdown and cream. Re-cover the slow cooker and let it cook for another 30 to 45 minutes. If your shrimp are big, chop them coarsely during this time, but little, whole shrimp will look prettier, of course!

Stir in the Ketatoes mix. Now stir in the shrimp and re-cover the pot. If your shrimp are pre-cooked, just give them 5 minutes or so to heat through. If they're raw, give them 10 minutes. Stir in the scallions and salt to taste. Thicken the broth with the guar or xanthan.

Yield: 5 servings

Each with 17 g protein, 7 g carbohydrate, 2 g dietary fiber, 5 g usable carbs.

Quick Green Chowder

1 package (10 ounces, or 280 g) frozen chopped spinach, thawed
2 cans (6½ ounces, or 185 g each) minced clams, including the liquid
1 cup (240 ml) half-and-half
1 cup (240 ml) heavy cream
1 cup (240 ml) water
Salt and pepper

Put the spinach, clams, half-and-half, cream, and water in a blender or food processor and purée.

Pour the mixture into a saucepan and bring to a simmer (use very low heat and don't boil!). Simmer for 5 minutes and add salt and pepper to taste.

(continued on page 206)

Yield: 4 servings

Each with 12 grams of carbohydrates and 2 grams of fiber, for a total of 10 grams of usable carbs and 29 grams of protein.

If you prefer, you can purée everything but the clams, adding them later so they stay in chunks.

Cheater's Chowder

This recipe is so called because you're cheating on the usual ingredients, and you sure are cheating on the cooking time! You are not, however, cheating on your diet. This filling soup is a meal in itself.

¼ **head cauliflower**
1 **medium turnip (just bigger than a tennis ball)**
3 **slices bacon**
½ **medium onion**
2 **cups (480 ml) half-and-half**
1 **can (10 ounces, or 280 g) minced clams**
Salt or Vege-Sal and pepper

Whack the cauliflower into a few good-size chunks and put it in your food processor with the S-blade in place. Peel the turnip, quarter it, and drop it in there, too. Pulse the processor until everything is chopped to a medium-fine consistency. Put the cauliflower and turnip in a microwaveable casserole dish with a lid, add a couple of tablespoons (30 ml) of water, cover, and microwave on high for 12 minutes.

While that's cooking, chop up the bacon—I snip mine up with cooking shears, right into the pot—and start frying it over medium-high heat in a large, heavy-bottomed saucepan, stirring from time to time.

Put that food processor bowl back on its base with the S-blade in place, throw in the half-onion, and pulse until it is chopped medium-fine. Dump the onion in with the bacon, which should be giving off some grease by now. Fry the onion and bacon together until the onion is translucent.

Pour the half-and-half and the clams into the pot—don't bother to drain the clams. Stir it and then let the whole thing come to a simmer, stirring from time to time.

When the cauliflower and turnips are done, add them to the pot, too—no need to drain. Stir them in, add salt or Vege-Sal and pepper to taste, let the soup simmer just another minute or two, and serve.

Yield: 3 servings

Each with 16 grams of carbohydrates and 1 gram of fiber, for a total of 15 grams of usable carbs and 31 grams of protein.

By the way, I tried running the nutritional analysis for this soup using heavy cream in place of the half-and-half. It only cut 1 gram of carb off each serving—but it added 175 calories. Not worth it, if you ask me.

Pantry Seafood Bisque

This soup is quick, easy, tasty, and what a gorgeous pale pink color! It's simple to double, of course, but it'll take a little longer for the larger quantity of half-and-half to heat through. You could microwave it to speed things along, if you like.

1 pint (480 ml) half-and-half
3 tablespoons (49.5 g) tomato paste
1 can (4 ounces, or 115 g) tiny shrimp, drained
1 can (6 ounces, or 170 g) flaked crab, drained
1 teaspoon dried dill weed
½ teaspoon lemon juice
Salt and pepper to taste

In a large saucepan over low heat, heat the half-and-half to just below a simmer. Whisk in the tomato paste and then stir in the shrimp, crab, dill, and lemon juice. Let the whole thing cook together for just a minute or two, add salt and pepper to taste, and serve.

Yield: 3 servings

Each with 11 grams of carbohydrates and 1 gram of fiber, for a total of 10 grams of usable carbs and 24 grams of protein. Each serving also has 254 milligrams of calcium!

Almost Lobster Bisque

Monkfish has long been known as "poor man's lobster," so I decided to use it in a classic lobster bisque. However, if your budget allows, feel free to use lobster tail in this recipe instead.

½ cup (120 ml) heavy cream
1 cup (240 ml) half-and-half
½ cup (120 ml) water
10-ounce (280-g) monkfish fillet
½ cup (120 ml) dry sherry
1½ teaspoons Dana's No-Sugar Ketchup
    (page 463) or other sugar-free ketchup
½ teaspoon Worcestershire sauce
½ teaspoon lemon juice
½ teaspoon salt or Vege-Sal
Guar or xanthan (optional)
1 scallion, finely sliced

First combine the cream, half-and-half, and water in a large, microwaveable dish. Microwave for 5 to 6 minutes on 70 percent power.

While the cream is heating, cut the monkfish fillet into bite-sized pieces. Bring the sherry to a simmer in a large, heavy-bottomed saucepan over medium-high heat. Add the monkfish, turn the heat down a little, and let the fish simmer in the sherry, stirring occasionally, for 4 to 5 minutes or until cooked through.

Stir in the cream, which should be hot by now. Stir in the ketchup, Worcestershire sauce, lemon juice, and salt, and heat it only to a simmer. If you'd like your bisque thicker, feel free to use guar or xanthan, but it's mighty nice the way it is. Ladle into dishes and top each serving with a scattering of sliced scallion.

Yield: 2 servings

Each with 10 grams of carbohydrates, a trace of fiber, and 26 grams of protein.

8

Sides

Cauliflower Purée (a.k.a. "Fauxtatoes")

This is a wonderful substitute for mashed potatoes with any dish that has a gravy or sauce. Feel free, by the way, to use frozen cauliflower instead; it works quite well here.

1 head cauliflower or 1½ pounds (680 g)
    frozen cauliflower
4 tablespoons (56 g) butter
Salt and pepper

Put the cauliflower in a microwaveable casserole dish with a lid, add a couple of tablespoons (30 ml) of water, and cover. Cook it on high for 10 to 12 minutes or until quite tender but not sulfur-y smelling. (You may steam or boil the cauliflower, if you prefer.) Drain it thoroughly and put it through the blender or food processor until it's well puréed. Add butter, salt, and pepper to taste.

Yield: At least 6 generous servings

Each with 5 grams of carbohydrates and 2 grams of fiber, for a total of 3 grams of usable carbs and 2 grams of protein.

The Ultimate Fauxtatoes

I'm not crazy about Ketatoes by themselves, but added to puréed-cauliflower Fauxtatoes, they add a potato-y flavor and texture that is remarkably convincing!

½ head cauliflower
½ cup (25 g) Ketatoes mix
½ cup (120 ml) boiling water
1 tablespoon (14 g) butter
Salt and pepper

Trim the bottom of the stem of your cauliflower and whack the rest of the head into chunks. Put them in a microwaveable casserole dish with a lid. Add a couple of tablespoons (30 ml) of water, cover, and microwave on high for 8 to 9 minutes.

While that's happening, measure your Ketatoes mix and boiling water into a mixing bowl and whisk together.

When the microwave beeps, pull out your cauliflower—it should be tender. Drain it well and put it in either your food processor, with the S-blade in place, or in your blender. Either way, purée the cauliflower until it's smooth. Transfer the puréed cauliflower to the mixing bowl and stir the cauliflower and Ketatoes together well. Add the butter and stir until it melts. Add salt and pepper to taste and serve.

Yield: 4 servings

Each with 10 g protein; 14 g carbohydrate; 8 g dietary fiber; 6 g usable carbs.

Chipotle-Cheese Fauxtatoes

1 large chipotle chile canned in adobo, minced;
    reserve 1 teaspoon sauce
½ cup (60 g) shredded Monterey Jack cheese
1 batch The Ultimate Fauxtatoes (page 209)

(continued on page 210)

Stir the minced chipotle, a teaspoon of the adobo sauce it was canned in, and the shredded cheese into the Ultimate Fauxtatoes. Serve immediately!

Yield: 4 servings

Each with 14 g protein; 14 g carbohydrate; 8 g dietary fiber; 6 g usable carbs.

Cheddar-Barbecue Fauxtatoes

My husband was crazy about these!

½ head cauliflower, cut into florets
½ cup (120 ml) water
½ cup (55 g) shredded cheddar cheese
2 teaspoons Classic Barbecue Rub (page 486)
**   or purchased barbecue rub**
2 tablespoons (10 g) Ketatoes mix

Put the cauliflower in your slow cooker, including the stem. Add the water. Cover the slow cooker, set it to high, and let it cook for 3 hours. (Or cook it on low for 5 to 6 hours.)

When the time's up, use a slotted spoon to scoop the cauliflower out of the slow cooker and into your blender or your food processor (have the S-blade in place) and purée it there, or you can drain off the water and use a hand-held blender to purée the cauliflower right in the pot. Either way, drain the cauliflower and purée it!

Stir in everything else until the cheese has melted.

Yield: 3 servings

Each with 8 g protein, 6 g carbohydrate, 3 g dietary fiber, 3 g usable carbs.

Italian Garlic and Herb Fauxtatoes

½ head cauliflower, cut into florets
½ cup (120 ml) chicken broth
1 teaspoon Italian seasoning
1 clove garlic, crushed
1 ounce (28 g) cream cheese
Guar or xanthan

Place the cauliflower in your slow cooker. Add the broth, Italian seasoning, and garlic. Cover the slow cooker, set it to low, and let it cook for 5 to 6 hours. (Or cook it on high for 3 hours.)

When the time's up, either remove the cauliflower with a slotted spoon and put it in your blender or food processor (with the S-blade in place) and purée it or drain the broth out of the slow cooker and use a hand-held blender to purée your cauliflower in the pot. Add the cream cheese and stir until melted.

The mixture will still be a little watery. Stir with a whisk as you use guar or xanthan to thicken it up a bit.

Yield: 3 servings

Each with 2 g protein, 2 g carbohydrate, 1 g dietary fiber, 1 g usable carbs.

Ranch and Scallion Fauxtatoes

This is great with anything with a barbecue flavor.

1 head cauliflower, cut into florets
1 cup (240 ml) water
1 cup (100 g) Ketatoes mix
6 teaspoons ranch-style dressing mix
4 scallions, thinly sliced

Place the cauliflower in your slow cooker with the water. Cover the slow cooker, set it to low, and let it cook for 5 hours. (Or cook it on high for 3 hours.)

When the time's up, the easiest thing to do is use a hand blender to purée the cauliflower right in the slow cooker. Don't bother to drain the water first. Whisk in the Ketatoes, ranch dressing mix, and scallions.

Yield: 6 servings

Each with 14 g protein, 23 g carbohydrate, 11 g dietary fiber, 12 g usable carbs.

Garlic-Onion Fauxtatoes

Our tester Maria said her kids were particularly impressed by this!

1 head cauliflower, cut into florets
½ cup (50 g) chopped onion
3 cloves garlic, crushed

⅔ cup (160 ml) water
⅔ cup (65 g) Ketatoes mix
3 tablespoons (42 g) butter

Place the cauliflower in your slow cooker. Add the onion, garlic, and water. Cover the slow cooker, set it to high, and let it cook for 2½ to 3 hours. (Or cook it on low for 5 to 6 hours.)

When the time's up, use a hand-held blender to purée the cauliflower, onion, and garlic right there in the slow cooker. Alternatively, scoop it all into a food processor to purée, but you'll want the water in the pot, so if you transfer the vegetables, put the purée back in the pot with the water when you're done. Now stir in the Ketatoes, butter, and add salt and pepper to taste.

Yield: 6 servings

Each with 9 g protein, 15 g carbohydrate, 7 g dietary fiber, 8 g usable carbs.

Bubble and Squeak

This is my decarbed version of a tradition Irish dish—and very tasty, too!

1 tablespoon (14 g) butter
2 cups (150 g) shredded cabbage
1 medium carrot, shredded
¾ cup (120 g) chopped onion
1 batch The Ultimate Fauxtatoes (page 209)
½ cup (60 g) shredded cheddar cheese

Preheat oven to 350°F (180°C, or gas mark 4).

(continued on page 212)

Melt the butter in a big, heavy skillet and sauté the veggies until the onion starts turning translucent and the cabbage has softened a bit.

Spray a 6-cup (1.4 L) casserole dish with nonstick cooking spray. Spread one-third of the Fauxtatoes on the bottom and then make a layer of half the cabbage mixture. Repeat the layers and finish with a layer of Fauxtatoes. Top with the cheese. Bake for 45 minutes and serve, scooping down through all the layers.

Yield: 6 servings

Each with 10 g protein; 14 g carbohydrate; 6 g dietary fiber; 8 g usable carbs.

Cauliflower Rice

I say thank you to Fran McCullough! I got this idea from her book *Living Low Carb*, and it's served me very well indeed.

½ head cauliflower

Simply put the cauliflower through your food processor, using the shredding blade. This gives a texture that is remarkably similar to rice. You can steam this or microwave it or even sauté it in butter. Whatever you do, though, don't overcook it!

Yield: This is about 3 cups (500 g), or at least 3 to 4 servings

Assuming 3 servings, each will have 5 g carbohydrate, 2 g of which will be fiber, for a usable carb count of 3 g; 2 g protein.

Cauliflower Rice Deluxe

This is higher-carb than plain cauliflower rice, but the wild rice adds a grain flavor that makes it quite convincing, and wild rice has about 25 percent less carbohydrate than most other kinds of rice do. I use this only for special occasions, but it's wonderful.

3 cups (500 g) cauliflower rice—about ½ head's worth
¼ cup (50 g) wild rice
¾ cup (180 ml) water

Cook your cauliflower rice as you please—I microwave mine for making this—taking care not to overcook it to mushiness; you want it just tender. Put the wild rice and water in a saucepan, cover it, and set it over the lowest heat until all the water is gone—at least half an hour, maybe a bit more. Toss together the cooked cauliflower rice and wild rice and season as you please.

Yield: 8 servings

Even with the wild rice, this has only 6 g carb, with 1 g fiber, for 5 g usable carb per ½ cup (85 g) serving.

Company Dinner "Rice"

This is my favorite way to season the cauliflower–wild rice blend above. It's a big hit at dinner parties!

1 small onion, chopped

1 stick (115 g) butter, melted

1 batch Cauliflower Rice Deluxe (page 212)

6 strips bacon, cooked until crisp, and crumbled

¼ teaspoon salt or Vege-Sal

¼ teaspoon pepper

½ cup (50 g) grated Parmesan cheese

Sauté the onion in the butter until it's golden and limp. Toss the Cauliflower Rice Deluxe with the sautéed onion and the bacon, salt, pepper, and cheese. Serve.

Yield: 8 servings

Each with 8 grams of carbohydrates and 2 grams of fiber, for a total of 6 grams of usable carbs and 5 grams of protein.

Saffron "Rice"

What a brilliant color! This looks so beautiful on your plate. It's good with any main dish that's a little fruity-spicy.

½ head cauliflower

1 teaspoon saffron threads

¼ cup (60 ml) water

½ medium onion, chopped

1 teaspoon minced garlic or 2 cloves garlic, crushed

2 tablespoons (28 g) butter

2 teaspoons chicken bouillon granules

¼ cup (30 g) chopped toasted almonds

Run the cauliflower through the food processor using the shredding blade. Put the cauliflower in a microwaveable casserole dish, add a couple of tablespoons (30 ml) of water, cover, and microwave on high for 7 minutes.

Start soaking the saffron threads in the water. While that's happening, sauté the onion and garlic in the butter over medium heat in a large, heavy skillet.

When the cauliflower is done, remove it from the microwave, drain it, and add it to the skillet. Pour in the water and saffron and stir in the chicken bouillon granules. Let the whole thing cook together for a minute or two while you chop the almonds. Stir the almonds into the "rice" and serve.

Yield: 5 servings of brilliantly yellow "rice"

Each with 4 grams of carbohydrates and 1 gram of fiber, for a total of 3 grams of usable carbs and 2 grams of protein.

Variation: Traditionally, saffron rice has raisins in it. If you can afford the extra carbohydrates—if, for instance, you're serving a very low-carb main dish—you can stir in 3 tablespoons (25 g) of raisins with the saffron and water. Each serving of this version will have 8 grams of carbohydrates and 1 gram of fiber, for a total of 7 grams of usable carbs and 2 grams of protein.

Saffron is the most expensive spice in the world and with good reason. Each saffron thread is the stamen of a particular kind of crocus flower. There are four per flower, and they all have to be plucked by hand with tweezers. It takes 50,000 of them to make a pound (455 g) of saffron! Luckily, small quantities of saffron make a big impact on a dish. Do look for saffron in a store that sells bulk spices—many natural food stores do. At least that way you're not paying extra for that little glass jar.

Japanese Fried "Rice"

½ head cauliflower, shredded
2 eggs
1 cup (75 g) snow pea pods, fresh
2 tablespoons (28 g) butter
½ cup (80 g) diced onion
2 tablespoons (16 g) shredded carrot
3 tablespoons (45 ml) soy sauce
Salt and pepper

Put the shredded cauliflower in a microwaveable casserole dish with a lid, add a couple of tablespoons (30 ml) of water, cover, and microwave on high for 6 minutes.

While that's happening, whisk the eggs, pour them into a skillet you've sprayed with nonstick cooking spray, and cook over medium-high heat. As you cook the eggs, use your spatula to break them up into pea-sized bits. Remove from skillet and set aside.

Remove the tips and strings from the snow peas and snip into ¼-inch (6-mm) lengths. (By now the microwave has beeped—take the lid off your cauliflower or it will turn into a mush that bears not the slightest resemblance to rice!)

Melt the butter in the skillet and sauté the pea pods, onion, and carrot for 2 to 3 minutes. Add the cauliflower and stir everything together well. Stir in the soy sauce and cook the whole thing, stirring often, for another 5 to 6 minutes. Add a little salt and pepper and serve.

Yield: 5 servings

Each with 4 g protein; 5 g carbohydrate; 1 g dietary fiber; 4 g usable carbs.

Chicken-Almond "Rice"

This is great for all of you who miss Rice-a-Roni and similar products. And it's terrific with a simple rotisserie chicken.

½ head cauliflower
½ medium onion, chopped
2 tablespoons (28 g) butter, divided
1 tablespoon (6 g) chicken bouillon granules
1 teaspoon poultry seasoning
¼ cup (60 ml) dry white wine
¼ cup (30 g) sliced or slivered almonds

Run the cauliflower through the food processor using the shredding blade. Put the cauliflower in a microwaveable casserole dish, add a couple of tablespoons (30 ml) of water, cover, and microwave on high for 7 minutes.

While that's cooking, sauté the onion in 1 tablespoon (14 g) of butter in a large, heavy skillet over medium-high heat.

When the cauliflower is done, pull it out of the microwave, drain it, and add it to the skillet with the onion. Add the chicken bouillon granules, poultry seasoning, and wine and stir. Turn the heat down to low.

Let that simmer for a minute or two while you sauté the almonds in the remaining tablespoon of butter in a small, heavy skillet. When the almonds are golden, stir them into the "rice" and serve.

Yield: 5 servings

Each with 4 grams of carbohydrates and 1 gram of fiber, for a total of 3 grams of usable carbs and 2 grams of protein.

Sunkist now puts out sliced, toasted almonds in various flavors, under the name "Almond Accents." Feel free to use these to vary this dish!

Lonestar "Rice"

½ **head cauliflower, shredded**
1 **tablespoon (15 ml) olive oil**
1 **tablespoon (14 g) butter**
¼ **cup (40 g) chopped onion**
1 **cup (100 g) sliced mushrooms**
½ **cup (40 g) snow pea pods, fresh, cut in**
  ½ **-inch (1.3-cm) pieces**
¼ **teaspoon chili powder**
2 **teaspoons beef bouillon granules or**
  concentrate

Put the cauliflower in a microwaveable casserole dish with a lid. Add a couple of tablespoons (30 ml) of water, cover, and microwave on high for 6 minutes.

While that's cooking, heat the olive oil and butter in a large skillet and sauté the onions, mushrooms, and snow peas. I like to use the edge of my spatula to break up the mushrooms into smaller pieces but leave the slices whole if you like them better that way—it's up to you. When the mushrooms have changed color and the snow peas are tender-crisp, drain your cooked cauli-rice and stir it in. Add the chili powder and beef bouillon, stir to distribute the seasonings well, and then serve.

Yield: 3 servings

Each with 2 g protein; 5 g carbohydrate; 1 g dietary fiber; 4 g usable carbs.

Beef and Bacon "Rice" with Pine Nuts

½ **head cauliflower**
4 **strips bacon**
½ **medium onion, chopped**
1 **tablespoon (15 ml) liquid beef bouillon**
  concentrate
2 **tablespoons (30 ml) tomato sauce**
2 **tablespoons (18 g) toasted pine nuts**
2 **tablespoons (7.6 g) chopped parsley**

Run the cauliflower through the food processor using the shredding blade, put it in a microwaveable casserole dish, add a couple of tablespoons (30 ml) of water, cover it, and cook it on high for 7 minutes.

While that's cooking, cut the bacon into little pieces—kitchen shears are good for this—and start the little bacon bits frying in a heavy skillet over medium-high heat. When a little grease has cooked out of the bacon, throw the onion into the skillet. Fry them until the onion is translucent and the bacon is browned and getting crisp.

By now the cauliflower should be done. Drain it and throw it in the skillet with the bacon and onion. Add the beef bouillon concentrate and tomato sauce and stir the whole thing up to combine everything—you can add a couple of tablespoons (30 ml) of water, if you like, to help the liquid flavorings spread.

Stir in the pine nuts and parsley (you can just snip it right into the skillet with clean kitchen shears) and serve.

Yield: 4 or 5 servings

(continued on page 216)

Assuming 4 servings, each will have 3 grams of carbohydrates and 1 gram of fiber, for a total of 2 grams of usable carbs and 4 grams of protein.

Venetian "Rice"

This is rich-tasting and slightly piquant.

½ **head cauliflower**
1 **tablespoon (15 ml) olive oil**
2 **tablespoons (28 g) butter**
1 **cup (100 g) sliced mushrooms**
3 **anchovy fillets, minced**
1 **clove garlic, crushed**
3 **tablespoons (18.8 g) grated Parmesan cheese**

Run the cauliflower through the shredding blade of your food processor. Put it in a microwaveable casserole dish with a lid, add a couple of tablespoons (30 ml) of water, cover, and cook on high for 5 to 6 minutes. When it's done, uncover immediately!

Combine the olive oil and butter in a big, heavy skillet over medium heat, swirling together as the butter melts. Add the mushrooms and sauté until they're soft and changing color. If your mushroom slices are quite large, you may want to break them up a bit with the edge of your spatula as you stir.

When the mushrooms are soft, stir in the minced anchovies and garlic. Add the cauli-rice, undrained—that little bit of water is going to help the flavors blend. Stir well to distribute all the flavors.

Stir in the Parmesan cheese and serve.

Yield: 3 to 4 servings

Each will have 4 g protein; 2 g carbohydrate; 1 g dietary fiber; 1 g usable carb.

Blue Cheese-Scallion "Risotto"

Since West Coasters call scallions "green onions," I toyed with calling this "Blue-Green 'Risotto.'" Making risotto out of cauliflower "rice" is one of the best ideas I've ever had!

½ **head cauliflower**
8 **scallions, thinly sliced**
⅔ **cup (100 g) diced green pepper**
1 **tablespoon (28 g) butter**
1 **tablespoon (15 ml) olive oil**
1 **teaspoon chicken bouillon granules**
¼ **cup (60 ml) dry white wine**
¼ **cup (30 g) crumbled blue cheese**
¼ **cup (25 g) grated Parmesan cheese**
2 **tablespoons (30 ml) heavy cream**

Put the cauliflower through the food processor using the shredding blade. Put it in a microwaveable casserole dish, add a couple of tablespoons (30 ml) of water, cover, and microwave on high for 7 minutes.

While that's cooking, slice the scallions and dice the pepper. In a large, heavy skillet over medium heat, start sautéing the scallions and pepper in the butter and oil.

When the microwave goes "ding," remove the cauliflower and drain it. When the green pepper is starting to get soft, add the cauliflower to the skillet and stir it in. Then stir in the bouillon, white wine, blue cheese, Parmesan cheese, and heavy cream. Cook for another 3 to 4 minutes and serve.

Yield: 5 servings

Each with 4 grams of carbohydrates and 1 gram of fiber, for a total of 3 grams of usable carbs and 4 grams of protein.

Mushroom "Risotto"

Man, this is good! One of the best side dishes I've ever come up with.

½ **head cauliflower**
3 **tablespoons (42 g) butter**
1 **cup (70 g) sliced mushrooms**
½ **medium onion, diced**
1 **teaspoon minced garlic or 2 cloves garlic**
2 **tablespoons (30 ml) dry vermouth**
1 **tablespoon (6 g) chicken bouillon granules**
¾ **cup (75 g) grated Parmesan cheese**
Guar or xanthan
2 **tablespoons (7.6 g) chopped fresh parsley**

Run the cauliflower through the food processor using the shredding blade. Put the cauliflower in a microwaveable casserole dish, add a couple of tablespoons (30 ml) of water, cover, and micro-wave on high for 7 minutes.

While the cauliflower is cooking, melt the butter in a large skillet over medium-high heat and add the mushrooms, onion, and garlic and sauté them all together.

When the cauliflower is done, pull it out of the microwave and drain it. When the mushrooms have changed color and are looking done, add

the cauliflower to the skillet and stir everything together. Stir in the vermouth, bouillon, and cheese and let the whole thing cook for another 2 to 3 minutes.

Sprinkle just a little guar or xanthan over the "risotto," stirring all the while, to give it a creamy texture. Stir in the parsley and serve.

Yield: 5 servings

Each with 4 grams of carbohydrates and 1 gram of fiber, for a total of 3 grams of usable carbs and 6 grams of protein.

Not-Quite-Middle-Eastern Salad

Here shredded cauliflower stands in for bulgar wheat instead of rice. This salad is incredibly delicious, incredibly nutritious, and quite beautiful on the plate. Plus it gets better after a couple of days in the fridge, so taking an extra few minutes to double the batch is definitely worth it.

½ **head cauliflower**
⅔ **cup (70 g) sliced stuffed olives***
7 **scallions, sliced**
2 **cups (40 g) triple-washed fresh spinach, finely chopped**
1 **stalk celery, diced**
1 **small ripe tomato, finely diced**
4 **tablespoons (15.2 g) chopped parsley**
¼ **cup (60 ml) olive oil**
1 **teaspoon minced garlic or 2 cloves garlic, crushed**

(continued on page 218)

1 tablespoon (15 ml) red wine vinegar
2 tablespoons (28 g) mayonnaise
Salt and pepper

Run the cauliflower through the food processor using the shredding blade, put it in a microwave-able casserole dish, add a couple of tablespoons (30 ml) of water, cover the dish, and cook it on high for just 5 minutes.

While that's cooking, put the olives, scallions, spinach, celery, tomato, and parsley in a large salad bowl.

When the cauliflower comes out of the microwave, dump it in a strainer and run cold water over it for a moment or two to cool it. (You can let the cauliflower cool uncovered instead, but it will take longer.) Drain the cauliflower well and dump it in with all the other vegetables. Add the oil, garlic, vinegar, and mayonnaise and toss. Add salt and pepper to taste, toss again, and serve.

Yield: 6 servings

Each with 5 grams of carbohydrates and 2 grams of fiber, for a total of 3 grams of usable carbs and 1 gram of protein.

*You can buy sliced stuffed olives in jars.

Hobo Packet

This cooks right on the grill along with your meat course—not even a mixing bowl to wash! It's really tasty, too.

½ **head cauliflower**
½ **medium onion**
1 **medium carrot**

1 **large rib celery**
½ **teaspoon salt**
½ **teaspoon pepper**
8 **slices bacon, cooked**
2 **tablespoons (28 g) butter**

Start a charcoal fire or preheat a gas grill.

Chop your cauliflower into smallish chunks. Coarsely chop the onion, slice the carrot about ¼ inch (6 mm) thick, and slice the celery about the same thickness.

Tear off a piece of heavy-duty aluminum foil about 18 inches (45 cm) long and lay it on the counter. Pile the vegetables in the middle. Sprinkle them with salt and pepper, crumble the cooked bacon on top, and dot with the butter. Fold the foil over the whole thing and fold the seam a few times to seal it well. Roll up the ends to seal them, too.

Throw the whole packet on the grill and cook about 12 to 15 minutes per side over a medium charcoal fire or gas grill. Pull the packet off the grill with tongs, put it on a plate to open it up, and serve.

Yield: 6 servings

Each serving will have 3 grams of carbohydrate and 1 gram of fiber, for a usable carb count of 2 grams; 3 grams protein.

Cauliflower Kugel

A kugel is a traditional Jewish casserole that comes in both sweet and savory varieties. This savory kugel makes a nice side dish with a simple meat course. It could also be served as a vegetarian main dish.

2 packages (10 ounces, or 280 g each) frozen
   cauliflower, thawed
1 medium onion, chopped
1 cup (225 g) cottage cheese
1 cup (120 g) shredded cheddar cheese
4 eggs
½ teaspoon salt or Vege-Sal
¼ teaspoon pepper
Paprika

Preheat the oven to 350°F (180°C, or gas mark 4).

Chop the cauliflower into ½ -inch (1.3-cm) pieces. Combine with the onion, cottage cheese, cheddar, eggs, salt, and pepper in a large mixing bowl and mix very well.

Spray an 8 × 8-inch (20 × 20-cm) baking pan with nonstick cooking spray and spread the cauliflower mixture evenly on the bottom. Sprinkle paprika lightly over the top and bake for 50 to 60 minutes or until the kugel is set and lightly browned.

Yield: 9 servings

Each with 5 grams of carbohydrates and 2 grams of fiber, for a total of 3 grams of usable carbs and 10 grams of protein.

Little Mama's Side Dish

This is just the thing with a simple dinner of broiled chops or a steak, and it's even good all by itself. It's beautiful to look at, too, what with all those colors.

4 slices bacon
½ head cauliflower
½ green pepper
½ medium onion
¼ cup (30 g) sliced stuffed olives*

Chop the bacon into small bits and start it frying in a large, heavy skillet over medium-high heat. (Give the skillet a squirt of nonstick cooking spray first.)

Chop the cauliflower into bits about ½ inch (1.3 cm). Chop up the stem, too; no need to waste it. Put the chopped cauliflower in a microwaveable casserole dish with a lid, add a couple of tablespoons (30 ml) of water, cover, and microwave for 7 minutes on high.

Give the bacon a stir, and then it's back to the chopping board. Dice the pepper and onion. By now some fat has cooked out of the bacon, and it is starting to brown around the edges. Add the pepper and onion to the skillet. Sauté until the onion is translucent and the pepper is starting to get soft.

By the time that confluence of events transpires, the cauliflower should be done. Add it to the skillet without draining and stir—the extra little bit of water is going to help to dissolve the yummy bacon flavor from the bottom of the skillet and carry it through the dish.

Stir in the olives, let the whole thing cook another minute while stirring, and then serve.

Yield: 4 or 5 servings

Assuming 5 servings, each will have 3 grams of carbohydrates and 1 gram of fiber, for a total of 2 grams of usable carbs and 2 grams of protein.

*You can buy sliced stuffed olives in jars.

Gratin of Cauliflower and Turnips

2 ½ cups (375 g) turnip slices
2 ½ cups (375 g) sliced cauliflower
1½ cups (360 ml) carb countdown dairy
    beverage
¼ cup (60 ml) heavy cream
¾ cup (90 g) blue cheese, crumbled
½ teaspoon pepper
½ teaspoon salt
1 teaspoon dried thyme
Guar or xanthan (optional)
¼ cup (25 g) grated Parmesan cheese

Preheat oven to 375°F (190°C, or gas mark 5).

Combine the turnips and cauliflower in a bowl, making sure they're pretty evenly interspersed.

In a saucepan over lowest heat, warm the carb countdown dairy beverage and heavy cream. When it's hot, add the blue cheese, pepper, salt, and thyme. Stir with a whisk until the cheese is melted. It's good to thicken this sauce just slightly with guar or xanthan.

Spray a casserole dish with nonstick cooking spray. Put about one-third of the cauliflower and turnip slices in the dish and pour one-third of the sauce evenly over them. Make two more layers of vegetables and sauce. Sprinkle the Parmesan cheese over the top. Bake for 30 minutes.

Yield: 6 servings

Each with 7 g protein; 8 g carbohydrate; 3 g dietary fiber; 5 g usable carbs.

Mushrooms in Sherry Cream

This is rich and flavorful and best served with a simple roast or the like.

8 ounces (225 g) small, very fresh mushrooms
¼ cup (60 ml) dry sherry
¼ teaspoon salt or Vege-Sal, divided
½ cup (115 g) sour cream
1 clove garlic
⅛ teaspoon pepper

Wipe the mushrooms clean and trim the woody ends off the stems.

Place the mushrooms in a small saucepan with the sherry and sprinkle with ⅛ teaspoon of salt.

Bring the sherry to a boil, turn the heat to low, cover the pan, and let the mushrooms simmer for just 3 to 4 minutes, shaking the pan once or twice while they're cooking.

In another saucepan over very low heat, stir together the remaining ⅛ teaspoon salt, sour cream, garlic, and pepper. You want to heat the sour cream through, but don't let it boil or it will separate.

When the mushrooms are done, pour off the liquid into a small bowl. As soon as the sour cream is heated through, spoon it over the mushrooms and stir everything around over medium-low heat. If it seems a bit thick, add a teaspoon or two of the reserved liquid.

Stir the mushrooms and sour cream together over low heat for 2 to 3 minutes, again making sure that the sour cream does not boil, and serve.

Yield: 3 servings

Each with 4 grams carbohydrates and 1 gram of fiber, for a total of 3 grams of usable carbs and 2 grams of protein.

Avocado Cream Portobellos

These are outstandingly delicious and look elegant on the plate, as well.

6 small portobello mushrooms (My grocery store has these under the name Baby Bellas.)
¼ cup (60 ml) olive oil
2 cloves garlic
1 tablespoon (4.2 g) dried thyme
2 dashes hot pepper sauce
1 small black avocado
3 tablespoons (45 g) sour cream
2 tablespoons (20 g) minced red onion
Salt
6 slices bacon

Start a charcoal fire or preheat a gas grill.

Remove the stems from your portobellos (save them to slice and sauté for omelets or to serve over steak!) and set the mushroom caps on a plate. Measure the olive oil and crush one of the cloves of garlic into it; then stir in the thyme and the hot pepper sauce. Using a brush, coat the portobello caps on both sides with the olive oil mixture.

Next, cut open the avocado, remove the pit, and scoop it into a small mixing bowl. Mash it with a fork. Stir in the sour cream, the onion, and the other clove of garlic, crushed. Add salt to taste.

Now we have to get your bacon cooking. Lay it on a microwave bacon rack or in a glass pie plate,

and cook it on high for 6 minutes (times may vary a bit depending on the power of your microwave).

While your bacon is cooking, go grill your mushrooms! Lay them on an oiled grill over well-ashed coals or over a gas grill set to medium to medium-low. Grill for about 7 minutes per side or until done through, basting frequently with the olive oil mixture—you'll also want a water bottle to put out flare-ups.

When your mushrooms are appealingly grilled, put them back on their plate and march them back to the kitchen. Check your bacon; if it's not crisp, give it another minute or two and then drain it. Divide the avocado mixture between the mushrooms, piling it high in a picturesque fashion. Crumble a slice of bacon over each stuffed mushroom and serve.

Yield: 6 servings

Each will have 9 grams of carbohydrate and 3 grams of fiber, for a usable carb count of 6 grams; 6 grams protein; 701 milligrams of potassium!

Cumin Mushrooms

This is a simply amazing accompaniment to steak made with the Many-Pepper Steak Seasoning (page 485). It also makes a killer omelet filling.

8 ounces (225 g) sliced mushrooms
1½ tablespoons (22 g) butter
1½ tablespoons (22 ml) olive oil
1 teaspoon ground cumin
¼ teaspoon pepper
2 tablespoons (30 g) sour cream

(continued on page 222)

Start sautéing the mushrooms in the butter and oil in a skillet over medium-high heat.

When they've gone limp and changed color, stir in the cumin and pepper. Let the mushrooms cook with the spices for a minute or two and then stir in the sour cream. Cook just long enough to heat through and serve.

Yield: 3 or 4 servings

Assuming 3 servings, each will have 4 grams of carbohydrates and 1 gram of fiber, for a total of 3 grams of usable carbs and 2 grams of protein.

Slice of Mushroom Heaven

This dish is rich enough to give Dean Ornish fits and is oh-so-good. Thanks to my friend Kay for the name!

4 tablespoons (56 g) butter
1 pound (455 g) mushrooms, sliced
½ medium onion, finely chopped
1 clove garlic, crushed
¼ cup (60 ml) dry white wine
1 teaspoon lemon juice
1 ½ cups (360 ml) half-and-half
3 eggs
1 teaspoon salt or Vege-Sal
¼ teaspoon pepper
3 cups (325 g) shredded Gruyère cheese, divided

Preheat the oven to 350°F (180°C, or gas mark 4).

Melt the butter in a heavy skillet over medium heat and begin frying the mushrooms, onion, and garlic. When the mushrooms are limp, turn the heat up a bit and boil off the liquid. Stir in the white wine and cook until that's boiled away, too.

Stir in the lemon juice and turn off the heat. Transfer the mixture to a large mixing bowl and stir in the half-and-half, eggs, salt, pepper, and 2 cups (215 g) of the cheese.

Spray an 8 × 8-inch (20 × 20-cm) baking pan with nonstick cooking spray and spread the mushroom mixture evenly over the bottom. Sprinkle the rest of the cheese on top and bake for 50 minutes or until the cheese on top is golden.

Yield: 9 generous servings

Each with 5 grams of carbohydrates and 1 gram of fiber, for a total of 4 grams of usable carbs and 13 grams of protein.

This dish is good hot, but I actually like it better cold—plus, when it's cold, it cuts in nice, neat squares. I think it makes a nice breakfast or lunch, and it's definitely a fine side dish. It would even make a good vegetarian main course.

Grilled Portobellos

4 large portobello mushrooms
½ green pepper
¼ small onion
1 clove garlic, crushed
¼ cup (60 ml) olive oil
Salt and pepper
¼ cup (25 g) grated Parmesan cheese

Start a charcoal fire or preheat a gas grill.

Remove the stems from your portobellos (save them to slice for omelets or to sauté to go on steak) and lay the caps on a plate.

Whack the green pepper and onion both into a few chunks and put them in your food processor with the S-blade in place. Add the garlic and pulse until everything is chopped fairly fine. Add the olive oil and pulse again.

Lay your portobellos gill-side down on a grill over a medium fire and brush with some of the oil in the green pepper mixture—just dip a brush into it. Let the mushrooms grill for 4 to 5 minutes. Turn them over and spoon the green pepper and onion mixture into them. Let them grill another 4 to 5 minutes. Watch for flare-ups from that olive oil! Remove to a serving plate, sprinkle with salt and pepper, and top each mushroom with 1 tablespoon (6.3 g) of Parmesan cheese. Serve.

Yield: 4 servings

Each serving will have 9 grams of carbohydrate and 2 grams of fiber, for a usable carb count of 7 grams; 6 grams of protein.

Mushrooms with Bacon, Sun Dried Tomatoes, and Cheese

Just looking at the ingredients in the title, you know you'll love this!

4 slices bacon
8 ounces (225 g) sliced mushrooms
½ teaspoon minced garlic or 1 clove fresh garlic
¼ cup (15 g) diced sun-dried tomatoes—about 10 pieces before dicing
2 tablespoons (30 ml) heavy cream
⅓ cup (26.7 g) shredded Parmesan cheese

Chop up the bacon or snip it up with kitchen shears. Start cooking it in a large, heavy skillet over medium-high heat. As some grease starts to cook out of the bacon, stir in the mushrooms.

Let the mushrooms cook until they start to change color and get soft. Stir in the garlic and cook for 4 to 5 more minutes. Stir in the tomatoes and cream and cook until the cream is absorbed.

Scatter the cheese over the whole thing, stir it in, let it cook for just another minute, and serve.

Yield: 3 or 4 servings

Assuming 4 servings, each will have 5 grams of carbohydrates and 1 gram of fiber, for a total of 4 grams of usable carbs and 6 grams of protein.

Zucchini-Mushroom Skillet

1 large or 2 medium zucchini
8 ounces (225 g) mushrooms
1 medium onion
½ cup (120 ml) olive oil
2 cloves garlic, crushed
½ teaspoon oregano
Salt

(continued on page 224)

Halve the zucchini lengthways and then cut into 1-inch (2.5-cm) sections. Wipe the mushrooms clean with a damp cloth and quarter them vertically. Halve the onion and cut it into slices about ¼ inch (6 mm) thick.

Heat the olive oil in a heavy skillet over medium-high heat. Add the zucchini, mushrooms, onion, and garlic and stir-fry until the zucchini and mushrooms are just barely tender and the onion is tender-crisp (about 10 minutes).

Stir in the oregano, add salt to taste, and serve.

Yield: 4 servings

Each with 7 grams of carbohydrates and 2 grams of fiber, for a total of 5 grams of usable carbs and 2 grams of protein.

Snow Peas, Mushrooms, and Bean Sprouts

The combination of flavors here is magical, somehow; these three vegetables seem to be made for each other.

3 tablespoons (45 ml) peanut oil
4 ounces (115 g) fresh snow peas
4 ounces (115 g) fresh mushrooms, sliced
4 ounces (115 g) fresh bean sprouts
1 teaspoon soy sauce

Heat the oil in a wok or heavy skillet over high heat. Add the snow peas and mushrooms and stir-fry until the snow peas are almost tender-crisp (3 to 4 minutes).

Add the bean sprouts and stir-fry for just another 30 seconds to 1 minute.

Stir in the soy sauce and serve.

Yield: 3 servings

Each with 7 grams of carbohydrates and 2 grams of fiber, for a total of 5 grams of usable carbs and 3 grams of protein.

Lemon-Parmesan Mushrooms

8 ounces (225 g) mushrooms
½ cup (120 ml) chicken broth
¼ cup (60 ml) lemon juice
½ cup (40 g) shredded Parmesan cheese
¼ cup (15.2 g) chopped fresh parsley

Wipe the mushrooms clean with a damp cloth or paper towel and put them in a slow cooker. Pour the broth and lemon juice over them. Cover the slow cooker, set it to low, and let it cook for 6 to 8 hours.

Remove the mushrooms from the slow cooker with a slotted spoon and put them on serving plates. Sprinkle with the Parmesan and parsley.

Yield: 4 servings

Each with 6 g protein, 5 g carbohydrate, 1 g dietary fiber, 4 g usable carbs.

Kolokythia Krokettes

These are rapidly becoming one of our favorite side dishes. They're Greek and very, very tasty. They make a terrific side dish with roast lamb or Greek roasted chicken.

3 medium zucchini, grated
1 teaspoon salt or Vege-Sal
3 eggs
1 cup (150 g) crumbled feta
1 teaspoon dried oregano
½ medium onion, finely diced
⅛ teaspoon pepper
3 tablespoons (15 g) soy powder or (32 g) rice protein powder
Butter

Mix the grated zucchini with the salt in a bowl and let it sit for an hour or so. Squeeze out and drain the liquid.

Mix in the eggs, feta, oregano, onion, pepper, and soy powder and combine well.

Spray a heavy skillet with nonstick cooking spray, add 1 tablespoon (14 g) of butter, and melt over medium heat. Fry the zucchini batter by the tablespoonful, turning patties once during cooking. Add more butter between batches, as needed, and keep the cooked krokettes warm. The trick to these is to let them get quite brown on the bottom before trying to turn them, or they tend to fall apart. If a few do fall apart, don't sweat it; the pieces will still taste incredible.

Yield: 6 servings

Each with 6 grams of carbohydrates and 2 grams of fiber, for a total of 4 grams usable carbs and 8 grams of protein.

Shave some time preparing the ingredients for this dish by running the zucchini and the onion through a food processor.

Zucchini-Crusted Pizza

This is like a somewhat-more-substantial quiche on the bottom and pizza on top.

3½ cups (440 g) shredded zucchini
3 eggs
⅓ cup (40 g) rice protein powder or (35 g) soy powder
1½ cups (175 g) shredded mozzarella, divided
½ cup (50 g) grated Parmesan cheese
A pinch or two of dried basil
½ teaspoon salt
¼ teaspoon pepper
Oil
1 cup (240 ml) sugar-free pizza sauce
Toppings as desired (sausage, pepperoni, peppers, mushrooms, or whatever you like)

Preheat the oven to 350°F (180°C, or gas mark 4).

Sprinkle the zucchini with a little salt and let it sit for 15 to 30 minutes. Put it in a strainer and press out the excess moisture.

Beat together the strained zucchini, eggs, protein powder, ½ cup (60 g) of mozzarella, Parmesan, basil, salt, and pepper.

(continued on page 226)

Spray a 9 × 13-inch (23 × 33-cm) baking pan with nonstick cooking spray and spread the zucchini mixture in it.

Bake for about 25 minutes or until firm. Brush the zucchini crust with a little oil and broil it for about 5 minutes until it's golden.

Next, spread on the pizza sauce and add the remaining 1 cup (120 g) of mozzarella and other toppings. (If you're using vegetables as toppings, you may want to sauté them a bit first.)

Bake for another 25 minutes and then cut into squares and serve.

Yield: 4 generous servings

Each with 14 grams of carbohydrates and 2 grams of fiber, for a total of 12 grams of usable carbs and 22 grams of protein. (Analysis does not include toppings.)

Lemon-Garlic Grilled Zucchini

This recipe has a sunny summer flavor!

6 smallish zucchinis
½ cup (120 ml) olive oil
¼ cup (60 ml) lemon juice
2 cloves garlic, crushed
Salt and pepper

Split your zucchinis in half lengthwise and cut off the stems. Put them in a large resealable plastic bag. Mix together the olive oil, lemon juice, and garlic and pour the mixture into the bag. Press out the air, seal the bag, turn it a few times to coat the zucchini, and throw it in the fridge until you need it.

When grilling time comes, pull out the bag, pour off the marinade into a bowl, and throw the zucchini on the grill. Baste them with the lemon dressing and grill them until they get soft and have brown grill marks. Sprinkle with salt and pepper and serve.

Yield: 6 servings

With the marinade, this comes to 7 grams of carbohydrate per serving, and 2 grams of fiber, but you'll discard much of that. I'd say 4 grams of carbohydrate, with those 2 grams of fiber, for a usable carb count of 2 grams; 2 grams protein.

Ratatouille

You pronounce this oh-so-French dish "rat-a-TOO-ee."

¾ cup (180 ml) olive oil
3 cups (450 g) chopped eggplant, cut into 1-inch cubes
3 cups (350 g) sliced zucchini
1 medium onion, sliced
2 green peppers, cut into strips
3 cloves garlic
1 can (14½ ounces, or 410 g) sliced tomatoes, undrained
1 can (4 ounces, or 115 g) sliced black olives, drained
1½ teaspoons dried oregano
½ teaspoon salt
¼ teaspoon pepper

Heat the oil in a heavy skillet over medium heat. Add the eggplant, zucchini, onion, peppers, and garlic.

Sauté for 15 to 20 minutes, turning with a spatula from time to time so all the vegetables come in contact with the olive oil. Once the vegetables are all starting to look about half-cooked, add the tomatoes (including the liquid), olives, oregano, salt, and pepper.

Stir it all together, cover, turn the heat to low, and let the whole thing simmer for 40 minutes or so.

Yield: 8 servings

Each with 11 grams of carbohydrates and 3 grams of fiber, for a total of 8 grams of usable carbs and 2 grams of protein.

You want to use your largest skillet for this dish—possibly even your wok, if you have one. This amount of veggies will cause even a 10-inch (25-cm) skillet to nearly overflow. And don't be afraid to toss in a little more olive oil if you need it while sautéing.

Eggplant Parmesan Squared

When you use Parmesan cheese instead of bread crumbs to "bread" the eggplant slices, it becomes Eggplant Parmesan Squared! This takes a little doing, but it's delicious, and it's easily filling enough for a main dish.

½ cup (60 g) low-carb bake mix or unflavored protein powder
2 or 3 eggs
1¼ to 1¾ cups (125 to 175 g) grated Parmesan cheese

1 large eggplant, sliced no more than ¼ -inch (6 mm) thick
Olive oil for frying
1 clove garlic, cut in half
1½ cups (360 ml) sugar-free spaghetti sauce
8 ounces (225 g) shredded mozzarella

Preheat the oven to 350°F (180°C, or gas mark 4).

Put the bake mix on a plate, break the eggs into a shallow bowl and beat well, and put 1 to 1½ cups (100 to 150 g) of Parmesan cheese on another plate.

Dip each eggplant slice in the bake mix so each side is well dusted.

Dip each "floured" slice of eggplant in the beaten egg and then in the Parmesan so that each slice has a good coating of the cheese. Refrigerate the "breaded" slices of eggplant for at least half an hour or up to an hour or two.

Pour ⅛ inch (3 mm) of olive oil in the bottom of a heavy skillet over medium heat. Add the garlic, letting it sizzle for a minute or two before removing. Now fry the refrigerated eggplant slices until they're golden brown on both sides (you'll have to add more olive oil as you go along.)

Spread ½ cup (120 ml) of spaghetti sauce in the bottom of a 9 × 11-inch (23 × 28-cm) roasting pan. Arrange half of the eggplant slices to cover bottom of pan. Cover with the mozzarella and top with the remaining eggplant. Pour on the rest of the spaghetti sauce and sprinkle the remaining Parmesan cheese on top. Bake for 30 minutes.

Yield: 6 servings

Each with 13 grams of carbohydrates and 4.5 grams of fiber, for a total of 8.5 usable carbs and 24 grams of protein.

(continued on page 228)

How many eggs and how much cheese you will need depends on how big your eggplant is.

Lemon Pepper Beans

I think this makes a particularly good side dish with chicken or fish.

1 bag (1 pound, or 455 g) frozen green beans, French cut or crosscut, thawed
¼ cup (60 ml) olive oil
1 clove garlic, crushed
1 tablespoon (15 ml) lemon juice
¼ teaspoon pepper

Over high heat, stir-fry the beans in the olive oil until they're tender-crisp. Stir in the garlic, lemon juice, and pepper. Cook just another minute and serve.

Yield: 4 servings

Each with 9 grams of carbohydrates and 3 grams of fiber, for a total of 6 grams of usable carbs and 2 grams of protein.

Country-Style Green Beans

Okay, truly country-style green beans are cooked for a billion hours with bacon or a ham hock, but these are much quicker. And this version tastes very good and down-home.

1 pound (455 g) frozen "cut" green beans
3 slices bacon
4 ounces (115 g) sliced mushrooms
½ tablespoon butter
1 tablespoon (15 ml) lemon juice

Put the beans in a microwaveable casserole dish with a lid, add a couple of tablespoons (30 ml) of water, cover, and microwave on high for 7 minutes.

Cut the bacon into little pieces and put it in a large, heavy skillet—I use kitchen shears to snip t right into the pan—and start cooking it over medium-high heat. When a little grease starts to cook out of the bacon, add the mushrooms and butter and cook it all together, stirring frequently, until the bacon is starting to get crispy and the mushrooms have softened and changed color.

Somewhere during this process, your microwave is going to go "ding!" When it does, go check the beans. Chances are they'll still be underdone in the center, so stir them up and give them another 4 to 5 minutes.

When the beans are tender-crisp, pull them out of the microwave, drain them, and stir them into the bacon and mushrooms. Stir in the lemon juice, let the whole thing cook together for just another minute or two to combine the flavors, and then serve.

Yield: 4 or 5 servings

Assuming 4 servings, each will have 10 grams of carbohydrates and 4 grams of fiber, for a total of 6 grams of usable carbs and 4 grams of protein.

Barbecue Green Beans

These are fab!

4 cups (600 g) cross-cut frozen green beans,
   unthawed
¼ cup (40 g) chopped onion
4 slices cooked bacon, drained and crumbled
⅓ cup (80 ml) low-carb barbecue sauce (see
   Chapter 13 or use purchased sauce)

Put the green beans in a slow cooker. Add the onion and bacon and then stir in the barbecue sauce. Cover the slow cooker, set it to high, and let it cook for 3 hours. (If you prefer, set it to low and let it cook for 5 to 6 hours.)

Yield: 6 servings

Each with 3 g protein, 8 g carbohydrate, 2 g dietary fiber, 6 g usable carbs.

Herbed Green Beans

3 tablespoons (42 g) butter
1 bag (1 pound, or 455 g) frozen, crosscut
   green beans, thawed
¼ cup (30 g) finely diced celery
¼ cup (40 g) finely diced onion
1 clove garlic, crushed
½ teaspoon dried rosemary, slightly crushed
½ teaspoon dried basil, slightly crushed
Salt

Melt the butter in a heavy skillet over medium heat. Add the beans, celery, onion, and garlic to the skillet and sauté until the beans are tender-crisp.

Stir in the rosemary and basil and sauté another minute or so. Add salt to taste and serve.

Yield: 4 servings

Each with 10 grams of carbohydrates and 4 grams of fiber, for a total of 6 grams of usable carbs and 2 grams of protein.

Stir-Fried Green Beans and Water Chestnuts

2 tablespoons (30 ml) oil
2 cups (300 g) frozen green beans, thawed
½ cup (100 g) canned water chestnuts, sliced
   or diced, drained
1 clove garlic, crushed
¼ cup (60 ml) chicken broth
1½ teaspoons soy sauce
Guar or xanthan

Heat the oil in a skillet or wok over high heat. Add the green beans and water chestnuts and stir-fry until the green beans are tender-crisp. Stir in the garlic, chicken broth, and soy sauce and let simmer for a couple of minutes; thicken the pan juices just a little with guar or xanthan and serve.

Yield: 3 servings

Each with 2 g protein; 10 g carbohydrate; 3 g dietary fiber; 7 g usable carbs.

Southern Beans

Southerners will be shocked to know that I never tasted green beans slowly cooked with bacon until I moved to southern Indiana, but I liked them right off. Around our house, this recipe is jokingly referred to as The Sacred Masonic Vegetable, because my husband's never been to a Masonic banquet that didn't feature beans cooked this way!

4 cups (600 g) frozen green beans, unthawed
⅓ cup (50 g) diced onion
¼ cup (30 g) diced celery
4 slices bacon, cooked and crumbled
1 tablespoon (15 ml) bacon grease
½ cup (120 ml) water

Place the beans in the slow cooker and stir in everything else. Cover the slow cooker, set it to low, and let it cook for 4 hours.

Yield: 6 servings

Each with 3 g protein, 7 g carbohydrate, 3 g dietary fiber, 4 g usable carbs.

Italian Bean Bake

If you're having a roast, simplify your life by serving this dish—it can cook right alongside the meat.

1 bag (1 pound, or 455 g) frozen Italian green beans, thawed
2 cans (8 ounces, or 225 g each) tomato sauce
¼ small onion, minced
1 clove garlic, crushed

1 teaspoon spicy brown or Dijon mustard
Pepper
½ cup (60 g) shredded mozzarella

Preheat the oven to 350°F (180°C, or gas mark 4).

Put the beans in an 8-cup (1.9-L) casserole dish.

Combine the tomato sauce, onion, garlic, mustard, and a dash of pepper in a mixing bowl; stir into the beans.

Bake for 1 hour or until the beans are tender. Then top with mozzarella and bake for another 3 to 5 minutes or until the cheese is melted. Serve.

Yield: 4 servings

Each with 12 grams of carbohydrates and 4 grams of fiber, for a total of 8 grams of usable carbs and 6 grams of protein.

If you're not serving a roast and you'd like to slice a half-hour off the baking time for this dish, microwave the beans until they're tender-crisp before you combine them with the sauce.

Tangy Beans

4 cups (600 g) frozen green beans, unthawed
¼ cup (40 g) chopped onion
¼ cup (30 g) chopped green bell pepper
¼ cup (60 ml) cider vinegar
2 tablespoons (3 g) Splenda
⅛ teaspoon black pepper

Combine everything in your slow cooker. Stir to distribute evenly. Cover the slow cooker, set it to low, and let it cook for 5 hours.

Serve with a pat of butter and a little salt.

Yield: 4 servings

Each with 2 g protein, 12 g carbohydrate, 4 g dietary fiber, 8 g usable carbs.

Greek Beans

2 tablespoons (30 ml) olive oil
½ small onion, finely minced
1 clove garlic, crushed
1 bag (1 pound, or 455 g) frozen, cut green beans, thawed
½ cup (120 ml) diced canned tomatoes
¼ cup (60 ml) beef broth or bouillon
¼ cup (60 ml) dry white wine

Heat the oil in a large, heavy skillet over medium heat. Add the onion and garlic and sauté for a minute or two.

Drain the beans and add them to the skillet, stirring to coat. Sauté the beans for 6 to 7 minutes, adding another tablespoon (15 ml) of oil if the skillet starts to get dry.

Stir in the tomatoes, broth, and wine. Turn up the heat to medium-high and let everything simmer until the beans are just tender-crisp and most of the liquid has cooked off (about 5 minutes).

Yield: 4 servings

Each with 11 grams of carbohydrates and 3 grams of fiber, for a total of 8 grams of usable carbs and 3 grams of protein.

Holiday Green Bean Casserole

You know that green bean casserole that mom serves every holiday? The one with the mushroom soup and the onion rings? It's pretty high carb. I'd rather have beans amandine, myself. But for you green bean casserole diehards—and I know that there are more than a few of you out there!—here's the new, decarbed version.

1 medium onion
¼ cup (30 g) low-carb bake mix or rice protein powder
¼ teaspoon salt or Vege-Sal
¼ teaspoon paprika
Oil for frying
4 cups (600 g) frozen green beans, cut style
1 can (4 ounces, or 115 g) mushrooms
2 tablespoons (20 g) minced onion
1 tablespoon (14 g) butter
1 cup (240 ml) heavy cream
½ teaspoon Worcestershire sauce
½ teaspoon chicken or beef bouillon concentrate
1 teaspoon soy sauce
Salt and pepper to taste
½ teaspoon guar or xanthan gum

Slice the onion thinly and separate into rings. Mix together the bake mix or protein powder, salt or Vege-Sal, and paprika. "Flour" the onion rings—the easiest way is to put the "flouring" mixture in a small paper sack and shake a few onion rings in it at a time. Heat about ¼ inch (6 mm) of oil in a heavy skillet over medium heat and fry the

(continued on page 232)

"floured" onion rings, turning once, until golden brown and crisp. Drain on absorbent paper. You can do this part well in advance, if you like.

When you're ready to make your casserole, preheat oven to 350°F (180°C, or gas mark 4) and start your green beans cooking—I like to microwave mine on high for about 7 or 8 minutes, but you can steam them if you prefer. While that's happening, drain the liquid off the mushrooms and reserve it. Sauté the mushrooms and the minced onion in the butter until the onion is limp and translucent. Now add the cream, the reserved mushroom liquid, the Worcestershire sauce, the bouillon concentrate, and the soy sauce and stir. Then add salt and pepper to taste.

Now you have a choice: you can either pour this mixture into a blender or use a hand blender. Either way, sprinkle the guar or xanthan over the top and run the blender just long enough to blend in the thickener and to chop the mushrooms a bit—but not to totally purée them; you want some bits of mushroom.

Okay, we're on the home stretch. Drain your cooked green beans, and put them in a 1½ -quart (1.4 L) casserole dish that you've sprayed with nonstick cooking spray. Stir in the mushroom mixture and half of those fried onions. Bake for 25 to 30 minutes and then top it with the rest of the fried onions and bake for another 5 minutes.

Yield: 6 servings

Each with 11 g carbohydrate and 4 g of fiber, for a usable carb count of 7 g; 6 g protein. For the record, this comes to just over half of the carb content of the original recipe—and just about the same calorie count.

Green Bean Casserole

28 ounces (785 g) frozen green beans, unthawed
1 cup (100 g) chopped mushrooms
¼ cup (35 g) roasted red pepper, diced
¼ cup (40 g) chopped onion
2 teaspoons dried sage
1 teaspoon salt or Vege-Sal
1 teaspoon pepper
½ teaspoon ground nutmeg
1 cup (240 ml) beef broth
1 teaspoon beef bouillon concentrate
½ cup (120 ml) heavy cream
Guar or xanthan
¾ cup (95 g) slivered almonds
1 tablespoon (14 g) butter

Combine the green beans, mushrooms, red pepper, and onion in a slow cooker.

In a bowl, mix together the sage, salt or Vege-Sal, pepper, nutmeg, broth, and bouillon. Pour the mixture over the vegetables. Stir the whole thing up. Cover the slow cooker, set it to low, and let it cook for 5 to 6 hours.

When the time's up, stir in the cream and thicken the sauce a bit with guar or xanthan. Re-cover the slow cooker and let it stay hot while you sauté the almonds in the butter until golden. Stir them into the beans.

Yield: 8 servings

Each with 7 g protein, 12 g carbohydrate, 4 g dietary fiber, 8 g usable carbs.

Green Beans a la Carbonara

Bacon, cheese, and garlic—if these three things won't get your family to eat green beans, nothing will. Another great recipe from the *Low Carb Success Calendar* by Vicki Cash, this has enough protein to be a main dish.

7 to 10 thick strips of bacon
1 teaspoon olive oil
½ small onion, chopped
1 clove garlic, minced
1 bag (1 pound, or 455 g) frozen green beans
6 eggs
3 tablespoons (45 ml) cream
½ teaspoon red pepper flakes
¼ teaspoon nutmeg
Salt and pepper
¾ cup (75 g) grated Parmesan cheese

Fry the bacon slices in a large, nonstick skillet over medium heat until they're not quite crisp. Drain on paper towels. Sauté the onion and garlic in the remaining bacon grease until brown.

Place the green beans in a 2-quart (1.9-L) microwave-safe bowl with 1 tablespoon (15 ml) of water. Cover and microwave on high for 10 minutes, turning bowl halfway through cooking.

While the beans are cooking, dice the bacon and add it to the onion and garlic in the skillet. Keep the skillet over low heat. Beat together the eggs, cream, pepper flakes, nutmeg, and salt and pepper to taste as if you were preparing scrambled eggs.

Turn the heat under the skillet up to medium. Add the egg mixture, hot green beans, and Parmesan to the skillet, stirring until the eggs are thoroughly cooked. Serve immediately.

Yield: 4 servings

Each with 12 grams of carbohydrates and 3 grams of fiber, for a total of 9 grams of usable carbs and 27 grams of protein.

Fried Brussels Sprouts

We've served these to company many times, and they're always a hit, even with people who think they don't like brussels sprouts. We didn't think we liked brussels sprouts, either, until our dear friends John and Judy Horwitz served them to us this way—and suddenly we were addicted.

1 pound (455 g) brussels sprouts (Fresh is best, but frozen will do.)
Olive oil
3 or 4 cloves garlic, crushed

If you're using fresh brussels sprouts, remove any bruised, wilted, or discolored outer leaves and trim the stems. If you're using frozen brussels sprouts, just thaw them.

In a heavy-bottomed pot or skillet, heat ½ inch (1.3 cm) of olive oil over medium heat. Add the brussels sprouts and fry them, stirring occasionally, until they are very dark brown all over—you really want them just about burned.

(continued on page 234)

For the last minute or so, add the garlic and stir it around well. Remove the skillet from the heat and serve the sprouts before the garlic burns. It's unbelievable!

Yield: Technically 4 servings, but my husband and I can easily eat a pound of these between the two of us.

Assuming you can bring yourself to share with 3 other people, you'll each get 10 grams of carbohydrates with 4 grams of fiber per serving, for a total of 6 grams of usable carbs and 4 grams of protein.

Nutty Brussels Sprouts

1 pound (455 g) brussels sprouts
½ cup (75 g) hazelnuts
6 tablespoons (84 g) butter, divided
4 slices bacon
¼ teaspoon salt or Vege-Sal
⅛ teaspoon pepper

Trim the stems of the brussels sprouts and remove any wilted or yellowed leaves. Thinly slice brussels sprouts using the slicing blade of a food processor.

Chop the hazelnuts to a medium texture in a food processor.

Melt 2 tablespoons (28 g) of the butter in a heavy skillet over medium heat and add the hazelnuts. Sauté, stirring frequently, for about 7 minutes or until golden. Remove from the skillet and set aside.

Cook the bacon, either using a separate skillet or the microwave. While the bacon is cooking, melt the remaining 4 tablespoons (56 g) of butter over medium-high heat in the same skillet you used for the hazelnuts. Add the sliced brussels sprouts and sauté, stirring frequently, for 7 to 10 minutes or until tender.

Stir in the toasted hazelnuts and the seasonings and transfer to a serving dish. Drain the bacon, crumble it over the top, and serve.

Yield: 4 servings

Each with 12 grams of carbohydrates and 5 grams of fiber, for a total of 7 grams of usable carbs and 8 grams of protein.

Orange Pecan Sprouts

My husband took a bite of these, pointed to his plate, and said, "You could make these again!" They're really wonderful.

1 pound (455 g) brussels sprouts
⅓ cup (40 g) chopped pecans
3 tablespoons (42 g) butter
1 teaspoon grated orange zest
3 tablespoons (45 ml) orange juice

Trim the stems of the brussels sprouts and remove any wilted outer leaves. Run the sprouts through the slicing blade of your food processor.

In a large, heavy skillet over medium-high heat, start sautéing the pecans in the butter. After about 2 minutes, add the brussels sprouts and sauté the two together, stirring every few minutes until the sprouts soften and start to have a few brown spots. While they're sautéing, you can grate the orange zest and squeeze the orange juice. (You could use bottled orange juice, but since you need the zest, too, fresh just makes sense.) When the sprouts are tender and flecked with brown, stir in the zest and juice, cook for just another minute, and serve.

Yield: 4 servings

Each with 12 grams of carbohydrates and 5 grams of fiber, for a total of 7 grams of usable carbs and 4 grams of protein.

Orange Mustard Glazed Sprouts

These are wonderful!

1 pound (455 g) brussels sprouts, halved
3 tablespoons (42 g) butter
2 tablespoons (30 ml) lemon juice
1½ teaspoons brown mustard
1 tablespoon (1.5 g) Splenda
½ teaspoon soy sauce
¼ teaspoon orange extract

Trim the stems of your brussels sprouts, remove any bruised leaves, and then slice each one in half.

Melt the butter in a large, heavy skillet over medium heat. Add brussels sprouts and sauté until they're just starting to get tender and develop a few brown spots.

While the sprouts are sautéing, mix together everything else. When the sprouts are nearly done, pour the mustard mixture into the skillet and stir to coat. Cook for another 2 to 3 minutes and serve.

Yield: 3 to 4 servings

Assuming 3 servings, each will have 5 g protein; 13 g carbohydrate; 5 g dietary fiber; 8 g usable carbs.

'Baga Fries

I'll bet you've never tried a rutabaga, and you're just guessing you're not going to like them. Well, everyone who tries these likes them.

2 pounds (910 g) rutabaga
3 to 4 tablespoons (42 to 56 g) butter
Salt

Peel your rutabaga and cut it into strips the size of big steak fries using a big, heavy knife with a sharp blade.

Steam the "fries" over boiling water in a pan with a tight lid until they're easily pierced with a fork but not mushy (about 10 to 15 minutes). You want them still to be al dente.

Melt the butter in a heavy-bottomed skillet over medium-high heat and fry the strips of rutabaga until they're browned on all sides. Sprinkle with salt and serve.

Yield: 6 servings

Each with 12 grams of carbohydrates and 4 grams of fiber, for a total of 8 grams of usable carbs and 2 grams of protein.

Glazed Turnips

These make wonderful substitute for potatoes with a roast.

**3 cups (450 g) chopped turnips, cut into small
   chunks**
2 tablespoons (28 g) butter
½ small onion
1 teaspoon Splenda
½ teaspoon liquid beef bouillon concentrate
⅛ teaspoon paprika

Steam or microwave the turnip chunks until tender—I steam mine in the microwave for about 7 minutes on high—and then drain.

Melt the butter in a heavy skillet over medium heat. Add the turnips and onion and sauté until the onion is limp.

Stir in the Splenda, bouillon concentrate, and paprika, coating all the turnips, and sauté for just another minute or two.

Yield: 6 servings

Each with 12 grams of carbohydrates and 3 grams of fiber, for a total of 9 grams of usable carbs and 2 grams of protein.

Mashed Garlic Turnips

This recipe is great with a steak, a roast, or chops.

**2 pounds (910 g) turnips, peeled and cut into
   chunks**
8 cloves garlic, peeled and sliced
2 tablespoons (28 g) butter
2 tablespoons (30 g) prepared horseradish
1 teaspoon salt or Vege-Sal
½ teaspoon pepper
⅛ teaspoon ground nutmeg
3 tablespoons (9 g) chopped fresh chives

Place the turnips and the garlic in a saucepan with a tight-fitting lid. Add water to fill about halfway, cover, and place over medium-high heat. Bring to a boil, turn down the heat, and simmer until quite soft (about 15 minutes). Drain the turnips and garlic very well.

Using a potato masher, mash the turnips and garlic together. Stir in the butter, horseradish, salt, pepper, and nutmeg and mix well. Just before serving, stir in the chives.

Yield: 6 servings

Each with 10 grams of carbohydrates and 2 grams of fiber, for a total of 8 grams of usable carbs and 2 grams of protein.

Balsamic Veggie Packet

My husband, no big fan of summer squash, really liked this.

2 medium turnips, peeled and cut into strips
½ medium onion, sliced
**1 medium yellow summer squash, halved
   lengthwise and sliced (You can substitute
   zucchini, if you prefer.)**

1 cup (70 g) broccoli florets
¼ cup (60 ml) olive oil
1 clove garlic, crushed
2 tablespoons (30 ml) balsamic vinegar
Salt and pepper

Start a charcoal fire or preheat a gas grill.

You'll need a big piece of heavy-duty foil. When you've got your vegetables cut up, heap them in the center of a piece of foil, jumbling them together. Mix the oil, garlic, and balsamic vinegar together. Make sure that the edges of the foil are turned up a bit and drizzle this mixture over the vegetables. Sprinkle salt and pepper over the whole thing. Then bring the opposite sides of the foil together and roll down to make a strong seam. Roll up the ends. Throw the whole thing on a medium grill for 12 minutes per side and then serve.

Yield: 5 to 6 servings

Assuming 5, each will have 7 grams of carbohydrate and 2 grams of fiber, for a usable carb count of 5 grams; 1 gram protein.

Turnips Au Gratin

This is sublime with top-quality Vermont cheddar cheese, but you can make it with any good, sharp cheddar.

2 pounds (910 g) turnips, peeled and thinly sliced
1 cup (240 ml) heavy cream
1 cup (240 ml) half-and-half
3 cups (340 g) shredded sharp cheddar cheese, divided

2 teaspoons prepared horseradish
¼ teaspoon ground nutmeg
½ medium onion, sliced
Salt and pepper

Preheat the oven to 350°F (180°C, or gas mark 4).

Steam the turnips until they're just tender. (I steam mine in the microwave for 7 minutes on high.)

While the turnips are cooking, combine the heavy cream and half-and-half in a saucepan over very low heat. Bring to a simmer.

When the cream is up to temperature, whisk in 2⅔ cups (300 g) of the cheese, a couple of tablespoons at a time. Stir each addition until it's completely melted before adding more. When all of the cheese is melted into the sauce, whisk in the horseradish and nutmeg. Turn off the heat.

Spray an 8 × 8-inch (20 × 20-cm) glass baking dish with nonstick cooking spray. Put about one-third of the turnips in the dish and scatter half of the sliced onion over it. Add another layer of one-third of the turnips, half of the onions, and the final third of the turnips on top. Pour the cheese sauce over the whole thing and scatter the last ⅓ cup (40 g) of cheese over the top. Bake for 30 to 40 minutes or until golden.

Yield: 6 servings

Each with 12 grams of carbohydrates and 2 grams of fiber, for a total of 10 grams of usable carbs and 17 grams of protein.

Jansonn's Temptation

This Swedish favorite is traditionally made with potatoes. I have no idea how this decarbed version compares, but it's utterly delicious in its own right. This is the natural side dish to serve with Swedish Meatballs (page 317).

2 turnips
½ head cauliflower
1 onion
2 tablespoons (28 g) butter
1 tablespoon (15 g) anchovy paste
¼ teaspoon salt, or Vege-Sal
¼ teaspoon pepper
½ cup (120 ml) heavy cream

Preheat oven to 400°F (200°C, or gas mark 6).

Peel the turnips and cut them into smallish strips—about the size of fast food French fries. Cut up the cauliflower, too—cut it in strips as much as possible (include the stem), but being cauliflower, it'll crumble some. That's fine. Combine the turnips and cauliflower and set aside.

Slice the onion quite thin. Melt the butter in a heavy skillet over medium heat and sauté the onion slices until they're limp and turning translucent.

Spray an 8 × 8-inch (20 × 20-cm) baking dish with nonstick cooking spray. Layer the turnip/cauliflower mixture and the onions in the baking dish.

Stir the anchovy paste, salt, and pepper into the cream until the anchovy paste is dissolved.

Pour this mixture over the vegetables. Bake for 45 minutes and then serve.

Yield: 5 servings

Each with 2 g protein; 6 g carbohydrate; 2 g dietary fiber; 4 g usable carbs.

Indian Cabbage

This is good with anything curried. This combination of seasonings works well with green beans, too.

Oil or butter
1 teaspoon black mustard seed
1 teaspoon turmeric
4 cups (280 g) shredded cabbage
1 teaspoon salt or Vege-Sal

Put a heavy skillet over medium heat. Add a few tablespoons (30 to 45 ml) of oil or butter (I like to use coconut oil) and then the mustard seed and the turmeric. Sauté together for just a minute.

Stir in the cabbage, add the salt or Vege-Sal, and stir-fry for a few minutes, combining the cabbage well with the spices.

Add a couple of tablespoons (30 ml) of water, cover, and let the cabbage steam for a couple more minutes until it is tender-crisp.

Yield: 4 servings

Each with 4 grams of carbohydrates and 2 grams of fiber, for a total of 2 grams of usable carbs and 1 gram of protein.

Bavarian Cabbage

This is great with the Sauerbrauten on page 401!

1 head red cabbage

1 medium onion, chopped

1 medium Granny Smith apple, chopped

6 slices cooked bacon, crumbled

2 teaspoons salt

1 cup (240 ml) water

3 tablespoons (4.5 g) Splenda

⅔ cup (160 ml) cider vinegar

3 tablespoons (45 ml) gin

Whack the head of cabbage in quarters and remove the core. Then whack it into biggish chunks. Put it in a big mixing bowl. Add the onion, apple, and bacon to the cabbage. Toss everything together. Transfer the mixture to a slow cooker. (This will fill a 3-quart cooker just about to overflowing! I barely got the top on mine.)

In a bowl, mix together the salt, water, Splenda, vinegar, and gin. Pour the mixture over the cabbage. Cover the slow cooker, set it to low, and let it cook for 6 to 8 hours.

Yield: 6 servings

Each with 2 g protein, 7 g carbohydrate, 1 g dietary fiber, 6 g usable carbs.

Sweet-and-Sour Cabbage

3 slices bacon

4 cups (280 g) shredded cabbage

2 tablespoons (30 ml) cider vinegar

2 teaspoons Splenda

In a heavy skillet, cook the bacon until crisp. Remove and drain.

Add the cabbage to the bacon grease and sauté it until tender-crisp.

Stir in the vinegar and Splenda, crumble in the bacon, and serve.

Yield: 4 servings

Each with 4 grams of carbohydrates and 2 grams of fiber, for a total of 2 grams of usable carbs and 2 grams of protein.

Dragon's Teeth

This hot stir-fried cabbage is fabulous. If you didn't think cabbage could be exciting, try this! Have the exhaust fan on or a window open when you cook this—when the chili garlic paste hits that hot oil, it may make you cough. It's worth it!

1 head Napa cabbage

¼ cup (66 g) chili garlic paste

1 teaspoon salt

2 teaspoons Splenda

2 teaspoons toasted sesame oil

2 tablespoons (30 ml) soy sauce

2 tablespoons (30 ml) peanut or canola oil

2 teaspoons rice vinegar

I like to cut my head of Napa cabbage in half lengthwise and then lay it flat-side down on the cutting board and slice it about ½-inch (1.3-cm)

(continued on page 240)

thick. Cut it one more time, lengthwise down the middle, and then do the other half of the head.

Mix together the chili garlic paste, salt, Splenda, toasted sesame oil, and soy sauce in a small dish and set by the stove.

In a wok or huge skillet over highest heat, heat the peanut or canola oil. Add the cabbage and start stir-frying. After about a minute, add the seasoning mixture and keep stir-frying until the cabbage is just starting to wilt—you want it still crispy in most places. Sprinkle in the rice vinegar, stir once more, and serve.

Yield: 4 servings

Each with 1g protein; 3 g carbohydrate; trace dietary fiber; 3 g usable carbs.

Thai Stir-Fried Cabbage

This exotic and tasty dish cooks lightning-fast, so make sure you have everything cut up, mixed up, and ready to go before you start stir-frying.

2 tablespoons (30 ml) lime juice
2 tablespoons (30 ml) Thai fish sauce (nam pla)
2/3 teaspoon red pepper flakes
Peanut, canola, or coconut oil
6 cups (420 g) finely shredded napa cabbage
6 scallions, sliced
2 cloves garlic, crushed
1/3 cup (23 g) unsweetened, flaked coconut
1/4 cup (30 g) chopped, dry-roasted peanuts

Mix together the lime juice, fish sauce, and red pepper flakes. Set aside.

In a wok or heavy-bottomed skillet, heat a few tablespoons (30 ml) of oil over high heat. Add the cabbage, scallions, and garlic and stir-fry for no more than 5 minutes or just until the cabbage is heated through.

Add the lime juice mixture to the cabbage and stir to coat. Let it cook just another minute and then stir in the coconut. Serve topped with peanuts.

Yield: 4 servings

Each with 13 grams of carbohydrates and 4 grams of fiber, for a total of 9 grams of usable carbs and 5 grams of protein.

Roasted Cabbage with Balsamic Vinegar

This is a simple way to cook a lot of cabbage!

1/2 head red cabbage
1/2 head cabbage
3 tablespoons (45 ml) olive oil
Salt and pepper
2 tablespoons (30 ml) balsamic vinegar

Preheat oven to 450°F (230°C, or gas mark 8).

Coarsely chop the two kinds of cabbage and separate the leaves. Put it in a good-sized roasting pan and toss it with the olive oil until it's coated all over. Sprinkle with salt and pepper and toss again.

Put the cabbage in the oven and roast for 15 to 20 minutes, stirring once or twice, until it's just browning around the edges but still not entirely limp. Sprinkle with the balsamic vinegar, toss again, and serve.

Yield: 5 to 6 servings

Assuming 5 servings, each will have trace protein; 1 g carbohydrate; trace dietary fiber; 1 g usable carb.

Blue Slaw

This is a really unusual twist on slaw.

4 cups (280 g) bagged coleslaw mix
3 tablespoons (45 g) plain yogurt
1 tablespoon (15 g) sour cream
¼ cup (60 g) mayonnaise
2 tablespoons (16 g) crumbled blue cheese

Just mix everything together—that's all!

Yield: 4 or 5 servings

Assuming 4 servings, each will have 5 grams of carbohydrates and 2 grams of fiber, for a total of 3 grams of usable carbs and 3 grams of protein.

If you want, you can streamline this further by substituting ½ cup (120 ml) bottled blue cheese dressing, but it's likely to have a little added sugar—not much, but a little.

Grilled Asparagus with Balsamic Vinegar

1 pound (455 g) asparagus
2 tablespoons (30 ml) olive oil
2 tablespoons (30 ml) balsamic vinegar
3 tablespoons (18.8 g) grated Parmesan cheese

Preheat an electric tabletop grill (or you can do this over your backyard grill!). Snap the ends off the asparagus where they break naturally. Put them on a plate and drizzle with the olive oil. Toss the asparagus a bit to make sure it's all coated with the oil.

Place the asparagus on your grill—you'll probably have to do it in two batches unless your grill is a lot bigger than mine. Set a timer for 10 minutes. (If grilling out of doors, just keep an eye on it and grill until it's tender with brown spots.)

If you've had to do two batches, put the first batch on a plate and cover it with a pot lid to keep it warm while the second batch cooks. When all the asparagus is done and all on the plate, drizzle with the balsamic vinegar. Roll it around to coat it and then top it with the Parmesan and serve.

Yield: 3 servings

Each with 6 g protein; 7 g carbohydrate; 2 g dietary fiber; 5 g usable carbs.

Asparagus with Aioli and Parmesan

Cold asparagus dipped in garlic sauce and cheese—It's so yummy!

2 pounds (910 g) asparagus
Aioli (page 479)
½ cup (50 g) grated Parmesan cheese

Break the ends off the asparagus where they snap naturally. Steam or microwave the asparagus for 3 to 4 minutes or just until the color brightens. (You want these even less done than tender-crisp.) Chill the asparagus.

At dinnertime, give each diner a couple of tablespoons (30 ml) of aioli and a little bit of Parmesan. Dip each asparagus stalk in the aioli, then in the Parmesan, and eat.

Yield: 4 servings

Each with 6 grams of carbohydrates and 2 grams of fiber, for a total of 4 grams of usable carbs and 5 grams of protein.

Asparagus with Curried Walnut Butter

1 pound (455 g) asparagus
4 tablespoons (56 g) butter
2 tablespoons (16 g) chopped walnuts
1 teaspoon curry powder

½ teaspoon cumin
1½ teaspoons Splenda

Snap the ends off of the asparagus where they want to break naturally. Put it in a microwaveable container with a lid or use a glass pie plate covered with plastic wrap. Either way, add a tablespoon or two (15 to 30 ml) of water and cover. Microwave on high for 5 minutes. Don't forget to uncover as soon as the microwave goes beep or your asparagus will keep cooking and be limp and sad!

While that's cooking, put the butter in a medium skillet over medium heat. When it's melted, add the walnuts. Stir them around for 2 to 3 minutes until they're getting toasty. Now stir in the curry powder, cumin, and Splenda and stir for another 2 minutes or so.

Your asparagus is done by now! Fish it out of the container with tongs, put it on your serving plates, and divide the Curried Walnut Butter between the three servings.

Yield: 3 servings

Each with 3 g protein; 5 g carbohydrate; 2 g dietary fiber; 3 g usable carbs.

Asparagus Bacon Bundles

This tastes great and has a cool-looking presentation, to boot!

1 pound (455 g) pencil-thin asparagus
7 slices bacon

Preheat an electric tabletop grill.

Snap the ends off the asparagus spears where they break naturally. Divide the asparagus into 7 bunches and wrap a slice of bacon in a spiral around each bunch. (In other words, don't let the bacon overlap itself but cover as much of the asparagus bundle as you can.)

Place the asparagus-bacon bundles on the grill. How many will fit will depend on how big your grill is; mine will just fit all 7. Close the grill and let them cook for 7 minutes or until the bacon is cooked through and serve.

Yield: 7 servings

Each with 2 grams of carbohydrates and 1 gram of fiber, for a total of 1 gram of usable carbs and 3 grams of protein.

Asparagus Pecandine

I never thought anything could be as good with asparagus as lemon butter is—and then I tried this.

5 tablespoons (70 g) butter
½ cup (60 g) chopped pecans
1½ teaspoons tarragon vinegar
1 pound (455 g) asparagus, steamed just until tender-crisp

Melt the butter in a heavy skillet over medium-high heat. Stir in the pecans and sauté, stirring frequently, for 5 to 7 minutes or until the pecans are golden and crisp. Stir in the tarragon vinegar.

Place the asparagus on serving plates and spoon the sauce over it. Serve immediately.

Yield: 4 servings

Each with 8 grams of carbohydrates and 4 grams of fiber, for a total of 4 grams of usable carbs and 4 grams of protein.

Grilled Sesame Asparagus

This is good with any of the Asian-influenced main courses in this book—or with anything else, for that matter.

1 pound (455 grams) asparagus
2 tablespoons (30 ml) soy sauce
2 tablespoons (30 ml) rice vinegar
1 tablespoon (15 ml) toasted sesame oil
1 jalapeño, finely minced
1 tablespoon sesame seeds

Have your charcoal or gas grill ready; the prep on this recipe doesn't take much time.

Snap the bottom off of each stalk of asparagus where it breaks naturally. Mix together the soy sauce, rice vinegar, sesame oil, and minced jalapeño in a bowl. (Now wash your hands! You must always wash your hands after handling hot peppers, or the next time you touch your eyes, nose, or mouth, you'll be sorry.)

Put the sesame seeds in a small, dry skillet, and shake them over medium-high heat until they start to make little popping sounds. Remove the pan from the heat.

(continued on page 244)

Okay, throw your asparagus on the grill, over a medium fire—it's a good idea to have a small-holed grill for this. Baste the asparagus with the soy sauce mixture as it grills and turn the asparagus a few times. Grill until the asparagus has brown spots and then remove to serving plates. Drizzle with the remaining soy sauce mixture, garnish with the toasted sesame seeds, and serve.

Yield: 4 servings

Each serving will have 4 grams of carbohydrate and 2 grams of fiber, for a usable carb count of 2 grams; 2 grams protein.

Asparagus with Sun-Dried Tomatoes

1 pound (455 g) asparagus
1 tablespoon (15 ml) olive oil
2 tablespoons (28 g) butter
2 tablespoons (20 g) minced red onion
½ clove garlic, crushed
2 tablespoons (10 g) sun-dried tomato halves, minced
2 teaspoons lemon juice

Snap the ends off of the asparagus where they want to break naturally. Put them in a microwaveable casserole dish with a lid, add a couple of tablespoons (30 ml) of water, and cover—but don't cook it yet. Make your sauce first.

In a medium skillet, heat the olive oil and the butter, swirling them together as the butter melts.

Add the onion, garlic, and sun-dried tomatoes to the oil and butter and sauté until the onion is soft, being careful not to brown the onions or garlic. Stir in the lemon juice. Turn off the heat.

Okay, back to your asparagus. Microwave it on high for just 5 minutes. Uncover it the second it's done! Divide it between 3 or 4 serving plates, spoon the sauce over it, and serve.

Yield: 3 to 4 servings

Assuming 3 servings, each will have 3 g protein; 10 g carbohydrate; 3 g dietary fiber; 7 g usable carbs.

Basic Artichokes

2 artichokes
¼ cup (60 ml) lemon juice

Using kitchen shears, snip the pointy tips off the artichoke leaves. Split the artichokes down the middle, top to bottom, and scrape out the chokes.

Fill a slow cooker with water, add the lemon juice, and put in the artichokes. Cover the slow cooker, set it to high, and let it cook for 3 to 4 hours. Drain the artichokes.

Serve the artichokes with the dipping sauce of your choice, such as lemon butter, mayonnaise, aioli, chipotle mayonnaise, or whatever you've got. If you have a big slow cooker, feel free to cook more artichokes!

Yield: 2 servings

Each with 4 g protein, 16 g carbohydrate, 7 g dietary fiber, 9 g usable carbs. Analysis does not include dipping sauces.

Fried Artichokes

This is one of the fastest ways I know to cook artichokes.

1 large artichoke
Olive oil
Lemon wedges
Salt

Cut about 1 inch (2.5 cm) off the top of your artichoke, trim the stem, and pull off the bottom few rows of leaves. Now slice it vertically down the center. You'll see the "choke"—the fuzzy, inedible part at the center. Using the tip of a spoon, scrape every last bit of this out (it pulls off of the yummy bottom part of the artichoke quite easily).

In a large, heavy skillet, heat 1 inch (2.5 cm) of olive oil over medium-high heat. When the oil is hot, add your cleaned artichoke, flat side down. Fry for about 10 minutes, turning over halfway through. It should be tender and just starting to brown a bit. Drain on paper towels or a brown paper bag.

Serve the artichoke halves with lemon wedges to squeeze over them and salt to sprinkle on them to taste.

Yield: 1 serving

13 grams of carbohydrates and a whopping 7 grams f fiber, for a total of 6 grams of usable carbs (a couple of teaspoons of lemon juice add just 1 more gram) and 4 grams of protein.

If you've never encountered a fresh artichoke, you'll probably be surprised to find that they're sort of fun to eat: You peel off the leaves, one by one, and drag the base of each one between your teeth, scraping off the little bit of edible stuff and the bottom of each leaf. When you've finished doing that and you have a big pile of artichoke leaves on your plate, use a fork and knife to eat the delectable heart.

Stir-Fried Spinach

Spinach originated in Asia, so stir-frying is a very traditional way of preparing it.

¼ cup (60 ml) peanut oil
2 pounds (910 g) fresh spinach, washed and dried
2 cloves garlic, crushed

Heat the oil in a heavy skillet or wok over high heat. Add the spinach and garlic, stir-fry for only a minute or two, and then serve.

Yield: 6 servings

Each with 6 grams of carbohydrates and 4 grams of fiber, for a total of 2 grams of usable carbs and 4 grams of protein.

Sicilian Spinach

3 tablespoons (42 g) butter
2 pounds (910 g) fresh spinach, washed and dried
1 clove garlic, crushed
1 or 2 anchovy fillets, finely chopped

(continued on page 246)

Heat the butter in a heavy skillet. Add the spinach and garlic and sauté until the spinach is just limp. Stir in the anchovies and serve.

Yield: 6 servings

Each with 5 grams of carbohydrates and 4 grams of fiber, for a total of just 1 gram of usable carbs and 5 grams of protein.

Not everyone likes anchovies, and if you're among those who don't, just leave them out.

Creamed Spinach

1 package (10 ounces, or 280 g) frozen, chopped spinach, thawed
¼ cup (60 ml) heavy cream
¼ cup (25 g) grated Parmesan cheese
1 clove garlic, crushed

Put all the ingredients in a heavy-bottomed saucepan over medium-low heat and simmer for 7 to 8 minutes.

Yield: 3 servings

Each with 5 grams of carbohydrates and 3 grams of fiber, for a total of 2 grams of usable carbs and 6 grams of protein.

Easy Garlic Creamed Spinach

This is about the easiest creamed spinach ever, and it's quite good too.

Two 10-ounce (280 g) boxes frozen chopped spinach, thawed, or two 10-ounce (280 g) bags triple-washed fresh spinach
1 tablespoon (14 g) butter
5.2-ounce (145 g) package creamy garlic-herb cheese (such as Boursin or Alouette)

If you're using fresh spinach, you might coarsely chop it. Melt the butter in a large, heavy skillet, and add the spinach. Cook, stirring, for 3 to 4 minutes—you want fresh spinach just barely wilted and frozen spinach just well-heated through.

Cut the cheese into a few chunks and add it to the skillet. Stir until the cheese is completely melted and then serve.

Yield: 6 servings

Each with 4 grams of carbohydrates and 3 grams of fiber, for a total of 1 gram of usable carbs and 4 grams of protein.

Greek Spinach

1 tablespoon (14 g) butter
¼ small onion, minced
1 package (10 ounces, or 280 g) frozen, chopped spinach, thawed
¼ cup (40 g) crumbled feta cheese
¼ cup (55 g) cottage cheese

Melt the butter in a heavy skillet over medium heat. Add the onion and let it sizzle for just a minute. Add the spinach and sauté, stirring now and then, for 5 to 7 minutes.

Add in the cheeses and stir until they start to melt. Let the spinach cook for another minute or so and then serve.

Yield: 3 servings

Each with 6 grams of carbohydrates and 3 grams of fiber, for a total of 3 grams of usable carbs and 7 grams of protein.

Sour Cream Spinach

My husband liked this so much, he ate the whole batch.

10-ounce (280-g) package frozen chopped spinach
¼ medium onion
2 tablespoons (28 g) butter
⅓ cup (75 g) sour cream
1 teaspoon cider vinegar

Unwrap the spinach and put it in a microwaveable casserole dish with a lid. Add a couple of tablespoons (30 ml) of water, cover, and cook it on high for 5 minutes.

Meanwhile, in a large, heavy skillet, start sautéing the onion in the butter over medium-high heat.

When the microwave goes "ding," check to see if the spinach is done—you want it good and hot all the way through but not cooked to death. If there's still a cold spot in the middle, stir it and put it back for another 2 minutes on high.

When the spinach is cooked and the onion is translucent, drain the spinach and stir it into the onion in the skillet, combining well. Stir in the sour cream and the vinegar, heat it through without letting it simmer, and then serve.

Yield: 3 servings

Each with 6 grams of carbohydrates and 3 grams of fiber, for a total of 3 grams of usable carbs and 4 grams of protein.

Sag Paneer

With the cottage cheese, this isn't totally authentic, but it's mighty tasty.

2 tablespoons (28 g) butter
1 teaspoon curry powder
1 package (10 ounces, 280 g) frozen, chopped spinach, thawed
1 teaspoon salt or Vege-Sal
⅓ cup (75 g) small-curd cottage cheese
2 teaspoons sour cream

Melt the butter in a heavy skillet over low heat and stir in the curry powder. Let the curry powder cook in the butter for 3 to 4 minutes.

Stir in the spinach and the salt. Cover the skillet and let the spinach cook for 4 to 5 minutes or until heated through.

Stir in the cottage cheese and sour cream and cook, stirring, until the cheese has completely melted.

Yield: 3 servings

Each with 5 grams of carbohydrates and 3 grams of fiber, for a total of 2 grams of usable carbs and 6 grams of protein.

Spinach Mushroom Kugel

I came up with this for a Passover column I wrote, but it's a great side dish for anyone, any time of year!

8 ounces (225 g) sliced mushrooms
1 medium onion, chopped
2 tablespoons (30 ml) olive oil
3 10-ounce (280 g) boxes frozen chopped
    spinach, thawed and drained
2 eggs
¾ cup (180 g) mayonnaise
1 teaspoon beef bouillon concentrate
2 tablespoons (20 g) almond meal
½ teaspoon guar or xanthan

Preheat oven to 350°F (180°C, or gas mark 4).

Sauté mushrooms and onion in the oil until the onion is translucent and the mushrooms soften. Transfer to a mixing bowl, reserving 9 mushroom slices for garnish, and add the spinach; mix well.

Stir together the eggs, mayonnaise, and bouillon concentrate until the concentrate dissolves. Stir into vegetables. Stir in the almond meal. Sprinkle half the guar or xanthan over the mixture and stir in well; repeat with the second half.

Spread evenly in a greased 8 × 8-inch (20 × 20-cm) baking dish. Decorate with reserved mushrooms. Bake for 1 hour. Cut in squares to serve.

Yield: 9 servings

Each with 6 g protein; 7 g carbohydrate; 3 g dietary fiber; 4 g usable carbs.

Soy Grilled Vidalias

I'm always so torn about onions. On the one hand, they're higher-carb than most vegetables. On the other hand, they're extremely nutritious and taste incredibly good—and they certainly aren't as high-carb as, say, a potato. So I grill onions, but I watch my portions.

2 large Vidalia onions
¼ cup (60 ml) soy sauce
1 clove garlic, crushed
2 teaspoons Splenda

Peel your onions and slice them pretty thickly—about ½ inch (1.3 cm) or a little thicker. Mix together everything else. Lay the onion slices in a grill basket or on a small-holed grill rack over a medium fire. Baste them with the soy sauce mixture and grill them until they're limp with brown spots; then serve.

Yield: 6 servings

If you can bring yourself to share these between 6 people, each of you will get 4 grams of carbohydrate and 1 gram of fiber, for a usable carb count of 3 grams; 1 gram protein.

You may well find that your slices fall apart into individual rings when you turn them. This doesn't bother me, but if it bothers you, here's a trick: before slicing your onions, pierce them with wooden or bamboo skewers (soak them in water for at least a half hour first) ½ inch (1.3 cm) apart and then slice between the skewers. Your slices will come out neatly skewered across the rings for easy turning.

Unbelievable Onion Rings

The thing you'll find hard to believe is that these are far lower-carb than the high-carb onion rings you get at restaurants! They're not dirt-low in carbs, but to me, onion rings are crack in food form, so being able to have a really good, reasonably low-carb onion ring now and then is a very big deal.

3 medium Vidalia onions
1 cup (115 g) Atkins Bake Mix
2 tablespoons Atkins Cornbread Mix
¼ cup (30 g) oat flour
1 teaspoon seasoned salt
2 eggs
12 ounces (360 ml) light beer (Michelob Ultra, Miller Lite, or Milwaukee's Best Light are lowest carb.)
Salt

Preheat a deep-fat fryer to 375°F (190°C).

Peel the onions and slice them fairly thick. Separate them into rings and set aside.

In a medium-size mixing bowl, combine the Atkins Bake Mix, Atkins Cornbread Mix, oat flour, and seasoned salt, stirring them together well. Add the eggs and the beer and whisk them in.

When the fat is up to temperature, dip the onion rings into the batter and then drop them (carefully!) into the hot fat. (Note: If you're using a deep-fat fryer, have your fry basket already submerged. If you put the batter-coated rings in the basket and then lower it, your onion rings will weld themselves to your fry basket and create a royal mess.) Fry until golden (you may have to turn them over to get both sides browned), drain on absorbent paper, sprinkle with salt, and devour!

Yield: 6 servings

Each with 14 grams of carbohydrate and 4 grams of fiber, for a usable carb count of 10 grams; 16 grams of protein. (By comparison, a serving of 8 to 9 restaurant onion rings averages about 30 grams of carbohydrate.)

Broccoli with Lemon Butter

I'm always bemused when I see frozen broccoli with lemon butter at the grocery store. I mean, how hard is it to add butter and lemon juice to your broccoli?

1 pound (455 g) frozen broccoli or 1 large head fresh broccoli
4 tablespoons (56 g) butter
1 tablespoon (15 ml) lemon juice

Steam or microwave the broccoli. When it's cooked, drain off the water and toss the broccoli with the butter and lemon juice until the butter is melted. That's it!

Yield: 4 servings

Each with 6 grams of carbohydrates and 3 grams of fiber, for a total of 3 grams of usable carbs and 3 grams of protein.

Broccoli Piquant

This is a country-style dish that's good with pork chops.

1 bag (1 pound, or 455 g) frozen broccoli
"cuts"
4 slices bacon
1 clove garlic, crushed
3 tablespoons (45 ml) cider vinegar

Steam or microwave the broccoli until just tender-crisp.

While the broccoli is cooking, fry the bacon until crisp, remove from the pan, and drain. Pour off all but a couple of tablespoons (30 ml) of the fat.

When the broccoli is cooked, drain and add it to the bacon fat in the skillet. Add the garlic and vinegar and stir over medium heat for a minute or two.

Crumble the bacon over the broccoli, stir for another minute or so, and serve.

Yield: 4 servings

Each with 7 grams of carbohydrates and 3 grams of fiber, for a total of 4 grams of usable carbs and 5 grams of protein.

Grilled Broccoli Salad

Before I made this salad, I'd never had grilled broccoli. It's wonderful!

1 head broccoli
2 tablespoons (30 ml) olive oil
¼ cup (60 ml) rice wine vinegar
¼ cup (60 ml) soy sauce
2 tablespoons (30 ml) toasted sesame oil
¼ cup (30 g) sesame seeds

Start a charcoal fire or preheat a gas grill.

Trim the bottom of the broccoli stem and cut into spears. Brush with a little of the olive oil and grill over a medium to medium-low fire until flecked with brown spots. Remove from the fire.

Put the grilled broccoli in a bowl and add the rest of the oil, the vinegar, the soy sauce, and the sesame oil. Stir to coat the broccoli and let the whole thing sit for at least a half hour or so.

Before serving, put the sesame seeds in a small, dry skillet and shake them over medium-high heat until they start to make little popping sounds. Add to your salad, toss, and serve at room temperature.

Yield: 4 to 5 servings

Assuming 4, each will have 12 grams of carbohydrate and 6 grams of fiber, for a usable carb count of 6 grams; 7 grams protein.

Broccoli Dijon

For the work involved—practically none—this is really great.

1 pound (455 g) frozen broccoli cuts or spears
¼ cup (60 ml) vinaigrette dressing (I use Paul Newman's Olive Oil and Vinegar.)
1 tablespoon (15 ml) Dijon mustard
3 scallions, sliced thin

I like to use broccoli cuts for this, but use spears or florets if that's what you have on hand; it'll be fine. If your broccoli is frozen in a clump, throw the bag on the floor, hard, a few times to break it up, or if it's a box, slam all sides of it against the counter. This will make sure it's separated and cooks evenly. Put your smashed-apart broccoli, still frozen, in a microwaveable casserole dish with a lid. Add a couple of tablespoons (30 ml) of water, cover, and cook on high for 7 minutes. It should be tender-crisp by then, but if there are still cold spots, stir it and give it another minute or two. Don't overcook!

While the broccoli is cooking, measure the dressing and the mustard into a bowl and whisk together.

Okay, the broccoli's done! Drain it and then pour the dressing over it and toss. Add the scallions, toss again, and serve immediately.

Yield: 3 to 4 servings

Assuming 3 servings, each will have 5 g protein; 9 g carbohydrate; 5 g dietary fiber; 4 g usable carbs.

Ginger Stir-Fry Broccoli

2 to 3 tablespoons (30 to 45 ml) peanut oil or other bland oil

2 cloves garlic, crushed

1 bag (1 pound, or 455 g) frozen broccoli "cuts," thawed

1 tablespoon (6 g) grated fresh ginger

1 tablespoon (15 ml) soy sauce

Heat the peanut oil in a wok or heavy skillet over high heat. Add the garlic and the broccoli and stir-fry for 7 to 10 minutes or until the broccoli is tender-crisp.

Stir in the ginger and soy sauce, stir-fry for just another minute, and serve.

Yield: 4 servings

Each with 7 grams of carbohydrates and 3 grams of fiber, for a total of 4 grams of usable carbs and 4 grams of protein.

Broccoli with Bacon and Pine Nuts

This is quite special. Don't cook your broccoli any longer than 2 hours!

1 pound (455 g) frozen broccoli, unthawed

1 clove garlic, crushed

3 slices cooked bacon, crumbled

1 tablespoon (14 g) butter

1 tablespoon (15 ml) oil

2 tablespoons (30 g) pine nuts (pignolia), toasted

Place the broccoli in a slow cooker. Stir in the garlic and crumble in the bacon. Cover the slow cooker, set it to low, and let it cook for 2 hours.

Before serving, stir in the butter and oil and top with the pine nuts.

Yield: 3 servings

Each with 8 g protein, 8 g carbohydrate, 5 g dietary fiber, 3 g usable carbs.

About Cooking Spaghetti Squash

If you've never cooked a spaghetti squash, you may be puzzled as to how to go about it, but it's really easy: Just stab it several times (to keep it from exploding) and put it in your microwave on high for 12 to 15 minutes. Then slice it open and scoop out and discard the seeds. Now take a fork and start scraping at the "meat" of the squash. You will be surprised and charmed to discover that it separates into strands very much like spaghetti, only yellow-orange in color.

Spaghetti squash is not a terribly low-carb vegetable, but it's much lower-carb than spaghetti, so it's a useful substitute in many recipes—especially casseroles. If you only need half of your cooked spaghetti squash right away, the rest will live happily in a resealable plastic bag in your fridge for 3 to 4 days until you do something else with it.

Spaghetti Squash Alfredo

We love this! My husband is an Alfredo fiend, so by using spaghetti squash instead of pasta, he gets his fix without all those additional carbs.

2 cups (450 g) cooked spaghetti squash, separated into strands

3 tablespoons (42 g) butter

3 tablespoons (45 ml) heavy cream

1 clove garlic, crushed

¼ cup (25 g) grated or shredded Parmesan cheese

Simply heat up your squash and stir in everything else. Stir until the butter is melted and serve!

Yield: 4 servings

Each with 4 grams of carbohydrates, a trace of fiber, and 3 grams of protein.

This makes a very nice side dish with some chicken sautéed in olive oil and garlic.

Spaghetti Squash Carbonara

This makes a very filling side dish.

8 slices bacon

4 eggs

¾ cup (75 g) grated Parmesan cheese

3 cups (675 g) cooked spaghetti squash, separated into strands

1 clove garlic, crushed

Fry the bacon until it's crisp. Remove it from the pan and pour off all but a couple tablespoons (30 ml) of grease.

Beat the eggs with the cheese and toss with the spaghetti squash. Pour the squash mixture into the hot fat in the skillet and add the garlic. Toss for 2 to 3 minutes over medium heat.

Crumble in the bacon, toss, and serve.

Yield: 6 servings

Each with 6 grams of carbohydrates and 1 gram of fiber, for a total of 5 grams of usable carbs and 11 grams of protein.

You can make this dish higher in protein by using a cup or two of diced leftover ham in place of the bacon. Brown the ham in olive oil, remove from the pan, cook the squash mixture in the oil, and then toss in the ham just before serving.

Spicy Sesame "Noodles" with Vegetables

This isn't terribly low-carb, but it sure can pull you out of the hole when you've got vegetarians coming to dinner.

3 cups (675 g) cooked spaghetti squash, separated into strands

¼ cup (60 ml) water

3 tablespoons (45 ml) soy sauce

5 tablespoons (75 g) tahini

1½ tablespoons (23 ml) rice vinegar

½ teaspoon red pepper flakes

1 tablespoon (9 g) sesame seeds

2 to 3 tablespoons (30 to 45 ml) peanut oil or other bland oil

1½ cups (105 g) mushrooms, thickly sliced

⅔ cup (100 g) diced green pepper

½ cup (60 g) diced celery

½ cup (80 g) chopped onion

¼ pound (115 g) snow peas, cut into 1-inch (2.5-cm) lengths

2 tablespoons (12 g) grated fresh ginger

2 cloves garlic, crushed

½ cup (55 g) cooked shrimp or diced leftover chicken, pork, or ham per serving (optional)

Place the spaghetti squash in a large mixing bowl.

In a separate bowl, combine the water, soy sauce, tahini, rice vinegar, and pepper flakes, mixing well. Pour over the spaghetti squash and set aside.

Place the sesame seeds in a small, heavy skillet over high heat and shake the skillet constantly until the seeds start to make little popping sounds and jump in the skillet. When that happens, immediately turn off the heat and shake the seeds out onto a small plate to cool. Set aside.

Just before you're ready to serve the dish, heat the oil in a large skillet or wok. Add the mushrooms, pepper, celery, onion, snow peas, ginger, and garlic and stir-fry over high heat for 7 to 10 minutes or until tender-crisp.

When the vegetables are done, add them to the large mixing bowl with the spaghetti squash mixture and toss until well combined.

Pile the squash mixture on serving plates. Top the meat-eaters' servings with the shrimp, chicken, pork, or ham (if using) and scatter sesame seeds over each serving.

Yield: 4 servings

Each with 19 grams of carbohydrates and 4 grams of fiber, for a total of 15 grams of usable carbs and 7 grams of protein. (Analysis does not include optional meat.)

(continued on page 254)

This is a great dish to make for guests because so much of it can be done ahead of time: You can prepare the "noodles" and the sesame seeds before your company arrives and then just stir-fry the vegetables and garnish the plates when it's time to eat.

Grilled Radicchio with Balsamic Vinaigrette

The grilling mellows the bitter edge of the radicchio, and the balsamic vinegar complements and enhances its newfound sweetness. I really love this!

¼ cup (60 ml) olive oil
2 tablespoons (30 ml) balsamic vinegar
1 clove garlic
1 dash salt
1 dash pepper
1 head radicchio

Mix together everything but the radicchio. Now, trim just the very bottom of the radicchio's stem and cut the whole thing in quarters from top to bottom (you want a bit of stem in each quarter, holding it together). Put the radicchio quarters on a plate and spoon some of the balsamic vinaigrette over them, letting it drizzle down between the leaves.

Now grill your radicchio, turning once or twice, until it's going limp and starting to brown. Then serve, drizzling it with a little more vinaigrette if you like.

Yield: 4 servings

Each serving will have 1 gram of carbohydrate and a trace of fiber, and a trace of protein.

Apple Walnut Dressing

This dressing has no grain of any kind in it, and it still tastes great. Serve with a simple poultry or pork dish.

4 tablespoons (56 g) butter
1 crisp, tart apple (I use a Granny Smith because I like the flavor, but one with a red skin would look prettier.)
2 large stalks celery
1 medium onion
1 cup (150 g) shelled walnuts
8 ounces (225 g) sliced mushrooms
¾ teaspoon salt or Vege-Sal
1½ teaspoons poultry seasoning

Melt the butter in a large, heavy skillet over medium heat.

Quarter the apple and trim out the core, whack each quarter in half (making eighths), and drop them in your food processor with the S-blade in place. Whack each stalk of celery into 4 or 5 big chunks and throw them in too. Quarter the onion, peel it, and throw it in and then dump in the walnuts. Pulse the food processor until everything's a medium consistency.

Dump this mixture, along with the mushrooms (which we're assuming you bought already sliced—if not, just chop them with everything else), into the butter in the skillet, turn the heat up to medium-high, and sauté everything for a minute or two, stirring. Then cover it and let it cook for 10 minutes, uncovering every 3 minutes or so to stir the whole thing again.

Stir in the salt and poultry seasoning, let it cook for another minute or two and serve.

Yield: 6 to 8 servings

Assuming 6 servings, each will have 9 grams of carbohydrates and 3 grams of fiber, for a total of 6 grams of usable carbs and 6 grams of protein.

Hush Puppies

I didn't know how this would work out, but it turned out very well indeed! You'll need a deep-fat fryer or at least a deep, heavy pot and a frying thermometer. My thanks to my Alabaman friend Kay for helping me get this recipe right. (She also tells me, a bit late, that hush puppies really go with fish fries, but hey, I got the idea from *Southern Living* magazine. I'm a Yankee, what do I know?)

⅔ **cup (80 g) Atkins Cornbread Mix**
2 tablespoons (15 g) Atkins Bake Mix
¼ **cup (30 g) rice protein powder**
1 teaspoon seasoned salt
½ **cup (120 ml) canola oil**
½ **cup (120 ml) water**
2 eggs
¼ **cup (40 g) finely minced onion**

Preheat a deep-fat fryer to 370°F (190°C).

In a medium-size mixing bowl, stir the Atkins Cornbread Mix, Atkins Bake Mix, rice protein powder, and salt together. In a 2-cup (480-ml)

glass measure, measure the oil, then the water (so that together the level is 1 cup). Break the eggs into the oil-and-water mixture and whisk the whole combination together. Stir the onion into the liquid ingredients. Then pour the oil mixture into the dry ingredients and stir the whole thing together with a few big strokes, just until everything's wet—don't overmix.

When your oil is up to temperature, drop the batter into the hot fat by the tablespoonful and fry until golden, just a few minutes. Drain on absorbent paper and serve hot.

Yield: 6 servings, at least!

Assuming 6, each serving will have 12 grams of carbohydrate and 3 grams of fiber, for a usable carb count of 9 grams; 17 grams of protein. (By comparison, a 5-pup serving of restaurant hush puppies will generally contain about 35 grams of carbohydrate.)

Low-Carb BBQ Baked Beans

In many parts of the country, baked beans are an indispensable side dish with any barbecue. Sadly, most beans are way too high carbohydrate for us. However, there is one sort of bean that is low-enough carb for us: black soybeans. You'll want to buy them canned, because soybeans take forever to cook soft—you can find them at the natural food store; a company called Eden cans them. They're sort of bland by themselves, but add onions, celery, etc., and they're fabulous.

(continued on page 256)

These aren't actually baked, I admit. I trust you'll forgive me. This makes only 4 servings, but it's very easy to double.

3 slices bacon
¼ cup (40 g) minced onion
¼ cup (30 g) minced celery
¼ cup (35 g) finely chopped green bell pepper
1 15-ounce (420-g) can black soybeans
3 tablespoons (45 ml) Dana's No-Sugar
    Ketchup (page 463)
2 tablespoons (3 g) Splenda
½ teaspoon blackstrap molasses
1 dash salt
1 dash pepper
1 dash hot pepper sauce

Chop up the bacon or snip it right into a saucepan with kitchen shears. Start it cooking over medium heat. When some grease has cooked out of the bacon, add the onion, celery, and green pepper. Sauté the vegetables in the bacon grease until soft.

Drain the canned black soybeans and dump them in with the vegetables. Stir in the ketchup, Splenda, molasses, salt, pepper, and hot sauce. Turn the heat to low, cover, and let the whole thing simmer for 15 minutes or so and then serve.

Yield: 4 servings

Each serving will have 11 grams of carbohydrate and 6 grams of fiber, for a usable carb count of 5 grams; 11 grams protein. (Bush's brand Barbecue Baked Beans have 32 grams of carbohydrate in a ½-cup (125 g) serving!)

Chili Lime Pumpkin

It's such a shame fresh pumpkin is available for only a couple of months in the autumn; it's so wonderful. This side dish is a tad high in carbs, but it's so unusual and so good I had to include it. Don't try shelling the seeds from the pumpkin you're cooking to complete the recipe—it's a tedious task! Just roast them and salt them as is and snack on them later.

1 little pumpkin, about 2 pounds (910 g)
2 tablespoons (28 g) butter
1 tablespoon (15 ml) oil
½ cup (120 g) shelled pumpkin seeds
    (pepitas)
1 teaspoon chili garlic paste
2 teaspoons lime juice

Whack your pumpkin in half and scoop out the seeds. Peel off the hard rind and then cut the flesh into slices about ¼-inch (6-mm) thick.

Put the butter and the oil in a big, heavy skillet over medium heat. Swirl them together as the butter melts. Now, lay the slices of pumpkin flat in the butter/oil mixture and sauté until they're lightly golden on both sides. They should be tender but still al dente. You'll need to do this in more than one batch; keep the stuff that's done warm on a plate under a pot lid.

While this is happening, toast your pepitas by stirring them in a dry skillet over medium-high heat until they swell a bit—about 4 to 5 minutes. Remove from the heat when they're done.

When the pumpkin's all cooked, put it all back in the skillet. Mix together the chili garlic paste and the lime juice and gently mix it in, coating all of the pumpkin slices.

Lay the pumpkin slices on serving plates, top each serving with a tablespoon of toasted pumpkin seeds, and serve.

Yield: 8 servings

Each with 2 g protein; 10 g carbohydrate; 1 g dietary fiber; 9 g usable carbs.

Cranberry-Peach Chutney

This is seriously kicked-up from regular cranberry sauce! It's a natural with curried poultry, but try it with any simple poultry or pork dish.

12 ounces (340 g) cranberries
1½ cups (300 g) diced peaches (I use unsweetened frozen peach slices, diced.)
1 clove garlic, minced
3 inches (7.5 cm) ginger, sliced into paper-thin rounds
1 lime, sliced paper-thin
1 ¼ cups (30 g) Splenda
1 cinnamon stick
1 teaspoon mustard seed
¼ teaspoon salt
¼ teaspoon orange extract
¼ teaspoon baking soda

Combine everything but the baking soda in a slow cooker. Cover the slow cooker, set it to low, and let it cook for 3 hours, stirring once halfway through.

When the time's up, stir in the baking soda and keep stirring until the fizzing subsides. Store in a tightly lidded container in the fridge. If you plan to keep it for long, freezing's a good idea.

Yield: Makes about 2½ cups, or 20 servings of 2 tablespoons

Each with trace protein, 8 g carbohydrate, 1 g dietary fiber, 7 g usable carbs.

Why baking soda? Because by neutralizing some of the acid in the cranberries, it lets you get away with less Splenda—and fewer carbs.

9

Fish and Seafood

Ceviche

Most countries in Latin America have a version of this classic dish, in which the fish is "cooked" in lime juice instead of by heat. This makes a posh appetizer or if you want to increase the serving sizes, a light main course. This is not only low-carb, it's also very low-calorie—and except for squeezing all those limes, very simple.

1½ pounds (680 g) fish fillets
8 limes
2 tomatoes
1 fresh jalapeño (optional)
1 black avocado
¼ red onion, diced
¼ cup (16 g) chopped fresh oregano
¼ cup (16 g) chopped fresh cilantro
Salt and pepper to taste

This dish lends itself to endless variation, but one thing remains constant: Everything must be perfectly fresh, especially the fish. Talk to the fish guy at your grocery store and tell him you'll be using the fish for ceviche (that's "seh-vee-chay"). Tell him you need fish that has never been frozen and choose from what he has, rather than going into the store with the idea of buying a particular kind of fish and ending up buying something that's been thawed. You can use seafood as well as fish fillets—shelled shrimp, scallops, baby squid, and chunks of lobster tail all lend themselves to this treatment. Or you can use fin fish like mackerel, red snapper, grouper, halibut, cod, or flounder. It is customary to use two to four kinds, rather than just one, but suit yourself.

Cut any fish fillets into serving-sized pieces. Put your fish or seafood in a glass or crockery dish. Squeeze 7 of your limes—you should have about 1¼ to 1½ cups (300 to 360 ml) lime juice—and pour the lime juice over the fish. Turn the fish to make sure it's completely coated. Cover the dish with piece of plastic wrap and refrigerate for 8 to 12 hours or overnight. If at all possible, it's best to turn the fish at least a few times during the marinating time to make sure it "cooks" evenly. Drain the fish or seafood and put it in a fresh bowl.

Cut the tomatoes in half across the equator and squeeze them gently to get rid of the seeds. Dice them fairly fine. Seed the jalapeño, if you're using it, and dice it fine, too. Cut the avocado in half, remove the seed, peel it, and cut it into dice as well. Put all of these vegetables and the diced red onion in the bowl with the fish. Throw in the fresh herbs, too. Squeeze the last lime over the whole thing, season with salt and pepper, toss gently, and serve.

Yield: 8 appetizer servings

Each with 16 g protein; 5 g carbohydrate; 2 g dietary fiber; 3 g usable carbs. This analysis assumes you discard all but about ¼ cup (60 ml) of the lime juice used to marinate the fish.

The Simplest Fish

Not only is this simple, but it's lightning-quick, too.

1 fillet (about 6 ounces, or 170 g) mild white fish
1 tablespoon (14 g) butter
1 tablespoon (3.8 g) minced fresh parsley
Wedge of lemon

(continued on page 260)

Melt the butter in a heavy-bottomed skillet over low heat. Add the fish fillets and sauté for 5 minutes on each side or until the fish is opaque and flakes easily, turning carefully.

Transfer to serving plates, top with the minced parsley, and serve with a wedge of lemon.

Yield: 1 serving

Trace of carbohydrates, no fiber, and 31 grams of protein.

Ginger Mustard Fish

4 (6 ounce, or 175 g) fish fillets, such as tilapia, cod, or orange roughy
4 tablespoons (56 g) butter
2 teaspoons minced garlic or 4 cloves garlic, crushed
2 teaspoons grated ginger
2 teaspoons spicy brown or Dijon mustard
1 tablespoon (15 ml) water

In a large, heavy skillet, start sautéing the fish in the butter over medium-low heat; 4 to 5 minutes per side should be plenty. Remove the fish to a plate.

Add the garlic, ginger, mustard, and water to the skillet and stir everything together well. Put the fish back in, turning it over once, carefully, to make sure both sides get acquainted with the sauce. Let it cook for another minute or so and then serve. Scrape the sauce out of the skillet over the fish.

Yield: 4 servings

Each with 1 gram of carbohydrates, a trace of fiber, and 31 grams of protein.

Aioli Fish Bake

1 fillet (about 6 ounces, or 170 g) of mild, white fish
2 tablespoons (30 ml) Aioli (page 479)
1 tablespoon (6.3 g) grated Parmesan cheese

Preheat the oven to 350°F (180°C, or gas mark 4).

Spray a shallow baking pan (a jelly roll pan is ideal) with nonstick cooking spray. Working right on the baking pan, spread a fillet thickly with Aioli and sprinkle ½ tablespoon of Parmesan over that. Turn the fillet over carefully and spread Aioli and sprinkle the remaining Parmesan on other side. Bake for 20 minutes and serve.

Yield: 1 serving

1 gram of carbohydrates, a trace of fiber, and 32 grams of protein.

Microwaved Fish and Asparagus with Tarragon Mustard Sauce

Microwaving is a great way to cook vegetables and a great way to cook fish—so it's a natural way to cook combinations of the two.

12 ounces (340 g) fish fillets—whiting, tilapia, sole, flounder, or any other mild white fish
10 asparagus spears
2 tablespoons (30 g) sour cream
1 tablespoon (15 g) mayonnaise
¼ teaspoon dried tarragon
½ teaspoon Dijon or spicy brown mustard

Snap the bottoms off the asparagus spears where they break naturally. Place the asparagus in a large glass pie plate, add 1 tablespoon (15 ml) of water, and cover by placing a plate on top. Microwave on high for 3 minutes.

While the asparagus is microwaving, stir together the sour cream, mayonnaise, tarragon, and mustard.

Remove the asparagus from the microwave, take it out of the pie plate, and set it aside. Drain the water out of the pie plate. Place the fish fillets in the pie plate and spread 2 tablespoons (30 ml) of the sour cream mixture over them. Re-cover the pie plate and microwave the fish for 3 to 4 minutes on high. Open the microwave, remove the plate from the top of the pie plate, and arrange the asparagus on top of the fish. Re-cover the pie plate and cook for another 1 to 2 minutes on high.

Remove the pie plate from the microwave and take the plate off. Place the fish and asparagus on serving plates. Scrape any sauce that's cooked into the pie plate over the fish and asparagus. Top each serving with the reserved sauce and serve.

Yield: 2 servings

Each with 4 grams of carbohydrates and 2 grams of fiber, for a total of 2 grams of usable carbs and 33 grams of protein.

This dish also packs in 949 mg of potassium!

Grilled Fish with Caper Sauce

This is more of a method for grilling a wide variety of fish fillets and adding a simple but elegantly piquant sauce. The main element of this recipe is the sauce. Ingredient amounts are not important, so you can vary to taste. The resulting mixture should be something you spoon over the fish, not a pourable sauce. (Our tester said he used 2 tablespoons of each of the following for 1 pound [455 g] of fish fillets, and it worked very well.) This is a very piquant sauce, not for the timid of palate, but most delicious!

As for grilling the fish, some people prefer to do it in the Spanish style of first sprinkling salt on the fillets, letting them sit for 15 minutes or so, rinsing and drying them, brushing them with olive oil, and grilling them on a cast-iron griddle. Swordfish and sea bass are wonderful this way; so are tilapia fillets (which are much cheaper).

Grilled fish of your choice
Garlic, finely chopped
Parsley, flat-leaf preferable, finely chopped (or half parsley, half cilantro)
Anchovies, finely chopped (if omitting, salt to taste)
Capers, drained

(continued on page 262)

Fresh lemon juice
Olive oil

Mix the garlic, parsley, anchovies, capers, lemon juice, and olive oil, spoon over grilled fish, and serve.

Yield: 4 servings

If sauce is made with the suggested 2 tablespoons of each ingredient and 1 pound (455 g) fish, each serving will have 23 g protein; 2 g carbohydrate; trace dietary fiber; 2 g usable carbs.

Chinese Steamed Fish

I made this with tilapia, and while it was quite tasty, it was also fragile. If you're willing to pay the difference for a firmer fish like orange roughy or cod, it will be easier to handle.

12 ounces (340 g) fish fillets
2 tablespoons (30 ml) dry sherry
1 tablespoon (15 ml) soy sauce
2 teaspoons grated ginger
½ teaspoon minced garlic or 1 clove garlic, crushed
1½ teaspoons toasted sesame oil
1 or 2 scallions, minced (optional)

Lay the fish fillets on a piece of heavy-duty aluminum foil and turn the edges of the foil up to form a lip.

Mix together the sherry, soy sauce, ginger, garlic, and sesame oil.

Fit a rack—a cake-cooling rack works nicely—into a large skillet. Pour about ¼ inch (6 mm) of water in the bottom of the skillet and turn the heat to high. Place the foil with the fish on it on the rack. Carefully pour the sherry mixture over the fish. Cover the pan tightly.

Cook for 5 to 7 minutes or until the fish flakes easily. Serve with minced scallions as a garnish, if desired.

Yield: 2 servings

Each with 2 grams of carbohydrates, no fiber, and 31 grams of protein.

Each serving has only 195 calories!

Baked Orange Roughy

1½ pounds (680 g) orange roughy fillets, cut into serving-sized pieces
1 teaspoon salt or Vege-Sal
Pepper
¼ medium onion, very thinly sliced
Juice of 1 lemon, or 2 tablespoons (30 ml) bottled lemon juice
¼ cup (56 g) butter, melted
Paprika
Minced fresh parsley (optional)

Preheat the oven to 325°F (170°C, or gas mark 3). Spray a shallow baking dish with nonstick cooking spray.

Arrange the fish in the prepared pan and sprinkle with salt and pepper to taste. Scatter the onion over the fish.

In a small bowl, combine the lemon juice and butter and pour over the fish and onions. Sprinkle with paprika.

Bake, uncovered, for 30 minutes. Sprinkle with parsley (if using) and serve.

Yield: 4 servings

Each with 2 grams of carbohydrates, a trace of fiber, and 25 grams of protein.

Orange Roughy Bonne Femme

This is my favorite fish recipe, and it's very, very simple to make. Kids will probably like it, too.

1½ pounds (680 g) orange roughy fillets
¼ cup (30 g) low-carb bake mix
Pinch of salt or Vege-Sal
3 to 4 tablespoons (42 to 56 g) butter

Mix the bake mix with the pinch of salt (about ⅛ teaspoon). Dip the fillets in the bake mix, covering them lightly all over.

Melt the butter in a heavy skillet over medium heat. Sauté the "floured" fillets in the butter for 5 to 7 minutes per side or until golden brown. Serve just as it is or with a squeeze of lemon juice.

Yield: 4 servings

Each with 1 gram of carbohydrates, no fiber, and 25 grams of protein.

Almond-Stuffed Flounder Rolls with Orange Butter Sauce

1 pound (455 g) flounder fillets, 4 ounces (115 g) each
4 tablespoons (56 g) butter, divided
2 tablespoons (30 ml) lemon juice
⅛ teaspoon orange extract
1 teaspoon Splenda
⅓ cup (45 g) almonds
¼ cup (40 g) minced onion
1 clove garlic, crushed
1½ teaspoons Dijon mustard
½ teaspoon soy sauce
¼ cup (15.2 g) minced fresh parsley, divided

Put 2 tablespoons (28 g) of the butter, the lemon juice, orange extract, and Splenda in a slow cooker. Cover the slow cooker, set it to low, and let it heat while you fix your flounder rolls.

Put the almonds in a food processor with the S-blade in place and grind them to a cornmeal consistency. Melt 1 tablespoon (14 g) of butter in a medium-size heavy skillet and add the ground almonds. Stir the almonds over medium heat for 5 to 7 minutes or until they smell toasty. Transfer them to a bowl.

Now melt the final tablespoon (14 g) of butter in the skillet and sauté the onion and garlic over medium-low heat until the onion is just turning translucent. Add them to the almonds and stir them in. Now stir in the mustard, soy sauce, and 2 tablespoons (7.6 g) of the parsley.

Lay the flounder fillets on a big plate and divide the almond mixture between them. Spread it over the fillets and then roll each one up and fasten it with a toothpick.

Take the lid off the slow cooker and stir the sauce. Place the flounder rolls in the sauce and spoon the sauce over them. Re-cover the pot and let the rolls cook for 1 hour. When they're done, spoon the sauce over the rolls and sprinkle the remaining parsley over them to serve.

Yield: 4 servings

Each with 24 g protein, 5 g carbohydrate, 2 g dietary fiber, 3 g usable carbs.

Baked Sole in Creamy Curry Sauce

This is simple, and the curry makes it a pretty yellow color.

2 pounds (910 g) sole fillets
1 cup (230 g) plain yogurt
½ cup (120 g) mayonnaise
1 tablespoon (15 ml) lemon juice
1 teaspoon curry powder

Preheat oven to 350°F (180°C, or gas mark 4).

Mix together everything but the sole fillets to make a sauce. Pat your fish fillets dry. Spray an 8 × 8-inch (20 × 20-cm) baking dish with nonstick cooking spray.

Now, spread each fillet with some of the sauce—you want to use up about half the sauce, total, in this process. As each fillet is spread with sauce, roll it up and place the roll, seam-side down, in the baking pan.

Spoon the rest of the sauce over and around the fish. Bake for 30 minutes and serve.

Yield: 6 servings

Each with 30 g protein; 2 g carbohydrate; trace dietary fiber; 2 g usable carbs.

Sautéed Sole in White Wine

This simple but elegant dish is very Italian.

1 pound (455 g) sole fillets
Salt and pepper
2 tablespoons (28 g) butter
1 tablespoon (15 ml) olive oil
¼ cup (60 ml) dry white wine
1 teaspoon dried oregano
3 tablespoons (15 g) shredded Parmesan cheese
3 lemon wedges

Pat the sole fillets dry with a paper towel and sprinkle them on both sides with a little salt and pepper. Lay them on a plate while you spray a big skillet with nonstick cooking spray and set it over medium heat. Add the butter and the olive oil to the skillet and swirl them together as the butter melts. When the fat is hot, lay the fillets in the pan and sauté them just a few minutes on each side, turning carefully.

Pour the wine into the skillet—pour it in around the edge rather than pouring it right over the fish. Sprinkle the oregano over the fish and let the fish simmer in the wine for 5 minutes—if it browns slightly on the bottom, all the better. Remove to serving plates, sprinkle each serving with a tablespoon (5 g) of Parmesan cheese, and serve with a lemon wedge to squeeze over it.

Yield: 3 servings

Each with 31g protein; 1 g carbohydrate; trace dietary fiber; 1 g usable carb.

Wine and Herb Tilapia Packets

This is a simple company fish dish.

1½ pounds (680 g) tilapia fillets, cut into 4 portions
4 tablespoons (56 g) butter, divided
½ cup (120 ml) dry white wine, divided
¼ cup (16 g) minced fresh herbs (chives, basil, oregano, thyme, or a combination of these), divided
Salt

Preheat the oven to 350°F (180°C, or gas mark 4).

Tear a piece of aluminum foil about 18 inches (45 cm) square for each fillet. Place a fillet in the center of the foil square and curl the edges of the foil up a little. Put 1 tablespoon (14 g) of butter, 2 tablespoons (30 ml) of wine, 1 tablespoon (4 g) of minced herbs, and just a little salt on the fillet.

Fold the foil up around the fish, rolling the edges down in the middle and at the ends so the packet won't leak in the oven. Repeat for all 4 servings.

Place the packets right on the oven shelf—there's no need for a pan—and bake for 35 minutes.

Yield: 4 servings

Each with 2 grams of carbohydrates and 1 gram of fiber, for a total of 1 gram of usable carbs and 31 grams of protein.

When it's time to serve dinner, simply place a packet on each plate and let diners open their own. That way, no one loses a drop of the yummy butter, wine, and herb sauce the fish cooked in.

Tilapia on a Nest of Vegetables

This meal is quite beautiful to look at and a fast one-dish dinner. You could substitute green pepper for either the red or the yellow, if you like.

1 pound (455 g) tilapia fillets
3 tablespoons (45 ml) olive oil
1 cup (150 g) red pepper, cut into thin strips
1 cup (150 g) yellow pepper, cut into thin strips
1½ cups (180 g) zucchini, cut in matchstick strips
1½ cups (180 g) yellow squash, cut in match-stick strips
1 cup (160 g) sweet red onion, thinly sliced
1 clove garlic, crushed

(continued on page 266)

Salt and pepper

¼ teaspoon guar or xanthan

Lemon wedges (optional)

Heat the olive oil in a heavy skillet over medium-high heat and sauté the peppers, zucchini, squash, onion, and garlic for just 2 to 3 minutes, stirring frequently.

Sprinkle the tilapia fillets lightly on either side with the salt and pepper and then lay them over the vegetables in the skillet. Cover, turn the heat to medium-low, and let the fish steam in the moisture from the vegetables for 10 minutes or until it flakes easily.

With a spatula, carefully transfer the fish to a serving platter and use a slotted spoon to pile the vegetables on top of the fish. Pour the liquid that has accumulated in the skillet into a blender and add the guar or xanthan. Run the blender for a few seconds and then pour the thickened juices over the fish and vegetables. To serve, spoon a mound of the vegetables onto each diner's plate and place a piece of the fish on top. A few lemon wedges are nice with this, but they're hardly essential.

Yield: 4 servings

Each with 11 grams of carbohydrates and 2 grams of fiber, for a total of 8 grams of usable carbs and 22 grams of protein.

Broiled Marinated Whiting

With a big salad and some crusty bread for the carb-eaters, this makes a nice, simple supper.

6 whiting fillets

½ cup (120 ml) olive oil

3 tablespoons (45 ml) wine vinegar

1 tablespoon (15 ml) lemon juice

1 teaspoon Dijon mustard

1 clove garlic, crushed

½ teaspoon dried basil

¼ teaspoon salt

¼ teaspoon pepper

Combine the oil, vinegar, lemon juice, mustard, garlic, basil, salt, and pepper and mix well.

Place the fillets in a large resealable plastic bag and pour in the oil mixture. Refrigerate for several hours, turning the bag over from time to time.

Preheat the broiler. Remove the fish from the marinade. Broil about 8 inches (20 cm) from the heat for 4 to 5 minutes per side or cook on a stovetop grill.

While the fish is cooking, put the leftover marinade in a saucepan, boil it briefly, and then serve it as a sauce.

Yield: 3 servings

Each with just over 1 gram of carbohydrates, no fiber, and 34 grams of protein.

If you're in a hurry or you just don't have all the ingredients to make this dish, use ¾ cup (180 ml) of store-bought vinaigrette dressing, instead.

Whiting with Mexican Flavors

I made this for lunch when a friend of my husband's was visiting town, and we all agreed it was one of the best things I've ever made.

4 whiting fillets
2 tablespoons (30 ml) lime juice, divided
¾ teaspoon chili powder
2 tablespoons (30 ml) oil
1 medium onion
2 tablespoons (30 ml) orange juice
½ teaspoon Splenda
¼ teaspoon ground cumin
¼ teaspoon dried oregano
1 tablespoon (15 ml) white wine vinegar
½ teaspoon hot pepper sauce
Salt and pepper

Lay the whiting fillets on a plate and sprinkle with 1 tablespoon (15 ml) of lime juice, turning to coat. Sprinkle the skinless sides of the fillets with chili powder.

Heat the oil in a heavy skillet over medium heat. Add the whiting fillets. Sauté for about 4 minutes per side, turning carefully, or until cooked through. Remove to a serving plate and keep warm.

Add the onions to the skillet and turn the heat up to medium-high. Sauté the onions for a couple of minutes until they begin to go limp. Stir in the remaining lime juice, orange juice, Splenda, cumin, oregano, vinegar, and hot pepper sauce. Cook them all together for a minute or two. Season with salt and pepper to taste. Spoon the onions over the fish and serve.

Yield: 4 servings

Each with 5 grams of carbohydrates and 1 gram of fiber, for a total of 4 grams of usable carbs and 17 grams of protein.

Each serving has only 162 calories!

Pan-Barbecued Sea Bass

This has a lot of flavor for something so quick and easy! Feel free to cook any firm-fleshed fish this way.

1 pound (455 g) sea bass fillets
1 tablespoon (8 g) Classic Barbecue Rub
    (page 486, or use purchased barbecue rub)
4 slices bacon
2 tablespoons (30 ml) lemon juice

Cut the sea bass fillets into serving portions. Sprinkle both sides liberally with the barbecue rub.

Spray a big, heavy skillet with nonstick cooking spray and place over medium-low heat. Using sharp kitchen shears, snip the bacon into small pieces, straight into the skillet. Stir it for a moment. As soon as a little grease starts to cook out of the bacon, clear a couple of spaces for the fish and put the fish in the pan. Cover and set your oven timer for 4 minutes.

When time is up, flip the fish, and stir the bacon around a bit, so it will cook evenly. Re-cover the pan and set the timer for another

(continued on page 268)

3 to 4 minutes. Peek at your fish at least once; you don't want to overcook it!

When the fish is flaky, remove to serving plates and top with the browned bacon bits. Pour the lemon juice in the skillet, stir it around, and pour over the fish. Serve.

Yield: 3 servings

Each with 31 g protein; 2 g carbohydrate; trace dietary fiber; 2 g usable carbs.

Sea Bass with Tapenade Cream Sauce

This is another one of those recipes that would impress the heck out of you at a restaurant but is very little trouble to make for yourself at home.

12 ounces (340 g) sea bass fillet
3 tablespoons (45 ml) olive oil, divided
¼ medium onion
½ teaspoon minced garlic or 1 clove garlic, crushed
2 tablespoons (30 ml) tapenade
1 tablespoon (15 ml) balsamic vinegar
1 teaspoon lemon juice
3 tablespoons (45 ml) heavy cream
Salt and pepper

Preheat the broiler.

If the bass is in one piece, cut it into two equal portions. Brush with 1 tablespoon (15 ml) of the olive oil and put it under a broiler set on high, 3 or 4 inches (7 to 10 cm) from the heat. The length of time the fish will need to broil will depend on its thickness. I use fillets about 1½ inch (4 cm) thick, and they take about 5 to 6 minutes per side.

While the fish is broiling, slice the quarter-onion in half lengthwise and then slice as thinly as possible. Put the rest of the olive oil in a medium skillet over medium heat and add the onion and garlic. Sauté together for 3 to 4 minutes.

Add the tapenade, stir in, and sauté for a few more minutes. (Remember that somewhere in here you'll need to turn the fish!)

Now, stir the vinegar and lemon juice into the mixture in your skillet and let it cook down for 1 to 2 minutes. Stir in the cream and let the whole thing cook down for another minute.

When the fish is done, place it on two serving plates. Season the sauce with salt and pepper to taste, spoon over the fish, and then serve.

Yield: 2 servings

Each with 4 grams of carbohydrates, a trace of fiber, and 32 grams of protein.

Zijuatenejo Sea Bass

1½ pounds (680 g) sea bass fillets
Salt and pepper
1 teaspoon ground cumin
2 tablespoons (30 ml) olive oil
Easy Orange Salsa (page 496)
¼ cup (16 g) chopped fresh cilantro

Cut your fish into individual portions, if needed. Sprinkle it on both sides with salt and pepper and the cumin. Heat the olive oil in a big heavy skillet over medium-low heat and throw in the fish. Give it 4 to 5 minutes per side or until opaque all the way through. Remove each portion to a serving plate; top each with 2 tablespoons (30 g) Easy Orange Salsa and 1 tablespoon (4 g) chopped cilantro.

Yield: 4 servings

Each with 32 g protein; 2 g carbohydrate; 1 g dietary fiber; 1 g usable carb.

Brined, Jerked Red Snapper

Have you had one too many meals of dried-out fish? Try brining it!

2 pounds (910 g) red snapper fillets
FOR THE BRINE:
⅓ cup (100 g) kosher salt
3 quarts (2.8 L) water
2 tablespoons Jerk Seasoning (page 484 or purchased)
FOR THE SEASONINGS:
4 cloves garlic, crushed
8 teaspoons olive oil
1 rounded tablespoon Jerk Seasoning (page 484 or purchased)
¼ cup (60 ml) lemon juice
4 teaspoons soy sauce
4 scallions, sliced

To make the brine: In a shallow, nonreactive container big enough to hold your fish fillets, dissolve the salt in the water—this is easier if the water's warm. Stir in the Jerk Seasoning. If you've used warm water, let it cool to no warmer than tepid before adding your fish fillets. Make sure they're submerged in the brine and let them sit for 1 to 2 hours in the fridge.

Okay, time's up. Start a charcoal fire or preheat a gas grill. Drain the brine off of your fish. In a rimmed plate or pie plate, mix together the garlic and olive oil and then stir in the Jerk Seasoning, lemon juice, and soy sauce. Reserve some marinade, lay the brined fillets in the rest of this marinade, and turn them over once or twice to coat. Let the fillets sit for 15 minutes or so. Then grill over a medium fire, 3–5 minutes per side. Baste both sides with the reserved seasoning mixture when you turn the fish.

When the fish is flaky, remove to serving plates and top each fillet with a sliced scallion.

Yield: 4 servings

Each serving will have 4 grams of carbohydrate and 1 gram of fiber, for a usable carb count of 3 grams (less if you use the Jerk Seasoning recipe); 41 grams protein.

Salmon with Lemon-Dill Butter

This is a classic flavor combination, and after you make this, you'll understand why.

(continued on page 270)

4 salmon steaks, each 1 inch thick

4 tablespoons (56 g) butter, softened

1 tablespoon (15 ml) lemon juice

1 teaspoon dry dill weed or 1 tablespoon
(3.3 g) minced fresh dill

Olive oil

Put the butter, lemon juice, and dill in a food processor with the S-blade in place. Pulse until well combined, scraping down the sides once or twice if necessary. (If you don't have a food processor, you can simply beat these things together by hand.) Chill.

About 15 minutes before dinner, preheat the broiler and rub each salmon steak on both sides with olive oil. Arrange the steaks on the broiler rack and broil 8 inches (20 cm) from high heat for 5 to 6 minutes per side or until the salmon flakes easily.

Place on the serving plates, top each steak with a tablespoon of the lemon-dill butter, and serve.

Yield: 4 very generous servings

Each with only a trace of carbohydrates, a trace of fiber, and about 34 grams of protein.

Salmon in Ginger Cream

This dish has all the goodness of salmon in an elegant sauce.

2 salmon fillets, 6 ounces (170 g) each, skin
still attached

2 tablespoons (28 g) butter

1 teaspoon minced garlic or 2 cloves garlic,
crushed

2 scallions, finely minced

2 tablespoons (8 g) chopped cilantro

¼ cup (60 ml) dry white wine

2 tablespoons (12 g) grated ginger

4 tablespoons (60 g) sour cream

Salt and pepper

Melt the butter in a heavy skillet over medium-low heat and start sautéing the salmon in it—you want to sauté it for about 4 minutes per side.

While the fish is sautéing, crush the garlic, mince the scallions, and chop the cilantro.

When both sides of the salmon have sautéed for 4 minutes, add the wine to the skillet, cover, and let the fish cook an additional 2 minutes or so until cooked through. Remove the fish to serving plates.

Add the garlic, scallions, cilantro, and ginger to the wine and butter in the skillet, turn the heat up to medium-high, and let them cook for a minute or two. Add the sour cream, stir to blend, and add salt and pepper to taste. Spoon the sauce over the fish and serve.

Yield: 2 servings

Each with 5 grams of carbohydrates and 1 gram of fiber, for a total of 4 grams of usable carbs and 36 grams of protein

This dish also has lots of EPA—the good fat that makes salmon so heart-healthy!

Salmon Stuffed with Lime, Cilantro, Anaheim Peppers, and Scallions

This is impressive for how simple it is, and it will feed a crowd.

1 whole salmon, cleaned and gutted, about 6 pounds (2.7 kg)
1 lime, sliced paper-thin
1 bunch cilantro, chopped
1 Anaheim chili pepper, cut in matchstick strips
3 scallions, sliced thin lengthwise
2 tablespoons (30 g) olive oil

This is simple. Preheat your oven to 350°F (180°C, or gas mark 4). Lay the salmon in a great big roasting pan you've sprayed with nonstick cooking spray. Now stuff everything else except the oil into the salmon, distributing everything evenly along the length of the body cavity.

I like to sew the salmon up, using a heavy needle and cooking twine. Now rub it with olive oil on both sides and throw it in the oven for 30 to 40 minutes. It's a good idea to stick a thermometer in the thick part of the flesh to see if it's done; it should read between 135°F and 140°F (about 60°C).

Cut into slices, with some of the stuffing in each serving.

Yield: 12 servings

Each with 45 g protein; 1 g carbohydrate; trace dietary fiber; 1 g usable carbs.

Lemon-Herb Stuffed Salmon

This is a great recipe to serve at a party since it will feed a dozen or more people. It will impress them, too!

1 whole salmon, cleaned and head removed, between 6 and 7 pounds (3 kg)
1 lemon, sliced as thinly as humanly possible
6 scallions, any wilted bits trimmed, and sliced very thinly lengthways
4 tablespoons (24 g) fresh oregano leaves, minced
1 tablespoon (2.4 g) fresh thyme leaves, stripped off their stems

First, start a charcoal fire or preheat a gas grill. If you're using charcoal, once the coals are ash-covered you'll want to use fireproof tongs to arrange them in a strip roughly the length and width of your fish. Either way, charcoal or gas, you'll want a medium-hot fire.

Lay the salmon out on a platter. Stuff the lemon slices into the body cavity, distributing them evenly along the length of the fish. Do the same with the scallions. Mix together the two herbs and stuff them into the body cavity as well.

Now, run toothpicks or skewers through the edges of the fish and use cooking twine to lace around the skewers to hold the edge of the fish closed. Or if you prefer, use a big needle and cooking twine to sew the salmon closed.

Slash the fish every couple of inches, down to the bone, to let the heat in. Now place the fish on an oiled grill over the fire and close the

(continued on page 272)

lid. After 15 to 20 minutes, turn the salmon very carefully, using two spatulas, and re-situate it over the fire.

Re-close the lid and give your salmon another 15 to 20 minutes. It's done when it flakes easily and an instant-read thermometer registers between 135°F and 140°F (60°C). Use your two spatulas to carefully remove the fish to a platter and serve.

Yield: 12 servings

Each serving will have just 1 gram of carbohydrate, a trace of fiber, and 49 grams of protein.

Lemon-Mustard Salmon Steaks

This is so simple and classic. The salmon comes out tender and moist.

2 salmon steaks (totaling about 1 pound, or 455 g)
2 tablespoons (28 g) butter
1 tablespoon (15 ml) lemon juice
1 teaspoon Dijon mustard
1 pinch salt or Vege-Sal
2 tablespoons (7.8 g) chopped fresh parsley

Combine the butter, lemon juice, mustard, and salt or Vege-Sal in a slow cooker. Cover the slow cooker, set it to low, and let it cook for 30 to 40 minutes. Stir together.

Now put the salmon steaks in the slow cooker and turn them once or twice to coat. Re-cover the slow cooker and let it cook for 1 hour. Spoon some of the pot liquid over the salmon and sprinkle with the parsley before serving.

Yield: 2 servings

Each with 46 g protein, 1 g carbohydrate, trace dietary fiber, 1 g usable carbs.

Feta-Spinach Salmon Roast

I saw something like this being sold for outrageous amounts of money in the fish case at the local grocery store, and I thought, "I can do that!"

3 ounces (85 g) cream cheese, softened
¾ cup (115 g) crumbled feta
2 scallions, thinly sliced, including the crisp part of the green
½ cup (10 g) fresh spinach, chopped
2 skinless salmon fillets of roughly equal size and shape, totaling ¾ pound (340 g)
Olive oil

Preheat the oven to 350°F (180°C, or gas mark 4).

Combine the cream cheese and feta, mashing and stirring with a fork until well blended. Add the scallions and spinach and combine well.

Spread the mixture evenly over one salmon fillet. (The filling will be about ¾ inch [2 cm] thick.) Top with the second salmon fillet. Brush both sides with olive oil, turning the whole thing over carefully with a spatula.

Place the loaf on a shallow baking pan and bake for 20 minutes. Slice carefully with a sharp, serrated knife.

Yield: 2 servings

Each with 5 grams of carbohydrates, a trace of fiber, and 45 grams of protein.

Buttered Salmon with Creole Seasonings

12 ounces (340 g) salmon fillet, in two or three pieces
1 teaspoon Creole Seasoning (page 485 or purchased)
¼ teaspoon dried thyme
4 tablespoons (56 g) butter
1 teaspoon minced garlic or 2 cloves garlic, minced

Sprinkle the skinless side of the salmon evenly with the Creole Seasoning and thyme. Melt the butter in a heavy skillet over medium-low heat and add the salmon, skin side down. Cook 4 to 5 minutes per side, turning carefully. Remove to serving plates, skin side down, and stir the garlic into the butter remaining in the pan. Cook for just a minute and then scrape all the garlic butter over the salmon and serve.

Yield: 2 or 3 servings

Assuming 2 servings, each will have 2 grams of carbohydrates and a trace of fiber, for a total of 2 grams of usable carbs and 35 grams of protein.

Orange Salmon Packets

1 pound (455 g) salmon fillets
¼ cup (60 g) plain yogurt
2 tablespoons (30 g) mayonnaise
¼ teaspoon orange extract
1 tablespoon (1.5 g) Splenda
1 tablespoon (15 ml) lemon juice
2 scallions, finely minced
1 tablespoon (3.8 g) parsley, finely minced

Preheat the oven to 425°F (220°C, or gas mark 7).

Combine the yogurt, mayonnaise, orange extract, Splenda, lemon juice, scallions, and parsley. Set aside.

If your salmon fillets have skin on them, remove it and cut the fish into 4 serving-sized pieces.

Tear 4 large squares of heavy-duty aluminum foil. Place each piece of salmon in the center of a square of foil and spoon 2 tablespoons (30 ml) of the sauce over it. Fold the foil up over the salmon, bringing the edges together, and roll the edges to make a tight seal. Roll up each end as well.

When all your salmon fillets are snug in their own little packets, bake them for 15 minutes. (You can put your salmon packets in a roasting pan if you're afraid they'll spring a leak, but I just put mine right on the oven rack.)

Place on individual serving plates, cut open, and serve. If you have a little sauce left over, serve it on the side.

Yield: 4 servings

Each with less than 2 grams of carbohydrates, a trace of fiber, and 24 grams of protein.

Orange-Sesame Salmon

1½ pounds (680 g) salmon fillet
¼ cup (60 ml) sesame oil
1 teaspoon orange extract
⅓ cup (80 ml) lemon juice
4 teaspoons Splenda
2 teaspoons Dijon mustard
2 teaspoons dried tarragon, crumbled

Cut the salmon into serving-sized pieces and lay it in a glass pie plate or any big plate with a rim.

Mix together everything else and pour it over the salmon fillets, turning them to coat. Stick the plate in the fridge and let the fish marinate for at least 30 minutes (an hour's fine).

Spray a big, heavy skillet with nonstick cooking spray and put it over medium heat. When it's hot, add the fish, reserving the marinade. Cook the salmon about 4 minutes on each side—you want it opaque almost all the way through. Then add the marinade and let the two cook together for another couple of minutes. Serve with the liquid from the pan scraped over the fish.

Yield: 4 servings

Each with 34 g protein; 2 g carbohydrate; trace dietary fiber; 2 g usable carbs.

Glazed, Grilled Salmon

Of all the ways I've cooked salmon, this drew the most praise.

12 ounces (340 g) salmon fillet, cut into
  2 or 3 serving-sized pieces
2 tablespoons (3 g) Splenda
1½ teaspoons dry mustard
1 tablespoon (15 ml) soy sauce
1½ teaspoons rice vinegar
¼ teaspoon blackstrap molasses, or the
  darkest molasses you can find

Mix together the Splenda, mustard, soy sauce, vinegar, and molasses in a small dish. Spoon out 1 tablespoon (15 ml) of this mixture and set it aside in a separate dish.

Place the salmon fillets on a plate and pour the larger quantity of the soy sauce mixture over it, turning each fillet so that both sides come in contact with the seasonings. Let the fish sit for a few minutes—just 2 or 3—with the skinless side down in the seasonings.

Now, you get to choose how you want to cook the salmon. I do mine on a stovetop grill, but you can broil it, cook it in a heavy skillet sprayed with nonstick cooking spray, cook it on an electric tabletop grill, or even do it on an outdoor grill. However you cook it, it will need about 5 minutes per side (or just 5 minutes total in an electric grill). If you choose a method that requires you to turn the salmon, turn carefully!

When the salmon is cooked through, remove it to serving plates and drizzle the reserved 1 tablespoon (15 ml) seasoning mixture over each piece before serving.

Yield: This makes 2 generous servings or 3 smaller ones

Assuming 2 servings, each will have 3 grams of carbohydrates, a trace of fiber, and 35 grams of protein.

Maple-Balsamic Glazed Salmon

This was amazingly popular with friends when I served it at a dinner party. Feel free to double this!

2 tablespoons (30 ml) extra-virgin olive oil
¼ cup (60 ml) sugar-free pancake syrup
2 cloves garlic, crushed
½ teaspoon salt
2 tablespoons (30 ml) balsamic vinegar
1 pound (455 g) salmon fillet

Start a charcoal fire or preheat a gas grill.

Mix together everything but the salmon and set aside half the mixture. Cut the salmon into 3 or 4 serving pieces (if you didn't buy it in serving-sized pieces), lay them on a plate, and brush both sides of each piece of salmon with half of the pancake-syrup mixture. Grill the salmon over well-ashed coals or over a gas grill set to medium-low about 5 minutes per side or until cooked through. Place on serving plates, drizzle with the reserved half of the syrup mixture, and serve.

Yield: 4 servings

Each serving will have 1 gram of carbohydrate, not including the polyols in the sugar-free pancake syrup; a trace of fiber; and 23 grams protein.

Salmon Patties

These are quick, easy, and from-the-pantry-shelf convenient. If you don't have scallions in the refrigerator, use a tablespoon or so of finely minced onion.

1 can (14¾ ounces, or 415 g) salmon
¼ cup (25 g) oat bran
1 egg
2 scallions, finely sliced
3 tablespoons (42 g) butter

Drain the salmon, place it in a mixing bowl, and mash it well. (Don't worry about any skin that may be in there; mash it right in.)

Add the oat bran, egg, and scallions and mix everything well. Form into 4 patties.

Melt the butter in a heavy skillet over medium heat. Sauté the patties in the butter, turning carefully, until they're quite golden on both sides (7 to 10 minutes per side).

Yield: 2 servings

Each with 9 grams of carbohydrates and 2 grams of fiber, for a total of 7 grams usable carbs and 47 grams of protein.

Not only do these patties have lots of healthy fish oils, they also contain half your day's requirement of calcium.

Orange Swordfish Steaks with Almonds

16 ounces (455 g) swordfish steak
¼ cup (60 ml) lemon juice

(continued on page 276)

2 tablespoons (30 ml) olive oil

½ teaspoon orange extract

2 teaspoons Splenda

2 tablespoons (28 g) butter

2 tablespoons (15 g) slivered almonds

Put the swordfish in a resealable plastic bag. Combine the lemon juice, olive oil, orange extract, and Splenda. Reserve some of the marinade and pour the rest into the bag. Seal the bag, pressing out the air as you go, and turn the bag once or twice to coat the fish. Throw it in the fridge. Let your fish marinate for an hour, turning it when you think of it.

Now, spray a skillet with nonstick spray and add half the butter. Melt over low heat and then add the swordfish steak. Pour off the marinade. Let the fish cook for 5 minutes and then turn it over and let it cook for another 5.

While the fish is cooking, melt the other half of the butter in a small skillet. Add the almonds and sauté, stirring frequently, until golden. If they're done before the fish is, remove from the heat.

When the 10 minutes of cooking time for the fish is up, add the reserved marinade to the pan. Let the fish cook another 2 to 3 minutes, turning once. Remove to a serving plate, pour the marinade over it, and top with the almonds. Serve.

Yield: 3 servings

Each with 31 g protein; 3 g carbohydrate; trace dietary fiber; 3 g usable carbs.

Panned Swordfish Steaks with Garlic and Vermouth

This dish is simple, fast, and elegant. And do you know how much you'd pay for this at a restaurant?

1 pound (455 g) swordfish steaks

Salt and pepper

1 tablespoon (15 ml) olive oil

¼ cup (60 ml) water

¼ cup (60 ml) dry vermouth

2 or 3 cloves garlic, crushed

3 to 4 tablespoons (11.4 to 15.2 g) minced parsley

Sprinkle the swordfish steaks lightly on both sides with salt and pepper.

Place a heavy skillet over high heat and add the olive oil. When the oil is hot, add the swordfish and sear on both sides (about 1 to 1½ minutes per side). Then add the water, vermouth, and garlic and turn down the heat to medium. Cover and let the fish simmer for 10 minutes.

Remove the fish to a serving platter or individual serving plates and keep warm. Turn the heat under the skillet to high and boil the pan juices hard for a minute or two until they're reduced to about ¼ cup (60 ml). Pour over the fish and top with parsley.

Yield: 3 servings

Each with 2 grams of carbohydrates, no fiber, and 32 grams of protein.

Swordfish Veracruz

This is so simple and quick—yet it's the sort of thing you'd pay big bucks for at a fancy restaurant. Salsa verde is a green salsa made from tomatillos. Look for it in the Mexican or international section of your grocery store.

24 ounces (680 g) swordfish steaks
½ cup (120 ml) ruby red grapefruit juice
   (I like to use fresh-squeezed.)
½ teaspoon ground cumin
1 tablespoon (15 ml) oil
¼ cup (65 g) salsa verde

Cut the swordfish into 4 servings and place on a plate with a rim. Mix together the grapefruit juice and the cumin. Reserve some marinade and pour the rest of it over the steaks, turning them to coat both sides. Let the swordfish steaks sit in the grapefruit juice for 5 minutes or so.

Spray a large, heavy skillet with nonstick cooking spray and place over medium heat. When the skillet is hot, add the oil and then the fish. Sauté for 4 minutes per side. Then pour in the reserved marinade and let the fish cook in it for another minute or two, turning once.

Place the fish on serving plates, top each serving with a tablespoon of salsa verde, and serve.

Yield: 4 servings

Each with 4 grams of carbohydrates, a trace of fiber, and 34 grams of protein.

Variation: You can expand this recipe a bit by serving the fish on a bed of avocado slices—split one avocado between the 4 servings—and sprinkling chopped fresh cilantro on top. This will take you up to 8 grams of carbohydrates per serving and 2 grams of fiber, for a total of 6 grams of usable carbs.

Curried Swordfish and Cabbage

I'll curry anything that stands still long enough! This is a fast and simple yet elegant meal, all made in one big skillet. But if you want to make more than 1 or 2 servings, you'll need to do it twice, or get a really, really huge skillet!

8 ounces (225 g) swordfish steak, 1½ inches
   (3.75 cm) thick
2 tablespoons (28 g) butter
1½ teaspoons curry powder
2 cups (150 g) shredded cabbage (You can
   used bagged coleslaw mix, if you like.)
¼ medium onion, sliced thin
1 clove garlic, crushed

Spray a big skillet with nonstick cooking spray. Melt the butter in it over low heat and add the curry powder. Let it cook for just a minute and then add the cabbage, onion, and garlic. Sauté the vegetables, stirring frequently, for 3 or 4 minutes.

Make a hole in the middle of the cabbage big enough to lay your swordfish steak on the pan. Cover the pan and set the oven timer for 5 minutes.

(continued on page 278)

When the timer beeps, turn the fish over and stir the cabbage. Re-cover the pan and set the timer for another 5 minutes. When time's up, serve the swordfish with the cabbage heaped around it.

Yield: 1 to 2 servings

Assuming 1, it will have 48 g protein; 13 g carbohydrate; 5 g dietary fiber; 8 g usable carbs.

Citrus-Ginger Mahi Mahi

1 pound (455 g) mahi mahi fillets
2 tablespoons (30 ml) lemon juice
¼ teaspoon orange extract
2 teaspoons soy sauce
½ teaspoon Splenda
1 tablespoon (6 g) grated ginger
1 tablespoon (15 ml) oil

This goes fast, so start a charcoal fire or preheat a gas grill before starting to prepare your food so you're not hanging around waiting for your fire to be ready.

On a plate with a rim or a glass pie plate, mix together everything but the fish. Lay the fish in the marinade and turn it over to coat. Let it sit for 15 to 30 minutes, at which point you want your grill to be medium-hot. Grill for just 5 to 6 minutes per side.

Yield: 2 to 3 servings

Assuming 2 servings, each will have 2 grams of carbohydrate—actually less, because you won't finish the marinade—a trace of fiber, and 41 grams protein.

Bacon-Wrapped Grilled Trout

This is simple and classic.

4 medium rainbow trout, cleaned, heads removed
8 sprigs fresh rosemary
8 slices bacon

Start a charcoal fire or preheat a gas grill.

Stuff the rosemary into the body cavities of the trout. Wrap each trout with 2 slices of bacon, covering as much of the skin of each fish as you can. Hold it in place with toothpicks you've soaked in water for a half hour or so. (It can be tough to get the toothpicks through the fish skin—use a metal skewer, a nut pick, or the point of a knife to assist, if needed.)

Grill over a medium fire, keeping down flare-ups with a water bottle, until the bacon is done and serve.

Yield: 4 servings

Each serving will have 1 gram of carbohydrate and a trace of fiber (which you'll get only if you eat the rosemary), and about 45 grams protein.

Truite au Bleu

This is more a method of preparation than a recipe, and it's a true classic. Expand or contract this recipe at will to serve however many diners you have.

Trout, cleaned and beheaded, but with the skin still on—about 10 ounces (280 g) per serving as a main course, or 5 or 6 ounces (140 to 170 g) per serving as a first course

Water

Cider vinegar

Bay leaves

Peppercorns or coarse cracked pepper

Salt or Vege-Sal

Butter

You'll need a pan big enough for the trout to lie flat—I generally do just one big trout, weighing about a pound (455 g), and the only pan I have where it can lie flat is my big soup pot. Use what you have, but it should be a pan that won't react with acid—stainless steel, enamelware, anodized aluminum, or stove-top glassware.

Next you make up a solution of water and vinegar, just enough to completely cover the trout. The proportions you want are roughly 3 or 4 parts water to 1 part vinegar. I find that 1½ quarts (1.4 L) of water and 1½ cups (360 ml) of vinegar are about right for my pan. Pour this solution in your pan and turn the heat to high.

Stir in 1 or 2 bay leaves, ½ tablespoon (3 g) of pepper per quart (litre), and 1 teaspoon (5 ml) of salt or Vege-Sal per quart (litre). Bring this mixture to a simmer.

Simply lower the trout into the simmering solution, reduce the heat to medium-low, and let the fish simmer for about 5 minutes. Lift the fish carefully out of the simmering solution and serve with a pitcher of melted butter to pour over the fish.

Yield: Servings will depend on how many fish you cook, of course.

The fish itself is carb-free, and of course most of the poaching solution is discarded—you can figure on no more than a gram of carbohydrates per serving, no fiber, and 59 grams of protein in a 10-ounce (280-g) trout.

Fried Catfish

I admit that without cornmeal this is somewhat inauthentic, but my catfish-loving spouse thought it was great. Catfish is among the least expensive fish, too, so this is a bargain to serve.

1 pound (455 g) catfish fillets

¼ cup (30 g) finely ground almonds

¼ cup (30 g) finely ground hazelnuts

2 tablespoons (16 g) rice protein powder

1½ teaspoons seasoned salt

1 egg

1 tablespoon (15 ml) water

Oil for frying (peanut, canola, or sunflower)

Lemon wedges

On a plate, combine the almonds, hazelnuts, protein powder, and seasoned salt, stirring well.

In a shallow bowl, beat the egg with the water.

Wash and dry the catfish fillets. Dip each one in the egg and then in the nut mixture, pressing it well into the fish.

If you have a deep fryer, by all means use it to fry your fish until it's a deep gold color (7 to 10 minutes). If you don't, use a large, heavy skillet. Pour 1 inch (2.5 cm) of oil into the skillet and put it over medium-high heat. Let it heat for at least 5 minutes; you don't want to put your fish in until the oil is up to temperature. (To test the oil, carefully put in one drop—no more—of water.

(continued on page 280)

It should sizzle, but not make the oil spit. If the oil spits, it's too hot. Turn the heat down and wait for it to cool a bit.)

When the oil is hot, put in your fish and fry it until it's a deep gold in color. If the oil doesn't completely cover the fish, you'll have to carefully turn it after about 5 minutes. (Figure 7 to 10 minutes total frying time.) Serve with lemon wedges.

Yield: Serves 3, unless one of them is my husband, in which case it may only serve 2

Assuming my husband isn't at your house (and if he is, I'd like to hear about it), each serving has 4 grams of carbohydrates and 1 gram of fiber, for a total of 3 grams of usable carbs and 30 grams of protein.

Citrus Catfish

Squeezing a little lemon over fish is a culinary classic—but this goes way beyond just lemon!

1½ pounds (680 g) catfish fillets
½ cup (120 ml) lemon juice
½ teaspoon orange extract
¼ cup (60 ml) soy sauce
2 tablespoons plus 2 teaspoons (4 g) Splenda
2 cloves garlic, crushed
¼ teaspoon pepper

Lay the fillets on a plate with a rim—a pie plate (or two) is ideal. Combine everything else, reserving some marinade for basting, and pour the rest over the fillets, turning to coat both sides. Let the fillets marinate for at least 15 minutes,

and a half hour won't hurt. Heat a gas grill or get a charcoal fire going in the meanwhile.

Make sure your grill is well oiled and grill the catfish over medium heat or well-ashed coals for about 5 minutes per side, basting it on both sides with the reserved marinade when you turn it—which you'll want to do carefully! When the fish is opaque and flaky, it's ready to serve.

Yield: 3 servings

6 grams of carb if you eat all of the marinade—I'd put it closer to 4 grams, a trace of fiber, and 29 grams of protein.

Indonesian Grilled Catfish

It's low-carb, low-fat, low-cal—this recipe is low in everything but flavor!

4 catfish fillets
¼ cup (60 ml) soy sauce
1 tablespoon (15 ml) rice wine vinegar
1 teaspoon Splenda
1 drop blackstrap molasses (If you keep your blackstrap molasses in a squeeze bottle, it's easy to measure just 1 drop.)
1 teaspoon grated ginger
1 clove garlic, crushed

Lay the catfish in a glass pie plate. Mix together everything else and pour over the catfish, turning to coat. Stash the whole thing in the fridge for at least a half hour, and a few hours would be great.

Flip the fish over halfway through to marinate both sides evenly.

Start a charcoal fire or preheat a gas grill. When marinating time is up, pull the fish out and throw it on a well-oiled grill over a medium fire. It shouldn't take more than 3 to 5 minutes per side to be flaky and done—turn it carefully!

Yield: 4 servings

Each serving will have 2 grams of carbohydrate, a trace of fiber, and 27 grams of protein.

This is good served with a cucumber salad. (See page 144.)

Lemon-Balsamic Catfish Kebabs

Catfish nuggets are often quite inexpensive, and they're great for making kebabs. Adjust the heat in this recipe by what sort of hot pepper sauce you use—Tabasco if you like it fairly mild or habañero or Scotch bonnet sauce if you like it spicy!

1 pound (455 g) catfish nuggets (If your grocery store doesn't have catfish nuggets, cut up fillets.)
2 cloves garlic, crushed
2 tablespoons (30 ml) lemon juice
1 tablespoon (15 ml) balsamic vinegar
1 teaspoon soy sauce
¼ teaspoon ground rosemary
¼ to ½ teaspoon hot pepper sauce
Olive oil

Mix together everything but the catfish and the olive oil in a bowl big enough to hold the catfish nuggets. When the marinade ingredients are blended, add the catfish nuggets and stir them up so they're coated.

Let them marinate for at least 30 minutes—during which time you can be soaking 3 or 4 bamboo skewers in water so they won't catch fire on the grill.

Okay, start your fire; you'll want it at medium or a little lower. Skewer the catfish nuggets, doubling the long ones if necessary to avoid floppy, dangling bits. Pack the nuggets fairly closely to avoid drying. Brush the kebabs with a little olive oil and make sure the grill is well oiled, too. Now grill the kebabs for about 4 to 5 minutes per side or until flaky and then serve.

Yield: 3 to 4 kebabs

Assuming 3 servings, each will have 2 grams of carbohydrate (actually less, because you won't eat every drop of the marinade), a trace of fiber, and 25 grams of protein.

Tuna Melt Casserole

Hey, we all grew up on tuna casserole. Here's one with no noodles for the low-carb grownups we've become.

1 can (6 ounces, or 170 g) albacore tuna, drained and mashed
1 teaspoon oil

(continued on page 282)

1 cup (115 g) shredded Cheddar cheese

3 slices (1½ ounces, or 42 g) processed American cheese

3 eggs

3 tablespoons (20 g) ground flaxseed meal or low-carb bake mix

1 teaspoon garlic powder

½ to 1 teaspoon salt

Preheat the oven to 400°F (200°C, or gas mark 6) and grease a 9-inch (23-cm) pie plate with the oil.

In a large bowl, combine the tuna, cheeses, eggs, flaxseed meal, garlic, and salt. Mix well.

Pour the tuna mixture into the prepared pie plate, pat down firmly, and bake for approximately 30 minutes or until browned and bubbly.

Yield: 3 servings

Each with 5 grams of carbohydrates and 3 grams of fiber, for a total of 2 grams of usable carbs and 38 grams of protein.

Tuna Steaks with Peach-Citrus Relish

The quantity of relish is small here to keep the carb count low—just enough to point up the flavor of the fish.

2 pounds (910 g) tuna steaks

1 ripe peach

1 tablespoon (15 ml) lime juice

¼ teaspoon orange extract

1 clove garlic, crushed

1 tablespoon (1.5 g) Splenda

½ tablespoon soy sauce

Olive oil

First peel the peach, cut it in half, remove the stone, and dice it small. Stir in the lime juice, orange extract, garlic, Splenda, and soy sauce. Set this aside—indeed, you can do this a few hours in advance if you like and refrigerate the relish until dinnertime. If you do this, get the relish out of the fridge before you get ready to grill the fish—it will have more flavor at room temperature.

When it's time to cook, either light a charcoal fire and let the coals burn down till they're ash-covered or set your gas grill to medium. Cut the tuna steaks into serving portions and rub each one lightly with olive oil. Make sure your grill is well oiled and grill the tuna no more than 3 to 5 minutes per side—it should still be red in the middle. (I learned this the hard way. Cook a tuna steak until it's pink all the way through, and it will be dry and tough.) Divide the relish between the portions and serve.

Yield: 4 servings

Each serving will have 4 grams of carbohydrate and 1 gram of fiber, for a usable carb count of 3 grams; and 53 grams protein.

California Tuna Fritters

This makes a quick and different supper out of simple canned tuna. You can make this into a few big tuna burgers, if you prefer, to cut a few minutes off the cooking time, but we really like these as little fritters.

12 ounces (340 g) canned water-pack tuna, drained

1 stalk celery

6 scallions

½ green pepper

2 tablespoons (7.6 g) chopped parsley

1 egg

1 tablespoon (15 ml) spicy brown mustard or Dijon mustard

⅓ cup (30 g) rice protein powder

4 to 5 tablespoons (56 to 70 g) butter, divided

Plunk the celery, scallions, pepper, parsley, egg, and mustard in a food processor with the S-blade in place and pulse until the vegetables are chopped to a medium-fine consistency. Add the tuna and rice protein powder and pulse to mix.

Spray a large, heavy skillet with nonstick cooking spray and place over medium-high heat. Melt 2 to 3 tablespoons (28 to 42 g) of butter in it and drop in the tuna mixture by the tablespoonful. Fry until brown, turn, and brown other side. It takes two batches to cook all of this mixture in my skillet; add the rest of the butter when you make the second batch. Serve with Easy Remoulade Sauce (page 476), which takes all of 2 or 3 minutes to make.

Yield: 4 or 5 servings

Assuming 5 servings, and not including the Easy Remoulade Sauce, each will have 5 grams of carbohydrates and 1 gram of fiber, for a total of 4 grams of usable carbs and 32 grams of protein.

Pantry Seafood Supper

This is convenient because as the name strongly suggests it uses seafood you've got sitting in your pantry. If you've got seafood sitting in your freezer, you can use it instead—just let it cook an extra 30 minutes or so to make sure it's thawed and cooked through.

1 can (6 ounces, or 170 g) tuna, drained

1 can (6 ounces, or 170 g) crab, drained

1 can (6 ounces, or 170 g) shrimp, drained

¼ cup (45 g) roasted red peppers jarred in oil, diced small (about 1 pepper)

⅓ cup (20.3 g) chopped parsley

1 cup (70 g) chopped mushrooms

¾ cup (180 ml) chicken broth

¾ cup (180 ml) dry white wine

2 tablespoons (20 g) minced onion

2 teaspoons dried dill weed

½ teaspoon paprika

½ teaspoon hot pepper sauce

1 cup (240 ml) Carb Countdown dairy beverage

¼ cup (60 ml) heavy cream

Guar or xanthan

Combine the red peppers, parsley, mushrooms, broth, wine, onion, dill, paprika, and hot pepper sauce in a slow cooker. Cover the slow cooker, set it to low, and let it cook for 3 to 4 hours.

When the time's up, stir in the Carb Countdown and cream and thicken the sauce to your liking with guar or xanthan. Now stir in the tuna, crab, and shrimp and let it cook for another 15 to 20 minutes.

(continued on page 284)

Now you have a choice: You can eat this as a chowder or you can serve it over Cauliflower Rice (page 212) or low-carbohydrate pasta—or even over spaghetti squash. It's up to you.

Yield: 4 servings

Each with 33 g protein, 4 g carbohydrate, 1 g dietary fiber, 3 g usable carbs.

Scampi!

1 pound (455 g) raw shrimp in the shell
½ cup (115 g) butter
¼ cup (60 ml) olive oil
3 cloves garlic, crushed
¼ cup (60 ml) dry white wine
¼ cup (15.2 g) minced fresh parsley

Melt the butter with the olive oil in a heavy skillet over medium-low heat. Add the garlic and stir it around.

Add the shrimp to the skillet. If they're room temperature, they'll take 2 to 3 minutes per side; frozen shrimp will take 4 to 5 minutes per side. Be careful not to overcook them.

Add the wine and simmer for another 1 to 2 minutes. Serve garnished with the parsley and put out plenty of napkins!

Yield: 3 servings

Each with 3 grams of carbohydrates, a trace of fiber, and 31 grams of protein.

Feel free to increase this recipe to however much your skillet can hold. This makes a great fast-and-easy company dinner; just add a salad and some crusty bread for the carb-eaters and call it a party.

Shrimp and Andouille Jambalaya

If you can't find andouille, just substitute the lowest-carb smoked sausage you can find.

2 cups (260 g) shelled, deveined, medium-size
**   shrimp (41/50 count)**
12 ounces (340 g) andouille sausage,
**   sliced ½ inch thick**
¼ cup (60 ml) olive oil
1⅓ cups (215 g) chopped onion
2 cloves garlic, crushed
1 large green pepper, diced
1 can (14½ ounces, or 410 g) diced tomatoes,
**   including liquid**
1 cup (240 ml) chicken broth
1 teaspoon dried thyme
6 cups (900 g) Cauliflower Rice (about one
**   good-size cauliflower; page 212)**
Salt and pepper
Hot pepper sauce

In a Dutch oven, start browning the andouille in the olive oil. When it's lightly golden on both sides, add the onion, garlic, and green pepper. Sauté the vegetables until the onion starts getting translucent.

Add the tomatoes, chicken broth, and thyme and bring to a simmer. Let it simmer for 20 minutes or so, uncovered, to blend the flavors.

Add the "rice" and simmer for another 15 minutes or until the cauliflower is starting to get tender.

Add the shrimp and simmer for another 5 minutes or so—just long enough to cook the shrimp. Add salt, pepper, and hot pepper sauce to taste and serve.

Yield: 6 servings

Each with 12 grams of carbohydrates and 4 grams of fiber, for a total of 8 grams of usable carbs and 32 grams of protein.

Cajun Skillet Shrimp

I threw this together when my husband brought a friend home for a quick lunch. This takes no more than 10 minutes, and it was a big hit.

2 cups (260 g) shelled, deveined shrimp (cooked or uncooked)
3 tablespoons (45 ml) olive oil
1 clove garlic, crushed
1 small onion, sliced
½ green pepper
½ yellow pepper
1 teaspoon Cajun seasoning

Heat the oil in a heavy skillet over medium-high heat. If your shrimp are uncooked, throw them in now along with the garlic, onion, and peppers and

stir-fry them all together until the shrimp are pink all the way through and the vegetables are just tender-crisp. If you're using cooked shrimp, sauté the vegetables first and then add the shrimp and cook just long enough to heat them through. (I threw mine in still frozen, and they were thawed and hot in just 4 to 5 minutes.)

Sprinkle the Cajun seasoning over everything. Stir it in and serve.

Yield: 2 servings

Each with 11 grams of carbohydrates and 2 grams of fiber, for a total of 9 grams of usable carbs and 28 grams of protein.

Curried Shrimp in Coconut Milk

This is so exotic!

1 pound (455 g) large shrimp, shelled (31/35 count)
14 ounces (425 ml) coconut milk
1½ tablespoons (9 g) curry powder
1 clove garlic, crushed
1 teaspoon chili garlic paste
1 tablespoon (15 ml) fish sauce
2 teaspoons Splenda
3 scallions, sliced thin
¼ cup (16 g) chopped cilantro

In a large, shallow pan, combine the coconut milk, curry powder, garlic, and chili garlic paste. Heat over medium-low and let simmer 7 to 10 minutes.

(continued on page 286)

Add shrimp, fish sauce, and Splenda. Stir and let simmer for 5 to 7 more minutes or until shrimp are pink all the way through.

Stir in the scallions, let simmer for another minute, and serve—spoon over Cauliflower Rice (page 212) if desired or eat as is. Top each serving with chopped cilantro.

Yield: 3 servings

Each with 29 g protein; 12 g carbohydrate; 4 g dietary fiber; 8 g usable carbs.

Shrimp Alfredo

I invented this for my Alfredo-obsessed husband, and he loves it.

2 cups (260 g) thawed small, frozen shrimp, cooked, shelled, and deveined
2 cups (500 g) frozen broccoli "cuts"
3 tablespoons (42 g) butter
3 cloves garlic, crushed
¾ cup (180 ml) heavy cream
¼ teaspoon guar or xanthan
1 cup (100 g) grated Parmesan cheese

Steam or microwave the broccoli until tender-crisp.

Melt the butter in a heavy skillet over medium heat and stir in the garlic. Drain the broccoli and add it to the skillet with the shrimp; stir to coat with garlic butter.

While the shrimp is heating through, put the cream in the blender, turn it to a low speed, and add the guar. Turn the blender off quickly so you don't make butter.

Pour the cream into the skillet and stir in the

Parmesan. Heat to a simmer and serve.

Yield: 3 servings

Each with 11 grams of carbohydrates and 4 grams of fiber, for a total of 7 grams of usable carbs and 30 grams of protein.

Easy Shrimp in Garlic Herb Cream Sauce

This seems too easy! You may use full-fat garlic and herb cheese—such as Boursin or Alouette—if you prefer. Your calorie count will go up but not your carb count.

1 pound (455 g) large shrimp, shelled (31/35 count)
2 tablespoons (28 g) butter
½ cup (115 g) light garlic and herb spreadable cheese
¼ cup (60 ml) heavy cream
4 tablespoons (15.2 g) chopped fresh parsley

Make sure your shrimp are shelled and ready to go. Melt the butter in a big skillet over medium heat and throw in the shrimp. Sauté for 2 to 3 minutes per side or until pink. Add the cheese and stir until it melts. Your sauce will look like a gloppy mess. Do not panic. Stir in the cream, and the whole thing will smooth out beautifully as you stir. Transfer to serving plates, top with parsley, and serve.

Yield: 3 servings

Each with 29 g protein; 3 g carbohydrate; 1 g dietary fiber; 2 g usable carbs.

Brined Lemon Pepper Shrimp

Brining shrimp makes them plumper and firmer—some say the texture resembles lobster. It adds flavor, too! I mean, what is sea water but a kind of brine? If you want to be terribly authentic, use sea salt!

FOR THE BRINE:

2 tablespoons (40 g) kosher salt or large-crystal sea salt

1 quart (960 ml) cold water

2 tablespoons (3 g) Splenda

¼ teaspoon blackstrap molasses

1 pound (455 g) shrimp in the shell—whatever size you like

FOR THE SEASONING:

2 cloves garlic

¼ cup (60 ml) olive oil

2 tablespoons (12 g) lemon pepper

To brine the shrimp: Dissolve the salt in the water. Stir in the Splenda and molasses. Now pour this mixture over the shrimp you've placed in a bowl or in a large resealable plastic bag. If you're using a bag, press out the air and seal it. Either way, make sure the shrimp are submerged. Let them sit in the brine for 30 to 45 minutes for medium-size shrimp or as much as an hour for really huge ones.

To cook: While your shrimp are brining, crush the garlic and pour the olive oil over it. That way, you'll have garlic-flavored olive oil by the time the shrimp are ready to cook.

Drain the brine off of the shrimp and pat them dry with a paper towel. Put the shrimp in a bowl, pour the garlic olive oil over them, and toss. Now sprinkle the lemon pepper over them and toss again.

You'll need a small-holed grill rack or a grill wok—I like to use a grill wok for this. Lift the shrimp out of the olive oil with a fork to let the excess oil drip off and put over a medium-hot fire. Grill quickly, turning two or three times, until pink all the way through—the timing will depend on the size of your shrimp, but it shouldn't take more than 6 or 7 minutes. If the olive oil causes flare-ups, keep them down with a squirt bottle.

Yield: 3 to 4 servings

Assuming 3, each serving would have 6 grams of carb—if you drank the brine (but you won't, of course). So figure no more than 4 grams per serving, a trace of fiber, and 31 grams of protein. (You'll actually get a little more protein if you cook big shrimp than if you cook little ones, because of the better shrimp-to-shell ratio.).

Variation: Brined Old Bay Shrimp. For the seasoning, use ¼ cup (60 ml) olive oil and 2 tablespoons (13 g) Old Bay Seasoning (look for this in the spice aisle). Drain the brined shrimp and pat them dry. Put them in a bowl, pour the olive oil over them, and toss. Sprinkle the Old Bay Seasoning over the shrimp and toss again. Finish as directed above.

(continued on page 288)

Yield: 3 to 4 servings.

Assuming 3, figure about 2 grams carbohydrate per serving, with no fiber, and 31 grams of protein.

Obscenely Rich Shrimp

This is a bit of trouble, and it's not cheap, so you'll probably only want to make it for company—but wow.

1 bag (14 ounces, or 400 g) frozen, cooked, shelled shrimp (small shrimp—51/60 count)

2 packages (10 ounces, or 280 g each) frozen chopped spinach

3 tablespoons (42 g) butter

1 pound (455 g) mushrooms, sliced

1 small onion, diced

2 teaspoons liquid beef bouillon concentrate

1½ cups (360 ml) heavy cream

1 cup (230 g) sour cream

1 cup (100 g) grated Parmesan cheese

1 cup (70 g) unsweetened flaked coconut

Preheat the oven to 350°F (180°C, or gas mark 4).

Cook the spinach; I put mine in a glass casserole dish, cover it, and microwave it on high for 7 minutes.

Meanwhile, melt the butter in a heavy skillet over medium heat and start sautéing the mushrooms and onions. When they're starting to get limp, break up the frozen shrimp a bit and add them to the skillet.

When the shrimp are thawed and the onions are quite limp and translucent, scoop out the vegetables and shrimp with a slotted spoon and put them aside in a bowl. Turn up the heat to medium-high. A fair amount of liquid will have accumulated in the bottom of the skillet; add the beef bouillon concentrate to it and boil the liquid until it's reduced to about one-third of its original volume.

Turn the heat back down to low, stir in the heavy cream, sour cream, and Parmesan and just heat it through (don't let it boil). Stir the shrimp and vegetables back into this sauce.

Rescue your spinach from the microwave and drain it well by putting it in a strainer and pressing it with the back of a spoon to make sure all the liquid is removed.

Spray a 10-cup (2.4-L) casserole dish with nonstick cooking spray and spread half of the spinach in the bottom of it. Put half of the shrimp mixture over that. Repeat the layers with the rest of the spinach and the rest of the sauce.

Top with the coconut and bake for 1½ hours.

Yield: 6 servings

Each with 15 grams of carbohydrates and 5 grams of fiber, for a total of 10 grams of usable carbs and 26 grams of protein. (Not to mention outrageous amounts of fat, but that doesn't bother us!)

Hot Paprika Shrimp

1 pound (455 g) large shrimp, shelled

¼ cup (60 ml) oil

4 teaspoons paprika

4 teaspoons chili garlic paste

4 cloves garlic, crushed

Just sauté the shrimp in the oil for about 5 minutes until it's pink. Sprinkle the paprika over it and stir in the chili garlic paste and garlic. Cook for another minute or so and serve.

Yield: 2 to 3 servings

Assuming 3, each will have 26 g protein; 4 g carbohydrate; 1 g dietary fiber; 3 g usable carbs.

Saigon Shrimp

This dish is vietnamese style—hot and a little sweet.

1 pound (455 g) large shrimp, shelled and deveined (31/35 count)

Scant ½ teaspoon salt

Scant ½ teaspoon pepper

1½ teaspoons Splenda

3 scallions

¼ cup (60 ml) peanut or canola oil

1½ teaspoons chili garlic paste

2 teaspoons minced garlic

Mix together the salt, pepper, and Splenda in a small dish or cup. Slice the scallions thinly and set them aside. Gather all the ingredients except the scallions together—the actual cooking of this dish is lightning-fast!

In a wok or heavy skillet over highest heat, heat the oil. Add the shrimp and stir-fry for 2 to 3 minutes or until they're about two-thirds

pink. Add the chili garlic paste and garlic and keep stir-frying. When the shrimp are pink all over and all the way through, sprinkle the salt, pepper, and Splenda mixture over them and stir for just another 10 seconds or so. Turn off the heat and divide the shrimp between 3 serving plates. Top each serving with a scattering of sliced scallion and serve.

Yield: 3 servings

Each with 2 grams of carbohydrates and 1 gram of fiber, for a total of 1 gram of usable carbs and 25 grams of protein.

This dish comes in at a low 288 calories a serving.

Shrimp and Artichoke "Risotto"

Not only is it lower carb and lower calorie to use cauli-rice to make "risotto," but it's tremendously quicker and easier, too. I adapted this recipe from one of Emeril's, and it's fabulous. You can use precooked or raw shrimp in this—since you're using the tiniest shrimp you can find, the cooking time is next to nothing anyway. Just make sure your shrimp are pink before you serve this—which should take approximately a minute and a half.

½ pound (225 g) extra small shrimp (61/70 count)

½ head cauliflower, shredded

½ cup (80 g) chopped onion

4 cloves garlic

(continued on page 290)

1 tablespoon (15 ml) olive oil

1 tablespoon (4.5 g) dried basil, or ¼ cup (10.6 g) chopped fresh basil

1 tablespoon (15 ml) lemon juice

1 teaspoon salt or Vege-Sal

½ teaspoon pepper

1 can (14 ounces, or 400 g) artichoke hearts, drained and chopped

1 teaspoon Creole Seasoning (page 485 or purchased)

½ cup (120 ml) heavy cream

¾ cup (75 g) grated Parmesan cheese

4 scallions, sliced, including the crisp part of the green shoot

Guar or xanthan

Put the cauliflower in a microwaveable casserole dish with a lid. Add a couple of tablespoons (30 ml) of water, cover, and microwave on high for 6 minutes.

While that's happening, throw the onion and garlic in a big, heavy skillet along with the olive oil. Sauté over medium-low heat until the microwave beeps—you want the onion to be turning translucent.

Okay, cauliflower's done. Pull it out, drain it, and add it to the onions and garlic. Stir in the basil, lemon juice, salt or Vege-Sal, pepper, chopped artichoke hearts, Creole Seasoning, shrimp, and cream. Let the whole thing simmer for a minute or two to blend the flavors. Stir in the Parmesan and scallions, thicken just until good and creamy with guar or xanthan, and serve.

Yield: 4 servings

Each with 22 g protein; 14 g carbohydrate; 2 g dietary fiber; 12 g usable carbs.

Noodleless Shrimp Pad Thai

This isn't terribly low in carbs—it's a maintenance dish, really—but I know that there are a lot of Thai food fans out there. So this is a lot lower-carb than Pad Thai with noodles, plus it's fast and incredibly tasty.

12 cooked, peeled shrimp

2 tablespoons (30 ml) Thai fish sauce

1 tablespoon (1.5 g) Splenda

2 tablespoons (30 ml) peanut oil or other bland oil

2 cloves garlic, smashed

2 eggs, beaten slightly

3 cups (675 g) cooked spaghetti squash, shredded

1½ cups (75 g) bean sprouts

2 tablespoons (16 g) dry-roasted peanuts, chopped

4 scallions, sliced

2 tablespoons (8 g) cilantro, chopped

1 lime, cut into wedges

Mix the fish sauce and Splenda and set the mixture aside.

Put the oil in a heavy skillet over medium-high heat and sauté the garlic for a minute. Add the shrimp and sauté for another minute. Add the fish sauce mixture.

Pour the beaten eggs into the skillet, let them set for 15 to 30 seconds, and then scramble. Stir in the spaghetti squash and bean sprouts, mixing with the shrimp and egg mixture. Cook until just heated through.

Place on serving plates. Top each serving with chopped peanuts, scallions, and cilantro and serve with a wedge of lime on the side.

Yield: 3 servings

Each with 19 grams of carbohydrates and 2 grams of fiber, for a total of 17 grams of usable carbs and 13 grams of protein.

If this carb count sounds way too high to you, keep in mind that regular Pad Thai usually has over 60 grams of carbohydrates per serving.

Shrimp in Sherry

This calls for 18 ounces (500 g) of shrimp because the big shrimp I get at my grocery run just about 1 ounce (30 g) apiece, and 6 big shrimp seemed a good serving size. But if you only have a pound of shrimp, don't sweat it.

18 ounces (500 g) extra jumbo shrimp—about an ounce (30 g) apiece—shelled (16/20 count)
3 tablespoons (45 ml) olive oil
3 tablespoons (45 ml) dry sherry
¼ teaspoon hot pepper sauce
Guar or xanthan

Have the shrimp shelled and ready to go. In a big skillet, sauté the shrimp in the olive oil over medium-high heat until they're pink almost all over. Add the sherry and hot pepper sauce and stir. Let cook another minute or two. Thicken the pan juices just a tiny bit with guar or xanthan and serve.

Yield: 3 servings

Each with 28 g protein; trace carbohydrate; trace dietary fiber; trace usable carb.

Shrimp Stewed in Curry Butter

Don't bother with napkins; put the roll of paper towels on the table—this is messy! It's delicious, though.

24 large, raw, "easy peel" shrimp (31/35 count)
6 tablespoons (84 g) butter
2 teaspoons curry powder
1 teaspoon minced garlic or 2 cloves garlic, crushed

Melt the butter in a large, heavy skillet over lowest heat. Stir in the curry powder and garlic and then add the shrimp in a single layer. Cook for 3 to 5 minutes per side or until the shrimp are pink all the way through. Transfer to serving plates and scrape the extra curry butter over them.

Yield: 2 servings

Each with 2 grams of carbohydrates, 1 gram of fiber (if you lick up every last drop of the curry-garlic butter), for a total of a bit less than 1 gram of usable carbs per serving and 15 grams of protein.

Spicy Shrimp in Beer and Butter

24 ounces (680 g) jumbo shrimp, shelled (21/25 count)

6 tablespoons (84 g) butter

¾ teaspoon salt

1½ teaspoons cayenne

¾ teaspoon dried thyme

½ teaspoon dried ground rosemary

½ teaspoon dried oregano

6 cloves garlic, crushed

1 tablespoon (15 ml) Worcestershire sauce

¾ cup (180 ml) light beer (I use Miller Lite or Milwaukee's Best Light.)

In a big, heavy skillet over very low heat, start melting the butter. As it melts, stir in the salt and the next 6 ingredients (through Worcestershire sauce). When the butter is all melted, add the shrimp—I like to use good, big ones about an ounce (28 g) apiece. Let the shrimp sauté 2 to 3 minutes per side, letting them get acquainted with the seasoned butter.

Now pour the light beer into the skillet. Cover the skillet and let the shrimp cook for 2 to 3 minutes. Uncover and let them cook for another 2 minutes or so.

Remove the shrimp to serving plates and turn up the heat under the skillet. Let the sauce boil hard until it's reduced by about half and then pour over the shrimp. Serve.

Yield: 3 to 4 servings

Assuming 3, each will have 38 g protein; 5 g carbohydrate; 1 g dietary fiber; 4 g usable carbs.

Shrimp in Brandy Cream

Wow—this dish is sheer elegance. And it's done in a flash!

1 pound (455 g) shrimp, shelled and deveined

4 tablespoons (56 g) butter

⅓ cup (80 ml) brandy

¾ cup (180 ml) heavy cream

Guar or xanthan (optional)

Sauté the shrimp in the butter over medium-high heat until cooked through—4 to 5 minutes. Add the brandy, turn up the heat, and let it boil hard for a minute or so to reduce. Stir in the cream and heat through. Thicken the sauce a bit with guar or xanthan if you like and then serve.

Yield: 3 or 4 servings

Assuming 3 servings, each will have 2 grams of carbohydrates, no fiber, and 26 grams of protein.

Sweet and Spicy Shrimp

1 pound (455 g) large shrimp, shelled (31/35 count)

2 tablespoons (30 ml) oil

½ teaspoon cayenne pepper

1½ teaspoons five-spice powder

2 cloves garlic, crushed

1 tablespoon (6 g) grated ginger

2 tablespoons (20 g) minced onion

2 tablespoons (30 ml) rice vinegar

2 tablespoons (3 g) Splenda

⅛ teaspoon blackstrap molasses

Salt and pepper

2 to 3 lime wedges

In a large, heavy skillet over medium-low, heat the oil and add the cayenne, five-spice powder, garlic, ginger, and onion. Stir for about 2 minutes or until fragrant, taking care not to let the garlic turn brown.

Stir in the rice vinegar, Splenda, and blackstrap molasses. Now add the shrimp and stir to coat with the seasonings. Sauté the shrimp, turning frequently, until they're pink all the way through. Season lightly with salt and pepper, transfer to serving plates, and serve with a lime wedge.

Yield: 2 to 3 servings

Assuming 2, each will have 38 g protein; 6 g carbohydrate; trace dietary fiber; 5 g usable carbs.

Sweet and Sour Shrimp

Adding the shrimp and snow peas at the last moment keeps them from becoming desperately overcooked.

1½ pounds (680 g) shrimp, shells removed

1 cup (220 g) peaches, peeled and cubed (Frozen unsweetened peaches work well. Just cut them into smaller chunks, about ½ inch, or 1.3 cm.)

½ cup (80 g) chopped onion

1 green bell pepper, diced

½ cup (60 g) chopped celery

½ cup (120 ml) chicken broth

2 tablespoons (30 ml) dark sesame oil

¼ cup (60 ml) soy sauce

2 tablespoons (30 ml) rice vinegar

¼ cup (60 ml) lemon juice

1 teaspoon red pepper flakes

1 tablespoon (1.5 g) Splenda

6 ounces (170 g) fresh snow pea pods, trimmed

⅓ cup (40 g) slivered almonds, toasted

Guar or xanthan

Put the peaches, onion, pepper, celery, broth, sesame oil, soy sauce, vinegar, lemon juice, red pepper flakes, and Splenda in a slow cooker and stir them together. Cover the slow cooker, set it to low, and let it cook for 4 hours. (Or you could cook it on high for 2 hours.)

When the time's up, turn the pot up to high while you trim the snow peas and cut them in 1-inch (2.5-cm) lengths. Stir them in and let it cook for 15 to 20 minutes. Now stir in the shrimp. If they're uncooked, give them 10 minutes or until they're pink through. If they're cooked already, just give them 5 minutes or so to get hot through.

You can serve this over rice for the carb-eaters in the family, of course. If you like, you can have yours on Cauliflower Rice (page 212), but this dish is high-carb enough already that I'd probably eat it plain.

Yield: 6 servings

Each with 27 g protein, 13 g carbohydrate, 3 g dietary fiber, 10 g usable carbs.

Coquilles St. Jacques

This is a seafood classic!

8 ounces (225 g) bay scallops
1 tablespoon (15 g) butter
1½ teaspoons minced onion
½ clove garlic, crushed
½ cup (35 g) chopped mushrooms
Salt and pepper
¼ cup (60 ml) dry white wine
½ cup (120 ml) heavy cream
Guar or xanthan
⅓ cup (40 g) shredded Gruyere

Preheat the broiler to low.

In a medium-size saucepan, melt the butter over medium-low heat. Add the onion and garlic and sauté for just a minute or so. Now add the mushrooms and sauté, stirring frequently, until mushrooms have changed color and are limp. Season a little with salt and pepper and add scallops and wine. Heat it to a bare simmer and let simmer just until scallops are opaque; do not overcook.

Using a slotted spoon, scoop out the scallops and mushrooms and divide between two large scallop shells or two ovenproof ramekins.

Turn up the heat under the liquid remaining in the saucepan and let it boil hard for just a minute or so to reduce. Turn heat back down and stir in cream. Now, using a whisk and the guar or xanthan, thicken the sauce up a bit. Add half the cheese and whisk until it's melted.

Divide the sauce between the two shells or ramekins and divide the remaining cheese between the two servings. Run the shells or ramekins under a low broiler about 4 inches (10 cm) from the heat until the tops have gotten golden—just 4 or 5 minutes. Serve.

Yield: 2 servings

Each with 26 g protein; 6 g carbohydrate; trace dietary fiber; 6 g usable carbs.

Scallops Vinaigrette

This recipe is fast and simple.

2 cups (350 g) bay scallops
2 tablespoons (20 g) minced onion
½ red bell pepper, cut in matchstick strips
4 teaspoons olive oil
¼ cup (60 ml) Italian salad dressing (I used Paul Newman's.)
Guar or xanthan

In a big skillet, sauté the onion and pepper in the olive oil for a couple of minutes. Add the scallops and sauté until they're white all the way through. Stir in the salad dressing and simmer for a couple of minutes. Thicken a little if you like and serve. Cauliflower Rice (page 212) is nice with this, though not essential.

Yield: 2 servings

Each with 40 g protein; 11 g carbohydrate; 1 g dietary fiber; 10 g usable carbs.

Lime-Basted Scallops

My seafood-loving husband thought these were some of the best scallops he'd ever had.

24 ounces (680 g) sea scallops
¼ cup (60 ml) lime juice
3 tablespoons (42 g) butter
2 cloves garlic
Guar or xanthan
¼ cup (16 g) chopped fresh cilantro

Put the lime juice, butter, and garlic in a slow cooker. Cover the slow cooker, set it to high, and let it cook for 30 minutes.

Uncover the slow cooker and stir the butter, lime juice, and garlic together. Now add the scallops, stirring them around to coat them with the sauce. Spread them in a single layer on the bottom of the slow cooker. (If the sauce seems to pool in one or two areas, try to cluster the scallops there. In my pot, the sauce liked to stay around the edges.) Re-cover the pot, set it to high, and let it cook for 45 minutes.

When the time's up, remove the scallops to serving plates. Thicken the pot liquid just a tiny bit with guar or xanthan and spoon the sauce over the scallops. Top each serving with 1 tablespoon (4 g) of cilantro.

Yield: 4 servings

Each with 29 g protein, 6 g carbohydrate, trace dietary fiber, 6 g usable carbs.

Stir-Fried Scallops and Asparagus

This stir-fry has a light, springlike flavor.

2 cups (350 g) bay scallops
10 asparagus spears
10 scallions
¼ cup (60 ml) canola oil
½ cup (60 g) shredded carrot
2 teaspoons soy sauce

Snap the bottoms off of the asparagus where the stalks break naturally. Slice on the diagonal into ½-inch (1.3-cm) pieces. Slice the scallions, too.

Heat the oil in a big skillet or in a wok, if you have one, over high heat.

Add the scallops, asparagus, scallions, and carrot. Stir-fry until the asparagus is tender-crisp and the scallops are cooked through. Stir in the soy sauce and serve.

Yield: 2 to 3 servings

Assuming 2, each will have 43 g protein; 18 g carbohydrate; 5 g dietary fiber; 13 g usable carbs.

Jalapeño Lime Scallops

I served this as a first course at a little dinner party, and everyone agreed they'd never had a better scallop dish, even at a restaurant. It's a sterling example of how a few perfect ingredients

(continued on page 296)

can combine to make something greater than the sum of the parts. By the way, you can use sea scallops instead of bay scallops if you like, but since they're bigger, they'll take longer to cook.

1½ pounds (680 g) bay scallops
4 tablespoons (56 g) butter
2 medium-size fresh jalapeños
3 tablespoons (45 ml) lime juice
3 tablespoons (12 g) chopped cilantro
Guar or xanthan

Melt the butter in a big, heavy skillet over medium heat. Add the scallops and sauté for a few minutes, stirring often. Meanwhile, split the jalapeños lengthwise and remove the stems, seeds, and ribs. Slice them lengthwise again, into quarters, and then slice them as thin as you can crosswise. Add to the skillet and sauté the jalapeños with the scallops until the scallops are cooked through—they should look quite opaque all over. (And wash your hands! You must always wash your hands after handling hot peppers or you'll be sorry the next time you touch your eyes, lips, or nose.)

Stir in the lime juice and cook for another minute while you chop the cilantro. Thicken the pan juices slightly with the guar or xanthan and divide the scallops between serving plates, spooning the pan juices over them. Scatter the cilantro on top and serve.

Yield: 4 main-dish servings or 6 first-course servings

Assuming 4 servings, each will have 6 grams of carbohydrates, a trace of fiber, and 29 grams of protein.

Scallops with Moroccan Spices

This dish is fast, easy, tasty, and different enough to be interesting! You can use bay scallops if you prefer, but I think the big sea scallops make for a more impressive presentation.

1 pound (455 g) sea scallops
2 tablespoons (30 ml) olive oil
2 tablespoons (28 g) butter
2 cloves garlic, crushed
1 teaspoon ground cumin
½ teaspoon ground ginger
2 teaspoons paprika
½ teaspoon hot pepper sauce
½ lemon
¼ cup (16 g) chopped fresh cilantro

In a big, heavy skillet, heat the olive oil and butter over medium heat and swirl them together. Add the garlic, let it cook for just a minute, and then add the cumin, ginger, paprika, and hot pepper sauce. Now add the scallops and sauté, stirring frequently for about 5 to 7 minutes or until they're opaque.

Squeeze the lemon over the scallops and transfer to 4 serving plates. Scatter 1 tablespoon (4 g) of cilantro over each plate and serve.

Yield: 4 servings

Each with 19 g protein; 5 g carbohydrate; trace dietary fiber; 5 g usable carbs.

Lemon-Maple Scallop Kebabs

These are bacon-wrapped scallops, but they're so different!

32 sea scallops (about a pound, or 455 g)
½ cup (120 ml) lemon juice
½ cup (120 ml) sugar-free pancake syrup
Barbecue rub—your choice; Classic Barbecue Rub (page 486) is good here
16 slices bacon

Put the scallops in a bowl. Mix together the lemon juice and pancake syrup, reserving some marinade for basting, and pour the rest over the scallops. Give them a stir. Then let them marinate for at least a half hour, and a few hours won't hurt—stir them now and again while they marinate.

At least 30 minutes before cooking time, put 4 bamboo skewers in water to soak. Get your grill going before you assemble your kebabs.

Okay, time to make kebabs. With a fork or slotted spoon, lift the scallops out of their Marinade. Pat them dry with a paper towel and put them on a plate. Sprinkle them liberally with the barbecue rub.

Cut the slices of bacon in half. Wrap each scallop around its circumference with a half-slice of bacon, piercing with a bamboo skewer to hold. Put 8 bacon-wrapped scallops on each skewer.

Grill, turning once or twice, over a medium-hot fire—have a water bottle on hand to put out flare-ups. Baste once or twice with the reserved lemon-maple marinade, using a clean utensil each time. Cook until the bacon is done and the scallops are fairly firm.

Yield: 4 servings

If you consumed all the marinade, you'd get 15 grams of carb per serving, not counting the polyols in the pancake syrup, but you're not going to. I'd give a generous estimate of 5 grams of carbohydrate per serving; 28 grams protein.

Broiled Orange Chili Lobster

If you ever manage to get tired of lobster with lemon butter or lobster with curried mayonnaise, try this.

4 lobster tails, split down the back of the shell
2 tablespoons (28 g) butter
1½ teaspoons chili garlic paste
¼ teaspoon orange extract
½ teaspoon Splenda
1 teaspoon lemon juice

Preheat the broiler.

The lobster tails should have their shells split along the back. Put them on a broiler rack.

Melt the butter and then stir in everything else. Baste the lobster tails with this mixture, being sure to get some down into the shell. Place the tails 5 to 6 inches (13 to 15 cm) under the broiler, set on high.

Broil for 7 to 8 minutes. Baste every couple of minutes with the butter mixture, using a clean utensil each time. End the basting about 2 minutes before the end of cooking time. Serve.

(continued on page 298)

Yield: 4 servings

Each with 53 g protein; 2 g carbohydrate; trace dietary fiber; 2 g usable carbs.

Oysters en Brochette

Oysters are an oddity in the world of animal protein because they actually contain a few carbs of their own. Still, they're quite nutritious (loaded with zinc), and many people love them. This makes an elegant appetizer or a very light supper.

16 large oysters
6 slices bacon
24 mushrooms
Butter (optional)
Lemon wedges (optional)

Preheat the broiler.

You'll either need metal skewers for this or you'll need to think far enough ahead to put 6 bamboo skewers in water to soak for a few hours before you begin cooking.

Either way, simply skewer a slice of bacon near the end and then skewer a mushroom. Fold the strip of bacon back over, skewering it again, add an oyster, and fold and skewer the bacon again—you're weaving the bacon in and out of the alternating mushrooms and oysters, see?

Lay the skewers on a broiler pan and broil them close to the heat with the broiler on low for about 10 minutes. Turn once or twice until the oysters are done and the bacon's getting crisp.

You can baste these with butter while they're broiling if you like, but it's not strictly necessary. Serve one skewer per person as a first course, with lemon wedges if you like.

Yield: 3 servings

Each with 8 grams of carbohydrates and 2 grams of fiber, for a total of 6 grams of usable carbs and 10 grams of protein.

Two Variations: My husband, who refers to mushrooms as "slime," likes these without the mushrooms. This cuts the carb count down to just 2 grams per serving.

If you'd like to impress the guests at your next party, you can cut strips of bacon in half and wrap each half-strip around an oyster, piercing with a toothpick to hold. Broil as directed above until the bacon gets crispy and serve hot. These are called Angels on Horseback—I have no idea why—and they're a classic hot appetizer. These will have just a trace of carbohydrates per piece.

10

Poultry

Drunken Chicken Wings

I'd call these Chinese-inspired except for the bourbon, which is all-American. How about calling it East-Meets-West?

20 whole chicken wings, or 40 drummettes
1 tablespoon (15 ml) fish sauce (nuoc mam or nam pla)
1 tablespoon (6 g) grated ginger
2 teaspoons black pepper
1 teaspoon chili garlic paste
¼ cup (6 g) Splenda
2 tablespoons (30 ml) sugar-free imitation honey
¼ cup (60 ml) bourbon

Throw your wings into a large resealable plastic bag. Mix together everything else. Reserve some of the marinade for basting and pour the rest over the wings. Press out the air, seal the bag, and toss it in the fridge. Let your wings live it up for at least a few hours.

When it's time to cook, light your grill; you'll want it medium-high. When the fire is ready pour off the marinade and arrange the wings on the grill. Grill for 7 to 10 minutes per side, basting often with the reserved marinade. Make sure you use clean utensils each time you baste to avoid cross-contamination. Serve.

Yield: You will, of course, have 20 wings or 40 drummettes—how many servings will depend on whether you're serving these as a main dish or an appetizer.

Whichever, each whole wing will have well under 1 gram of usable carbohydrate, and 9 grams of protein. Halve those figures for drummettes. Carb count does not include polyol in sugar-free honey.

Roast Chicken with Balsamic Vinegar

This has wonderfully crunchy skin and a sweet-and-tangy sauce to dip bites of chicken in.

1 cut up broiler-fryer
Bay leaves
Salt or Vege-Sal
Pepper
3 to 4 tablespoons (45 to 60 ml) olive oil
3 to 4 tablespoons (42 to 56 g) butter
½ cup (60 ml) dry white wine
3 tablespoons (45 ml) balsamic vinegar

Preheat the oven to 350°F (180°C, or gas mark 4).

Tuck a bay leaf or two under the skin of each piece of chicken. Sprinkle each piece with salt and pepper and arrange them in a roasting pan.

Drizzle the chicken with olive oil and dot them with the same amount of butter. Roast in the oven for 1½ hours, turning each piece every 20 to 30 minutes. (This makes for gloriously crunchy, tasty skin.)

When the chicken is done, put it on a platter and pour off the fat from the pan. Put the pan over medium heat and pour in the wine and balsamic vinegar. Stir this around, dissolving the tasty brown stuff stuck to the pan to make a sauce. Boil this for just a minute or two, pour into a sauceboat or a pitcher, and serve with the chicken. Discard the bay leaves before serving.

Yield: 4 servings

Each with 2 grams of carbohydrates, a trace of fiber, and 44 grams of protein.

Orange-Five-Spice Roasted Chicken

This is my way of combining my love of Chinese food with the current trend toward citrus flavors. It's good, too!

3 pounds (1.4 kg) chicken thighs
¼ cup (60 ml) soy sauce
2 tablespoons (30 ml) canola or peanut oil
1 tablespoon (15 ml) lemon juice
1 tablespoon (15 ml) white wine vinegar
1 tablespoon (1.5 g) Splenda
2 tablespoons (40 g) low-sugar orange marmalade
2 teaspoons five-spice powder

Place the chicken in a big resealable plastic bag. Mix together everything else. Reserve some of the marinade for basting and pour the rest into the bag. Seal the bag, pressing out the air as you go. Turn the bag to coat the chicken and throw it in the fridge. Let it sit for at least a couple of hours, and longer is fine.

Preheat your oven to 375°F (190°C, or gas mark 5). Haul the chicken out of the fridge, pour off the marinade, and arrange the chicken in a baking pan. Roast your chicken for 1 hour and baste 2 or 3 times with the reserved marinade, making sure to use a clean utensil each time you baste to avoid cross-contamination.

Yield: 5 to 6 servings

Assuming 6, each will have 32 g protein; 3 g carbohydrate; trace dietary fiber; 3 g usable carbs—and that's assuming you end up consuming all of the marinade.

Greek Roasted Chicken

Many carry-out places do a brisk business in chickens roasted Greek-style, and it's no wonder why—they're terrific. But the best-kept secret about those roasters is that they're as easy as can be to make at home.

3 to 4 pounds (1.4 to 1.8 kg) of chicken (whole, split in half, cut-up broiler-fryer, or cut-up parts of your choice)
¼ cup (60 ml) lemon juice
½ cup (120 ml) olive oil
½ teaspoon salt
¼ teaspoon pepper

Wash the chicken and pat it dry with paper towels.

Combine the lemon juice, olive oil, salt, and pepper and stir them together well. If you're using a whole chicken, rub it all over with some of this mixture, making sure to rub plenty inside the body cavity as well. If you're using cut-up chicken, put it in a large resealable plastic bag, pour the marinade over it, and seal the bag.

Let the chicken marinate for at least an hour or as long as a day.

(continued on page 302)

At least 1 hour before you want to serve the chicken, pull it out of the bag. You can either grill your chicken or you can roast it in a 375°F (190°C, or gas mark 5) oven for about 1 hour. Either way, cook it until the juices run clear when it's pierced to the bone.

Yield: 5 servings

Each with less than 1 gram of carbohydrates, a bare trace of fiber, and 52 grams of protein.

If you have a rotisserie, this is a terrific dish to cook in it. Follow the instructions that come with your unit for cooking times.

Absolutely Classic Barbecued Chicken

You'll notice that this is remarkably similar to the Absolutely Classic Barbecued Ribs (page 435), the only difference being that it's chicken!

3 pounds (1.4 kg) cut-up chicken (on the bone, skin on—choose light or dark meat, as you prefer)
⅓ cup (40 g) Classic Barbecue Rub (page 486)
½ cup (120 ml) chicken broth
½ cup (120 ml) oil
½ cup (120 ml) Kansas City Barbecue Sauce (page 467)
Wood chips or chunks, soaked for at least 30 min

Get your grill going, setting it up for indirect smoking.

While the grill's heating, sprinkle the chicken with all but a tablespoon of the rub. Combine the reserved rub with the chicken broth and oil to make a mop.

When your fire is ready, place the chicken over a drip pan, add the wood chips or chunks, and close the grill. Let it smoke for half an hour before you start to baste it with the mop. Then mop it every time you add more chips or chunks, using a clean utensil each time you baste. Smoke the chicken for about 90 minutes or until an instant-read thermometer registers 180°F (85°C). When the chicken is just about done, baste the skin side with the Kansas City Barbecue Sauce and move it over the fire, skin-side down, for 5 minutes or so. Baste the other side with the sauce using a clean utensil, turn it over, and give it another 5 minutes over the fire. Boil the remainder of the sauce and serve with the chicken.

Feel free to use this same basic method with any rub and any sauce!

Yield: 5 servings

Each serving will have 9 grams of carbohydrate and 1 gram of fiber, for a usable carb count of 8 grams; 35 grams protein.

Korean Barbecued Chicken

Hot, spicy, garlicky, and a little sweet—this chicken is truly wonderful. And unlike classic American barbecued chicken, this is actually grilled, so it cooks faster than the slow-smoked variety.

2 pounds (910 g) chicken pieces

2 tablespoons (33 g) chili garlic paste

3 tablespoons (45 ml) dry sherry

1 tablespoon (15 ml) soy sauce

4 cloves garlic, crushed

1½ tablespoons (23 ml) toasted sesame oil

1 tablespoon (6 g) grated ginger

2 scallions, minced

2 teaspoons black pepper

1 tablespoon (1.5 g) Splenda

Put the chicken in a large resealable plastic bag. Mix together everything else. Reserve some marinade for basting and pour the rest over the chicken. Press out the air, seal the bag, and toss it in the fridge. Let your chicken marinate for several hours.

When it's time to cook, fire up the grill. You'll want it at medium to medium-high. When the grill is ready for cooking, remove the chicken from the bag and pour off the marinade. Cook the chicken skin-side up for about 12 to 15 minutes, keeping the grill closed except when basting. Turn it skin-side down and let it grill for 7 to 9 minutes, again with the grill closed. Turn it skin-side up again and let it grill until the juices run clear when pierced to the bone and an instant-read thermometer registers 180°F (85°C). Baste several times with the reserved marinade while cooking, making sure to use a clean utensil each time you baste. Discard remaining marinade and serve chicken.

Yield: 4 servings

With all the marinade, each serving would have 4 grams of carbohydrate and 1 gram of fiber, but you won't consume all the marinade; I'd count no more than 3 grams per serving; 30 grams of protein.

Orange-Tangerine Up-the-Butt Chicken

Once someone figured out that standing a chicken up on a beer can made for a perfectly roasted chicken, soda-can chicken was inevitable!

1 3½ to 4-pound (1.6 to 1.8 kg) whole roasting chicken

1 teaspoon salt or Vege-Sal

1 teaspoon Splenda

1 drop blackstrap molasses (It helps to keep your molasses in a squeeze bottle.)

1 teaspoon chili powder

3 tablespoons (60 g) low-sugar orange marmalade

1 12-ounce (360-ml) can tangerine Diet-Rite soda, divided (Make sure the can is clean!)

2 to 3 teaspoons oil

1 teaspoon spicy brown mustard

Prepare your grill for indirect cooking—if you have a gas grill, light only one side; if you're using charcoal, pile the briquettes on one side of the grill and light.

Remove the neck and giblets from the chicken. Rinse the chicken and pat it dry with paper towels.

In a small bowl combine the salt or Vege-Sal, Splenda, molasses, and chili powder. Spoon out half the mixture (1½ teaspoons) into a bowl and reserve; rub the rest inside the cavity of your chicken.

(continued on page 304)

Stir the low-sugar orange marmalade into the reserved seasoning mixture. Open the can of tangerine soda and pour out 2/3 cup (160 ml). Put ¼ cup (60 ml) of the soda you poured off into the marmalade/seasoning mixture and stir it in—you can drink the remainder of the soda you poured off or throw it away. Now, using a church-key-type can opener, punch several more holes around the top of the can. Spray the can with nonstick cooking spray and set it in a shallow baking pan. Carefully place the chicken down over the can, fitting the can up into the cavity of the chicken. Rub the chicken with the oil.

Okay, you're ready to cook! Make sure you have a drip pan in place. Set the chicken, standing upright on its soda can on the side of the grill not over the fire and spread the drumsticks out a bit, making a tripod effect. Close the grill and cook the chicken at 250°F (130°C) or so for 75 to 90 minutes or until the juices run clear when it's pricked to the bone. You can also use a meat thermometer—it should register 180°F (85°C).

While the chicken is roasting, add the mustard to the marmalade/soda/seasoning mixture and stir the whole thing up. Use this mixture to baste the chicken during the last 20 minutes or so of roasting.

When the chicken is done, carefully remove it from the grill—barbecue gloves come in handy here or use heavy hot pads and tongs. Twist the can to remove it from the chicken and discard. Let the chicken stand for 5 minutes before carving. In the meantime, heat any leftover basting sauce to boiling—and serve as a sauce with the chicken.

Yield: 5 servings

Each serving will have 5 grams of carbohydrate and a trace of fiber. Assuming a 3½-pound (1.6-kg) chicken, each serving will have 40 grams of protein.

Cinnachick

This is really unusual and wonderful!

1 broiler-fryer, cut up—about 2½ to 3 pounds (1.1 to 1.4 kg)
½ cup (120 ml) dry sherry
3 tablespoons (45 ml) sugar-free imitation honey
3 tablespoons (4.5 g) Splenda
2 teaspoons ground cinnamon
1 teaspoon curry powder
1 clove garlic, crushed
½ teaspoon salt

Just combine everything but the chicken, reserving some marinade for basting, and pour the rest over the chicken in a shallow, nonreactive pan or a resealable plastic bag. If you're using a bag, press out the air and seal it. Put the chicken in the fridge and let it marinate for anywhere from a few hours to all day.

Then heat your grill—medium-high for a gas grill or well-ashed coals in a charcoal grill. Grill the chicken bone-side down for about 12 minutes and then turn it and grill it for 7 or 8 minutes skin-side down. Keep the hood closed except when turning the chicken or fighting off flare-ups with your squirt bottle. Turn it again and grill until juices run clear when the chicken is pierced to the bone. Baste the chicken frequently with the reserved marinade using a clean utensil each time you baste.

Yield: 4 servings

Each with 4 grams of carbohydrate, not counting the polyols in the imitation honey; 1 gram fiber. These figures, however, assume you'll consume all of the marinade, which you won't—so I'd guess no more than 2 grams per serving; 36 grams of protein.

Balsamic-Mustard Chicken

1 broiler-fryer chicken, about 3 pounds (1.4 kg), cut up, or whatever chicken parts you like
2 tablespoons (33 g) chili garlic paste
½ cup (120 ml) spicy brown mustard
¼ cup (60 ml) balsamic vinegar
¼ cup (60 ml) olive oil

Put the chicken parts in a large, heavy resealable plastic bag. Combine everything else and whisk together well. Reserve some marinade for basting and then pour the rest into the bag with the chicken, press out the air, and seal the bag. Throw the bag in the fridge and let the chicken marinate for anywhere from a few hours to all day.

When it's time to cook, light your charcoal or gas grill; you'll want a medium to medium-high fire. When the grill is ready, pull the chicken out of the marinade using tongs and place it on a plate. Pour off the marinade.

Now put the chicken on the grill skin-side up and grill it for 12 to 15 minutes. Turn it and let it grill for 7 to 9 minutes skin-side down. Turn it again and cook for another 5 to 10 minutes or until the juices run clear when it's pierced to the bone and an instant-read thermometer reads 180°F (85°C). Baste frequently with the reserved marinade using a clean utensil each time you baste. Keep the grill closed except when basting or turning the chicken.

Yield: 5 to 6 servings

Assuming 6 servings, if you consumed all the marinade, each would have 3 grams of carbohydrate and a trace of fiber, but actually you'll get less than that. Assuming 6 servings, each will have 30 grams of protein.

Spatchcocked (or UnSpatchcocked) Chicken with Vinegar Baste

Treating chicken to an acidic baste or marinade of some kind is a time-honored way of bringing out the flavor of our favorite fowl. This baste also adds some heat and complex spiciness—yum! What the heck is "spatchcocked" chicken? It's a chicken that's been cut along the backbone and opened up flat for easier grilling.

3½ pounds (1.6 kg) chicken—either whole or cut up
1 cup (240 ml) cider vinegar
3 teaspoons chili powder
2 tablespoons (3 g) Splenda
1 teaspoon cayenne
1 teaspoon paprika

(continued on page 306)

1 teaspoon dry mustard
1 teaspoon black pepper
½ teaspoon cumin
½ teaspoon salt

Technically, you're supposed to cut along both sides of the backbone and remove it entirely, but that's too much work for me, so I just let my chicken look uneven. I know this sounds hard, but if you have good poultry or kitchen shears—my Martha Stewart shears from Kmart work just fine—it takes all of about a minute and a half. Make the cut along the bottom side of the chicken, grab either side of the cut, and pull the chicken open. Press down on the breastbone until you hear a slight crack. Now you have a flat chicken you can lay on a grill.

Or you can just not bother. I'm describing the process because it's terribly, terribly trendy in grilling circles right now, and anyway, whole chickens are often quite cheap. However, I think it's easier just to use a cut-up chicken, you know? The baste works just as well with the parts, and you don't have to carve.

Either way, start by lighting your grill; you'll want it at medium heat. While the grill is heating, combine everything but the chicken.

Grill the chicken starting skin-side up, and keeping the grill closed except when basting or dealing with flare-ups, grill for 15 minutes, basting frequently with the vinegar mixture using a clean utensil each time. Turn skin-side down and grill for 7 to 9 minutes, still basting; then turn skin-side up again and continue grilling until juices run clear when chicken is pierced to the bone or an instant-read thermometer registers 180°F (85°C). Serve.

Yield: 5 servings

Even with all of the basting liquid you'd get only 5 grams of carb, with 1 gram of fiber, or 4 grams of usable carb per serving—but you won't consume all of the basting liquid. Count no more than 2 grams per serving; 40 grams of protein.

Sherry-Mustard-Soy Marinated Chicken

3½ to 4 pounds (1.6 to 1.8 kg) cut-up chicken
¼ cup (6 g) Splenda
3 tablespoons (45 ml) olive oil
3 tablespoons (45 ml) sherry
1 tablespoon (15 ml) mustard
1 tablespoon (15 ml) soy sauce
1 tablespoon (6.3 g) black pepper
½ tablespoon Worcestershire sauce
¼ cup (40 g) minced onion
1 clove garlic, crushed
2 tablespoons (30 ml) water

Combine everything but the chicken, mixing well. Put the chicken either in a shallow, nonreactive pan or in a large resealable plastic bag. Reserve some marinade for basting and pour the rest of the marinade over the chicken. If it's in a pan, turn it once or twice to coat. If it's in a bag, press out the air, seal the bag, and turn it a few times to coat the chicken. Either way, stick the chicken in the fridge and let it marinate for at least 1 or 2 hours, and longer won't hurt.

When the chicken is ready to grill, have the gas grill set to medium or the charcoal covered with white ash. Grill the chicken bone-side down for 10 to 12 minutes with the lid closed (but check now and then for flare-ups!), basting with the reserved marinade once or twice using a clean utensil each time you baste. Turn the chicken over with tongs and grill skin-side down for 6 to 7 minutes, again with the grill closed, but check now and then for flare-ups. Turn the chicken back to bone-side down, baste it one more time, and grill with the lid closed for another 5 to 10 minutes until the juices run clear when the chicken is pierced to the bone or until an instant-read thermometer reads 180°F (85°C).

Yield: 5 to 6 servings

Assuming 6, and assuming you consumed all the marinade, each serving would have 4 grams of carb and 1 gram of fiber, for a usable carb count of 3 grams. Since you won't consume all of the marinade, however, I'd count 2 grams per serving; 34 grams protein.

Tarragon Chicken

1 cut up broiler-fryer
2 tablespoons (28 g) butter
1 teaspoon salt or Vege-Sal
Pepper
3 tablespoons (4.8 g) dried tarragon leaves
1 clove garlic, crushed
½ cup (120 ml) dry white wine

If your chicken is in quarters, cut the legs from the thighs and the wings from the breasts. (It will fit in your skillet more easily this way.)

Melt the butter in a heavy skillet over medium-high heat and brown the chicken, turning it once or twice, until it's golden all over.

Pour off most of the fat and sprinkle the chicken with the salt and just a dash of pepper. Scatter the tarragon over the chicken, crushing it a little between your fingers to release the flavor, and then add the garlic and the wine.

Cover the skillet, turn the heat to low, and simmer for 30 minutes, turning the chicken at least once. Spoon a little of the pan liquid over each piece of chicken when serving.

Yield: 4 servings

Each with 2 grams of carbohydrates, a trace of fiber, and 44 grams of protein.

San Diego Chicken

A version of this recipe appeared in my local paper, and though it looked tasty, it was way too high-carb for us. I played around with it, cut out a lot of the carbs, and ended up with this recipe—fruity and tomato-y and yummy.

3 pounds (1.4 kg) cut-up chicken
1 8-ounce (220 ml) can tomato sauce
1 tablespoon (15 ml) lemon juice
1 tablespoon (15 ml) lime juice
⅛ teaspoon lemon extract
½ teaspoon orange extract
3 tablespoons (4.5 g) Splenda
3 tablespoons (45 ml) white wine vinegar (If you don't have any on hand, I'm sure cider vinegar would taste fine—different, but fine.)
2 cloves garlic, crushed
1 teaspoon Italian seasoning
1 teaspoon hot pepper sauce

(continued on page 308)

Mix together everything but the chicken pieces. Place the chicken pieces in a large resealable plastic bag and pour the tomato sauce mixture over it. Seal the bag, pressing out the air as you go, and turn to coat all the chicken pieces. Let your chicken marinate for at least a few hours, and I'm betting a day wouldn't hurt a bit.

When you're ready to cook: Get your grill ready—charcoal covered with white ash or gas grill set to medium. Pull the chicken out of the marinade and pour the marinade out of the bag and into a saucepan. Go throw the chicken on the grill, bone-side down. Close the lid and set a timer for 13 to 15 minutes.

While the chicken is grilling, put that pan of marinade over the heat and let it come to a boil. Now, go check your chicken for flare-ups—I keep a squeeze bottle of water by the grill to keep these at bay. You want your chicken cooked, not charred!

Has the timer gone "ding?" Turn the chicken using a pair of tongs. Set your timer for another 13 to 15 minutes. When time's up, turn it skin-side up again and pierce a piece to the bone to make sure all the juices are running clear. If there's any pink in the juices, let the chicken cook another few minutes.

When it's done, serve each piece with a little of that marinade you boiled spooned over the top. Enjoy!

Yield: 6 servings

Each serving will have 5 grams of carbohydrate and 1 gram of fiber, for a usable carb count of 4 grams; 29 grams of protein.

I use serious Jamaican scotch bonnet hot sauce in this, and it isn't scorch-your-mouth hot, just nicely spicy. If you want to, you can crank the heat up or down by either using more or less hot pepper sauce or using hotter or less-hot pepper sauce.

Curried Chicken

4 or 5 chicken quarters, cut up and skinned
1 medium onion
1 tablespoon (28 g) butter
1 rounded (6 g) tablespoon curry powder
1 cup (240 ml) heavy cream
3 or 4 cloves of garlic, crushed
½ cup (120 ml) water

Preheat the oven to 375°F (190°C, or gas mark 5).

Arrange the chicken in a shallow baking pan. Chop the onion and scatter it over the chicken.

Melt the butter in a small, heavy skillet and sauté the curry powder in it for a couple of minutes—just until it starts to smell good.

Mix together the cream, garlic, water, and sautéed curry powder and pour this over the chicken. Bake it uncovered for 1 hour to 1 hour and 20 minutes, turning the chicken over every 20 to 30 minutes so that the sauce flavors both sides.

To serve, arrange the chicken on a platter. Take the sauce in the pan (it will look dreadful and sort of curdled up, but it will smell like heaven) and scrape it all into your blender. Blend it with a little more water or cream, if necessary, to get a nice, rich, golden sauce. Pour it over the chicken and serve.

Yield: 4 generous servings

Each with 6 grams of carbohydrates and 1 gram of fiber, for a total of 5 grams of usable carbs and 42 grams of protein.

Pizza Chicken

This recipe is basically a skillet cacciatore, except for the mozzarella—that's what makes it Pizza Chicken.

3 chicken quarters, either legs or thighs
1 to 2 tablespoons (15 to 30 ml) olive oil
1 can (8 ounces, or 225 g) plain tomato sauce
1 can (4 ounces, or 115 g) mushrooms, drained
½ cup (120 ml) dry red wine
1 green pepper, chopped
1 small onion, chopped
1 or 2 cloves garlic, crushed, or 1 to 2 tea-
** spoons jarred chopped garlic in oil**
1 to 1½ teaspoons dried oregano
3 ounces (85 g) shredded mozzarella cheese
Parmesan cheese (optional)

Strip the skin off the chicken and cut the leg and thigh quarters in two at the leg joint.

Warm the olive oil in a big, heavy skillet and brown the chicken in it over medium heat.

Pour in the tomato sauce, mushrooms, and wine. Add the green pepper, onion, garlic, and oregano. Cover the whole thing, turn the heat to its lowest setting, and forget about it for 45 minutes to 1 hour.

When the chicken is cooked through, remove the pieces from the skillet and put them on the serving plates. If the sauce isn't good and thick by now, turn up the heat to medium-high and let the sauce boil down for a few minutes.

While the sauce is thickening, sprinkle the shredded mozzarella over the chicken and warm each plate in the microwave for 20 to 30 seconds on 50 percent power to melt the cheese. (Your microwave may take a little more or a little less time.)

Spoon the sauce over each piece of chicken and serve. Sprinkle a little Parmesan cheese over your Pizza Chicken, if you like.

Yield: 3 servings

Each with 16 grams of carbohydrates and 4 grams of fiber, for a total of 12 grams of usable carbs and 49 grams of protein.

Chicken Tenders

These are good for when you're having fast-food cravings or the kids are nagging for "normal" food. You really can make these in 15 minutes—because the pieces are small, they cook very quickly.

1 pound (455 g) boneless, skinless chicken
** breast**
1 egg
1 tablespoon (15 ml) water
¾ cup (85 g) low-carb bake mix
½ teaspoon salt
¼ teaspoon pepper
⅓ cup (80 ml) oil

(continued on page 310)

Cut the chicken breasts into pieces about 1 inch (2.5 cm) wide and 2 inches (5 cm) long. Beat the egg with the water in a bowl. On a plate, combine the bake mix with the salt and pepper. Heat the oil in a heavy skillet over medium-high heat.

Dip each chicken piece in the egg wash, roll it in the seasoned bake mix, and drop it in the hot oil. Fry these until golden all over and serve with one of the dipping sauces in the Sauces and Seasonings chapter (page 462).

Yield: 4 servings

Each with 5 grams of carbohydrates and 2 grams of fiber, for a total of 3 grams of usable carbs (exclusive of the dipping sauces) and 40 grams of protein.

Chicken Sancocho

This delicious, fresh-tasting Caribbean chicken stew/soup is not a quick recipe, but it's not terribly complicated, either. It's great to make over the weekend when you're getting other things done; you'll just check in with your food every so often. And it reheats like a dream! Sadly, the fresh pumpkin needed to make it is only available for a few months in autumn, but then this makes a great chilly-evening supper anyway!

1 whole chicken, about 5 to 5½ pounds (2.3 to 2.5 kg)

FOR THE MARINADE:
4 tablespoons (60 ml) lime juice
1½ cups (180 g) diced celery
1 large ripe tomato
1 medium onion
1 medium green pepper

½ tablespoon (2.3 g) poultry seasoning
½ teaspoon ground nutmeg
1 tablespoon ground cumin

FOR THE STEW:
1 quart (960 ml) chicken broth
1 large carrot, sliced
1½ cups (210 g) cubed rutabaga
1½ cups (175 g) cubed fresh pumpkin
1 small turnip, cubed
1 cup (150 g) cauliflower florets and stems, cut in small chunks
3 cups (225 g) shredded cabbage—Prepared coleslaw mix works nicely.
1 teaspoon to 1 tablespoon hot pepper sauce, or to taste—Use Caribbean Scotch bonnet sauce if you can get it!

Remove any giblets from the chicken's body cavity and place the chicken in a soup pot.

To make the marinade: Put all the marinade ingredients in a food processor with the S-blade in place (you'll want to cut everything in big chunks first and peel the onion and core the pepper and all) and pulse until you have a coarse slurry. Pour this mixture over the chicken and use clean hands to rub it all over, including into the body cavity. Stick the whole pot in the fridge and let the whole thing sit overnight, turning the chicken over once or twice in that time if you think of it.

To make the stew: The next day, pull the pot with the chicken out of the refrigerator, put it on the stove, and pour the chicken broth over the chicken. Cover it, put the whole thing over medium heat, bring it to a simmer, turn it down to low, and let it simmer for an hour. Turn it off and let the pot sit on the stovetop and cool.

When cooled, remove the chicken from the broth (big tongs work well for this), put it on a platter, and set it aside. Skim the excess fat from the broth and skim out the vegetables that were in the marinade—I used a Chinese skimmer for this, but you could just pour it through a sieve if you like. Be sure to press any broth out of the vegetables and back into the pot before you discard them!

Put the pot of skimmed broth back on the stove and turn the heat beneath it to medium-high. Stir in the carrot, rutabaga, pumpkin, and turnip and let the whole thing simmer for a half an hour. While that's cooking, remove the skin from the chicken and discard it. Then remove the meat from the bones, discard the bones, and cut the meat into bite-sized pieces. About 20 minutes before serving time, stir the chicken, the cauliflower, and the cabbage into the pot, along with the hot pepper sauce. Add water if needed, so that the broth is level with the top of the meat and vegetables. Simmer for 20 minutes and serve.

Yield: 8 servings

Each with 41 g protein; 13 g carbohydrate; 3 g dietary fiber; 10 g usable carbs—but that figure is actually a tad high, since you discard some of the vegetables. I'd call it 8 g per serving. There's lots of beta carotene and calcium, too.

Spicy Peanut Chicken

This takes 10 minutes to put together and only another 15 to cook. It's hot and spicy—quasi-Thai.

2 or 3 boneless, skinless chicken breasts
1 teaspoon ground cumin
½ teaspoon ground cinnamon
2 to 3 tablespoons (30 to 45 ml) olive or peanut oil for sautéing (I think peanut is better here.)
½ smallish onion, thinly sliced
1 can (14½ ounces, 410 g) diced tomatoes, undrained
2 tablespoons (32 g) natural peanut butter
1 tablespoon (15 ml) lemon juice
2 cloves garlic, crushed
Fresh jalapeño, cut in half and seeded

On a saucer or plate, stir the cumin and cinnamon together and then rub into both sides of chicken breasts.

Put the oil in a heavy skillet over medium heat and add the chicken and sliced onion. Brown the chicken a bit on both sides.

While that's happening, put all the liquid and half the tomatoes from the can of tomatoes in a blender or food processor along with the peanut butter, lemon juice, garlic, and jalapeño. (Wash your hands after handling that hot pepper or you'll be sorry the next time you touch your eyes!) Blend or process until smooth.

Pour this rather thick sauce over the chicken (which you've turned at least once by now, right?), add the rest of the canned tomatoes, cover, turn the heat to low, and let it cook for 10 to 15 minutes or until the chicken is cooked through.

Yield: About 3 servings

Each with 14 grams of carbohydrates and 1 gram of fiber, for a total of 13 grams of usable carbs and 26 grams of protein.

Some like it hot, and some like it a little bit less so. So when you're buying your ingredients, choose a little jalapeño or a big one, depending on how hot you like your food. I use a big one, and it definitely makes this dish hot. And don't forget, there's no law against using only half a jalapeño.

Cashew-Crusted Chicken

Since cashews are a relatively high-carb nut, this is just a light coating—but it's very flavorful. You can find raw cashews at most natural food stores.

1½ pounds (680 g) boneless, skinless chicken breast
⅔ cup (90 g) raw cashew pieces
¼ teaspoon salt
½ teaspoon pepper
¼ teaspoon paprika
1 egg
2 to 3 tablespoons (28 to 42 g) butter

First, put the cashew pieces in a food processor with the S-blade in place and grind them to a fine texture. Dump them out onto a plate and add the salt, pepper, and paprika, mixing the whole thing well. Set aside.

Pound the chicken breasts until they're ½ inch (1.3 cm) thick all over. Cut into 4 servings if necessary.

Break the egg into another plate with a rim around it. (A pie plate would work well.) Now, dip each chicken breast piece into the egg and then into the cashew mixture, coating both sides.

Melt the butter in a heavy skillet over medium to medium-high heat and add the chicken. Sauté until it's golden on both sides and cooked through about 5 minutes per side.

Yield: 4 servings

Each with 6 grams of carbohydrates and 1 gram of fiber, for a total of 5 grams of usable carbs and 33 grams of protein.

Slow Cooker Chicken Mole

Chicken mole is the national dish of Mexico, and I'm crazy about it. On my honeymoon in Mexico, I bought a container of chicken mole at the deli at the local grocery store and kept it in the hotel room fridge to heat up in the microwave! Here's a slow cooker version.

3 pounds (1.4 kg) skinless chicken thighs
1 can (14½ ounces, or 411 g) tomatoes with green chiles
½ cup (80 g) chopped onion
¼ cup (30 g) slivered almonds, toasted
3 cloves garlic, crushed
3 tablespoons (17 g) unsweetened cocoa powder
2 tablespoons (18 g) raisins
1 tablespoon (9 g) sesame seeds
1 tablespoon (1.5 g) Splenda
¼ teaspoon ground cinnamon
¼ teaspoon ground nutmeg
¼ teaspoon ground coriander
¼ teaspoon salt

Guar or xanthan

2 tablespoons (15 g) slivered almonds, toasted

Put the tomatoes, onion, ¼ cup (30 g) almonds, garlic, cocoa powder, raisins, sesame seeds, Splenda, cinnamon, nutmeg, coriander, and salt in a blender or food processor and purée coarsely.

Place the chicken in a slow cooker. Pour the sauce over it. Cover the slow cooker, set it to low, and let it cook for 9 to 10 hours.

Remove the chicken from the slow cooker with tongs. Thicken the sauce to taste with guar or xanthan. Serve the sauce over the chicken. Top with the 2 tablespoons (15 g) almonds.

Yield: 8 servings

Each with 37 g protein, 8 g carbohydrate, 2 g dietary fiber, 6 g usable carbs.

Easy Mexicali Chicken

How simple is this? Yet you know the whole family will like it. Just remember to read the labels to get the lowest-carb salsa.

1½ pounds (680 g) boneless, skinless chicken breast

2 tablespoons (30 ml) oil

4 ounces (115 g) Monterey Jack, pepper Jack, or shredded Mexican cheese blend

½ cup (130 g) mild, medium, or hot salsa, as you prefer

Pound the chicken breasts to ½ inch (1.3 cm) thick and divide into portions, if needed.

Place a large, heavy skillet over medium-high heat, add the oil, and sauté the chicken breasts for about 5 minutes or until the bottom is golden. Turn and sauté for another 3 to 4 minutes. Top the chicken with the cheese, turn the heat down to medium-low, cover the skillet, and let the whole thing cook for another 3 to 4 minutes or until the cheese is melted.

While the cheese is melting, put the salsa in a microwaveable dish and cook it for a minute at 50 percent power.

Remove the chicken to serving plates, top with the salsa, and serve. You could add a dollop of sour cream if you like or maybe some chopped fresh cilantro, but it's not really necessary.

Yield: 4 or 5 servings

Assuming 4 servings, each will have 2 grams of carbohydrates and 1 gram of fiber, for a total of 1 gram of usable carbs and 45 grams of protein. Analysis does not include sour cream.

Chicken with Raspberry-Chipotle Sauce

Oh my—this is wonderful. My only regret about this recipe is that the Raspberry-Chipotle Sauce loses its brilliant ruby color during the long, slow cooking. But the flavor definitely remains.

(continued on page 314)

Consider using this simple sauce uncooked as a condiment on roasted poultry or pork. If you can't find raspberry syrup at a local coffee shop, you can order it online.

3 pounds (1.4 kg) chicken
6 teaspoons adobo seasoning
2 tablespoons (30 ml) oil
1 cup (110 g) raspberries
¼ cup (60 ml) raspberry-flavored sugar-free coffee flavoring syrup (I used Atkins brand, but Da Vinci would be fine, too.)
1 chipotle chile canned in adobo sauce
1 tablespoon (15 ml) white wine vinegar
¼ cup (16 g) chopped fresh cilantro (optional)

Sprinkle the chicken all over with the adobo seasoning.

In a big, heavy skillet, heat the oil over medium-high heat and then brown the chicken all over. Transfer the chicken to a slow cooker.

In a blender or food processor with the S-blade in place, combine the raspberries, raspberry-flavored coffee syrup, chipotle, and vinegar. Process until smooth. Pour the mixture evenly over the chicken. Cover the slow cooker, set it to low, and let it cook for 6 hours.

Stir the sauce before serving it over the chicken. Sprinkle a little cilantro over each piece of chicken, if desired.

Yield: 5 servings

Each with 35 g protein, 5 g carbohydrate, 2 g dietary fiber, 3 g usable carbs.

Crispy Skillet BBQ Chicken

Add some slaw made from bagged coleslaw mix, and supper is served.

1½ pounds (680 g) boneless, skinless chicken breast
Sprinkle-on barbecue dry rub or "soul" seasoning
½ cup (40 g) crushed barbecue-flavor pork rinds
2 tablespoons (30 ml) oil

One at a time, pound the chicken breasts until they're about ½ inch (1.3 cm) thick all over. If necessary, cut the breasts into 4 servings. Sprinkle both sides of each piece liberally with the seasoning. Then sprinkle each side of each serving with 1 tablespoon of the pork rind crumbs and press them onto the surface with a clean palm.

Heat the oil in a large, heavy-bottomed skillet over medium-high heat. Add the chicken breasts and sauté for 5 to 6 minutes per side or until crispy and cooked through. Serve. This is great with any sort of salad or coleslaw as a side.

Yield: 4 servings

This has no carbs to speak of (maybe a tiny trace from the seasoning), no fiber, and 44 grams of protein per serving. Analysis does not include side dishes.

Slow Cooker Chicken Guadeloupe

This isn't authentically anything, but it borrows its flavors from the Creole cooking of the Caribbean.

1 cut-up broiler-fryer chicken, about
    3½ pounds (1.5 to 2 kg), or whatever
    chicken parts you prefer
½ medium onion, chopped
2 teaspoons ground allspice
1 teaspoon dried thyme
¼ cup (60 ml) lemon juice; bottled is fine
1 can (14 ounces, or 400 g) diced tomatoes
    with chilies
1 shot (3 tablespoons, or 45 ml) dark rum
Guar or xanthan
Salt and pepper

Just throw the chicken, onion, allspice, thyme, lemon juice, chilies, and rum in a slow cooker, set it to low, and let it cook for 5 to 6 hours. Fish out the chicken carefully—it'll be sliding from the bone! Thicken up the stuff in the pot with the guar or xanthan, add salt and pepper to taste, and serve over the chicken.

Yield: 5 or 6 servings

Assuming 5 servings, each will have 6 grams of carbohydrates and 1 gram of fiber, for a total of 5 grams of usable carbs and 35 grams of protein.

Skillet Chicken Florentine

My husband took one bite of this and said, "This is going to get you a lot of new readers!" I know of no other dish that's so quick and easy, yet so incredibly good.

Olive oil
2 or 3 boneless, skinless chicken breasts
1 package (10 ounces, or 280 g) frozen
    chopped spinach, thawed
2 cloves garlic, crushed
¼ cup (60 ml) heavy cream
¼ cup (25 g) grated Parmesan cheese

Warm a little olive oil in a heavy skillet and brown the chicken breasts over medium heat to the point where they just have a touch of gold. Remove the chicken from the skillet.

Add a couple more tablespoons of olive oil, the spinach, and the garlic, and stir for 2 to 3 minutes. Stir in the cream and cheese and spread the mixture evenly over the bottom of the skillet. Place the chicken breasts on top, cover, turn the heat to low, and let simmer for 15 minutes.

Serve chicken breasts with the spinach on top.

Yield: 3 servings

Each with 5 grams of carbohydrates and 3 grams of fiber, for a total of 2 grams of usable carbs and 33 grams of protein.

Chicken Cacciatore

Here's a slow cooker version of an old favorite. It's easy, too—what I call a dump-and-go recipe.

6 skinless chicken leg and side quarters (about 3 lbs/1.5 kg)
2 cups (480 ml) no-sugar-added spaghetti sauce (I use Hunt's.)
1 can (8 ounces, or 225 g) whole mushrooms, drained
2 teaspoons dried oregano
½ cup (80 g) chopped onion
1 green bell pepper, diced
2 cloves garlic, crushed
¼ cup (60 ml) dry red wine
Guar or xanthan (optional)

Simply put everything except the guar or xanthan in a slow cooker and stir it up to combine. Cover the slow cooker, set it to low, and let it cook for 7 hours.

When the time's up, remove the chicken with tongs and put it in a big serving bowl. Thicken the sauce up a little with the guar or xanthan if it needs it and ladle the sauce over the chicken.

If you like, you can serve this over Cauliflower Rice (page 212), spaghetti squash, or even low-carb pasta, but I'd probably eat it as is.

Yield: 6 servings

Each with 42 g protein, 11 g carbohydrate, 4 g dietary fiber, 7 g usable carbs. Analysis does not include side dishes.

Chicken and Artichoke Skillet

This is quick and easy enough for a weeknight but elegant enough for company.

4 boneless, skinless chicken breasts
3 tablespoons (42 g) butter, divided
1 can (14 ounces, or 400 g) quartered artichoke hearts, drained
½ red bell pepper, cut into strips
1 medium onion, sliced
1 clove garlic, crushed
¼ cup (60 ml) dry white wine
1 teaspoon dried thyme

Melt 2 tablespoons (28 g) of butter in a heavy skillet over medium heat and sauté the chicken breasts until they're golden (5 to 7 minutes per side). Remove from the skillet.

Melt the remaining tablespoon of butter and toss the artichoke hearts, pepper, onion, and garlic into the skillet. Sauté for 3 minutes or so, stirring frequently.

Pour the wine into the skillet and sprinkle the thyme over the vegetables. Place the chicken breasts over the vegetables, turn the heat to medium low, cover, and simmer for 10 minutes.

Yield: 4 servings

Each with 8 grams of carbohydrates and 4 grams of fiber, for a total of 4 grams of usable carbs and 26 grams of protein.

Chicken with Thyme and Artichokes

This dish is sort of a classic, yet it's very little work.

1½ pounds (680 g) boneless, skinless chicken thighs

2 tablespoons (30 ml) olive oil

½ cup (120 ml) dry white wine

1 tablespoon (15 ml) lemon juice

1 teaspoon chicken bouillon concentrate

2 teaspoons dried thyme

1 clove garlic, crushed

¼ teaspoon pepper

13 ounces (370 grams) canned artichoke hearts, drained

Guar or xanthan

In a big, heavy skillet, brown the chicken in the oil over medium-high heat until golden on both sides. Transfer to a slow cooker.

In a bowl, stir together the wine, lemon juice, bouillon, thyme, garlic, and pepper. Pour the mixture over the chicken. Place the artichokes on top. Cover the slow cooker, set it to low, and let it cook for 6 hours.

Scoop out the chicken and artichokes with a slotted spoon. Thicken the liquid left in the pot with just enough guar or xanthan to make it the thickness of half-and-half.

Serve the chicken and artichokes, plus the sauce, over Cauliflower Rice (page 212).

Yield: 4 servings

Each with 42 g protein, 7 g carbohydrate, trace dietary fiber, 7 g usable carbs. Analysis does not include Cauliflower Rice.

Chicken with Asparagus and Gruyère

1½ pounds (680 g) boneless, skinless chicken breast

1 tablespoon (14 g) butter

1 pound (455 g) asparagus

1 tablespoon (15 ml) dry white wine

1 tablespoon (15 ml) lemon juice

Salt and pepper

4 ounces (115 g) gruyère, thinly sliced

First, pound the chicken breasts until they're ¼ inch (6 mm) thick all over. Cut into 4 portions.

Melt the butter in a large, heavy skillet over medium-high heat and start browning the chicken.

While that's happening, snap the ends off the asparagus where they break naturally. Put the asparagus in a microwaveable casserole dish or lay it in a glass pie plate. Add a couple of tablespoons (30 ml) of water and cover. (Use plastic wrap or a plate to cover if you're using a pie plate.) Microwave on high for 3 to 4 minutes.

When the chicken is golden on both sides, add the wine and the lemon juice to the skillet and turn the chicken breasts to coat both sides. Season lightly with salt and pepper. Turn the heat to medium-low and let the chicken continue to cook until the asparagus is done microwaving.

(continued on page 318)

Remove the asparagus from the microwave and drain. Lay the asparagus spears over the chicken, dividing equally between the portions. Cover each with gruyère and cover the skillet with a tilted lid. Continue cooking a few minutes just until the cheese is melted. Serve.

Yield: 4 servings

Each with 3 grams of carbohydrates and 1 gram of fiber, for a total of 2 grams of usable carbs and 38 grams of protein.

Tuscan Chicken

This is fabulous Italian chicken!

4 pounds (1.8 kg) skinless chicken thighs
1 tablespoon (15 ml) olive oil
½ cup (80 g) chopped onion
1 red bell pepper, cut into strips
1 green bell pepper, cut into strips
1 can (15 ounces, or 420 g) black soybeans, drained
1 can (14½ ounces, or 410 g) crushed tomatoes
½ cup (120 ml) dry white wine
1 teaspoon dried oregano
1 clove garlic, crushed
1 teaspoon chicken bouillon concentrate

In a big, heavy skillet, brown the chicken in the oil over medium-high heat. Meanwhile, put the onion, peppers, and soybeans in a slow cooker. Place the chicken on top of the vegetables and beans.

In a bowl, stir together the tomatoes, wine, oregano, garlic, and bouillon. Pour the mixture over the chicken. Cover the slow cooker, set it

to low, and let it cook for 6 to 7 hours. Add salt and pepper to taste.

Yield: 8 servings

Each with 31 g protein, 10 g carbohydrate, 5 g dietary fiber, 5 g usable carbs.

Italian Chicken with White Wine, Peppers, and Anchovy

Don't be afraid of the anchovy paste in this sauce. There's no fishy taste to the recipe; it's just mellow and complex.

3 pounds (1.4 kg) chicken pieces
¼ cup (60 ml) olive oil
3 cloves garlic
1 cup (240 ml) dry white wine
1 tablespoon (15 g) anchovy paste
2 medium tomatoes, chopped
1 large green bell pepper, chopped
Salt and pepper

In a Dutch oven, over medium heat, brown the chicken in the olive oil. When the chicken is golden all over, remove to a plate and set aside. Pour off the fat.

Now add the garlic, white wine, and anchovy paste to the Dutch oven and stir until the anchovy paste is dissolved. Add the tomatoes and green pepper.

Sprinkle salt and pepper over the chicken and plunk it back into the Dutch oven. Cover, set to lowest heat, and let simmer for 40 minutes. If you like, you can thicken the liquid in the pot a little before serving, but don't thicken it too much.

Yield: 5 servings

Each with 36 g protein; 5 g carbohydrate; 1 g dietary fiber; 4 g usable carbs.

Italian Chicken and Vegetables

2 pounds (910 g) skinless chicken breasts
2 pounds (910 g) skinless chicken thighs
½ head cabbage, cut in wedges
1 medium onion, sliced
8 ounces (225 g) sliced mushrooms
2 cups (480 ml) no-sugar-added spaghetti sauce (I use Hunt's.)
Guar or xanthan (optional)
Grated Parmesan cheese

Put the cabbage, onion, and mushrooms in a slow cooker. Place the chicken on top of the vegetables. Pour the spaghetti sauce over the top.

Cover the slow cooker, set it to low, and let it cook for 6 hours. Thicken the sauce with guar or xanthan if needed and serve with Parmesan cheese.

Yield: 6 servings

Each with 46 g protein, 4 g carbohydrate, 1 g dietary fiber, 3 g usable carbs.

Parmesan Chicken Breasts

You might recognize this recipe as being quite similar to Wicked Wings. However, Wicked Wings take well over an hour, and this is quite quick.

1½ pounds (680 g) boneless, skinless chicken breast
1 cup (100 g) grated Parmesan cheese*
4 teaspoons dried oregano
1 teaspoon garlic powder
1 teaspoon paprika
1 teaspoon pepper
2 eggs
4 tablespoons (56 g) butter

Pound the chicken breasts until they're ¼ inch (6 mm) thick and cut into 6 portions. Set aside.

Combine the cheese with the oregano, garlic, paprika, and pepper on a plate.

On another plate or in a shallow bowl, beat the eggs. Dip the chicken in the egg and then the cheese mixture, coating both sides well.

Melt the butter in a heavy skillet over medium-low heat (higher heat will scorch the cheese) and sauté for 4 to 5 minutes per side or until cooked through.

Yield: 6 servings

Each with 2 grams of carbohydrates and 1 gram of fiber, for a total of 1 gram of usable carbs and 33 grams of protein.

*Use the Parmesan cheese in the round, green shaker for this.

Saltimbocca

Who says all Italian food involves pasta?

4 boneless, skinless chicken breasts
¼ pound (115 g) prosciutto or good boiled
ham, thinly sliced
40 leaves fresh or dry sage (Fresh is
preferable.)
2 tablespoons (28 g) butter
2 tablespoons (30 ml) olive oil
½ cup (120 ml) dry white wine

Place a chicken breast in a large, heavy, resealable plastic bag and pound it until it's ¼ inch (6 mm) thick. Repeat with the remaining chicken breasts.

Once all your chicken breasts are pounded thin, place a layer of the prosciutto on each one, scatter about 10 sage leaves over each one, and roll each breast up. Fasten with toothpicks.

Melt the butter with the olive oil in a heavy skillet over medium heat. Add the chicken rolls and sauté, turning occasionally, until golden all over.

Add the wine to the skillet, turn the heat to low, cover the skillet, and simmer for 15 minutes.

Remove the chicken rolls to a serving plate and cover to keep warm. Turn the heat up to high and boil the liquid in the skillet hard for 5 minutes to reduce. Spoon over the chicken rolls and serve.

Yield: 4 servings

Each with 2 grams of carbohydrates, no fiber, and 37 grams of protein.

Middle Eastern Skillet Chicken

3 boneless, skinless chicken breasts
3 tablespoons (45 ml) olive oil
1 medium onion, chopped
½ teaspoon ground coriander
1 teaspoon ground cumin
¼ teaspoon ground cinnamon
½ teaspoon turmeric
¼ teaspoon black pepper
1 tablespoon (6 g) freshly grated ginger
1 can (14½ ounces, or 410 g) diced tomatoes
2 cloves garlic, crushed
1 cup (240 ml) chicken broth

Cut the chicken breasts into cubes. Heat the olive oil over medium heat in a heavy skillet and add the chicken and onions.

Sauté for a couple of minutes and then stir in the coriander, cumin, cinnamon, turmeric, and pepper. Cook until the chicken is white all over.

Add the ginger, tomatoes, garlic, and broth; stir. Cover, turn the heat to low, and simmer for 15 minutes.

Yield: 3 servings

Each with 14 grams of carbohydrates and 1 gram of fiber, for a total of 13 grams of usable carbs and 26 grams of protein.

Aegean Chicken

The minute I told my sister about this, she started hounding me for the recipe.

1½ pounds (680 g) boneless, skinless chicken breast
¼ cup (60 ml) olive oil
4 ounces (115 g) kasseri cheese, sliced
8 tablespoons (120 ml) tapenade
¼ cup (60 ml) dry white wine
2 cloves garlic

One at a time, pound the chicken breasts until they're ¼ inch (6 mm) thick all over. Cut the breasts into 6 servings, if necessary. Sauté them in the olive oil over medium-high heat. When they're turning golden on the bottom, turn them and lay the slices of kasseri over them. Let them cook another 2 to 3 minutes or until the cheese is starting to melt. Spread the tapenade over the breasts and add the wine to the skillet. Let the whole thing cook for another minute or two, just to warm the tapenade and make sure the chicken is cooked through. Remove the chicken to serving plates, add the garlic to the wine left in the skillet, stir the whole thing and let it boil for a minute or so, and pour it over the chicken before serving.

Yield: 6 servings

Each with just 2 grams of carbohydrates, a trace of fiber, and 40 grams of protein.

Greek Chicken with Yogurt

3 pounds (1.4 kg) chicken pieces
2 tablespoons (30 ml) lemon juice
Salt and pepper
3 tablespoons (42 g) butter
1 medium onion, sliced
2 cloves garlic, crushed
½ cup (120 ml) dry white wine
1 cup (240 ml) chicken broth
½ teaspoon ground rosemary
1 cup (230 g) plain yogurt
Guar or xanthan

Rub the chicken with the lemon juice and sprinkle it with salt and pepper.

Melt the butter in a big, heavy skillet over medium-high heat and brown the chicken all over. When the chicken is brown, remove it from the skillet, pour off the fat, and put the chicken back.

Add the onion, garlic, wine, chicken broth, and rosemary to the skillet. Cover, turn the heat to low, and let the whole thing simmer for 30 minutes or so.

When time's up, pull the skillet off the heat and uncover. Let it cool for about 10 minutes. Remove the chicken to a serving platter. Whisk the yogurt into the sauce in the skillet, stirring until it smoothes out. Thicken a bit with guar or xanthan and serve over the chicken.

Yield: 5 to 6 servings

Assuming 5, each will have 38 g protein; 6 g carbohydrate; trace dietary fiber, 6 g usable carbs.

Chicken Kampama

This dish is Greek chicken, simmered in red wine, tomatoes, and spices. If all you've had is Greek roasted chicken (which is wonderful, by the way!), try this!

3 pounds (1.4 kg) cut-up chicken
2 tablespoons (28 g) butter
2 tablespoons (30 ml) olive oil
1 cup (160 g) chopped onion
1 cup (240 g) canned diced tomatoes
4 tablespoons (66 g) tomato paste
¼ cup (60 ml) dry red wine
1 clove garlic, crushed
¼ teaspoon ground allspice
½ teaspoon ground cinnamon
¼ cup (60 ml) chicken broth

In a big, heavy skillet, brown the chicken all over in the butter and olive oil. When it's golden, remove from the pan and pour off all but about 1 tablespoon (15 ml) of the fat.

In that fat, sauté the onion a bit. When it's golden, add the tomatoes, tomato paste, wine, garlic, allspice, cinnamon, and chicken broth. Stir it all together and bring to a simmer.

Add the chicken back to the skillet, turn the heat to the lowest setting, cover, and cook for 30 minutes. Uncover and simmer for another 30 minutes and then serve.

Yield: 6 servings

Each with 30 g protein; 8 g carbohydrate; 1 g dietary fiber; 7 g usable carbs.

Picnic Chicken

1 cut up broiler-fryer
⅔ cup (160 ml) apple cider vinegar
3 tablespoons (45 ml) oil
2 teaspoons salt
¼ teaspoon pepper

Combine the vinegar, oil, salt, and pepper. Reserve some marinade for basting and pour the rest over the chicken in a large resealable plastic bag. Marinate for at least an hour; more time wouldn't hurt.

Preheat the broiler to high. Take the chicken out of the marinade and broil it about 8 inches (20 cm) from the flame. Baste it with the reserved marinade every 10 to 15 minutes while cooking using a clean utensil each time you baste. Give it about 25 minutes per side or until cooked through. (Pierce it to the bone; the juices should run clear, not pink.) You may need to rearrange the chicken pieces on your broiler rack to get them to cook evenly so they're all ready at the same time.

Yield: 4 servings

Each with 3 grams of carbohydrates per serving if you consumed all the marinade, but of course you don't, so each serving has less than 1 gram of carbohydrates, no fiber, and 44 grams of protein.

You may be wondering why this is called Picnic Chicken—it's because come summer, if you really were going on a picnic, you could bring the bag of chicken and reserved marinade along in the cooler and grill it at the park or the beach. What a treat!

Chicken Paprikash

Making my Paprikash with real sour cream is one of the great joys of low-carbing!

1 cut-up broiler-fryer
3 tablespoons (42 g) butter
1 small onion
2 tablespoons (12.6 g) paprika
½ cup (120 ml) chicken broth
1 cup (230 g) sour cream
Salt or Vege-Sal and pepper

Melt the butter in a heavy skillet and brown the chicken and onions over medium-high heat.

In a separate bowl, stir the paprika into the chicken broth. Pour the mixture over the chicken.

Cover the skillet, turn the heat to low, and let it simmer for 30 to 45 minutes.

When the chicken is tender and cooked through, remove it from the skillet and put it on a serving platter. Stir the sour cream into the liquid left in the pan and stir until smooth and well blended. Heat through but do not let it boil or it will curdle. Season with salt and pepper to taste and serve this gravy with the chicken.

Yield: 4 servings

Each with 7 grams of carbohydrates and 1 gram of fiber, for a total of 6 grams of usable carbs and 53 grams of protein.

Be sure to serve plenty of Cauliflower Purée (page 209) with it to smother in the extra gravy!

Deviled Chicken

1 cut-up broiler-fryer
4 tablespoons (56 g) butter
½ cup (12 g) Splenda
¼ cup (60 ml) spicy brown mustard
1 teaspoon salt
1 teaspoon curry powder

Preheat the oven to 375°F (190°C, or gas mark 5).

Melt the butter in a shallow roasting pan. Add the Splenda, mustard, salt, and curry powder and stir until well combined.

Roll the chicken pieces in the butter mixture until coated and then arrange them skin side up in the pan. Bake for 1 hour.

Yield: 4 servings

Each with 5 grams of carbohydrates, a trace of fiber, and 44 grams of protein.

Pollo en Jugo de Naranja (Mexican Chicken in Orange Juice)

The recipe I adapted this from was terribly high-carb, including a cup of orange juice and a lot more raisins. The decarbed version is delicious!

(continued on page 324)

3 pounds (1.4 kg) cut-up chicken, whatever
 you like—I like legs and thighs.
Salt and pepper
2 tablespoons (30 ml) oil
1 orange
¼ cup (30 g) slivered almonds, toasted
1 tablespoon (15 ml) lemon juice
2 tablespoons (20 g) raisins
¼ cup (40 g) chopped onion
1 clove garlic, crushed
⅔ cup (160 g) canned diced tomatoes,
 undrained
¼ cup (60 ml) dry sherry
1 bay leaf
¼ cup (15.2 g) snipped fresh parsley
½ teaspoon dried thyme
½ teaspoon dried oregano
Guar or xanthan gum (optional)

Sprinkle the chicken pieces with a little salt and pepper. In a large, heavy skillet, heat the oil and brown the chicken until it's lightly golden all over.

While that's happening, grate the zest of the orange and reserve. If your almonds aren't toasted, this is a good time to do that too—simply stir them in a small, heavy, dry skillet over medium heat until they start to turn golden and then set aside.

When the chicken is browned, pour off any excess fat. Squeeze in the juice of the orange, adding any pulp that may squeeze out. Add all remaining ingredients, including the reserved orange zest, cover the pan, turn the heat to low, and let the whole thing simmer for 45 to 50 minutes or until chicken is tender. Remove chicken to a serving platter.

Remove the bay leaf and thicken the sauce a bit with guar or xanthan, if you like; serve with the chicken.

Yield: 5 to 6 servings

Assuming 6, each will have 31 g protein; 9 g carbohydrate; 2 g dietary fiber; 7 g usable carbs.

Key Lime Chicken

This is an unusual—and good!—combination of flavors.

1 cut-up broiler-fryer
½ cup (120 ml) lime juice
½ cup (120 ml) olive oil
1 tablespoon (10 g) grated onion
2 teaspoons tarragon
1 teaspoon seasoned salt
¼ teaspoon pepper

Arrange the chicken pieces on the broiler rack, skin side down.

In a bowl, combine the lime juice, oil, onion, tarragon, salt, and pepper. Reserve some of this mixture in another small bowl. Brush the chicken well with the marinade.

Broil the chicken about 8 inches (20 cm) from the heat for 45 to 50 minutes, turning the chicken and basting with the reserved lime mixture every 10 minutes or so, using a clean utensil each time you baste.

Yield: 4 servings

Each with 4 grams of carbohydrates, a trace of fiber, and 44 grams of protein.

Lemon Mustard Herb Chicken

24 ounces (680 g) boneless, skinless chicken breast

⅓ cup (80 ml) lemon juice

⅓ cup (80 ml) spicy brown mustard

1 tablespoon (4 g) rubbed sage

1½ teaspoons dried thyme

3 cloves garlic, crushed

3 scallions

This is quick and easy. Just mix together the lemon juice, mustard, sage, thyme, and garlic. Put the chicken breasts on a plate and spread this mixture over both sides. Let it sit for ten minutes, and a little more won't hurt.

Heat up an electric tabletop grill and throw the chicken breast in. Set your oven timer for 5 minutes. Slice up the scallions, including the crisp part of the green. When the timer goes off, put the chicken on a serving plate, scatter the scallions over it, and serve.

Yield: 3–4 servings

Each with 53 g protein; 8 g carbohydrate; 1 g dietary fiber; 7 g usable carbs.

Sweet Lemon-Brined and Glazed Chicken Breast

Like the convenience of boneless, skinless chicken breasts but find they often come out bland and dry? With this recipe, they'll be plump, moist, and flavorful even if you overcook them a little!

1½ pounds (680 g) boneless, skinless chicken breast

FOR THE BRINE:

1 tablespoon (15 g) kosher salt

16 ounces (475 ml) lemon-flavored Fruit₂O

1 tablespoon (15 ml) soy sauce

1 clove garlic

1 dash hot pepper sauce

FOR THE GLAZE:

2 tablespoons (30 ml) lemon juice

1 tablespoon DiabetiSweet or other polyol-based sweetener

½ tablespoon soy sauce

1 clove garlic

Cut the chicken breasts into 4 portions, if needed.

To make the brine: Dissolve the salt in the Fruit₂O. (Heating the Fruit₂O will help the salt dissolve.) Then stir in the rest of the brine ingredients. Pour over the chicken breasts in a shallow, nonreactive dish small enough that the breasts are submerged and stick the whole thing in the fridge.

Three to 4 hours later, get your grill going. When the coals are well ashed or the gas grill is heated to medium, pull the chicken out of the fridge and drain off the brine. Make sure your grill is well oiled and grill the chicken about 7 to 10 minutes per side or until an instant-read thermometer registers 180°F (85°C).

(continued on page 326)

To make the glaze: While the chicken is grilling, combine the glaze ingredients in a small saucepan and simmer for just 1 to 2 minutes. Brush over the chicken during the last few minutes of grilling. If there's any glaze left over, drizzle it over the chicken before serving.

Yield: 4 servings

Each serving will have 2 grams carbohydrate, a trace of fiber, and 38 grams protein. Carb count does not include polyol sweetener.

Chicken Piccata

Meat cooked "piccata" is traditionally floured first, but with all this flavor going on, who'll miss it?

4 boneless, skinless chicken breasts
¼ cup (60 ml) olive oil
1 clove garlic, crushed
1 tablespoon (15 ml) lemon juice, or the juice of ½ lemon
½ cup (120 ml) dry white wine
1 tablespoon (9 g) capers, chopped
3 tablespoons (11.4 g) fresh parsley, chopped

Place a chicken breast in a large, heavy, resealable plastic bag and pound it until it's ¼ inch (6 mm) thick. Repeat with the remaining chicken breasts.

Heat the olive oil in a large, heavy skillet over medium-high heat. Add the chicken; if it doesn't all fit at the same time, cook it in two batches, keeping the first batch warm while the second batch is cooking. Cook the chicken until it's done through (3 to 4 minutes per side).

Remove the chicken from the pan. Add the garlic, lemon juice, white wine, and capers to the pan, stirring it all around to get the tasty little brown bits off the bottom of the pan. Boil the whole thing hard for about 1 minute to reduce it a little.

Put the chicken back in the pan for another minute, sprinkle the parsley over it, and serve.

Yield: 4 servings

Each with 1 gram of carbohydrates, a trace of fiber, and 29 grams of protein.

Variation: Pork Piccata. Make this variation just like Chicken Piccatta, only substitute 4 good, big pork steaks, chops, or thinly sliced pork butt (1 to 1½ pounds [455 to 680 g] of meat total) for the chicken breasts. (Cut the bones out of the pork steaks or chops and discard.)

Yield: 4 servings, each with 1 gram of carbohydrates, a trace of fiber, and 26 grams of protein.

Lemon-Pepper Chicken and Gravy

1 cut-up broiler-fryer
1¼ teaspoons lemon pepper, divided
1¼ teaspoons onion powder, divided
1 teaspoon salt
¼ cup (60 ml) chicken broth
½ cup (120 ml) heavy cream
1½ teaspoons spicy brown or Dijon mustard

Preheat the oven to 375°F (190°C, or gas mark 5).

Sprinkle the chicken pieces with 1 teaspoon of lemon pepper, 1 teaspoon of onion powder, and the salt. Arrange in a roasting pan and roast, basting once or twice, for about 1 hour or until the juices run clear when the chicken is pierced.

Remove the chicken from the roasting pan and skim off the excess fat, leaving just the brown drippings. Place the roasting pan over low heat, add the chicken broth to the pan, and stir, scraping up the tasty brown bits off the bottom of the pan. When the broth is simmering, add the cream, the rest of the lemon pepper and onion powder, and the mustard. Stir well, heat through, and pour over the chicken.

Yield: 4 servings

Each with 2 grams of carbohydrates, a trace of fiber, and 44 grams of protein.

Lemon-Rosemary Chicken

This is a very classic flavor combination.

1 pound (455 g) boneless, skinless chicken breast
¼ cup (60 ml) olive oil
2 tablespoons (30 ml) lemon juice
2 cloves garlic, crushed
1 tablespoon (3.6 g) dried rosemary, crushed a bit

Mix together everything but the chicken. Put the chicken breasts in a shallow dish. Reserve some marinade for basting and pour the rest the olive oil/lemon mixture over the chicken. Turn the breasts over once or twice to coat them. (We're not doing this in a bag because we're going to marinate the chicken for only a short time.)

Now, go start your grill. You'll want it at medium heat. When it's ready, throw the chicken on the grill and cook for about 7 minutes per side, basting with the reserved olive oil/lemon mixture a few times using a clean utensil each time you baste.

I like to heat any leftover marinade until it boils hard and then spoon just a little over each breast while serving.

Yield: 3 servings

Even if you consumed all the marinade, which you won't, you'd get only 2 grams of carb per serving, 1 gram of which would be fiber. 34 grams protein.

Chicken Breasts L'Orange

Chicken combines so well with all sorts of fruit flavors, and this dish is sure to be a hit with the whole family.

1½ pounds (680 g) boneless, skinless chicken breast
¼ cup (60 ml) oil
⅓ cup (80 ml) orange juice
2 tablespoons (3 g) Splenda
2 teaspoons cider vinegar

(continued on page 328)

¼ teaspoon blackstrap molasses

1 teaspoon spicy brown or Dijon mustard

1 teaspoon minced garlic or 2 cloves garlic, crushed

Salt and pepper

Cut the chicken breasts into 4 portions and brown them in the oil in a large, heavy skillet over high heat. While that's happening, mix together the orange juice, Splenda, vinegar, molasses, mustard, and garlic.

When the chicken is light golden on both sides, add the orange juice mixture to the skillet. Simmer the chicken for another 7 to 8 minutes, turning once. Season with salt and pepper to taste and serve.

Yield: 4 servings

Each with 4 grams of carbohydrates, a trace of fiber, and 38 grams of protein.

Orange Teriyaki Chicken

This has been officially rated "Very Easy and Very Good!"

2 pounds (910 g) boneless, skinless chicken breasts, cubed

16 ounces (455 g) frozen Oriental vegetable mixture, unthawed

¾ cup (180 ml) chicken broth

2 tablespoons (30 ml) Low-Carb Teriyaki Sauce (page 465) or purchased low-carb teriyaki sauce

1 teaspoon chicken bouillon concentrate

1 tablespoon (20 g) low-sugar orange marmalade

¼ teaspoon orange extract

2 tablespoons (30 ml) lemon juice

1 teaspoon Splenda

1 teaspoon dry mustard

½ teaspoon ground ginger

Guar or xanthan

Pour the vegetables into a slow cooker. Place the chicken on top.

In a bowl, combine the broth and the next 8 ingredients (through ginger), stirring well. Pour the mixture over the chicken and vegetables. Cover the slower cooker, set it to low, and let it cook for 4 to 5 hours.

Before serving, thicken the sauce a bit with guar or xanthan.

Serve over Cauliflower Rice (page 212), if desired. Or for the carbivores, you can serve it over brown rice, lo mein noodles, or plain old spaghetti.

Yield: 6 servings

Each with 36 g protein, 7 g carbohydrate, 2 g dietary fiber, 5 g usable carbs. Analysis does not include side dishes.

Citrus Chicken

Don't look at this list of ingredients and turn the page! This is actually easy—just make a marinade, marinate your chicken, and while the chicken's roasting, cook down the marinade for a sauce. Since you put the chicken in to marinate long before dinnertime, the actual oh-my-God-it's-already-six-and-the-kids-are-screaming cooking time is quite short—just 20 to 30 minutes.

FOR THE CHICKEN:

3 pounds (1.4 kg) cut-up chicken

¼ cup (40 g) minced onion

2 cloves garlic, crushed

½ cup (120 ml) lemon juice

½ teaspoon orange extract

1 tablespoon (15 ml) soy sauce

1 tablespoon (15 ml) rice vinegar

¼ cup (6 g) Splenda

1 tablespoon (6 g) grated ginger

1 tablespoon (15 ml) brown mustard

2 tablespoons (30 ml) canola or peanut oil

1 tablespoon (15 ml) sesame oil

FOR THE SAUCE:

1 cup (240 ml) chicken broth

2 teaspoons spicy brown mustard

2 teaspoons Splenda

1 teaspoon beef bouillon concentrate

Guar or xanthan

To make the chicken: Combine the onion, garlic, lemon juice, orange extract, soy sauce, rice vinegar, ¼ cup (6 g) Splenda, ginger, and 1 tablespoon (15 g) mustard. Put the chicken in a big resealable plastic bag. Reserve some marinade for basting and add the rest to the bay. Seal the bag, pressing out the air as you go. Turn the bag a few times to coat the chicken. Throw the bag in the fridge for at least a few hours, and all day won't hurt a bit.

Okay, time to cook! Set your oven for 500°F (250°C, or gas mark 10). (Yes, I do mean 500°F!) Pull the chicken out of the fridge and pour off the marinade into a saucepan. Arrange the chicken in a roasting pan. Now mix together the canola and sesame oils and brush the chicken well all over with the mixture. When the oven is up to temperature, put the chicken in and set a timer for 20 minutes.

To make the sauce: Put the saucepan with the marinade over medium-high heat, and add the chicken broth, the final 2 teaspoons of mustard, the final 2 teaspoons of Splenda, and the beef bouillon concentrate. Boil this mixture hard, until it's reduced by half. Thicken just a little—you want it about the texture of cream.

When the oven timer goes off, check the chicken. Pierce a piece to the bone—if the juices run clear, it's done. If the juices are pink, give it another five minutes and check again. When the chicken is done, serve with the sauce.

Yield: 6 servings

Each with 30 g protein; 4 g carbohydrate; trace dietary fiber; 4 g usable carbs.

Seriously Spicy Citrus Chicken

You could cut back on the red pepper flakes if you'd like to make Moderately Spicy Citrus Chicken.

1½ pounds (680 g) boneless, skinless chicken breast

¼ cup (60 ml) olive oil

½ cup (120 ml) lime juice

¼ cup (60 ml) lemon juice

1 tablespoon plus 1 teaspoon (12 g) red pepper flakes

1 tablespoon plus 1 teaspoon (11.2 g) minced garlic

1 tablespoon plus 1 teaspoon (8 g) grated ginger

(continued on page 330)

¼ cup (6 g) Splenda

4 scallions, finely sliced

2 tablespoons (8 g) chopped cilantro

Cut the chicken into 4 servings, if necessary. Sauté the chicken in the olive oil over medium-high heat, covering the pan but tilting the lid. While it's sautéing, mix together the lime juice, lemon juice, red pepper flakes, garlic, ginger, and Splenda. After the chicken has turned golden on both sides (about 4 to 5 minutes per side), pour the lime juice mixture into the skillet and turn the breasts over to coat both sides. Sauté for another 2 to 3 minutes on each side and then move the chicken to serving plates, scraping the liquid from the pan over the chicken. Scatter sliced scallions and chopped cilantro over each portion and serve.

Yield: 4 servings

Each with 8 grams of carbohydrates and 1 gram of fiber, for a total of 7 grams of usable carbs and 32 grams of protein.

Citrus Spice Chicken

3 pounds (1.4 kg) skinless chicken thighs

⅓ cup (78 ml) lemon juice

2 tablespoons (3 g) Splenda

½ teaspoon orange extract

½ cup (120 ml) Dana's No-Sugar Ketchup (page 463) or purchased low-carb ketchup

2 tablespoons (40 g) low-sugar orange marmalade

½ teaspoon ground cinnamon

½ teaspoon ground allspice

⅛ teaspoon ground cloves

¼ teaspoon cayenne

In a bowl, stir together the lemon juice, Splenda, orange extract, ketchup, marmalade, cinnamon, allspice, cloves, and cayenne.

Put the chicken in a slow cooker and pour the sauce over it. Cover the slow cooker, set it to low, and let it cook for 6 hours.

Serve with Cauliflower Rice (page 212).

Yield: 5 servings

Each with 31 g protein, 2 g carbohydrate, trace dietary fiber, 2 g usable carbs. Analysis does not include Cauliflower Rice.

Apricot-Bourbon Chicken

I like the Saffron "Rice" (page 213) as a side with this.

2 pounds (910 g) boneless, skinless chicken breasts

3 tablespoons (42 g) butter, divided

½ cup (60 g) chopped pecans

¼ cup (80 g) low-sugar apricot preserves

¼ cup (60 ml) bourbon

2 tablespoons (30 ml) plain tomato sauce

2 teaspoons spicy brown or Dijon mustard

½ teaspoon minced garlic or 1 clove garlic, crushed

¼ cup (40 g) minced onion

3 scallions, thinly sliced

First, pound the chicken breasts until they're ½ inch (1.3 cm) thick all over and cut into 6 portions. Brown them in 2 tablespoons (28 g) of butter in a large, heavy skillet over high heat.

While the breasts are browning, melt the last tablespoon of butter in a small, heavy skillet and stir in the pecans. Stir them over medium-high heat for a few minutes until they begin to turn golden. Remove from the heat and reserve.

Stir together the preserves, bourbon, tomato sauce, mustard, garlic, and onion. When the chicken is light golden on both sides, pour this mixture into the skillet. Turn the chicken over once or twice to coat both sides with the sauce. Cover with a tilted lid and let it simmer for about 5 minutes or until cooked through.

Serve with the sauce spooned over each portion and top each with the toasted pecans and sliced scallions.

Yield: 6 servings

Each with 7 grams of carbohydrates and 1 gram of fiber, for a total of 6 grams of usable carbs and 35 grams of protein.

Apricot-Rosemary Glazed Chicken Breasts

This is a very speedy meal, especially if you have a gas grill, and it's very good!

4 boneless, skinless chicken breasts—1½ to 2 pounds (680 to 910 g) total
2 tablespoons (40 g) low-sugar apricot preserves
2 teaspoons ground rosemary
2 teaspoons lemon juice
2 cloves garlic, crushed

First, light a charcoal fire or start heating a gas grill. You'll want medium heat.

Simply combine everything but the chicken breasts in a bowl and mix well. Divide the mixture into 2 bowls, reserving the second bowl for basting. Cut the chicken breasts into serving-sized portions if needed. Start the chicken breasts grilling over medium heat, brushing the side facing up with apricot mixture. After about 7 minutes, brush with the apricot mixture again, turn, and brush with the glaze again. Grill another 7 minutes or so, brushing a couple of times with the reserved apricot glaze and using a clean utensil each time you baste.

When the breasts are cooked through, serve. If there's any apricot glaze remaining, you can heat it thoroughly in the microwave—make sure it boils hard!—and spoon it over the breasts before serving.

Yield: 4 servings

Each serving will have 4 grams of carbohydrate and a trace of fiber. Assuming 1½ pounds (680 g) of chicken, each serving will have 38 grams of protein.

Chicken-Almond Stir-Fry

Serve this tasty stir-fry over brown rice for the carb-eaters in your family and enjoy yours straight.

3 large boneless, skinless chicken breasts, cut into ½-inch (1.3-cm) cubes

2 tablespoons (30 ml) soy sauce

¼ cup (60 ml) dry sherry

1 clove garlic, smashed

1 inch (2.5 cm) or so fresh ginger, grated

¼ teaspoon guar (optional)

Peanut oil (Canola or coconut oil would work, too.)

⅓ cup (40 g) slivered almonds

1½ cups (110 g) snow peas, cut in half

1½ cups (105 g) mushrooms, sliced

15 scallions, cut into pieces about 1 inch (2.5 cm) long

¼ cup (50 g) sliced water chestnuts (optional; They increase the carb count, but they're tasty.)

There's one hard-and-fast rule with stir-fries: Make sure all your ingredients are chopped, sliced, and grated before you begin cooking. Once your ingredients are ready, stir together the soy sauce, sherry, garlic, and ginger. (If you're using the guar, put these seasonings through the blender with the guar.)

Heat a couple of teaspoons of the peanut oil in a wok or large, heavy skillet over high heat. Add the almonds and stir-fry them until they're light golden. Remove and set aside.

Heat another couple of tablespoons (30 ml) of oil in the pan and add the snow peas, mushrooms, scallions, and water chestnuts (if using) to the pan. Stir-fry for about 5 minutes or until just barely tender-crisp. Remove from the pan and set aside.

Heat another couple of tablespoons (30 ml) of oil in the pan and add the chicken. Stir-fry for 5 to 7 minutes or until done; there should be no pink left.

Return the vegetables to the skillet and add the soy sauce/sherry mixture. Toss everything together well. Cover and simmer for 3 to 4 minutes. Top with the almonds and serve.

Yield: 3 servings

Each with 18 grams of carbohydrates and 6 grams of fiber, for a total of 12 grams of usable carbs and 36 grams of protein.

Thai-ish Chicken Basil Stir-Fry

If all you've had are Chinese stir-fries, you'll find this an interesting change.

3 boneless, skinless chicken breasts cut into ½-inch (1.3-cm) cubes

2 tablespoons (30 ml) Thai fish sauce

2 tablespoons (30 ml) soy sauce

1 teaspoon Splenda

¼ teaspoon guar or xanthan

2 teaspoons dried basil

1½ teaspoons red pepper flakes

Peanut, canola, or coconut oil

2 cloves garlic, crushed

1 small onion, sliced

1½ cups (225 g) frozen, crosscut green beans, thawed

Combine the fish sauce, soy sauce, Splenda, and guar or xanthan in a blender. Blend for several seconds, then turn off the blender and add the basil and red pepper flakes, and set aside.

Heat a few tablespoons (30 ml) of oil in a wok or heavy skillet over high heat. When the oil is hot, add the garlic, chicken, and onion and stir-fry for 3 to 4 minutes. Add the green beans and continue to stir-fry until the chicken is cooked through.

Stir the fish sauce mixture into the stir-fry, turn the heat to medium, cover, and let it simmer for 2 to 3 minutes (the beans should be tender-crisp).

Yield: 3 servings

Each with 13 grams of carbohydrates and 3 grams of fiber, for a total of 10 grams of usable carbs and 31 grams of protein.

Thai Chicken Bowls

This was a big hit with Maria's family!

8 boneless, skinless, boneless chicken thighs, cubed (a little over 2¼ lbs/1 kg)
2 cloves garlic, crushed
½ cup (80 g) chopped onion
2 stalks celery, sliced
2 teaspoons grated ginger
1 teaspoon five-spice powder
½ teaspoon salt
1 tablespoon (15 ml) lemon juice
1 teaspoon hot pepper sauce (optional)
28 ounces (850 ml) chicken broth
1 head cauliflower
Guar or xanthan

6 tablespoons (35 g) sliced scallions
6 tablespoons (24 g) chopped cilantro

Place the chicken in a slow cooker. Top with the garlic, onion, celery, ginger, five-spice powder, salt, and lemon juice.

In a bowl, combine the hot pepper sauce, if using, with the broth and pour it into the slow cooker. Cover the slow cooker, set it to low, and let it cook for 5 to 6 hours.

Okay, it's almost supper time. Run the cauliflower through the shredding blade of your food processor to make cauli-rice. Put the cauli-rice in a microwaveable casserole dish with a lid, add a couple of tablespoons (30 ml) of water, cover, and microwave on high for 6 minutes.

Thicken up the sauce in the slow cooker with a little guar or xanthan to about the texture of heavy cream.

Okay, the cauli-rice is done! Uncover it immediately, drain, and divide it into 6 bowls. Divide the chicken mixture, ladling it over the cauli-rice. Top with the scallions and cilantro.

Yield: 6 servings

Each with 20 g protein, 4 g carbohydrate, 1 g dietary fiber, 3 g usable carbs.

Curried Chicken with Coconut Milk

The day I first made this my cleaning crew was here, and they couldn't stop talking about how great it smelled. It tastes even better! Find

(continued on page 334)

coconut milk in the Asian section of big grocery stores or at Asian markets. It comes in regular or light, and they generally have the same carb count, so choose whichever you prefer.

3 pounds (1.4 kg) skinless chicken thighs
½ cup (80 g) chopped onion
2 cloves garlic, crushed
1½ tablespoons (8 g) curry powder
1 cup (240 ml) coconut milk
1 teaspoon chicken bouillon concentrate
Guar or xanthan

Put the chicken in a slow cooker. Place the onion and garlic over it.

In a bowl, mix together the curry powder, coconut milk, and bouillon. Pour the mixture over the chicken and vegetables in the slow cooker. Cover the slow cooker, set it to low, and let it cook for 6 hours.

When the time's up, remove the chicken and put it on a platter. Thicken the sauce to a gravy consistency with guar or xanthan.

You'll want to serve this with Cauliflower Rice (page 212) to soak up the extra curry sauce. It's too good to miss!

Yield: 5 servings

Each with 32 g protein, 6 g carbohydrate, 2 g dietary fiber, 4 g usable carbs.

Thai Grilled Chicken

1½ pounds (680 g) boneless, skinless chicken breast

¼ cup (60 ml) coconut milk (You can find this in cans at Asian markets or in grocery stores with a good international section.)
2 tablespoons (30 ml) fish sauce (nuoc mam or nam pla)
2 tablespoons (30 ml) lime juice
2 teaspoons Splenda
2 cloves garlic
½ teaspoon turmeric

Combine everything but the chicken and stir well. Pour it over the chicken in a large resealable plastic bag. Press out the air, seal the bag, and toss it in the fridge for 1 or 2 hours, and all day won't hurt.

When dinnertime rolls around, light a grill. When the grill is hot, cook the chicken for about 7 minutes per side or until cooked through. Serve with Thai Peanut Sauce (below).

Yield: 5 servings

Each serving will have no more than 3 grams of carbohydrate before adding the peanut sauce—and once again, actually a bit less because of the marinade that gets thrown away—31 grams of protein. Analysis does not include the Thai Peanut Sauce.

Thai Peanut Sauce
½ teaspoon hot pepper sauce
1 tablespoon (6 g) grated ginger
1 clove garlic, crushed
2 scallions, sliced, including the crisp part of the green
⅓ cup (80 g) natural peanut butter
⅓ cup (80 ml) coconut milk
2 tablespoons (30 ml) fish sauce (nam pla or nuoc mam)

1½ tablespoons (23 ml) lime juice

2 teaspoons Splenda

Put everything in a blender or a food processor with the S-blade in place and process until smooth.

Yield: Makes roughly 1 cup (240 ml), or 8 servings of 2 tablespoons each.

4 grams of carbohydrate per serving, and 1 gram of fiber, for a usable carb count of 3 grams; 3 grams of protein.

Chili-Lime Chicken

This was a big hit at our annual Toastmasters Bash at the Lake.

3 pounds (1.4 kg) chicken pieces—either a cut-up broiler/fryer or whatever parts you like (I used thighs.)

1 tablespoon (16.5 g) chili garlic paste

2 cloves garlic, crushed

1 tablespoon (6 g) grated ginger

¼ cup (60 ml) soy sauce

½ cup (120 ml) lime juice

3 tablespoons (4.5 g) Splenda

Place the chicken in a big resealable plastic bag. Mix together everything else, pour it into the bag with the chicken, press out the air, and seal the bag. Throw the bag in the fridge and let the chicken marinate for at least a few hours, and more won't hurt.

When it's time to cook, fire up the grill—you'll want medium to medium-high heat. Just drain the marinade off the chicken and throw it on the grill

skin-side up when it's ready. Close the grill and keep it closed until it's time to turn the chicken, unless you suspect a flare-up. Cook for about 12 to 15 minutes, turn skin-side down and cook another 7 to 9 minutes, and then turn skin-side up again. Let it cook until the juices run clear when it's pierced to the bone and an instant-read thermometer registers 180°F (85°C). Then serve!

Yield: 6 servings

If you consumed all of the marinade, you'd get 5 grams of carb and a trace of fiber per serving, but since you discard most of it, you won't get anywhere near that much—I'd count no more than 1 to 2 grams per serving. Assuming 6 servings, each will have 30 grams of protein.

Thai Hot Pot

This recipe takes a few more steps than some, but the results are worth it! If you can't get Southeast Asian fish sauce, you can substitute soy sauce.

1½ pounds (680 g) boneless, skinless chicken thighs

1 medium carrot, sliced

1 medium onion, sliced

1 clove garlic, crushed

14 ounces (425 ml) coconut milk

1 tablespoon (6 g) grated ginger

2 tablespoons (30 ml) fish sauce (nam pla or nuoc mam) or soy sauce

1 tablespoon (15 ml) lime juice

2 teaspoons Splenda

½ teaspoon hot pepper sauce

(continued on page 336)

⅓ cup (85 g) natural peanut butter

1 pound (455 g) shrimp, shelled

1 cup (75 g) fresh snow pea pods, cut into
  ½-inch (1.3-cm) pieces

Guar or xanthan

6 cups (720 g) Cauliflower Rice (page 212)

⅓ cup (40 g) chopped peanuts

Put the chicken in your slow cooker and add the carrot, onion, and garlic.

In a blender, combine the coconut milk, ginger, fish sauce or soy sauce, lime juice, Splenda, hot pepper sauce, and peanut butter and blend until smooth. Pour the sauce over the chicken and vegetables, using a rubber scraper to make sure you get all of it! Cover the slow cooker, set it to low, and let it cook for 8 hours.

Stir in the shrimp and snow peas, re-cover the slow cooker, and turn it up to high. Cook for 10 minutes or until the shrimp are pink all the way through.

Thicken the sauce slightly with guar or xanthan. Serve over the Cauliflower Rice (or brown rice for the carb-eaters). Top each serving with the peanuts.

Yield: 6 servings

Each with 33 g protein, 19 g carbohydrate, 7 g dietary fiber, 12 g usable carbs. Analysis does not include Cauliflower Rice.

Singing Chicken

This is another Vietnamese dish, and it is definitely for those who enjoy breathing fire. I'm a big fan of hot food, and this dish had me sweating by halfway through the meal. It's delicious! Broccoli goes nicely with this.

1½ pounds (680 g) boneless, skinless chicken
  breast, cut crosswise into thin slices*

2 to 3 tablespoons (30 to 45 ml) vegetable oil,
  preferably peanut

1 tablespoon (6 g) grated ginger

1 teaspoon minced garlic or 2 cloves garlic,
  crushed

2 tablespoons (3 g) Splenda

¼ cup (60 ml) soy sauce

1 teaspoon fish sauce (nuoc mam)

¾ cup (180 ml) dry white wine

1 fresh jalapeño, or 2 or 3 little red chilies,
  finely minced

1 teaspoon pepper

Guar or xanthan

Have the chicken sliced, the ingredients measured, the pepper minced, and everything standing by and ready to go before starting to cook—once you start stir-frying, this goes very quickly.

Put a wok or heavy skillet over high heat. Add the oil, let it heat for a minute or so, and then add the ginger and garlic. Stir for 1 minute to flavor the oil. Add the chicken and stir-fry for 1 to 2 minutes. Add the Splenda, soy sauce, fish sauce, white wine, jalapeño, and pepper, stirring often, for 7 to 8 minutes or until the chicken is cooked through. Thicken the pan juices very slightly with guar or xanthan and serve.

Yield: 3 or 4 servings

Assuming 4 servings, each will have 4 grams of carbohydrates, a trace of fiber, and 39 grams of protein.

*This is easiest if the meat is half-frozen.

Chicken Vindaloo

I made this at a local campground over Memorial Day Weekend, and it was a huge hit with fellow campers. It's exotic and wonderful.

6 pounds (2.7 kg) boneless, skinless chicken thighs
1 medium onion, chopped
5 cloves garlic, crushed
¼ cup (24 g) grated ginger
4 teaspoons purchased garam masala
1 teaspoon ground turmeric
¼ cup (60 ml) lime juice
¼ cup (60 ml) rice vinegar
½ cup (120 ml) chicken broth
1 teaspoon salt

Put the chicken, onion, and garlic in a slow cooker.

In a bowl, stir together the remaining ingredients. Pour the mixture over the chicken. Cover the slow cooker, set it to low, and let it cook for 6 to 7 hours.

Serve with Major Grey's Chutney (page 496).

Yield: 12 servings

Each with 46 g protein, 2 g carbohydrate, trace dietary fiber, 2 g usable carbs. Analysis does not include Chutney.

Chicken in Creamy Horseradish Sauce

Don't think that just because this has horseradish it's really strong. The sauce is mellow, subtle, and family-friendly.

4 pounds (1.8 kg) cut-up chicken
1 tablespoon (14 g) butter
1 tablespoon (15 ml) olive oil
¾ cup (180 ml) chicken broth
1½ teaspoons chicken bouillon concentrate
1 tablespoon (15 g) prepared horseradish
4 ounces (115 g) cream cheese, cut into chunks
¼ cup (60 ml) heavy cream
Guar or xanthan (optional)

In a big, heavy skillet, brown the chicken in the butter and oil over medium-high heat. Transfer the chicken to a slow cooker.

In a bowl, stir together the broth, bouillon, and horseradish. Pour the mixture over the chicken. Cover the slow cooker, set it to low, and let it cook for 6 hours.

When the time's up, remove the chicken with tongs and put it on a platter. Melt the cream cheese into the sauce in the slow cooker. Stir in the cream. Thicken the sauce with guar or xanthan if you think it needs it. Add salt and pepper to taste.

I think this would be good with Fauxtatoes (page 209) and green beans.

Yield: 8 servings

Each with 30 g protein, 1 g carbohydrate, trace dietary fiber, 1 g usable carbs. Analysis does not include side dishes.

Black and Bleu Chicken

This is quick and easy and very good. Why use only three chicken breasts? Because that's what fits in my skillet! Once they were pounded out thin, they just barely squeezed in there together. If you want to increase this recipe, you'll need two skillets—but it will still be quick and very good!

3 boneless, skinless chicken breasts
Cajun seasoning, purchased or homemade
3 tablespoons (42 g) butter
¼ pound (115 g) blue cheese, crumbled

Start a large, heavy-bottomed skillet heating over medium-high heat. In the meanwhile, one at a time, place each chicken breast in a heavy resealable plastic bag. Use a meat tenderizing hammer, a regular hammer, or whatever blunt object comes to hand (I use a 3-pound dumbbell!) to pound each breast until it's about ¼ inch (6 mm) thick all over—this should take about 30 seconds per breast. Sprinkle both sides of each pounded breast with the Cajun seasoning. Melt the butter in the skillet and add the chicken breasts. Sauté for 4 to 5 minutes per side or until cooked through. When they're just about done, sprinkle the crumbled blue cheese over the chicken breasts, dividing it evenly between all three. Cover the skillet for a minute more to let the cheese melt and serve.

Yield: 3 servings

Each with 36 g protein; 2 g usable carbs; a trace of fiber.

Chicken with Root Vegetables, Cabbage, and Herbs

I think of this as being a sort of French Country dish. Of course, I've never been to the French countryside, so what do I know? It's good, though, and you don't need another darned thing with it.

5 pounds (2.3 kg) chicken
1½ tablespoons (23 ml) olive oil
1½ tablespoons (21 g) butter
2 medium turnips, cut into ½-inch (1.3-cm) cubes
2 medium carrots, cut into ½-inch (1.3-cm) slices
1 medium onion, cut into ¼-inch (6 mm) half-rounds
1 head cabbage
4 cloves garlic, crushed
½ teaspoon dried rosemary
½ teaspoon dried thyme
½ teaspoon dried basil
2 bay leaves, crumbled

In a big, heavy skillet, brown the chicken on both sides in the oil and butter over medium-high heat.

When the chicken is browned all over, remove it to a plate and reserve. Some extra fat will have accumulated in the skillet. Pour off all but a couple of tablespoons (30 ml) and then add the turnips, carrots, and onion. Sauté them, scraping the tasty brown bits off the bottom of the skillet as you stir, until they're getting a touch of gold, too.

Transfer the sautéed vegetables to a slow cooker.

Cut the cabbage into eighths and put it on top of the vegetables. Arrange the chicken on top of the cabbage. Sprinkle the garlic over the chicken and vegetables, making sure some ends up on the chicken and some down among the vegetables. Sprinkle the rosemary, thyme, basil, and bay leaves into the slow cooker, making sure some gets down into the vegetables. Season with salt and pepper. Cover the slow cooker, set it to low, and let it cook for 6 to 7 hours.

Yield: 8 servings

Each with 36 g protein, 6 g carbohydrate, 2 g dietary fiber, 4 g usable carbs.

Chicken with Camembert and Almonds

4 boneless, skinless chicken breasts
6 tablespoons (84 g) butter, divided
8 ounces (225 g) Camembert
⅓ cup (40 g) slivered almonds
4 scallions, thinly sliced

Place a chicken breast in a large, heavy, resealable plastic bag and pound it until it's ¼ inch (6 mm) thick. Repeat with the remaining chicken breasts.

Melt 4 tablespoons (56 g) of the butter in a heavy skillet over medium heat. Sauté the chicken until it's golden on the first side.

While the first side of the chicken is cooking, divide the cheese into four equal portions, peel off the white rind, and thinly slice each portion.

Flip the chicken and lay a portion of cheese over each chicken breast.

Melt the remaining 2 tablespoons (28 g) of butter in a small skillet and add the almonds. Stir until they're lightly golden.

When the second side of the chicken is golden and the cheese is melted, place each breast on a serving plate and divide the almonds evenly over them. Scatter a sliced scallion over each breast and serve.

Yield: 4 servings

Each with 4 grams of carbohydrates and 2 grams of fiber, for a total of 2 grams of usable carbs and 43 grams of protein.

If you're the type of person who likes to multitask, this recipe is for you. If you can slice and peel the cheese while the first side of the chicken cooks and get the almonds toasting. You should be able to get the almonds done just in time to move hot almonds onto just-done chicken breasts.

Slow Cooker Brewery Chicken and Vegetables

There are plenty of vegetables in here, so you don't need a thing with it, except maybe some bread for the carb-eaters in the family. And the gravy comes out a beautiful color!

(continued on page 338)

2½ to 3 pounds (1.3 to 1.4 kg) cut-up chicken (I use leg and thigh quarters, cut apart at the joints.)

8 ounces (225 g) turnips (two turnips roughly the size of tennis balls), peeled and cut into chunks

2 stalks celery, sliced

1 medium carrot, sliced

½ medium onion, sliced

1 tablespoon (15 ml) chicken bouillon concentrate

12 ounces (360 ml) light beer

1 can (14½ ounces, or 410 g) tomatoes with green chiles

Guar or xanthan (optional)

Put the turnips, celery, carrot, onion, bouillon, and chicken in a slow cooker. Pour the beer and the tomatoes over the lot. Cover the slow cooker, set it to low, and let it cook for 8 to 9 hours.

When the time's up, remove the chicken with tongs and place it on a serving platter. Then use a slotted spoon to scoop out the vegetables. Put 1½ cups (360 ml) of them in a blender and pile the rest on and around the chicken on the platter. Scoop out 1½ to 2 cups (360 to 480 ml) of the liquid left in the slow cooker and put it in the blender with the vegetables. Purée the vegetables and broth and thicken the mixture a little more with the guar or xanthan, if it seems necessary. Add salt and pepper to taste and serve as a sauce with the chicken and vegetables.

Yield: 5 servings

Each with 30 g protein, 10 g carbohydrate, 2 g dietary fiber, 8 g usable carbs.

Sort-of-Ethiopian Chicken Stew

The slow cooker method is hardly authentic, but the flavors come from an Ethiopian recipe—except that the Ethiopians would use a lot more cayenne! Increase it if you like really hot food.

1 cut-up broiler-fryer, about 3 pounds (1.4 kg)

1 medium onion, chopped

1 teaspoon cayenne

1 teaspoon paprika

½ teaspoon pepper

½ teaspoon grated ginger

2 tablespoons (30 ml) lemon juice

½ cup (120 ml) water

Guar or xanthan

Place the everything but the guar or xanthan in a slow cooker. Cover the slow cooker, set it to low, and let it cook for 5 to 6 hours.

If you'd like to make this really stewlike, you can pick the meat off the bones when it's done (which will be very easy), thicken the gravy with guar or xanthan, and then stir the chicken back into the liquid. Or you can just serve the gravy over the chicken. Take your pick.

Yield: 5 servings

Each with 34 g protein, 3 g carbohydrate, 1 g dietary fiber, 2 g usable carbs.

Stewed Chicken with Moroccan Seasonings

This is almost a Moroccan *tagine*, but all the recipes I've seen call for some sort of starch. So I ditched the starch and just kept the seasonings, which are exotic and delicious.

3½ to 4 pounds (1.6 to 1.8 kg) chicken, cut up
¼ cup (60 ml) olive oil
1 medium onion, thinly sliced
2 cloves garlic, crushed
¾ cup (180 ml) chicken broth
½ teaspoon ground coriander
½ teaspoon ground cinnamon
½ teaspoon paprika
½ teaspoon ground cumin
1 teaspoon ground ginger
½ teaspoon pepper
¼ teaspoon cayenne
1 tablespoon (1.5 g) Splenda
1 tablespoon (16.5 g) tomato paste
1 teaspoon salt or Vege-Sal

Heat the oil in a Dutch oven over medium heat and brown the chicken in the oil.

When the chicken is golden all over, remove it from the Dutch oven and pour off the fat. Put the chicken back in the Dutch oven and scatter the onion and garlic over it.

Combine the broth and the next 10 ingredients (through salt) and whisk together well. Pour over the chicken, cover the Dutch oven, and turn the heat to low. Let the whole thing simmer for a good 45 minutes.

Uncover the chicken and let it simmer for another 15 minutes or so to let the juices concentrate a bit. Serve each piece of chicken with some of the onion and juices spooned over it.

Yield: 4 generous servings

Each with 6 grams of carbohydrates and 1 gram of fiber, for a total of 5 grams of usable carbs and 58 grams of protein.

Chicken Stew

This dish is a nice change from the usual beef stew. It's light, flavorful, and your whole meal in one pot.

1½ pounds (680 g) boneless, skinless chicken
    thighs, cut into 1-inch (2.5-cm) cubes
2 tablespoons (30 ml) olive oil, divided
8 ounces (225 g) sliced mushrooms
1 medium onion, sliced
3 cups (345 g) zucchini slices
4 cloves garlic, crushed
1 can (14 ounces, or 400 g) tomato wedges
¾ cup (180 ml) chicken broth
1 teaspoon chicken bouillon concentrate
1 tablespoon (3 g) poultry seasoning
Guar or xanthan

In a big, heavy skillet, heat 1 tablespoon (15 ml) of the oil. Brown the chicken until it is golden all over. Transfer the chicken to a slow cooker.

(continued on page 342)

Heat the remaining 1 tablespoon (15 ml) of oil in the skillet and sauté the mushrooms, onion, and zucchini until the mushrooms change color and the onions are translucent. Transfer them to the slow cooker, too. Add the garlic and tomatoes to the slow cooker.

Put the broth and bouillon in the skillet and stir them around to dissolve any flavorful bits sticking to the skillet. Pour into the slow cooker. Sprinkle the poultry seasoning over the mixture. Cover the slow cooker, set it to low, and let it cook for 4 to 5 hours. When the time's up, thicken the liquid in the slow cooker with guar or xanthan.

Yield: 6 servings

Each with 11 g protein, 12 g carbohydrate, 2 g dietary fiber, 10 g usable carbs.

Yassa

This chicken stew comes from Senegal. Traditionally it is quite hot, so feel free to increase the cayenne if you like!

6 pounds (2.7 kg) chicken, cut up
3 large onions, thinly sliced
6 cloves garlic, crushed
½ cup (120 ml) lemon juice
1½ teaspoons salt
½ teaspoon cayenne, or more to taste
¼ cup (60 ml) oil
8 cups (960 g) Cauliflower Rice (page 212)

In a slow cooker, combine the onions, garlic, lemon juice, salt, and cayenne. Add the chicken and toss so that all the chicken comes in contact with the seasonings. Cover your slow cooker and refriger-

ate overnight. (It's a good idea to stir this a few times if you think of it, though I don't expect you to get up in the middle of the night to do it!)

Using tongs, remove the chicken from the marinade. Pat it dry with paper towels and set it aside.

In a big, heavy skillet, heat the oil over medium-high heat. Place the chicken skin side down and cook it until the skin is browned. (You'll need to do this in batches, unless your skillet is a lot bigger than mine!) Don't bother browning the other side of the chicken.

Transfer the chicken back to the slow cooker with the marinade. Cover the slow cooker, set it to low, and let it cook for 5 to 6 hours.

Remove the chicken from the slow cooker with tongs. Put the chicken on a platter, cover it with foil, and put it in a warm place.

Ladle the onions and liquid out of the slow cooker into the skillet and turn the heat to high. Boil this hard, stirring often, until most of the liquid has evaporated. (You want the volume reduced by more than half.) Serve the chicken, onions, and sauce over the Cauliflower Rice.

Yield: 8 servings

Each with 45 g protein, 11 g carbohydrate, 3 g dietary fiber, 8 g usable carbs.

Chicken and Dumplings

This takes some work, but boy, is it comfort food. You could make this with leftover turkey instead if you prefer. If you do that, put the cubed, cooked turkey in about 5 to 6 hours into the initial cooking time.

1½ pounds (680 g) boneless, skinless chicken thighs, cut into 1″ cubes

2 medium carrots, sliced

1 medium onion, chunked

2 medium turnips, cut into ½-inch (1.3-cm) cubes

1½ cups (225 g) frozen green beans, cross-cut

8 ounces (225 g) sliced mushrooms

1½ cups (360 ml) chicken broth

1 teaspoon poultry seasoning

3 teaspoons chicken bouillon concentrate

½ cup (120 ml) heavy cream

Guar or xanthan

Dumplings (page 343)

In a slow cooker, combine the carrots, onion, turnips, green beans, mushrooms, and chicken.

In a bowl, mix together the broth, poultry seasoning, and bouillon. Pour the mixture over the chicken and vegetables. Cover the slow cooker, set it to low, and let it cook for 6 to 7 hours.

When the time's up, stir in the cream and thicken the gravy to a nice consistency with guar or xanthan. Add salt and pepper to taste. Re-cover the slow cooker and turn it to high.

While the slow cooker is heating up (it'll take at least 30 minutes), make the Dumplings, stopping before you add the liquid. Wait until the gravy in the slow cooker is boiling. Then stir in the buttermilk to the Dumpling dough and drop it by spoonfuls over the surface of the chicken and gravy. Re-cover the slow cooker and let it cook for another 25 to 30 minutes.

Yield: 8 servings

Each with 36 g protein, 14 g carbohydrate, 4 g dietary fiber, 10 g usable carbs (calculations include the dumplings).

Dumplings

Feel free to use this with other meat-and-gravy dishes if you like! (These instructions require gravy to boil the Dumplings in.)

¾ cup (90 g) ground almonds, or "almond meal"

½ cup (65 g) rice protein powder

¼ cup (25 g) wheat gluten

2 tablespoons (28 g) butter

2 tablespoons (30 ml) coconut oil

½ teaspoon salt

2 teaspoons baking powder

½ teaspoon baking soda

¾ cup (180 ml) buttermilk

Put everything but the buttermilk into a food processor with the S-blade in place. Pulse the food processor to cut in the butter. (You want it evenly distributed in the dry ingredients.) Dump this mixture into a mixing bowl.

Check to make sure your gravy is boiling. (If it isn't, have a quick cup of tea until it is.) Now pour the buttermilk into the dry ingredients and stir it in with a few swift strokes. (Don't over-mix; you just want to make sure everything's evenly damp.) This will make a soft dough. Drop by spoonfuls over the boiling gravy, cover the pot, and let it cook for 25 to 30 minutes.

Yield: 12 servings

Each with 14 g protein, 4 g carbohydrate, 1 g dietary fiber, 3 g usable carbs.

Chunky Chicken Pie

This is a fair amount of work, but it's certainly comfort food for a cold winter night!

1½ pounds (680 g) dark meat chicken, no skin, but on the bone

1 quart (960 ml) water

1 tablespoon (15 ml) chicken bouillon concentrate

1 pound (455 g) frozen California-blend vegetables

1 cup (70 g) sliced mushrooms

1 cup (240 ml) Carb Countdown dairy beverage or half-and-half

½ teaspoon poultry seasoning

Guar or xanthan

Salt and pepper

1 batch Buttermilk Drop Biscuits (page 120)

Plunk chicken in a big saucepan and add the water and chicken bouillon concentrate. Cover it, turn the heat to low, and let the whole thing simmer for 60 to 90 minutes.

Fish the chicken out with a fork or tongs and set it on a plate until cool enough to handle. In the meantime, add the California-blend vegetables and the sliced mushrooms to the broth—I actually cut mine up a little more, but you can leave everything in really big chunks if you prefer. Let this simmer for 25 to 30 minutes or until the vegetables are tender but not mushy.

While that's happening, strip the chicken off the bones. Discard the bones and cut the meat into bite-sized pieces. Reserve.

Okay, your vegetables are cooked. Stir in the Carb Countdown dairy beverage and poultry seasoning. Thicken with guar or xanthan to make a rich gravy consistency. Now add salt and pepper to taste and stir in the chicken. Turn off the heat.

Preheat the oven to 475°F (240°C, or gas mark 9) and then make a batch of Buttermilk Drop Biscuit dough, stopping right before you add the buttermilk to the dry ingredients.

Spray a 2-quart (1.9-L) casserole dish with nonstick cooking spray. When the oven is up to temperature, turn the heat back on under the chicken and vegetable mixture and bring it back to a boil. While that's heating, stir the buttermilk into the biscuit dough. Now, pour the boiling chicken mixture into the casserole dish and spoon the dough over the top. Don't worry about covering every single millimeter of the gravy with the dough; it'll spread a bit. Just spoon it on pretty evenly, and it'll be fine. Put it in the oven immediately and bake for 10 to 12 minutes or until golden and then serve.

Yield: 6 servings

Each with 48 g protein; 13 g carbohydrate; 5 g dietary fiber; 8 g usable carbs.

Mom's 1960s Chicken, Redux

Back in the 1960s my mom would make a dish for company with chicken breasts, wrapped in bacon, laid on a layer of chipped beef, topped with a sauce made of sour cream and cream of mushroom soup. It tasted far more sophisticated than it sounds and never failed to draw raves from dinner party guests. This is my attempt to de-carb and slow-cooker-ize the same dish—without the carb-filled cream of mushroom soup.

2 pounds (910 g) boneless, skinless chicken breasts

2¼ ounces (62 g) dried beef slices (aka "chipped beef")

6 slices bacon

1 cup (70 g) sliced mushrooms

1 tablespoon (14 g) butter

1 cup (240 ml) heavy cream

1 teaspoon beef bouillon concentrate

1 pinch onion powder

1 pinch celery salt

¼ teaspoon pepper

Guar or xanthan

1 cup (230 g) sour cream

Paprika

Line the bottom of a slow cooker with the dried beef.

Place the bacon in a glass pie plate or on a microwave bacon rack and microwave for 3 to 4 minutes on high. Drain the bacon and reserve. (What you're doing here is cooking some of the grease off of the bacon without cooking it crisp.)

Cut the chicken into 6 servings. Wrap each piece of chicken in a slice of bacon and place it in the slow cooker on top of the dried beef.

In a big, heavy skillet, sauté the mushrooms in the butter until they're soft. Add the cream and bouillon and stir until the bouillon dissolves. Stir in the onion powder, celery salt, and pepper and then thicken with guar or xanthan until the mixture reaches a gravy consistency. Stir in the sour cream.

Spoon this mixture over the chicken breasts and sprinkle with a little paprika. Cover the slow cooker, set it to low, and let it cook for 5 to 6 hours.

To serve, scoop up some of the dried beef and sauce with each bacon-wrapped piece of chicken.

Yield: 6 servings

Each with 41 g protein, 4 g carbohydrate, trace dietary fiber, 4 g usable carbs.

Chicken Liver Sauté

The worst possible thing you can do to liver of any kind is overcook it, which makes chicken livers an ideal candidate for a super-fast gourmet supper. The cauliflower rice is optional with this, but it takes very little extra time, adds only 1 gram of extra carbs to a serving, and makes this seem more like a meal.

8 ounces (225 g) chicken livers

½ head cauliflower (optional)

4 ounces (115 g) sliced mushrooms

¼ medium onion

1 tablespoon (14 g) butter

½ teaspoon minced garlic or 1 clove garlic, crushed

½ teaspoon ground rosemary*

¼ cup (60 ml) dry sherry

½ teaspoon lemon juice

(continued on page 346)

Salt and pepper

Guar or xanthan

If you want cauliflower rice to serve the chicken livers on, make that first. Run the cauliflower through the shredding blade of your food processor, put it in a microwaveable casserole dish with a lid, add a couple of tablespoons (30 ml) of water, cover it, and microwave it on high for 7 minutes. If the cauliflower is done cooking before you're quite done with your livers, remove the lid. This will let the steam out and stop the cooking. Otherwise you'll get a white mush that bears little resemblance to rice or even cauliflower.

Okay, you're ready to deal with the livers. Cut each liver into 3 or 4 chunks. I'm assuming you bought presliced mushrooms, but if you didn't, slice them now. Take the onion quarter, cut it in half again (making two eighths), and then slice it as thin as you can. Melt the butter in a large, heavy skillet over medium-high heat. Add the livers, mushrooms, onions, and garlic, and stir-fry until the mushrooms are starting to change color and most of the pink is gone from the livers. Add the rosemary, sherry, lemon juice, and a little salt and pepper and let it all simmer for just 1 to 2 minutes. Thicken the pan liquid slightly with guar or xanthan and serve, with or without cauliflower rice.

Yield: 2 servings

Without the cauliflower rice, each serving will have 8 grams of carbohydrates and 1 gram of fiber, for a total of 7 grams of usable carbs and 22 grams of protein. If you serve it with the cauliflower rice, each serving will have 10 grams of carbohydrates and 2 grams of fiber, for a total of 8 grams of usable carbs and 22 grams of protein.

*You can use a teaspoon of dried rosemary needles instead, and it will taste good, but you'll have little tough needles in your food.

Chicken Liver and "Rice" Casserole

I'm a big fan of chicken livers, and they're highly nutritious. No, the liver does not contain every toxin eaten by the animal during its life. The liver processes and removes this stuff. It doesn't just hold on to it forever.

1 pound (455 g) chicken livers, cut into bite-sized pieces

1 stick butter

1 small onion, chopped

1 rib celery, including leaves, diced

1 bay leaf, crumbled fine

½ teaspoon dried thyme

½ teaspoon salt or Vege-Sal

½ teaspoon seasoned salt

4 cups Cauliflower Rice Deluxe (page 212)

¼ cup (25 g) grated Parmesan cheese

Preheat oven to 375°F (190°C, or gas mark 5).

Melt the butter in a heavy skillet over medium heat and sauté the onion, celery, bay leaf, thyme, salt, and seasoned salt.

When the onion is golden, add the chicken livers and cook for another 5 minutes, stirring frequently. Toss the vegetables and livers together with the Cauliflower Rice Deluxe.

Spray a good-sized casserole dish (10 cups [2.4 L] or so) with nonstick cooking spray and dump the liver and "rice" mixture into the casserole dish. Sprinkle the top with the Parmesan cheese and bake the whole thing uncovered for 15 minutes.

Yield: 5 servings

Each with 16 grams of carbohydrates and 3 grams of fiber, for a total of 13 grams usable carbs and 21 grams of protein.

Curried Chicken "Pilau"

Back in my low-fat, high-carb day, I made a three-grain curried chicken pilau that was our very favorite supper. I hadn't had it since the day I went low carb—but this is a really convincing decarbed version and far faster to cook. Don't omit the garnishes: chutney, chopped peanuts, and crumbled bacon. They're what make the dish!

1 pound (455 g) boneless, skinless chicken breast, cut in ½-inch (1.3-cm) cubes
½ cup (80 g) chopped onion
2 cloves garlic, crushed
2 tablespoons (12 g) curry powder
1 tablespoon (14 g) butter
½ cup (40 g) fresh snow pea pods (measure them after you cut them up!)
½ head cauliflower
2 teaspoons chicken bouillon concentrate
¼ cup (60 ml) hot water

In a big, heavy skillet over medium heat, start the onion, garlic, curry powder, and chicken sautéing in the butter. Remember to stir it once in a while during the sautéing process.

While that's happening, pinch the ends off of your snow peas, pull off any strings, and cut them into ½-inch (1.3-cm) pieces. Run the cauliflower through the shredding blade of your food processor—but this time, you're not going to microwave your cauli-rice. Just hang on to it. In a cup or small bowl, dissolve the bouillon in the water.

When the chicken is white all over and the onion is translucent, stir in the cauli-rice and the dissolved bouillon, making sure everything is well combined—you want the chicken and curry flavors throughout the whole dish. Cover, turn the heat to low, and let it cook for 4 to 5 minutes. Uncover, add the snow peas, and stir again. Re-cover and let cook for another 4 to 5 minutes. Then check to see how your cauli-rice is—you want it just barely tender, but not mushy. When it reaches that state, serve with Major Grey's Chutney (page 496), crumbled bacon, and chopped salted peanuts.

Yield: 3 to 4 servings

Assuming 3, each will have 36 g protein; 8 g carbohydrate; 3 g dietary fiber; 5 g usable carbs. Analysis does not include garnishes.

Chicken "Risotto" alla Milanese

This is my decarbed version of a very famous Italian dish—and it's quick and easy enough for a weeknight supper. My husband loved this—but then, any food with butter, cream, and cheese, especially all three, is pretty much his ideal.

(continued on page 348)

1 pound (455 g) boneless, skinless chicken
  breast

½ head cauliflower

3 tablespoons (42 g) butter

¾ cup (120 g) chopped onion

4 cup (60 ml) dry white wine

2 teaspoons chicken bouillon concentrate

¼ teaspoon saffron threads

1 clove garlic, crushed

¼ cup (60 ml) heavy cream

Guar or xanthan

Salt and pepper

½ cup (40 g) shredded Parmesan cheese

First, run the cauliflower through the shredding blade of your food processor. Put it in a micro-waveable casserole dish with a lid, add a couple of tablespoons (30 ml) of water, cover, and microwave on high for 5 or 6 minutes. Uncover as soon as the microwave beeps!

Cut the chicken breast in ½-inch (1.3-cm) cubes. Melt the butter in a big, heavy skillet over medium to medium-high heat and start sautéing the chicken and onion.

When the chicken is white all over and the onion is softened, stir in the wine, bouillon concentrate, saffron threads, and garlic. Stir it around until the bouillon concentrate dissolves.

Drain the cauli-rice and throw it in the skillet. Stir it around to blend all the flavors and let the whole thing cook for 2 to 3 minutes. Stir in the heavy cream and cook for another minute. If you want the whole thing a little creamier, use just a little guar or xanthan, but I didn't bother. Season with salt and pepper to taste.

Spoon onto plates or into bowls, top each serving with 3 tablespoons (15 g) Parmesan, and serve.

Yield: 3 servings

Each with 30 g protein; 5 g carbohydrate; 1 g dietary fiber; 4 g usable carbs.

Lettuce Wraps

These are currently a hot appetizer at Asian restaurants, and they're delicious—but the restaurant version usually contains an unaccept-able amount of sugar. Serve these as an appe-tizer if you like, but I like them as a light supper. Even if you have to make the Asian Dipping Sauce too, this will take you all of 15 minutes.

1 pound (455 g) ground chicken

1 can (8 ounces, or 225 g) water chestnuts,
  drained

1 cup (70 g) sliced mushrooms

5 scallions, roots and limp shoot removed,
  cut into 2 or 3 pieces each

3 tablespoons (45 ml) soy sauce

2 tablespoons (3 g) Splenda

½ teaspoon blackstrap molasses

1½ teaspoons minced garlic or 3 cloves of
  garlic, crushed

1½ teaspoons rice vinegar

3 tablespoons (45 ml) oil

Guar or xanthan

Iceberg or leaf lettuce

Asian Dipping Sauce (page 478)

Place the water chestnuts, mushrooms, and scallions in a food processor with the S-blade in place. Pulse just enough to chop everything to a medium consistency.

Combine the soy sauce, Splenda, blackstrap molasses, garlic, and rice vinegar. Set aside.

Heat the oil in a wok or large skillet over highest heat. Add the chicken and stir-fry, breaking it up as it cooks. When about half of the pink is gone from the chicken, add the chopped vegetables and stir-fry everything together for a few more minutes. When the chicken is cooked through, stir in the soy sauce mixture and let everything cook together for just another minute or so. Thicken the pan juices just a little with guar or xanthan and serve.

To eat this, you wrap spoonfuls of the meat mixture in lettuce leaves, dip the rolls in the Asian Dipping Sauce, and then eat them by hand. The tidiest way to do this is to take a whole, firm head of iceberg lettuce and slice a good 2-inch (5-cm) thick slab off the side, making lettuce "cups"—you can do this all over the head, leaving the inside of the head for salad. However, there's no reason not to use leaf lettuce if you prefer it.

Yield: Figure this is 6 servings as an appetizer

Each with 10 grams of carbohydrates and 2 grams of fiber, for a total of 8 grams of usable carbs (exclusive of the dipping sauce) and 25 grams of protein, which is a pretty filling appetizer!

If you figure this is 4 servings as a main course, each with 15 grams of carbohydrates and 3 grams of fiber, for a total of 12 grams of usable carbs (again, exclusive of the dipping sauce) and 37 grams of protein.

Chicken Burritos

Wow—This is easy, delicious, low-carb, low-calorie, and reheats easily. What more do you want from a recipe?

2½ pounds (1.1 kg) boneless, skinless chicken thighs

5 cloves garlic, crushed

2 tablespoons (15.6 g) chili powder

2 tablespoons (30 ml) olive oil

2 tablespoons (30 ml) lime juice

1 teaspoon salt

1 large jalapeño, minced, or 2 teaspoons canned jalapeños

12 6-inch (15-cm) low-carb tortillas

1 cup (20 g) shredded lettuce

1 cup (115 g) shredded cheddar cheese

⅔ cup (180 g) light sour cream

¾ cup (195 g) salsa

½ cup (32 g) chopped fresh cilantro (optional)

Place the chicken in a slow cooker.

In a bowl, mix the garlic, chili powder, oil, lime juice, salt, and jalapeño together. Pour over the chicken and stir to coat. Cover the slow cooker, set it to low, and let it cook for 10 hours. (Or cook on high for 5 hours.)

When the time's up, stir the mixture with a fork to reduce the chicken to a big pot of tasty chicken shreds. Fill each tortilla with ⅓ cup chicken (75 g) and top with lettuce, cheese, 1 tablespoon (15 g) sour cream, a generous tablespoon salsa, and a sprinkling of cilantro, if desired. Wrap and devour!

This is a great meal for a family that has some low-carbers and some non–low-carbers—just give them regular or (preferably) whole wheat flour tortillas. The chicken keeps well in the fridge, and it reheats quickly in the microwave for a fast snack. (I find that 45 seconds on 70 percent power is about right for a ⅓-cup serving.)

Yield: 12 servings

(continued on page 350)

Each with 22 g protein, 14 g carbohydrate, 9 g dietary fiber, 5 g usable carbs.

Seriously Simple Chicken Chili

The name says it all!

2 pounds (910 g) boneless, skinless chicken breasts
1 jar (16 ounces, or 455 g) prepared salsa
1 tablespoon (7.8 g) chili powder
1 teaspoon chicken bouillon concentrate
3 ounces (85 g) shredded Monterey Jack cheese
6 tablespoons (90 g) light sour cream

Put the chicken in a slow cooker.

In a bowl, stir together the salsa, chili powder, and bouillon, making sure the bouillon dissolves. Pour the mixture over the chicken. Cover the slow cooker, set it to low, and let it cook for 7 to 8 hours.

When the time's up, shred the chicken with a fork. Serve topped with the cheese and sour cream.

Yield: 6 servings

Each with 39 g protein, 6 g carbohydrate, 2 g dietary fiber, 4 g usable carbs.

Turkey Tetrazzini

You'll thank me for this recipe the weekend after Thanksgiving!

3 cups (330 g) diced leftover turkey
2 tablespoons (28 g) butter
1 small onion, diced
2 4-ounce (115 g) cans mushrooms, drained
1 cup (240 ml) heavy cream
1 cup (240 ml) half-and-half
2 teaspoons chicken bouillon concentrate
2 tablespoons (30 ml) dry sherry
1 teaspoon guar or xanthan (It's optional, but it makes the sauce thicker.)
¾ cup (75 g) grated Parmesan cheese
3 cups (675 g) cooked spaghetti squash, scraped into strings

Over medium heat, melt the butter in a heavy skillet and start the onions and the mushrooms sautéing in it. While that's cooking, combine the cream, half-and-half, bouillon concentrate, sherry, and guar, if you're using it, in a blender and blend it for just ten seconds or so to combine. Go back and stir the vegetables! When the onion is limp and translucent, transfer half of the vegetables into the blender, add the Parmesan cheese, and blend for another 20 seconds or so to purée the vegetables. Combine this cream sauce with the spaghetti squash, the rest of the vegetables, and the turkey and mix everything well. Put in a 10-cup (2.4-L) casserole dish that you've sprayed with nonstick cooking spray. Bake uncovered at 400°F (200°C, or gas mark 6) for 20 minutes or until bubbly.

Yield: 6 to 8 servings

Assuming 6, each will have 7 g carbohydrate; trace fiber; 24 g protein; 7 g usable carbs.

This tetrazzini is wonderful; everyone who tries it loves it. However, if you have some folks in your family who are going to be unhappy about spaghetti squash, here's what you do: use half spaghetti squash and half spaghetti. Mix half of the sauce with the turkey. Divide the other half of the sauce and the un-puréed mushrooms and onions between 1½ cups (340 g) spaghetti squash and 1½ cups (105 g) cooked spaghetti. Put the spaghetti squash at one end of your casserole dish and the spaghetti at the other end (it helps to use a rectangular casserole dish!). Then make a groove down the middle of the whole thing, lengthwise and pour the turkey mixture into the groove. Bake according to the instructions above.

Low-Carb Microwave Pasticcio

This has become my sister's standby recipe for potlucks and other casserole occasions.

FOR THE PASTICCIO:
1 pound (455 g) ground turkey
½ medium onion, chopped
1 clove garlic, crushed
¾ teaspoon ground cinnamon
⅛ teaspoon ground nutmeg
1 cup (250 g) ricotta cheese
¼ cup (15.2 g) chopped fresh parsley
¼ teaspoon salt or Vege-Sal
⅛ teaspoon pepper

FOR THE SAUCE:
2 tablespoons (28 g) butter
½ teaspoon salt or Vege-Sal
1½ cups (360 ml) heavy cream
½ cup (50 g) grated Parmesan cheese
2 cups (450 g) cooked spaghetti squash

To make the pasticcio: In a microwave-safe casserole dish, combine the onion and garlic; place the turkey on top. Microwave this uncovered for 5 minutes at full power. Stir it up a bit, breaking up the ground turkey in the process. Microwave the turkey and onion mixture for another 3 minutes or until the turkey is cooked through.

Break up the turkey some more—you want it well crumbled—and drain off the fat. Stir in the cinnamon and nutmeg and microwave it for just another minute to blend the flavors. Transfer the turkey mixture to a bowl and set aside.

In a separate bowl, combine the ricotta cheese, parsley, and salt and pepper; set aside.

To make the sauce: In yet another bowl or a measuring cup (okay, you need both a microwave and a dishwasher for this to be a convenient recipe!) combine the butter, salt, cream, and cheese to make the sauce.

Spray a microwave-safe casserole dish with nonstick cooking spray. In the dish, layer half of the spaghetti squash, then half the turkey mixture, then half the ricotta mixture, and then half the sauce. Repeat the layers, ending with the sauce.

Microwave the pasticcio at full power for 6 to 8 minutes or until it's bubbly and hot all the way through. Let it sit for 5 minutes or so and serve.

Yield: 6 servings

Each with 7 grams of carbohydrates, a trace of fiber, and 22 grams of protein.

Homestyle Turkey Loaf

If you haven't eaten a lot of ground turkey, you may find it's a nice change from meat loaf made from ground beef.

1 pound (455 g) ground turkey
½ cup (40 g) crushed pork rinds
1 rib celery, finely chopped
1 small onion, finely chopped
½ cup (45 g) finely chopped apple
1½ tablespoons (23 ml) Worcestershire sauce
2 teaspoons poultry seasoning
1 teaspoon salt or Vege-Sal
1 egg

Preheat the oven to 350°F (180°C, or gas mark 4).

Combine all the ingredients in a big bowl and with clean hands squeeze it together until it's very well combined.

Spray a loaf pan with nonstick cooking spray and pack the turkey mixture into the pan. Bake for 50 minutes.

Yield: 5 servings

Each with 5 grams of carbohydrates and 1 gram of fiber, for a total of 4 grams of usable carbs and 32 grams of protein.

Turkey Loaf with Thai Flavors

Ground turkey is cheap, low-carb, and low-calorie—and by itself just plain boring. So jazz it up by adding some Thai flavors.

2 pounds (910 g) ground turkey
1 medium onion, chopped
1 can (4½ ounces, or 130 g) mushroom slices, drained
4 cloves garlic, crushed
2 tablespoons (30 ml) lemon juice
4 tablespoons (60 ml) lime juice, divided
4 teaspoons chili paste
3 tablespoons (18 g) grated ginger
1½ tablespoons (30 ml) fish sauce
1½ tablespoons (23 ml) soy sauce
1½ teaspoons pepper
½ cup (40 g) pork rind crumbs (Run some pork rinds through your food processor.)
½ cup (32 g) chopped fresh cilantro
½ cup (115 g) mayonnaise

Place the turkey in a big mixing bowl.

Place the onion, mushrooms, and garlic in a food processor. Pulse until everything is chopped medium-fine. Add it to the turkey.

Add the lemon juice, 2 tablespoons (30 ml) of the lime juice, the chili paste, ginger, fish sauce, soy sauce, pepper, pork rind crumbs, and cilantro to the bowl. Mix it around with clean hands until it is well blended.

Spray a rack or a collapsible-basket-type steamer with nonstick cooking spray and place it in your slow cooker. Add 1 cup (240 ml) of water under the rack. If the holes in the rack are pretty large, cover it with a sheet of foil and pierce it all over with a fork. Take two 18-inch (45-cm) squares of foil, fold them into strips about 2 inches (5 cm) wide, and criss-cross them across the rack or steamer, running the ends up the sides of the slow cooker. (You're making a sling to help lift the meat loaf out of the slow cooker.) Place the meat mixture on the rack or steamer and form it into an evenly-domed loaf. Cover the slow cooker, set it to low, and let it cook for 6 hours.

When the time's up, use the strips of foil to gently lift the loaf out of the slow cooker and place it on a platter.

In a bowl, mix together the mayonnaise and the remaining 2 tablespoons (30 ml) lime juice. Cut the loaf into wedges and serve it with the lime mayonnaise.

Yield: 8 servings

Each with 25 g protein, 5 g carbohydrate, 1 g dietary fiber, 4 g usable carbs.

Turkey Feta Burgers

1 pound (455 g) ground turkey
2 tablespoons (20 g) minced red onion
1 teaspoon dried oregano
1 clove garlic, crushed
¾ cup (90 g) crumbled feta cheese
¼ cup (25 g) chopped kalamata olives
2 tablespoons (20 g) sun-dried tomatoes, packed in oil, chopped

Plunk everything in a mixing bowl and with clean hands smoosh it all together until it's very well blended. Form into four burgers—the mixture will be pretty soft, so you may want to chill them for a while before cooking.

Preheat an electric tabletop grill. When it's hot, add the burgers and cook for 6 minutes. That's it!

Yield: 4 servings

Each with 24 g protein; 4 g carbohydrate; 1 g dietary fiber; 3 g usable carbs.

Thai Turkey Burgers

1 pound (455 g) ground turkey
1 tablespoon (15 ml) lemon juice
1 tablespoon (15 ml) lime juice
½ cup (60 g) grated carrot
2 teaspoons chili paste
4 scallions, minced
2 tablespoons (8 g) chopped cilantro
1 teaspoon fish sauce
1 batch Chili Lime Mayo (page 479)

This is very straightforward. Preheat an electric tabletop grill. Then dump everything except the Chili Lime Mayo in a bowl, smoosh it all together really well with clean hands, and make three burgers—the mixture will be pretty soft. When the grill is hot, slap the burgers in it and cook for 5 minutes. Top with Chili Lime Mayo and serve.

Yield: 3 servings

Each with 27 g protein; 6 g carbohydrate; 1 g dietary fiber; 5 g usable carbs.

Asian Turkey Burgers

Ground turkey is handy, but by itself it can be bland. Here's a good way to liven it up.

1 pound (455 g) ground turkey
¼ cup (40 g) minced onion
3 tablespoons (11.4 g) chopped fresh parsley
2 tablespoons (30 ml) Worcestershire sauce
2 tablespoons (20 g) minced green bell pepper
1 tablespoon (15 ml) soy sauce
1 tablespoon (15 ml) cold water
1 tablespoon (6 g) grated fresh ginger
¼ teaspoon pepper
2 cloves garlic, crushed

Combine all the ingredients in a big bowl and with clean hands squeeze it together until it's very well combined.

Divide into three equal portions and form into burgers about ¾ inch (2 cm) thick.

Spray a skillet with nonstick cooking spray and place over medium-high heat. Cook the burgers for about 5 minutes per side until cooked through.

Yield: 3 servings

Each with 5 grams of carbohydrates and 1 gram of fiber, for a total of 4 grams of usable carbs and 27 grams of protein.

Turkey Chorizo with Eggs

Here's how to turn a pound of ground turkey into a quick-and-easy Mexican dinner!

1 pound (455 g) ground turkey
2 tablespoons (30 ml) olive oil
4 cloves garlic, crushed
2 teaspoons dried oregano
½ teaspoon ground cinnamon
½ teaspoon ground cloves
1 teaspoon pepper
2 tablespoons (30 ml) dry sherry
1 teaspoon Splenda
1 teaspoon salt or Vege-Sal
8 eggs
1 cup (240 g) canned diced tomatoes, drained
¼ cup (40 g) minced onion

Start the turkey browning in the olive oil, crumbling it as you go. When it's mostly browned, add the garlic, oregano, cinnamon, cloves, and pepper. Cook it for 2 or 3 more minutes and then stir in the sherry, Splenda, and salt or Vege-Sal. Remove from the heat.

Now scramble the eggs and stir in the tomatoes and onion. Put the skillet back on the heat, pour the eggs over the turkey, and scramble until the eggs are set.

Yield: 4 servings

Each with 32 g protein; 8 g carbohydrate; 1 g dietary fiber; 7 g usable carbs.

Sloppy Toms

This is an easy way to add interest to a pound of plain old ground turkey. You can serve this on low-carb rolls, if you can get them locally. I prefer to serve it over cauli-rice or in omelets—even better!

1 pound (455 g) ground turkey

1 tablespoon (15 ml) olive oil

⅓ cup (55 g) chopped onion

1 clove garlic, crushed

1 Anaheim chili pepper, diced

½ cup (120 ml) Dana's No-Sugar Ketchup (page 463)

1 tablespoon (15 ml) yellow mustard

2 tablespoons (30 ml) cider vinegar

1 tablespoon (1.5 g) Splenda

1 tablespoon (15 ml) Worcestershire sauce

In a big, heavy skillet, start browning and breaking up the ground turkey in the olive oil. Throw in the onion, garlic, and diced pepper.

When all the pink is gone from the turkey, stir in the ketchup, mustard, vinegar, Splenda, and Worcestershire sauce. Simmer the whole thing for 5 minutes before serving.

Yield: 4 to 5 servings

Assuming 5, each will have 17 g protein; 10 g carbohydrate; 2 g dietary fiber; 8 g usable carbs. Analysis does not include cauli-rice or low-carb rolls.

Braised Turkey Wings with Mushrooms

Turkey wings are my favorite cut of turkey for the slow cooker. They fit in easily, they come in good individual serving sizes, and they taste great.

3¼ pounds (1.5 kg) turkey wings

¼ cup (60 ml) olive oil

½ cup (120 ml) chicken broth

1 teaspoon chicken bouillon concentrate

1 teaspoon poultry seasoning

1 tablespoon (16.5 g) tomato paste

1 cup (70 g) sliced mushrooms

½ medium onion, sliced

½ cup (115 g) sour cream

In a big, heavy skillet, brown the turkey all over in the oil over medium-high heat. Transfer the turkey to a slow cooker.

In a bowl, stir together the broth, bouillon, poultry seasoning, and tomato paste. Pour the mixture over the turkey. Add the mushrooms and onion. Cover the slow cooker, set it to low, and let it cook for 6 to 7 hours.

When the time's up, remove the turkey from the slow cooker with tongs. Whisk the sour cream into the sauce and serve the sauce over the turkey.

Yield: 3 servings

Each with 41 g protein, 6 g carbohydrate, 1 g dietary fiber, 5 g usable carbs.

Lemon-Glazed Turkey Cutlets

Turkey cutlets—slices of turkey breast less than ¼ inch (6 mm) thick—are good for cooks in a hurry because they take almost no time to cook through. They're pretty bland by themselves, however, and can easily turn dry and tough. But they take beautifully to this tart-sweet lemon glaze.

3 turkey cutlets, about 4 ounces (115 g) each
1 tablespoon (15 ml) olive oil
1 tablespoon (15 ml) lemon juice
1 tablespoon (15 ml) dry sherry
2 teaspoons Splenda
½ teaspoon soy sauce
Guar or xanthan
3 scallions, finely sliced

In a large, heavy skillet over medium heat, brown the cutlets in the oil. While that's happening, mix together the lemon juice, sherry, Splenda, soy sauce, and just a sprinkle of guar or xanthan to thicken the mixture. When the cutlets have just a touch of golden color on each side, pour the lemon juice mixture into the skillet and turn the cutlets over once to coat both sides. Turn the heat to medium-low, cover, and let the cutlets simmer for just a few more minutes until the sauce reduces a little.

Serve with any glaze left in the pan scraped over the cutlets and a sliced scallion scattered over each.

Yield: 2 or 3 servings

Assuming 2 servings, each will have 4 grams of carbohydrates and 1 gram of fiber, for a total of 3 grams of usable carbs and 37 grams of protein.

Mustard-Pecan Turkey Cutlets

Of all the things I've tried with turkey cutlets, this is my husband's favorite. The mustard-mayo coating keeps these from getting dry.

3 turkey breast cutlets, about 4 ounces (115 g) each
½ cup (60 g) shelled pecans
1 tablespoon (15 ml) spicy brown or Dijon mustard
3 tablespoons (45 g) mayonnaise
1½ tablespoons (21 g) butter

Place the pecans in a food processor with the S-blade in place and pulse until they're ground medium-fine. (Alternately, you could buy the pecans already ground.)

Mix together the mustard and mayonnaise, blending well.

Lay the turkey cutlets on a plate and spread half of the mustard and mayonnaise mixture on one side. Sprinkle half of the ground pecans over the mustard and mayonnaise and press lightly with the back of a spoon to help them stick.

Spray a large, heavy skillet with nonstick cooking spray. Place over medium-high heat. Melt the butter and add the cutlets, pecan side down. Sauté for about 4 minutes. With the cutlets still in the pan, spread the remaining mustard-mayo mixture on the uncoated sides and sprinkle the rest of the pecans over that, once again pressing them in a bit with the back of a spoon. Flip the cutlets carefully, doing your best not to dislodge the crust. Sauté for another 5 minutes and serve. Scrape any yummy toasted pecans that are stuck to the skillet over the cutlets before serving.

Yield: 2 or 3 servings

Assuming 2 servings, each will have 4 grams of carbohydrates and 2 grams of fiber, for a total of 2 grams of usable carbs and 39 grams of protein.

Turkey with Mushroom Sauce

3 pounds (1.4 kg) boneless, skinless turkey breast (in one big hunk, not thin cutlets)
2 tablespoons (28 g) butter
¼ cup (15.2 g) chopped fresh parsley
2 teaspoons dried tarragon
½ teaspoon salt or Vege-Sal
¼ teaspoon pepper
1 cup (70 grams) sliced mushrooms
½ cup (120 ml) dry white wine
1 teaspoon chicken bouillon concentrate
Guar or xanthan (optional)

In a big, heavy skillet, sauté the turkey in the butter until it's golden all over. Transfer the turkey to a slow cooker.

Sprinkle the parsley, tarragon, salt or Vege-Sal, and pepper over the turkey. Place the mushrooms on top.

In a bowl, mix the wine and bouillon together until the bouillon dissolves. Pour it over the turkey. Cover the slow cooker, set it to low, and let it cook for 7 to 8 hours.

When the time's up, remove the turkey and put it on a platter. Transfer about half of the mushrooms to a blender and add the liquid from the slow cooker. Blend until the mushrooms are puréed. Scoop the rest of the mushrooms into the dish you plan to use to serve the sauce, add the liquid, and thicken further with guar or xanthan, if needed.

Yield: 8 servings

Each with 34 g protein, 1 g carbohydrate, trace dietary fiber, 1 g usable carbs.

Orange Blossom Turkey Breast

This is very moist and tasty! It's wonderful left over too, especially made into turkey salad.

1 turkey breast, bone in, about 5 pounds (2.3 kg)
½ cup (120 ml) white wine vinegar
½ teaspoon orange extract
¼ cup (60 ml) sugar-free imitation honey
¼ cup (6 g) Splenda
¼ cup (60 ml) yellow mustard
2 tablespoons (30 ml) soy sauce
3 cloves garlic
Wood chips or chunks, soaked for at least 30 minutes

(continued on page 358)

For this recipe, it's really nice to have a meat injector—basically a big hypodermic syringe used for injecting meat with various flavors. They're pretty easy to find and even easier to use! If you don't have one, this is still a great marinade, but it won't penetrate the meat quite so much.

Mix together everything but the turkey breast. Put the breast in a nonreactive bowl that's fairly deep and narrow. Reserve some marinade for basting and pour the rest the marinade over the turkey. Stick the whole thing in the fridge and let the breast marinate all day or even overnight, turning it now and then. If you have a meat injector, suck up some marinade with it and inject the breast all over with the marinade.

When the time comes to cook, set up a grill for indirect cooking—pile the charcoal to the side, or light only one gas burner. Have plenty of wood chips or chunks soaking! Place a drip pan under the grill under where you're placing the turkey, add the wood chips or chunks, and put the turkey on the grill. Smoke the turkey for about 1¾ to 2 hours, replacing the wood chips or chunks whenever the smoke stops and maintaining the grill temperature at about 225°F (110°C). Baste the turkey now and then with the reserved marinade, using a clean utensil each time you baste. The turkey is done when a meat thermometer stuck in the thickest part of the breast (but not touching the bone) registers 170°F (80°C). Remove from the grill and let the breast sit for 10 minutes before carving.

Yield: 8 to 10 servings

Assuming 8 servings, each would have 9 grams of carbohydrate (not counting the polyols in the imitation honey) if you consumed all of the marinade. Since you won't, figure closer to 4 or 5 grams per serving; 57 grams of protein.

Mediterranean Marinated Turkey Legs

Turkey legs are a convenient cut to grill or barbecue. They cook relatively quickly and are a nice one-serving size—they taste great, too!

3 turkey legs
½ cup (120 ml) olive oil
⅓ cup (80 ml) red wine vinegar
3 cloves garlic
1 tablespoon (15 ml) lemon juice
Wood chips or chunks, soaked for at least
   30 minutes

Put the turkey legs in a big resealable plastic bag. Mix everything else together. Reserve some marinade for basting and pour the rest into the bag, press the air out of the bag, and turn the bag a few times to coat. Stash in the fridge and let the turkey legs marinate for several hours.

Okay, it's cooking time! Get a charcoal or gas grill going; you'll want a medium fire. Pour the marinade off. Add the wood chips or chunks to the grill. Smoke the legs over indirect heat in a closed grill. Baste every 15 minutes or so with the reserved marinade, using a clean utensil each time you baste. Turn and then close the grill again. They'll take about an hour.

Yield: 3 servings, 1 leg per person

Even if you used all the marinade you'd get only 3 grams of carbohydrate per serving, with a trace of fiber. As it is, I'd count no more than 2 grams, and maybe 1. About 47 grams of protein—it depends on the size of your legs!

Chipotle Turkey Legs

This dish has a spicy, rich Southwestern flavor.

3 turkey legs

1½ teaspoons cumin

1 teaspoon chili powder

1 teaspoon dried, powdered sage

1 teaspoon minced garlic or 2 cloves garlic, crushed

½ teaspoon red pepper flakes

¼ teaspoon turmeric

1 or 2 canned chipotle chilies in adobo sauce, plus a couple of teaspoons of the sauce they come in

8 ounces (225 ml) tomato sauce

1 tablespoon (15 ml) Worcestershire sauce

Guar or xanthan

6 tablespoons (45 g) shredded queso quesadilla (optional)*

Plunk the turkey legs in a slow cooker. (If you can fit more, feel free. My slow cooker will only hold 3.) Put the cumin, chili powder, sage, garlic, red pepper flakes, turmeric, chipotles, tomato sauce, and Worcestershire sauce in the blender, run it for a minute, and then pour the mixture over the turkey legs. Cover, turn the slow cooker to low, and leave it for 5 to 6 hours.

When it's done, remove each turkey leg to a serving plate, thicken the juices in the pot with guar or xanthan, and spoon over the turkey legs. If you like, sprinkle 2 tablespoons (7 g) of shredded cheese over each turkey leg and let it melt for a minute or two before serving.

Yield: 3 servings

Each with 8 grams of carbohydrates and 2 grams of fiber, for a total of 6 grams of usable carbs and—depending on the size of the turkey legs—40 to 50 grams of protein.

Chipotle peppers are smoked jalapeños. They're very different from regular jalapeños, and they're quite delicious. Look for them, canned in adobo sauce, in the Mexican foods section of big grocery stores. Since you're unlikely to use the whole can at once, you'll be happy to know that you can store your chipotles in the freezer, where they'll live happily for months and stay pliable enough that you can peel one off when you want to use it. Queso quesadilla is a mild, white Mexican cheese. Monterey Jack is an acceptable substitute.

Cranberry-Peach Turkey Roast

This fruity sauce really wakes up the turkey roast!

3 pounds (1.4 kg) turkey roast

2 tablespoons (30 ml) oil

½ cup (80 g) chopped onion

1 cup (110 g) cranberries

¼ cup (6 g) Splenda

3 tablespoons (45 ml) spicy mustard

¼ teaspoon red pepper flakes

1 peach, peeled and chopped

If your turkey roast is a Butterball like mine, it will be a boneless affair of light and dark meat rolled into an oval roast, enclosed in a net sack. Leave it in the net for cooking so it doesn't fall apart.

(continued on page 360)

In a big heavy skillet, heat the oil and brown the turkey on all sides. Transfer the turkey to a slow cooker.

In a blender or food processor with the S-blade in place, combine the onion, cranberries, Splenda, mustard, red pepper, and peach. Run it until you have a coarse purée. Pour the mixture over the turkey. Cover the slow cooker, set it to low, and let it cook for 6 to 7 hours.

Remove the turkey to a platter, stir up the sauce, and ladle it into a sauce boat to serve with the turkey. You can remove the net from the turkey before serving, if you like, but I find it easier just to use a good sharp knife to slice clear through the netting and let diners remove their own.

Yield: 8 servings

Each with 31 g protein, 4 g carbohydrate, 1 g dietary fiber, 3 g usable carbs.

Tequila Citrus Game Hens

2 Cornish game hens
½ cup (120 ml) lime juice
½ cup (120 ml) lemon juice
¼ teaspoon orange extract
1 tablespoon (1.5 g) Splenda
1 cup (240 ml) tequila
¼ medium onion, minced fine
¼ cup (60 ml) olive oil
2 tablespoons (30 ml) Worcestershire sauce
1 whole jalapeno, seeded and minced fine
**Wood chips or chunks, soaked for at least
    30 minutes**

I like to put everything but the hens in a blender and whiz everything up (and don't forget to wash your hands after handling that jalapeno!). Put the hens in a nonreactive container just big enough to hold them. Reserve some marinade for basting and pour the rest of it over the hens. Turn them once or twice to make sure that the hens are coated and make sure some marinade gets inside the body cavities. Stick the whole thing in the fridge for at least 3 or 4 hours, and all day won't hurt a bit.

A couple of hours before dinnertime, get the grill going for indirect cooking (put the coals on one side of the grill or light only one side). Add the wood chips or chunks and place the hens on the grill. Baste the hens every 30 minutes or so with the reserved marinade using a clean utensil each time. Smoke the hens for about 2½ hours or until their leg joints move freely. An instant-read thermometer inserted into the thickest part of the meat (but not touching the bone) should register 180 to 185°F (85°C). Remove the birds from the grill and allow them to sit for 5 to 10 minutes before carving.

While those birds are resting, bring the reserved marinade to a boil, and boil it hard for at least 3 or 4 minutes. Thicken it a little with guar or xanthan, if you like, and serve as a sauce with the hens.

Yield: This is 2 hefty but elegant whole-bird servings, or 4 more reasonable but less pictur-esque servings.

Assuming 2 servings, you'll get 16 grams of carbohy-drate and 1 gram of fiber—if you consume all of the marinade. If you just have a spoonful or two, you can figure on getting 2 or 3 grams of usable carb; 59 grams of protein.

Sesame Orange Duck

Duck is unbelievably rich—but what a special-occasion treat! If you'd like, you can cook chicken the same way, for a less-expensive, lower-calorie dish.

1 duck, cut into 4 servings

¼ cup (60 ml) soy sauce

2 tablespoons (40 g) low-sugar orange marmalade

¼ teaspoon orange extract

2 teaspoons Splenda

2 cloves garlic

2 teaspoons grated ginger

2 tablespoons (30 ml) white wine vinegar

4 tablespoons (32 g) sesame seeds

Before we get to the recipe, let's talk about cutting up the duck. My grocery store didn't have duck in stock, so I asked them to order a couple for me. They came in whole and frozen. I let my duck thaw, and it then took me about 5 minutes to cut it up using my trusty Kmart shears—not a big deal. However, if you'd prefer, you could ask the nice meat guys at your grocery store if they could order you a cut-up duck, or alternately, let the duck thaw there and cut it up for you. If you choose this last option, however, don't take your duck home and refreeze it—just arrange for it to be ready to pick up the day you want to cook it.

Okay, time to cook your duck! Light a charcoal fire or preheat a gas grill. Mix together the soy sauce, orange marmalade, orange extract, Splenda, garlic, ginger, and vinegar in a bowl. Tear off 4 sheets of heavy-duty aluminum foil, each big enough to wrap one of your pieces of duck. Put a piece of duck on a piece of foil and bend up the edges enough that the sauce won't run off. Spoon about 1 tablespoon (15 ml) of sauce over the piece of duck, smear it around a little with the back of the spoon, and wrap the foil around the piece of duck—fold opposite edges to the middle, roll down, and then roll the ends in. Repeat with the remaining 3 pieces of duck and pieces of foil.

Grill the duck packets over a medium fire for about 40 minutes, turning halfway through.

In the meantime, toast the sesame seeds by putting them in a small, dry skillet and shaking them over a hot burner until they start to make little popping sounds. Remove from heat.

Okay, 40 minutes is up. Retrieve the duck from the grill and carefully unwrap each piece. Put the unwrapped duck back on the grill skin-side down for 5 minutes or until the skin is crisp. Remove to serving plates, top each with 1 tablespoon (8 g) of sesame seeds, and serve.

Yield: 4 servings

Each serving will have 4 grams of carbohydrate and 1 gram of fiber, for a usable carb count of 3 grams; 39 grams of protein.

11

Beef

Bleu Burger

⅓ **pound (150 g) hamburger patty**
1 **tablespoon (8 g) crumbled blue cheese**
1 **teaspoon finely minced sweet red onion**

Cook the burger by your preferred method. When it's almost done to your liking, top with the bleu cheese and let it melt. Remove from the heat, put it on plate, and top with onion.

Yield: 1 serving

Only a trace of carbohydrates, no fiber, and 27 grams of protein.

Chipotle Cheeseburgers

These are truly great; my husband and I couldn't stop talking about how well this recipe worked out! Of course, since I have to keep cooking new stuff, we won't get to eat these again till 2012. But still, they're just amazing.

2 **pounds (910 g) ground beef**
6 **chipotle chiles canned in adobo sauce, minced**
½ **cup (32 g) chopped cilantro**
2 **cloves garlic, crushed**
¼ **cup (40 g) minced onion**
½ **teaspoon salt**
6 **ounces (170 g) Monterey Jack cheese, sliced**

Plunk everything but the cheese into a big bowl and use clean hands to mush everything together until very well blended. Form into 6 burgers about 1 inch (2.5 cm) thick. Put your burgers on a plate and stick them in the fridge to chill for a good hour—it makes them easier to handle on the grill.

Get your fire going—you'll want your gas grill on medium or a little lower or well-ashed charcoal. Grill the burgers for a good 7 to 10 minutes per side or until juices run clear, keeping down flare-ups with a water bottle. When the burgers are almost done, top with the cheese and let it melt. Serve with Chipotle Sauce (page 477).

Yield: 6 servings

Exclusive of Chipotle Sauce, each serving will have 1 gram of carbohydrate and 1 gram of fiber, for a usable carb count of 0 grams; 33 grams protein.

Smothered Burgers

This is a delicious burger smothered in mushrooms and onions—mmmm!

4⅓-**pound (150 g) hamburger patties**
2 **tablespoons (28 g or 30 ml) butter or olive oil**
½ **cup (80 g) sliced onion**
½ **cup (35 g) sliced mushrooms**
Dash of Worcestershire sauce

Cook the burgers by your preferred method. While the burgers are cooking, melt the butter or heat the oil in a small, heavy skillet over medium-high heat. Add the onion and mushrooms and sauté until the onions are translucent. Add a dash of Worcestershire sauce, stir, and spoon over the burgers.

(continued on page 364)

Yield: 4 servings

Each with just 2 grams of carbohydrates, at least a trace of fiber, and 27 grams of protein.

Crunchy Peking Burgers

FOR BURGERS:
1 pound (455 g) ground beef
½ cup (100 g) canned water chestnuts, drained
2 scallions
¼ cup (60 ml) soy sauce
2 tablespoons (30 ml) dry sherry
1 teaspoon Splenda
1 teaspoon minced garlic or 2 cloves garlic, crushed
½ teaspoon grated ginger

FOR SAUCE:
1½ tablespoons (30 g) low-sugar apricot preserves
1 teaspoon soy sauce
¼ teaspoon grated ginger

Preheat an electric tabletop grill.

Chop the water chestnuts a bit and slice the scallions. Put them in a mixing bowl with all the other burger ingredients and use clean hands to mix them well. Form into 4 burgers and put them on the grill. Cook for 5 minutes.

While the burgers are cooking, mix together the preserves, soy sauce, and ginger in a small dish. When the burgers are done, top each with a teaspoon of sauce and serve.

Yield: 4 servings

Each with 7 grams of carbohydrates and 1 gram of fiber, for a total of 6 grams of usable carbs and 20 grams of protein.

Mexiburgers

⅓ pound (150 g) hamburger patty
1 ounce (28 g) jalepeño Jack or Monterey Jack cheese
1 tablespoon (16 g) salsa

Cook the burger by your preferred method. When it's almost done to your liking, melt the cheese over the burger. Top with salsa and serve.

Yield: 1 serving

2 grams of carbohydrates, a trace of fiber, and 27 grams of protein.

Paprika Burgers

Looking for something new to do with the eternal hamburger, I thought of the middle European flavors of Stroganoff and paprikash and invented this burger.

2 pounds (910 g) ground beef
½ cup (80 g) minced onion
2 tablespoons (13.8 g) paprika
2 tablespoons (33 g) tomato paste
2 tablespoons (30 ml) Worcestershire sauce
2 teaspoons salt
Sour cream or plain yogurt (optional)

Throw everything in a bowl and use clean hands to smoosh it all together until well blended. Form into 6 burgers and put them on a plate. Stash them in the fridge to chill for an hour.

Okay, light your grill—set your gas grill to medium or a little lower or wait until your charcoal has burned down to well-ashed coals. Throw the burgers on the grill and cook for 7 to 10 minutes per side, keeping down flare-ups with a water bottle. Serve these with a dollop of sour cream or plain yogurt on top, if you like, to keep the Mitteleuropa theme going.

Yield: 6 servings

Exclusive of sour cream or yogurt, each will have 4 grams of carbohydrate and 1 gram of fiber, for a usable carb count of 3 grams; and 28 grams protein. 1 tablespoon (15 g) sour cream will add 1 gram of carbohydrate, 0 grams fiber, and a trace of protein. 1 tablespoon of plain yogurt (15 g) will add 1 gram of carbohydrate (less, if you go by the GO-Diet's count of 4 grams of carbohydrate per cup), 0 grams fiber, and 1 gram protein.

Blue Bacon Burgers

Here's a bacon cheeseburger with the bacon and cheese cooked in!

1⅓ pounds (600 g) ground chuck
4 tablespoons (30 g) blue cheese, crumbled
4 tablespoons (60 ml) blue cheese salad dressing
4 tablespoons (40 g) minced red onion
6 slices cooked bacon, crumbled

Assemble everything in a mixing bowl. Use clean hands to smoosh everything together well. Form into 4 to 6 burgers. It's good to chill these for 30 minutes before cooking, but it's not essential.

I like to cook my burgers in an electric tabletop grill for about 5 to 6 minutes. You could also cook these for about 5 minutes per side under the broiler, in a hot skillet, or on your grill outside.

Yield: 4 to 6 servings

Assuming 4, each will have 32 g protein; 2 g carbohydrate; trace dietary fiber, 2 g usable carbs.

Poor Man's Poivrade

This dish has a real peppery bite—it's not for the timid!

⅓ pound (150 g) hamburger patty
1 tablespoon (6.3 g) coarse cracked pepper
1 tablespoon (14 g) butter
2 tablespoons (30 ml) dry white wine, dry sherry, or dry vermouth

Roll the raw hamburger patty in the pepper until it's coated all over.

Fry the burger in the butter over medium heat until it's done to your liking.

Remove the burger to a plate. Add the wine to the skillet and stir it around for a minute or two, until all the nice brown crusty bits are scraped up. Pour this over the hamburger and serve.

(continued on page 366)

Between 4 and 6 grams of carbohydrates per serving (depending on whether you use wine, sherry, or vermouth—wine is lowest, vermouth is highest) and 2 grams of fiber, for a total of 2 to 4 grams of usable carbs and 27 grams of protein.

Bacon Chili Burgers

Here's something interesting to do with your ground beef when you're weary of plain burgers!

1 pound (455 g) ground chuck
2 tablespoons (33 g) chili garlic paste
¼ cup (40 g) minced onion
6 slices bacon, cooked and drained

Put the ground chuck, chili garlic paste, and onion in a mixing bowl. Crumble the bacon into the bowl as well. Now, use clean hands to smoosh everything together until it's well mixed. Form into 3 burgers. Put them on a plate and chill for half an hour or so—this isn't strictly necessary, but it makes them easier to handle.

Now you can cook your burgers—I like to give mine 6 minutes in an electric tabletop grill, but you can broil them for 4 to 5 minutes per side or even cook them on your grill outdoors.

Yield: 3 servings

Each with 31 g protein; 2 g carbohydrate; trace dietary fiber; 2 g usable carbs.

Pizza Burger

⅓ pound (150 g) hamburger patty
1 tablespoon (15 ml) sugar-free jarred pizza sauce
2 tablespoons (15 g) shredded mozzarella cheese

Cook the burger by your preferred method. When it's almost done to your liking, top with pizza sauce, then mozzarella. Cook until the cheese is melted and serve.

Yield: 1 serving

With (depending on your brand of pizza sauce) no more than 2 grams of carbohydrates, no fiber, and 28 grams of protein.

One of the lowest-carb nationally distributed brands of spaghetti sauce is Hunt's Classic. It has 7.5 grams of carbs per ½-cup (120-ml) serving, of which 4 g is fiber, for an effective carb count of just 3.5 grams.

Ultra Meat Sauce

This is spaghetti without the spaghetti, as it were.

1½ pounds (680 g) ground beef
1 small onion, diced
1 clove garlic crushed
1 green pepper, diced
1 can (4 ounces, or 115 g) mushrooms, drained
2 cups (480 ml) low-carb spaghetti sauce

Brown and crumble the ground beef in a large, heavy skillet. As the grease starts to collect in the skillet, add the onion, garlic, green pepper, and mushrooms. Continue cooking until pepper and onion are soft.

Pour off the excess grease. Stir in the spaghetti sauce and serve.

Yield: 5 servings

Each with (if you use the lowest-carbohydrate spaghetti sauce) 11 grams of carbohydrates and 4.6 grams of fiber, for a total of 6.4 grams of usable carbs and 25 grams of protein.

This is a good supper for the family, because again, it's easy to add carbs for those who want them—you eat your very meaty meat sauce with a good sprinkling of Parmesan cheese, and you let the carb-eaters have theirs over spaghetti. Serve a big salad with it, and there's dinner.

Skillet Stroganoff

1 pound (455 g) ground beef
1 medium onion, diced
1 clove garlic, crushed
1 can (4 ounces, or 115 g) mushrooms, drained
1 teaspoon liquid beef broth concentrate
2 tablespoons (30 ml) Worcestershire sauce
1 teaspoon paprika
¾ cup (180 g) sour cream
Salt or Vege-Sal and pepper to taste

Brown and crumble the ground beef in a heavy skillet over medium heat. Add the onion and garlic as soon as there's a little grease in the bottom of the pan and cook until all pinkness is gone from the ground beef.

Drain the excess grease. Add the mushrooms, broth concentrate, Worcestershire, and paprika. Stir in the sour cream and then add salt and pepper to taste. Heat through, but don't let it boil. This is great as-is, but you may certainly serve it over noodles for the non-low-carb set.

Yield: 3 servings

Each with 9 grams of carbohydrates and 2 grams of fiber, for a total of 7 grams of usable carbs and 28 grams of protein.

Ground Beef "Helper"

When your family starts agitating for the "normal" food of yore, whip up this recipe.

1 pound (455 g) lean ground beef or ground turkey
½ cup (75 g) chopped green pepper
½ cup (80 g) chopped onion
½ cup (60 g) diced celery
2 cans (8 ounces [225 g] each) tomato sauce
2 cloves garlic, crushed; 1 teaspoon minced garlic; or ½ teaspoon garlic powder
½ teaspoon Italian seasoning
2 cups (220 g) shredded cheddar or Monterey Jack cheese, divided
1 box (about 1¾ ounces, or 50 g) low-carb pasta
⅓ cup (80 ml) water
Salt and pepper to taste

(continued on page 368)

Preheat the broiler.

In a large, oven-safe skillet, brown the meat with the pepper, onion, and celery. Drain off the grease.

Add the tomato sauce, garlic, seasoning, 1 cup (110 g) of the cheese, pasta, water, and salt and pepper to taste. Cover and simmer over low heat for 10 minutes. Turn on the broiler to preheat during last the few minutes of cooking time.

Stir well. Spread the remaining 1 cup (110 g) of cheese over the top and broil until the cheese starts to brown.

Yield: 6 servings

Each with 11 grams of carbohydrates and 2 grams of fiber, for a total of 9 grams of usable carbs and 36 grams of protein.

Hamburger Chop Suey

1 pound (455 g) ground round or other very lean ground beef

2 tablespoons (30 ml) oil

1 medium onion, sliced

2 cups (140 g) sliced mushrooms

2 stalks celery, thinly sliced on the diagonal

½ green pepper, diced

½ teaspoon minced garlic or 1 clove garlic, crushed

2 cups (100 g) bean sprouts

⅓ cup (80 ml) soy sauce

½ teaspoon liquid beef bouillon concentrate

In a wok or large skillet over high heat, start browning the beef in the oil and breaking it up. When it's about halfway browned, add the onion, mushrooms, celery, green pepper, and garlic. Continue breaking up the meat while stir-frying the vegetables. When all the pink is gone from the beef and the vegetables are almost tender-crisp, add the bean sprouts, soy sauce, and beef bouillon concentrate. Continue stir-frying until the bean sprouts are just barely starting to wilt and then serve.

Yield: 4 servings

Each with 8 grams of carbohydrates and 2 grams of fiber, for a total of 6 grams of usable carbs and 24 grams of protein.

Ground Beef Stir-Fry

This looks like a lot of instructions, but it actually goes together rather quickly. It's good when you're missing Chinese food, which is generally full of added sugar and starch.

1 pound (455 g) ground beef

2 tablespoons (30 ml) soy sauce, divided

3 tablespoons (45 ml) dry sherry, divided

1 or 2 cloves garlic, crushed

Peanut oil or other bland oil for stir-frying

½ cup (60 g) coarsely chopped walnuts

2 cups (300 g) frozen crosscut green beans, thawed, or 2 cups (500 g) frozen broccoli "cuts," thawed

1 medium onion, sliced

1½ teaspoons grated fresh ginger

Remember the Law of Stir-Frying: Have everything chopped, thawed, sliced, and prepped before you start cooking! In a bowl, combine 1 tablespoon (15 ml) soy sauce, 1½ tablespoons (23 ml) sherry, and the garlic. Add the ground beef and with clean hands mix the flavorings into the meat.

Heat 2 to 3 tablespoons (30 to 45 ml) oil in a wok or large, heavy skillet over high heat. Put the walnuts in the skillet and fry for a few minutes until crispy. Drain and put aside.

Using the same oil, stir-fry bite-sized chunks of the ground beef mixture until cooked through. Lift out the beef and drain.

Pour the oil and fat out of the skillet and put in a few tablespoons (30 ml) of fresh oil. Heat it up over high heat and then add the green beans, onion, and ginger. Stir-fry until the vegetables are tender-crisp.

Add the beef back to the pan and stir everything up. Stir in the remaining soy sauce and sherry and another clove of crushed garlic if you like.

Serve without rice for you and on top of rice for the carb-eaters in the family. Sprinkle the toasted walnuts on top of each serving and pass the soy sauce at the table for those who like more.

Yield: 3 servings

Each with 19 grams of carbohydrates and 6 grams of fiber, for a total of 13 grams of usable carbs and 34 grams of protein.

Meatza!

Here's a dish for all you pizza-lovers, and I know you are legion. Just add a salad and you have a supper that will please the whole family.

1½ pounds (680 g) ground beef or ¾ pound (340 g) each ground beef and Italian-style sausage

1 small onion, finely chopped

1 clove garlic, crushed

1 teaspoon dried oregano or Italian seasoning (optional)

8 ounces (220 ml) sugar-free pizza sauce

Parmesan or Romano cheese (optional)

8 ounces (225 g) shredded mozzarella

Toppings (peppers, onions, mushrooms, or whatever you like)

Olive oil (optional)

Preheat the oven to 350°F (180°C, or gas mark 4).

In a large bowl and with clean hands, combine the meat with the onion, garlic, and oregano or Italian seasoning (if using). Mix well.

Pat the meat mixture out in an even layer in a 9 × 12-inch (23 × 30-cm) baking pan. Bake for 20 minutes. Remove from oven and set broiler to high.

When the meat comes out, it will have shrunk a fair amount because of the grease cooking off. Pour off the grease and spread the pizza sauce over the meat. Sprinkle the Parmesan or Romano cheese on the sauce (if using) and then distribute the shredded mozzarella evenly over the sauce.

Top with whatever you like: green peppers, banana peppers, mushrooms, olives, or anchovies.

(continued on page 370)

I love broccoli on pizza, and thawed frozen broccoli "cuts" work perfectly. You could also use meat toppings, such as sausage and pepperoni, but they seem a little redundant, since the whole bottom layer is meat.

Drizzle the whole thing with a little olive oil (if using; it's really not necessary).

Put your Meatza! 4 inches (10 cm) below a broiler set on high. Broil for about 5 minutes or until the cheese is melted and starting to brown.

Yield: 6 servings

Each with about 5 grams of carbohydrates per serving, only a trace of fiber, and 27 grams of protein. (This is based on using sugar-free pizza sauce and only cheese, no other toppings.)

If you haven't been able to find a pizza sauce that doesn't have sugar, you might combine an 8-ounce (225 g) can of tomato sauce with a crushed clove of garlic and some oregano.

Joe

This is our favorite one-dish skillet supper. It's flexible, too; don't worry if you use a little less or a little more ground beef or one more or one fewer egg. It'll still come out great.

1½ pounds (680 g) ground beef
1 package (10 ounces, or 280 g) frozen chopped spinach
1 medium onion, chopped
1 or 2 cloves garlic, crushed
5 eggs
Salt and pepper

In a heavy skillet over medium heat, begin browning the ground beef.

While the beef is cooking, cook the spinach according to the package directions (or 5 to 7 minutes on high in the microwave should do it).

When the ground beef is half cooked, add the onion and garlic and cook until the beef is completely done. Pour off the extra fat.

Drain the spinach well—I put mine in a strainer and press it with the back of a spoon—and stir it into the ground beef.

Mix the eggs well with a fork and stir them in with the beef and spinach. Continue cooking and stirring over low heat for a few more minutes, until the eggs are set. Season with salt and pepper to taste and serve.

Yield: 6 servings

Each with 4 grams of carbohydrates and 2 grams of fiber, for a total of 2 grams of usable carbs and 25 grams of protein.

My sister likes a little Parmesan cheese sprinkled over her Joe, and I surely wouldn't argue about a little thing like that!

Sloppy José

This is so easy it's almost embarrassing, and the kids will probably like it. Different brands of salsa vary a lot in their carb contents, so read labels carefully.

1 pound (455 g) ground beef
1 cup (240 g) salsa (mild, medium, or hot, as you prefer)
1 cup (115 g) shredded Mexican-style cheese

In a large skillet, crumble and brown the ground beef and drain off the fat.

Stir in the salsa and cheese and heat until the cheese is melted.

Yield: About 4 servings

Each with 4 grams of carbohydrates and 1 gram of fiber, for a total of 3 grams of usable carbs and 27 grams of protein.

Variation: Mega Sloppy José. Try adding another ½ cup (120 ml) salsa and another ½ cup (60 g) cheese. **Yield:** 4 servings

Each with 6 grams of carbohydrates and 2 grams of fiber, for a total of 4 grams of usable carbs and 30 grams of protein.

This is good with a salad or even on a salad. Of course, if you have carb-eaters around, they'll love the stuff on some corn tortillas.

All-Meat Chili

Some folks consider tomatoes in chili to be anathema, but I like it this way. Don't look funny at that cocoa powder, by the way. It's the secret ingredient!

2 pounds (910 g) ground beef
1 cup (160 g) chopped onion
3 cloves garlic, crushed
1 can (14½ ounces, or 410 g) tomatoes with green chilies
1 can (4 ounces, or 110 ml) plain tomato sauce
4 teaspoons ground cumin
2 teaspoons dried oregano

2 teaspoons unsweetened cocoa powder
1 teaspoon paprika

Brown and crumble the beef in a heavy skillet over medium-high heat. Pour off the grease and add the remaining ingredients. Stir to combine.

Turn the heat to low, cover, and simmer for 30 minutes. Uncover and simmer for another 15 to 20 minutes or until the chili thickens a bit. Serve with grated cheese, sour cream, chopped raw onion, or other low-carb toppings.

Yield: 6 servings

Each with 7 grams of carbohydrates and 2 grams of fiber, for a total of 5 grams of usable carbs and 27 grams of protein. Analysis does not include toppings.

It's easy to vary this recipe to the tastes of different family members. If some people like beans in their chili, just heat up a can of kidney or pinto beans and let them spoon their beans into their own serving. If you like beans in your chili, buy a can of black soybeans at a natural food store; there are only a couple of grams of usable carbs in a couple of tablespoons. And of course, if you like your chili hotter than this, just add crushed red pepper, cayenne, or hot pepper sauce to take things up a notch.

Firehouse Chili

Here's a crowd-pleaser! I served this on a rainy afternoon at our local campground and made a lot of friends! You could halve this, but you'd be left with a half a can of soybeans. You know you'll eat it up, so why bother?

(continued on page 372)

2 pounds (910 g) ground chuck

1½ cups (240 g) chopped onion

4 cloves garlic, crushed

3 tablespoons (23 g) chili powder

3 teaspoons paprika

4 teaspoons ground cumin

¼ cup (60 ml) Dana's No-Sugar Ketchup
(page 463) or purchased low-carb ketchup

2 tablespoons (33 g) tomato paste

1 can (14½ ounces, or 410 g) diced tomatoes

12 ounces (360 ml) light beer

1 teaspoon Splenda

2½ teaspoons salt

1 can (15 ounces, or 425 g) black soybeans

In a big, heavy skillet, brown and crumble the beef over medium-high heat. Drain it and place it in a slow cooker. Add the remaining ingredients. Stir everything up. Cover the slow cooker, set it to low, and let it cook for 8 hours.

This is good with shredded cheese and sour cream. What chili isn't? But it also stands on its own very well.

Yield: 10 servings

Each with 21 g protein, 12 g carbohydrate, 4 g dietary fiber, 8 g usable carbs. Analysis does not include toppings.

Spanish "Rice"

Okay, this isn't really Spanish. It's not even authentically Mexican. And of course it's not rice. But it is passingly like the "Spanish Rice" my mom used to throw together to make a quick, one-dish meal out of hamburger! Feel free to used canned,

diced tomatoes without the chilies if you don't like spicy food, although this is really quite mild.

1 pound (455 g) ground round or other very
lean ground beef

1 to 2 tablespoons (15 to 30 ml) oil

½ head cauliflower

½ green pepper, chopped

½ medium onion, chopped

1 teaspoon minced garlic

1 can (14½ ounces, or 410 g) diced tomatoes
with green chilies

½ teaspoon ground cumin

1 teaspoon Worcestershire sauce

¼ cup (60 ml) water

Salt and pepper

In a large skillet, start browning the beef in the oil over medium-high heat. Meanwhile, run the cauliflower through the shredding blade of a food processor. Put the cauliflower in a microwavable casserole dish, add a tablespoon or two (15 to 30 ml) of water, cover, and microwave on high for just 5 minutes.

Go back to the beef and start breaking it up. When you've got just a little fat in the pan, add the pepper and onion and sauté them, too. When all the pink is gone from the meat, add the garlic, tomatoes, cumin, Worcestershire sauce, and water and bring the whole thing to a simmer. Stir in the cauliflower "rice," cover, and let the whole thing simmer for 3 to 5 minutes. Season with salt and pepper to taste and serve.

Yield: 4 or 5 servings

Assuming 4 servings, each will have 7 grams of carbohydrates and 1 gram of fiber, for a total of 6 grams of usable carbs and 23 grams of protein.

Southwestern Stuffed Peppers

This was one of those recipes you just come up with out of what's in the house at the time—and it turned out so well, I'd be willing to go buy the ingredients to make it!

1 pound (455 g) ground beef

½ cup (80 g) chopped onion

1 clove garlic, crushed

1 can (14½ ounces, or 410 g) tomatoes with green chilies, divided

1 egg

½ cup (120 ml) half-and-half

½ cup (70 g) pork rind crumbs

1 teaspoon ground cumin

1 teaspoon salt or Vege-Sal

½ teaspoon pepper

3 big, nicely shaped green peppers

Preheat oven to 350°F (180°C, or gas mark 4)

In a large bowl combine the ground beef, onion, garlic, ½ cup (120 g) of the tomatoes with chilies, the egg, half-and-half, pork rind crumbs, and seasonings. Use clean hands to combine everything well. Cut the peppers in half from top to bottom and scoop out the seeds and core. Form the meat mixture into 6 equal balls and press each into a pepper half, mashing it down a little to fill the peppers. Arrange peppers in a baking pan as you stuff them. Spoon the remaining tomatoes over the top and bake for 75 to 90 minutes.

Yield: This makes 6 servings from 1 pound (455 g) of ground beef, which is pretty impressive! It's filling, too.

Each serving has 9 g carbohydrate; 2 g fiber; for a usable carb total of 7 g; 27 g protein.

Thai Beef Lettuce Wraps

This is fast to make, yet it's interestingly exotic. And it's fun to eat wrapped-up stuff, whether you use tortillas or lettuce leaves!

1 pound (455 g) ground round

1 teaspoon red pepper flakes

½ cup (80 g) chopped onion

1 clove garlic

1 medium yellow pepper, diced (If you don't have a yellow one, a green or red one will do!)

¼ cup (60 ml) lemon juice

2 teaspoons chopped fresh mint

1 teaspoon beef bouillon granules

½ head cauliflower, shredded

1 tablespoon (15 ml) fish sauce (nuoc mam or nam pla)

2 teaspoons soy sauce

½ cup (60 g) chopped peanuts

½ cucumber, diced small

16 lettuce leaves

In a big, heavy skillet, start browning and crumbling the ground round along with the red pepper flakes.

When the beef is browned, tilt the pan and spoon off any fat that's accumulated.

Stir in the onion, garlic, pepper, lemon juice, mint, and beef bouillon granules. Stir until the bouillon dissolves. Turn the heat to low and let the whole thing simmer.

(continued on page 374)

While that's happening, put the cauliflower in a microwaveable casserole dish with a lid, add a couple of tablespoons (30 ml) of water, cover, and microwave on high for 6 minutes.

By the time the cauliflower's done, the pepper and onion should be tender. Drain the cauli-rice and stir it into the beef mixture. Stir in the fish sauce and soy sauce, too.

Put the peanuts and the cucumber in small dishes. Arrange 4 good-sized lettuce leaves on each of 4 plates and spoon a mound of the meat mixture next to them.

To eat, spoon some of the meat mixture into a lettuce leaf and sprinkle with cucumber and peanuts. Wrap in the lettuce and eat as you would a burrito.

Yield: 4 servings

Each with 28 g protein; 12 g carbohydrate; 3 g dietary fiber; 9 g usable carbs.

Unstuffed Cabbage

Stuffed cabbage is a perennial favorite, but it's time consuming! Here's a recipe that gives you all the flavor of stuffed cabbage at breakneck speed. Do use very lean ground beef for this recipe—it saves you the time needed to drain off the grease.

1½ pounds (680 g) ground round or other very lean ground beef
1 medium onion, chopped
1 teaspoon minced garlic or 2 cloves garlic, crushed

½ head cabbage, coarsely chopped
1 can (8 ounces, or 225 g) tomato sauce
2 tablespoons (30 ml) lemon juice
½ teaspoon pepper
½ teaspoon ground nutmeg
½ teaspoon ground cinnamon
1 teaspoon salt

Start the ground beef cooking in a heavy skillet over high heat; spread it out to cover the bottom of the pan so it cooks quicker.

While the ground beef is browning, chop the onion and crush the garlic. Plunk them in the pan with the ground beef and stir it up using a spatula to turn it over and break it up so that it cooks evenly. Cover the pan and let it continue cooking.

Meanwhile, chop the cabbage coarsely. Stir this into the beef mixture a bit at a time—it will come close to overwhelming your skillet, unless yours is bigger than mine. Again, take care to turn everything over to keep it cooking evenly. Re-cover the pan.

Continue to stir the meat mixture to keep it cooking evenly, covering in between stirrings. When the cabbage is starting to wilt, stir in the tomato sauce, lemon juice, pepper, nutmeg, cinnamon, and salt. Re-cover, let the whole thing simmer for 5 minutes, and then serve.

Yield: 5 servings

Each with 7 grams of carbohydrates and 2 grams of fiber, for a total of 5 grams of usable carbs and 25 grams of protein.

Homestyle Meat Loaf

1 pound (455 g) ground chuck
2 tablespoons (15 g) oat bran
1 egg
¼ cup (60 ml) vegetable juice, such as V8
¼ cup (40 g) minced onion
½ cup plus 1 tablespoon (135 g) Dana's No-Sugar Ketchup (page 463), divided
3 teaspoons spicy mustard, divided
½ teaspoon salt or Vege-Sal
¼ teaspoon pepper
3 tablespoons (4.5 g) Splenda
½ teaspoon blackstrap molasses

Preheat the oven to 350°F (180°C, or gas mark 4).

Plop the ground chuck, oat bran, egg, vegetable juice, onion, 1 tablespoon (15 ml) ketchup, 1 teaspoon spicy mustard, salt, and pepper into a big mixing bowl and use clean hands to smoosh it all together really well. Pack it into a loaf pan to mold it and then turn it out onto the broiler rack. Bake for 1 hour.

Twenty minutes before it's done, combine the remaining ½ cup (120 ml) ketchup, the Splenda, blackstrap molasses, and the other 2 teaspoons of mustard. Brush over the meat loaf to glaze and return to oven to finish baking.

Yield: 4 to 5 servings

Assuming 5, each will have 19 g protein; 8 g carbohydrate; 1 g dietary fiber; 7 g usable carbs.

Mexicali Meat Loaf

1 pound (455 g) ground beef
1 pound (455 g) mild pork sausage
1 cup (80 g) crushed plain pork rinds
1 can (4½ ounces, or 130 g) diced mild green chilies
1 medium onion, finely chopped
8 ounces (225 g) Monterey Jack cheese, cut into ¼- to ½-inch (0.6- to 1.3-cm) cubes or shredded
¾ cup (195 g) salsa (mild, medium, or hot, as desired)
1 egg
2 or 3 cloves garlic, crushed
2 teaspoons dried oregano
2 teaspoons ground cumin
1 teaspoon salt or Vege-Sal

Preheat the oven to 350°F (180°C, or gas mark 4).

Combine all the ingredients in a really big bowl and then with clean hands knead it all until it's thoroughly blended.

Dump it out on a clean broiler rack and form into a loaf—it'll be a big loaf—about 3 inches (7.5 cm) thick. Bake for 1½ hours.

Yield: 8 servings

Each with 5 grams of carbohydrates and 1 gram of fiber, for a total of 4 grams of usable carbs and 28 grams of protein.

Do chop the onion quite fine for your meat loaves. If it's in pieces that are too big, it tends to make the loaf fall apart when you cut it. The Mexicali Meat Loaf may crumble a bit anyway because it's quite tender.

Chili-Glazed Meat Loaf

FOR THE MEAT LOAF:
1 pound (455 g) ground chuck
¼ cup (30 g) minced green bell pepper
¼ cup (30 g) shredded carrot
⅓ cup (55 g) minced onion
1 egg
2 tablespoons (30 ml) Dana's No-Sugar Ketchup (page 463)
1 teaspoon chili garlic paste
2 tablespoons (15 g) oat bran
¼ teaspoon dried oregano
¼ teaspoon dried basil
½ teaspoon salt or Vege-Sal
¼ teaspoon pepper

FOR THE GLAZE:
¼ cup (60 ml) Dana's No-Sugar Ketchup
1 tablespoon (1.5 g) Splenda
¼ teaspoon blackstrap molasses
1 teaspoon apple cider vinegar
1 tablespoon (15 ml) olive oil
½ teaspoon chili garlic paste

Preheat oven to 350°F (180°C, or gas mark 4).

To make the meat loaf: First, put the pepper, carrot, and onion in a big mixing bowl. Add the remaining meat loaf ingredients. Using clean hands, smoosh everything together until it's all very well mixed. Pack it into a loaf pan to mold it and then turn the meat loaf out onto a broiler rack. Bake for 50 to 60 minutes.

To make the glaze: Combine the glaze ingredients in a small bowl. About 20 to 30 minutes before baking time is up, take the meat loaf out of the oven and spread the glaze over it. Return it to the oven until it's done.

Yield: 4 to 5 servings

Assuming 5, each will have 19 g protein; 8 g carbohydrate; 2 g dietary fiber; 6 g usable carbs.

Low-Carb Swiss Loaf

I adapted this from a recipe that had a whole pile of bread crumbs and a cup of milk in it. I simply left them out, and I've never missed them.

2½ pounds (1.1 kg) ground beef
5 ounces (140 g) Swiss cheese, diced small or grated
2 eggs, beaten
1 medium onion, chopped
1 green pepper, chopped
1 small rib celery, chopped
1 teaspoon salt or Vege-Sal
½ teaspoon pepper
½ teaspoon paprika

Preheat the oven to 350°F (180°C, or gas mark 4).

With clean hands combine all the ingredients in a large bowl until the mixture is well blended.

Pack the meat into one large loaf pan or two small ones. Turn out onto a broiler rack. Bake a large loaf for 1½ to 1¾ hours. Bake two small loaves for 1¼ hours.

Yield: 8 servings

Each with 3 grams of carbohydrates and 1 gram of fiber, for a total of 2 grams of usable carbs and 30 grams of protein.

I turn the loaf out of the pan and onto a broiler rack to bake so the excess fat runs off—not because I'm afraid of fat, but because I like it better that way. If you like, though, you could bake yours right in the pan, and it would probably be a bit more tender.

Zucchini Meat Loaf Italiano

The inspiration for this meat loaf was a recipe in an Italian cookbook. The original recipe was for a "zucchini mold," and it had only a tiny bit of meat in it. I thought to myself, "How could adding more ground beef be a problem here?" And I was right; it's very moist and flavorful.

1½ pounds (680 g) ground beef
3 tablespoons (45 ml) olive oil
2 medium zucchini, chopped (about 1½ cups, or 190 g)
1 medium onion, chopped
2 or 3 cloves garlic, crushed
2 tablespoons (7.6 g) snipped fresh parsley
1 egg
¾ cup (75 g) grated Parmesan cheese
1 teaspoon salt
½ teaspoon pepper

Preheat the oven to 350°F (180°C, or gas mark 4).

Heat the olive oil in a skillet and sauté the zucchini, onion, and garlic in it for 7 to 8 minutes.

Let the vegetables cool a bit and then put them in a big bowl with the beef, parsley, egg, cheese, salt, and pepper. Using clean hands, mix the ingredients thoroughly.

Take the rather soft meat mixture and put it in a big loaf pan, if you like, or form the loaf right on a broiler rack so the grease will drip off. (Keep in mind that if you do it this way, your loaf won't stand very high—it'll be about 2 inches [5 cm] thick.)

Bake for 75 to 90 minutes or until the juices run clear but the loaf is not dried out.

Yield: 5 servings

Each with 3 grams of carbohydrates and 1 gram of fiber, for total of 2 grams of usable carbs and 29 grams of protein.

My Grandma's Standby Casserole

Okay, my grandma used egg noodles instead of spaghetti squash, but it tastes good this way, too. This is handy for potlucks and such.

1 pound (455 g) ground beef
2 tablespoons (28 g) butter
1 clove garlic, crushed
1 teaspoon salt
Dash pepper
2 cans (8 ounces, or 225 g each) plain tomato sauce
6 scallions
3 ounces (85 g) cream cheese
1 cup (230 g) sour cream
3 cups (675 g) cooked spaghetti squash
½ cup (60 g) shredded cheddar cheese

(continued on page 378)

Preheat the oven to 350°F (180°C, or gas mark 4).

Brown the ground beef in the butter. Pour off the grease and stir in the garlic, salt, pepper, and tomato sauce.

Cover, turn the heat to low, and simmer for 20 minutes.

While the meat is simmering, slice the scallions, including the crisp part of the green, and combine with the cream cheese and sour cream. Blend well.

In the bottom of a 6-cup (1.4-L) casserole dish, layer half the spaghetti squash, half the scallion mixture, and half the tomato-beef mixture; repeat the layers. Top with the cheddar and bake for 20 minutes.

Yield: 5 servings

Each with 15 grams of carbohydrates and 2 grams of fiber, for a total of 13 grams of usable carbs and 23 grams of protein.

Comfort Food Casserole

This is one of those meal-in-a-bowl sorts of things that just somehow seem comforting. I've found that slow cooking really brings out the best in turnips. They end up remarkably like potatoes.

1½ pounds (680 g) ground round
1 tablespoon (15 ml) oil
1 medium onion, chopped
4 cloves garlic, crushed
4 stalks celery, diced

1 cup (240 ml) beef broth
1 teaspoon beef bouillon concentrate
½ teaspoon salt or Vege-Sal
1 teaspoon pepper
2 teaspoons dried oregano
1 teaspoon dry mustard
2 tablespoons (33 g) tomato paste
4 ounces (115 g) cream cheese
3 turnips, cubed
¾ cup (85 g) shredded cheddar cheese

In a big, heavy skillet, brown and crumble the beef over medium-high heat. Pour off the fat and transfer the beef to a slow cooker.

Add the oil to the skillet and reduce the heat to medium-low. Add the onion, garlic, and celery and sauté until they're just softened. Add the broth, bouillon, salt or Vege-Sal, pepper, oregano, dry mustard, and tomato paste and stir. Now add the cream cheese, using the edge of a spatula to cut the cream cheese into chunks. Let this mixture simmer, stirring occasionally, until the cream cheese is melted. Meanwhile, add the turnips to the slow cooker.

When the cream cheese has melted into the sauce, pour the sauce into the slow cooker. Stir until the ground beef and turnips are coated. Cover the slow cooker, set it to low, and let it cook for 6 hours. Serve with cheddar cheese on top.

Yield: 6 servings

Each with 35 g protein, 12 g carbohydrate, 3 g dietary fiber, 9 g usable carbs.

Spicy Orange Meatballs

1 pound (455 g) ground round

1 teaspoon Worcestershire sauce

½ teaspoon salt or Vege-Sal

¼ teaspoon pepper

¼ medium onion, minced fine

¼ teaspoon chili powder

1 clove garlic, crushed

1 egg

½ cup (120 ml) Dana's No-Sugar Ketchup (page 463)

2 tablespoons (30 ml) Worcestershire sauce

2 tablespoons (40 g) low-sugar orange marmalade

1 pinch cayenne

½ teaspoon chili powder

¼ teaspoon orange extract

2 tablespoons (30 ml) lemon juice

2 tablespoons (30 ml) white vinegar

1½ tablespoons (2.25 g) Splenda

½ cup (120 ml) beef broth

Guar or xanthan

Plunk the ground round into a mixing bowl and add the next 7 ingredients (through the egg). Using clean hands, smoosh everything together until
it's well blended and then form 1-inch (2.5-cm) meatballs. You should have about 40 of them.

Spray a big skillet with nonstick cooking spray and put it over medium heat. Add the meatballs and let them brown all over. Remove them to a plate and pour off the grease.

Add the ketchup and the next 9 ingredients (through the beef broth) into the skillet and whisk it all together over medium heat until it's smooth.

Thicken just a little with guar or xanthan. Put the meatballs back in the skillet, turning to coat with the sauce, and simmer for 10 minutes.

You can serve this as is or over Cauliflower Rice (page 212). They are also very good as a party nibble; keep them in a chafing dish and have a supply of toothpicks on hand for spearing.

Yield: 3 servings

Each with 32 g protein; 6 g carbohydrate; trace dietary fiber; 6 g usable carbs. Analysis does not include Cauliflower Rice.

Cranberry Meatballs

1½ pounds (680 g) ground beef

1 egg

½ cup (80 g) minced onion

¾ teaspoon salt or Vege-Sal

¼ teaspoon pepper

1 teaspoon dry mustard

1 can (8 ounces, or 225 g) tomato sauce

½ cup (50 g) cranberries

3 tablespoons (4.5 g) Splenda

1 tablespoon (15 ml) lime juice

¼ cup (60 ml) water

In a big bowl, combine the ground beef, egg, minced onion, salt or Vege-Sal, pepper, and mustard. Using clean hands, smoosh everything until well combined. Form into meatballs about 1½ inches (3.75 cm) in diameter.

(continued on page 380)

Put everything else in a food processor with the S-blade in place and pulse until the cranberries are chopped fairly fine.

Now spray a big, heavy skillet with nonstick cooking spray and put it over medium-high heat. Brown the meatballs all over. Pour off the fat and add the cranberry mixture. Turn the burner to low, cover, and simmer for 30 minutes. Serve over Cauliflower Rice (page 212) if you want something to sop up the sauce, but they're fine alone.

Yield: 4 to 5 servings

Assuming 4, each will have 31 g protein; 8 g carbohydrate; 2 g dietary fiber; 6 g usable carbs. Analysis does not include Cauliflower Rice.

Swedish Meatballs

This traditional Swedish favorite usually has mashed potatoes in it, but the Ketatoes mix works very well. Serve this with Jansson's Temptation (page 238) for a Swedish feast! Or keep these warm in a chafing dish, with a supply of toothpicks, for a great hot appetizer.

1 pound (455 g) ground chuck
¼ large onion, minced
6 tablespoons (20 g) Ketatoes mix
⅓ cup (80 ml) heavy cream
1 tablespoon (15 ml) water
1 egg
½ teaspoon salt or Vege-Sal
¼ teaspoon pepper
2 tablespoons (7.6 g) minced parsley
2 tablespoons (28 g) butter

Assemble everything but the butter in a mixing bowl. Using clean hands, smoosh it all together until it's very well blended. Form into meatballs about 1 inch (2.5 cm) in diameter.

Put the meatballs in a heavy skillet over medium heat. Melt the butter and brown the meatballs all over—you'll have to do this in a couple of batches unless your skillet is a lot bigger than mine!

You can serve these as is, and they're very nice. Or if you like, you can pour another cup (240 ml) of heavy cream over them, let them simmer for 10 minutes or so, and serve them over Ultimate Fauxtatoes (page 209), or even keep them hot in a chafing dish and serve them as a hot appetizer.

Yield: Assuming this is dinner, not an appetizer, it's 4 servings

Each with 30 g protein; 12 g carbohydrate; 6 g dietary fiber; 6 g usable carbs. (Analysis does not include adding the extra 1 cup [240 ml] of cream. Add about 1.5 g carbs per serving if you use the cream. Analysis also does not include Fauxtatoes.)

Ropa Vieja

This is a basic recipe for Mexican shredded beef that can be used in many ways. The name means "old clothes," and it refers to the shredded texture of the meat.

2 pounds (910 g) boneless beef roast (Chuck or round is good.)
1 carrot, cut in chunks
1 onion, sliced ¼ inch (6 mm) thick
1 stalk celery, whacked into 3 or 4 pieces
Water

Place the beef, carrot, onion, and celery in a Dutch oven or a slow cooker. Add just enough water to cover. If using a slow cooker, set to low; if using a Dutch oven, cover and set on very low heat. Either way, let the beef and vegetables simmer until the beef wants to fall apart when you stick a fork in it—about 3 to 4 hours on the stove and at least 7 or 8 hours in a slow cooker. When the beef is very tender, turn off the heat and let it cool in the broth.

Now, fish the beef out of the broth and put it on a big plate. Using clean hands or two forks, shred it until it's a big pile of little beef threads. Now you're ready to use this very tasty beef in a number of ways. Be sure and save the broth, too.

Yield: 5 servings

Each with 29 g protein; 4 g carbohydrates; 1 g fiber; 3 usable carbs (if you eat all of the vegetables).

Ropa Vieja Hash

This is a great Mexican take on hash. It's bound to be popular with the family!

4 cups (800 g) Ropa Vieja (page 380)
1 cup (150 g) turnip, diced small
1 cup (150 g) cauliflower, diced small
1 medium onion, diced
1 pasilla chili, diced, or 1 green bell pepper, diced
Red pepper flakes to taste
1 clove garlic, crushed
2 tablespoons (30 ml) oil
1 cup (240 ml) Ropa Vieja broth (page 381)
1 cup (64 g) chopped cilantro

First, put the turnip and cauliflower in a microwaveable container with a lid, add a tablespoon (15 ml) or so of water, cover, and cook it on high for 7 minutes.

While that's happening, start sautéing the onion, pepper, red pepper flakes, and garlic in the oil over medium heat. After a couple of minutes, add the Ropa Vieja and stir everything together. Continue sautéing for about 10 minutes, stirring often, at which time your turnip and cauliflower will be ready to add to the skillet.

So add them! Stir them in and keep sautéing! Give it another 5 minutes or so and then add 1 cup (240 ml) of the broth and some of the vegetables from the Ropa Vieja. Stir this into the hash, chopping up the boiled vegetables with the edge of your spatula or spoon.

Let everything cook, stirring from time to time, until the broth has evaporated and the whole thing is fairly dry. Serve topped with cilantro.

Yield: 5 servings

Each with 24 g protein; 9 g carbohydrate; 3 g dietary fiber; 6 g usable carbs.

Basil Beef Stir-Fry

Basil in stir-fries is a Thai touch, but this isn't hot, like most Thai food is.

1 pound (455 g) boneless chuck
½ cup (120 ml) peanut oil or other bland oil
6 scallions, including the crisp part of the green, cut into 1-inch (2.5-cm) lengths

(continued on page 382)

2 teaspoons dried basil or 2 tablespoons
(5.4 g) chopped fresh basil
1 tablespoon (15 ml) soy sauce
¼ teaspoon Splenda
Pepper

Thinly slice the beef across the grain.

Put the oil in a wok or heavy skillet over high heat. When it's hot, add the beef and stir-fry for a minute or two. Add the scallions and stir-fry for another 3 to 4 minutes or until all the pink is gone from the beef.

Add the basil, soy sauce, Splenda, and pepper to taste and toss with the beef, cooking just another minute or so.

Yield: 3 servings

Each with 3 grams of carbohydrates and 1 gram of fiber, for a total of 2 grams of usable carbs and 25 grams of protein.

Sesame Orange Beef

This is an unusual sort of stir-fry!

1 pound (455 g) beef chuck
2 teaspoons dark sesame oil
¾ cup (180 ml) white wine vinegar
2 tablespoons (3 g) Splenda
1 teaspoon orange extract, divided
1 tablespoon (15 ml) soy sauce
3 tablespoons (45 ml) peanut or canola oil
½ medium onion, sliced

½ cup (60 g) shredded carrots
2 cups (300 g) frozen cross-cut green beans, thawed
Guar or xanthan

Slice the beef thin across the grain and put it in a large resealable plastic bag. Combine the sesame oil, white wine vinegar, Splenda, and ½ teaspoon of the orange extract and pour over the beef. Press the air out of the bag, seal, and turn it over a few times to coat the beef. Throw the bag in the fridge for a few hours, and all day won't hurt. This would be a good time to pull the green beans out of the freezer to thaw, too!

Okay, it's dinnertime. Pull the beef out of the fridge and pour off the marinade into a little bowl. Stir the soy sauce and the rest of the orange extract into the marinade bring it to a boil, and have this waiting by the stove.

Put a big, heavy skillet or a wok, if you have one, over highest heat and add the oil. When it's hot, throw in the beef and stir-fry it until all the pink is gone. Remove from the skillet to a bowl or plate. Add a little more oil, if needed, and let it heat. Throw in the onion, carrots, and green beans and stir-fry until they're just tender-crisp. Add the beef back to the skillet or wok, stir in the boiled marinade, thicken a tiny bit with guar or xanthan if you think it needs it, and serve alone or over Cauliflower Rice (page 212).

Yield: 4 servings

Each with 20 g protein; 10 g carbohydrate; 2 g dietary fiber; 8 g usable carbs. Analysis does not include Cauliflower Rice.

Inauthentic Bulgogi Steak

True bulgogi is a popular Korean dish made with very thin sheets of sliced beef. That's time-consuming, so we're using good old steak, and boy, the results are spectacular!

1½ pounds (680 g) tender, well-marbled steaks, ½ inch (1.3 cm) thick—sirloin, rib eye, strip, whatever you like

¼ medium onion

2 teaspoons minced garlic or 4 cloves garlic, peeled

¼ cup (60 ml) soy sauce

2 tablespoons (3 g) Splenda

1 teaspoon pepper

A few dashes hot pepper sauce

2 tablespoons (30 ml) toasted sesame oil

Preheat the broiler.

Put the onion, garlic, soy sauce, Splenda, pepper, hot pepper sauce, and sesame oil in a food processor with the S-blade in place and run it until the onion is pulverized. Reserve some of this liquid for basting.

Place the steaks on a plate and pour the remaining seasoning mixture over them, turning them so that they're coated on both sides. Let the steaks sit for a minute and then place them on a broiler rack. Broil the steaks as close to the heat as possible until they're done to your liking—4½ to 5 minutes per side is right for me. When you're turning the steaks, baste with some of the reserved seasoning mixture, using a clean utensil each time.

Yield: 4 servings

Calculations show 4 grams per serving and a trace of fiber, but that would only be true if you consumed all of the seasoning mixture, which you won't. Figure closer to 2 grams of carbs and 26 grams of protein.

Beef and Artichoke Skillet

This is different and good. Because quite a lot of the carbs in artichokes are in the form of inulin, a very low-impact carb, this is even easier on your blood sugar than the carb count would suggest.

1½ pounds (680 g) boneless beef—Sirloin or chuck are fine.

8 slices bacon

½ medium onion, thinly sliced

2 tablespoons (30 ml) olive oil

¼ cup (60 ml) cider vinegar

1 tablespoon (1.5 g) Splenda

½ teaspoon pepper

½ teaspoon minced garlic or 1 clove garlic, crushed

1 can (14 ounces, or 400 g) quartered artichoke hearts, drained

Lay the bacon on a microwave bacon rack or in a glass pie plate. Microwave on high for 8 minutes.

While the bacon is cooking, slice the beef as thinly as you can and then cut across the strips a couple of times so they're no more than 2 to 3 inches (5 to 7 cm) long. (This is easiest if the meat is partly frozen.) Slice up the onion now, too.

(continued on page 384)

Heat the oil in a large, heavy skillet over high heat and start stir-frying the beef and onion. When the pink is gone from the beef, add the vinegar, Splenda, pepper, garlic, and artichoke hearts and let the whole thing simmer for 5 minutes or so.

Check on the bacon while the beef is simmering. If it's not crisp yet, cook it another minute or so.

Divide the beef mixture between 6 serving plates or bowls and crumble about a strip and a half of bacon over each portion before serving.

Yield: 6 servings

Each with 9 grams of carbohydrates and 4 grams of fiber, for a total of 5 grams of usable carbs and 23 grams of protein.

Balsamic-Olive Beef Kebabs

1 pound (455 g) beef round roast, trimmed
½ cup (120 ml) olive oil
¼ cup (60 ml) balsamic vinegar
1 clove garlic, crushed
About 16 stuffed green olives
½ medium onion
Salt and pepper

Cut the beef into cubes about 1½ inches (4 cm) square. Put them in a nonreactive bowl or in a large resealable plastic bag. Combine the olive oil, balsamic vinegar, and garlic. Reserve some marinade for basting and pour the rest over the beef cubes. If you're using a bowl, stir the whole thing up to coat the cubes. If you're using a resealable plastic bag, press out the air, seal it, and turn it a few times to coat. Either way, throw the beef in the fridge and let it marinate for at least a few hours. If you're going to use bamboo skewers, this is a good time to put them in water to soak, too.

When it's time to cook, first get a fire going. You'll want to set a gas grill on medium or let coals get well covered with ash.

Now, pull out the beef cubes, the olives, and the half onion. Cut the onion half into quarters. Separate the onion into its separate layers. Drain the marinade off of the beef cubes. Skewer a beef cube, then an olive, then a layer of onion, then a beef cube, and so forth. Build all three skewers evenly. Sprinkle the kebabs lightly with salt and pepper.

Fire ready? Throw the kebabs on the grill and cook for about 7 to 10 minutes per side. Baste a few times with the reserved marinade, using a clean utensil each time. You want them cooked through but still a little pink in the center.

Yield: 3 servings

Each serving will have 5 grams of carbohydrate and 1 gram of fiber, for a usable carb count of 4 grams; 34 grams of protein.

Beef Carbonnade

2 pounds (910 g) beef round, cut into 1-inch (2.5-cm) cubes
2 tablespoons (30 ml) olive oil
1 large onion, sliced

2 medium carrots, cut 1 inch (2.5 cm) thick

2 turnips, cubed

12 ounces (360 ml) light beer

¼ cup (60 ml) red wine vinegar

3 tablespoons (4.5 g) Splenda

¼ teaspoon blackstrap molasses

1 cup (240 ml) beef broth

2 teaspoons beef bouillon concentrate

3 cloves garlic, crushed

2 teaspoons dried thyme

2 teaspoons Worcestershire sauce

½ teaspoon pepper

2 bay leaves

Guar or xanthan

In a big, heavy skillet over high heat, sear the beef all over in the oil. Place the beef in a slow cooker. Add the onion, carrots, and turnips and stir everything around a bit.

In a bowl, mix together the beer, vinegar, Splenda, molasses, broth, bouillon, garlic, thyme, Worcestershire sauce, and pepper. Pour the mixture into the slow cooker. Throw the bay leaves on top. Cover the slow cooker, set it to low, and let it cook for 8 hours.

When the time's up, remove the bay leaves and add guar or xanthan to thicken the sauce a bit.

You can serve this as is, or to be more traditional, serve it over Fauxtatoes (page 209).

Yield: 6 servings

Each with 34 g protein, 10 g carbohydrate, 2 g dietary fiber, 8 g usable carbs. Analysis does not include Fauxtatoes.

Pepper Steak with Whiskey Sauce

1 pound (455 g) steak, 1¼ inches (3 cm) thick—Rib eye, sirloin, or T-bone would all be fine.

2 tablespoons (28 g) butter, divided

2 tablespoons (20 g) minced onion

1 cup (240 ml) beef broth

½ teaspoon beef bouillon granules

¼ teaspoon pepper

1 clove garlic

1½ ounces (45 ml) bourbon

Guar or xanthan

1½ teaspoons coarsely ground pepper

1 tablespoon (15 ml) oil

Melt 1 tablespoon (14 g) butter in a medium saucepan and add the onion. Sauté 4 or 5 minutes until it's just turning golden. Add beef broth, bouillon granules, pepper, garlic, and bourbon and let the whole thing boil until it's reduced by about half. Thicken just a little with guar or xanthan—you want it about the texture of heavy cream—right before you serve the steak.

While the sauce is cooking down, sprinkle the pepper evenly over both sides of the steak and press it into the surface. Put a big, heavy skillet over medium-high heat and add remaining butter and oil. As soon as the butter and oil are hot, throw in the steak. Assuming the steak is 1¼ inches (3 cm) thick, I think 6½ minutes per side is about right—that gives me a steak that's medium-rare—but cook it to your liking. Serve with the whiskey sauce.

(continued on page 386)

Yield: 3 servings

Each with 26 g protein; 3 g carbohydrate; trace dietary fiber; 3 g usable carbs.

Southwestern Steak

I adore steak and I adore guacamole—the combination is fantastic.

**1½ to 2 pounds (680 to 910 g) well-marbled
    steak (sirloin, rib eye, or the like),
    1 to 1½ inches (2.5 to 3 cm) thick**
Olive oil
Guacamole (page 59)
Salt and pepper

Rub a couple of teaspoons of olive oil on either side of the steak.

Arrange your broiler so you can get the steak so close that it's almost but not quite touching the broiling element. (I have to put my broiler pan on top of a skillet turned upside down to do this.) Turn the broiler to high and get that steak in there. Leave the oven door open—this is crucial. For a 1-inch (2.5-cm) thick steak, set the oven timer for 5 to 5½ minutes; for a 1½-inch (3-cm) thick steak, you can go up to 6 minutes.

When the timer beeps, quickly flip the steak, and set the timer again. Check at this point to see if your time seems right. If you like your steak a lot rarer or more well-done than I do or if you have a different brand of broiler, you may need to adjust how long you broil the second side for.

When the timer goes off again, get that steak out of there quickly and put it on a serving plate. Spread each serving of steak with a heaping tablespoon of guacamole and sprinkle with salt and pepper to taste.

Yield: The number of servings will depend on the size of your steak

The guacamole will add 4 grams of carbohydrates and 1 gram of fiber, for a total of 3 grams of usable carbs. You'll also get 275 milligrams of potassium.

Salisbury Steak

Talk about your old-time comfort food! Our tester said she'd happily pay for this in a restaurant.

2 pounds (910 g) ground round
¼ cup (25 g) oat bran
¼ cup (20 g) crushed pork rinds
4 tablespoons (60 ml) heavy cream, divided
½ cup (80 g) minced onion, divided
**1½ tablespoons (22.5 ml) Worcestershire
    sauce, divided**
½ teaspoon salt or Vege-sal
¼ teaspoon pepper
8 ounces (225 g) sliced mushrooms
1 cup (240 ml) beef broth
½ teaspoon beef bouillon granules
1 clove garlic
1 teaspoon tomato paste
½ cup (120 ml) Carb Countdown dairy beverage
Guar or xanthan
Salt and pepper to taste

Preheat oven to 300°F (150°C, or gas mark 2).

In a big mixing bowl, combine the ground round, oat bran, pork rind crumbs, 2 tablespoons (30 ml) of the heavy cream, ¼ cup (40 g) of the minced onion, 1 tablespoon (15 ml) Worcestershire sauce, ½ teaspoon salt, and ¼ teaspoon pepper. Using clean hands, smoosh these together until they're well-blended. Form into 6 oval patties. Brown them on either side in a hot skillet and then remove to a baking dish.

Pour off all but about 1 tablespoon (15 ml) grease from the skillet. Add the mushrooms and remaining ¼ cup (40 g) onion to the skillet and sauté until the mushrooms soften.

Add the beef broth, beef bouillon granules, garlic, and tomato paste and stir until the bouillon and tomato paste blend in. Now stir in the Carb Countdown and the remaining 2 tablespoons (30 ml) cream. Thicken to a gravy consistency with guar or xanthan, stir in the remaining ½ tablespoon (7.5 ml) Worcestershire sauce, and season with salt and pepper to taste.

Pour the gravy over the patties, distributing the mushrooms evenly. Bake for 1 hour. Serve with Fauxtatoes (page 209) for that gravy!

Yield: 6 servings

Each with 35 g protein; 7 g carb; 1 g dietary fiber; 6 grams usable carbs. Analysis does not include Fauxtatoes.

Chuckwagon Steak

2 to 2½ pounds (910 g to 1.1 kg) boneless beef chuck steak, 1½ to 2 inches (4 to 5 cm) thick
2 teaspoons meat tenderizer

1 cup (240 ml) olive oil
¼ cup (60 ml) cider vinegar
⅔ cup (160 ml) lime juice

Sprinkle half the tenderizer evenly over one side of the chuck and pierce the meat all over with a fork. Turn it over and repeat on the other side using the other teaspoon of tenderizer.

Now, put the meat in a flat, shallow, nonreactive pan that fits it fairly closely or in a big resealable plastic bag. Mix together the rest of the ingredients and pour them over the steak. If you're using a bag, press out the air, seal it up, and turn it a few times to coat the whole piece of meat. If you're using a pan, turn the meat to coat it. Stick the whole thing in the fridge, and let the meat marinate for at least several hours, turning it a few times.

When dinnertime rolls around (or actually a bit beforehand), get a grill going—you'll want your charcoal to be white or your gas grill on medium or a touch higher. Just pull the steak out and grill it—about 12 minutes per side puts it at about the degree of doneness I like, but you cook it to your liking; then slice it across the grain.

This is great plain, but it's also a good choice to serve with the Cilantro Chimichurri (page 476).

Yield: 6 servings

If you consumed all of the marinade, each serving would have 3 grams of carbohydrate and a trace of fiber, but of course, you drain the marinade off. I'd count no more than 1 gram of carbohydrate per serving, and I suspect that's a generous estimate; 30 grams of protein. Analysis does not include Cilantro Chimichurri.

Steak Diane

12-ounce (340 g) steak, ½ inch (1.3 cm)
  thick—Use rib eye, sirloin, strip, or whatever
  you like.
2 tablespoons (28 g) butter
3 scallions, finely minced
1 tablespoon (3.8 g) minced parsley
1½ teaspoons minced garlic
1 tablespoon (15 ml) brandy
2 tablespoons (30 ml) dry sherry
1½ teaspoons Worcestershire sauce

In a heavy skillet over medium-high heat, sauté
the steak in the butter—figure 5 to 6 minutes
per side. While that's happening, mince up the
scallions and parsley.

When the steak is done to your liking, remove
it to a platter and keep it warm.

Turn the heat down to medium. Add the
scallions, parsley, and garlic and sauté in the
butter for a minute or so. Add the brandy, sherry,
and Worcestershire sauce, turn the heat back up,
and boil hard while stirring to scrape any nice
brown bits off the bottom of the pan. Let it boil
for a minute or so to reduce, pour it over the
steak, and serve.

Yield: 2 servings

Each with 3 grams of carbohydrates and 2 grams of
fiber, for a total of just 1 gram of usable carbs and
25 grams of protein.

Uptown Chuck

2 to 2½ pounds (910 g to 1.1 kg) boneless
  chuck steak, 1½ to 2 inches (4 to 5 cm)
  thick

2 teaspoons meat tenderizer
½ cup (120 ml) canola oil
¼ cup (60 ml) soy sauce
½ cup (120 ml) dry red wine
1 tablespoon (6 g) grated ginger
2 teaspoons curry powder
2 tablespoons (30 ml) Dana's No-Sugar
  Ketchup (page 463)
¼ teaspoon pepper
1 teaspoon hot pepper sauce

Sprinkle half the tenderizer over one side of the
steak, pierce it all over with a fork, turn it, and
repeat with the rest of the tenderizer. This one
works best with a shallow, flat, nonreactive pan.
Place the steak in the pan. Mix everything else
together, reserving some marinade for basting.
Pour the rest over the steak and then turn the
steak over to coat both sides with the marinade.
Stick the whole thing in the fridge and let it
marinate, turning it over when you think of it,
for at least several hours, and overnight is
even better.

Start a charcoal fire or preheat a gas grill.
Once you have your grill going and your coals are
white or your gas grill is heated, grill the steak
for about 12 minutes per side or to your liking,
basting a few times with the reserved marinade
and using a clean utensil each time you baste.
Slice across the grain and serve.

Yield: 6 servings

3 grams of carbohydrate per serving, but again,
that assumes you consume all of the marinade.
I'd count no more than 1 gram per serving;
25 grams of protein.

Steak with Brandy-Stilton Cream Sauce

This is decadent beyond belief and absolutely magnificent. Stilton, if you haven't tried it, is a very strong blue cheese from England. If you can't find it, use whatever blue cheese you've got kicking around, and I'm sure it will be fine.

1 pound (455 g) beef rib eye steak, 1¼ inches (3 cm) thick (or use any tender, broilable cut)
1 tablespoon (15 ml) olive oil
2 tablespoons (30 ml) brandy
½ cup (120 ml) heavy cream
2 ounces (55 g) Stilton cheese, crumbled

In a big, heavy skillet over medium-high heat, start pan-broiling the steak in the olive oil. About 6 minutes per side is right for my tastes, but do it to your preferred degree of doneness. When the steak is done, remove to a platter and keep t warm!

Remove the pan from the heat and carefully pour in the brandy. Return the pan to the stove and stir the brandy around, dissolving all the brown bits stuck to the skillet. Now pour in the cream and stir. Add the Stilton and stir until it's melted and the sauce smoothes out. Pour over the steak and serve.

Yield: 3 servings

Each with 26 g protein; 1 g carbohydrate; 0 g dietary fiber; 1 g usable carb.

Costa Brava Steak

I was surprised that this traditional, anchovy-based Spanish sauce was not particularly fishy—just rich, mellow, and complex.

12 to 16 ounces (340 to 455 g) steak, ½ to ¾ inch thick (1 to 2 cm)—rib eye, sirloin, strip, anything tender and fit for broiling
⅓ cup (50 g) shelled walnuts
3 anchovy fillets
½ teaspoon red wine vinegar or sherry vinegar
⅓ cup (80 ml) olive oil

Start the steak broiling as close as possible to the heating element. Set your timer to remind you when to turn it—for a steak ½-inch (1 cm) thick, 5 minutes per side is about right for my tastes.

While the steak is broiling, put the walnuts, anchovies, and vinegar in a food processor with the S-blade in place. Pulse to chop everything together—unless your machine is smaller than mine, the mixture will end up out against the walls of the processor bowl pretty quickly!

Scrape down the sides of the processor to get the mixture back into the path of the blade. Put the top back on, turn the processor on, and slowly pour in about half of the olive oil. If necessary, scrape down the sides of the processor again at this point and then turn it back on and add the rest of the oil.

When both sides of the steak are done, spread this sauce over the steak. Turn the broiler to low, put the steak back under it for just a minute and then serve.

(continued on page 390)

Yield: The number of servings will depend on the size of your steak

Assuming a 12-ounce (340 g) steak, I'd call it 2 servings, each with 3 grams of carbohydrates and 1 gram of fiber, for a total of 2 grams of usable carbs and 31 grams of protein.

Portobello Fillets

Here's a very simple way to make those wonderful but pricey little fillets mignon seem bigger, while impressing the heck out of your company. Add a big tossed salad and a loaf of crusty bread for the carb eaters, and you've got an elegant meal that takes practically no work.

4 fillets mignon, about 5 ounces (140 g) each
4 large portobello mushrooms
1 cup (240 ml) balsamic vinaigrette dressing
Olive oil for brushing

Lay the portobellos in a shallow baking dish, gill-side up, and pour the balsamic vinaigrette over them. Turn them over once or twice to make sure they're thoroughly coated in the dressing and then let them sit for 10 to 15 minutes.

Okay, now you're going to multitask: Heat the broiler to high and brush the steaks with a little olive oil. Also heat up an electric tabletop grill.

Start the fillets broiling close to the heat—I'd probably give them about 5 to 5½ minutes per side, but cook them to your own preference. When you turn them over, put the marinated mushrooms in the electric grill. Let them cook for about 5 minutes. Your steak and your mushrooms should be done right about the same moment!

Put each mushroom on a plate and put a fillet on top of each. Serve piping hot.

Yield: 4 servings

Each with 28 g protein; 9 g carbohydrate; 2 g dietary fiber; 7 g usable carbs. However, this analysis assumes you consume all of the balsamic vinaigrette, while in actuality some will be left in the dish you marinated the mushrooms in. So you'll actually get fewer carbs than this.

Feel free to cut a larger steak into individual portions to serve on your mushrooms, if you prefer. Those fillets just come exactly the right size. Do, however, use a good thick steak for this—at least 1¼ inches (3 cm).

Ginger Marinated Chuck

I have a yummy pot roast recipe that calls for tomatoes, cider vinegar, and ginger, so this idea was a natural.

2 pounds (910 g) boneless chuck,
    1½ to 2 inches (4 to 5 cm) thick
2 teaspoons meat tenderizer
¼ cup (60 ml) Dana's No-Sugar Ketchup
    (page 463)
¼ cup (60 ml) vinaigrette dressing (I use Paul
    Newman's.)
2½ tablespoons (3.8 g) Splenda
½ teaspoon blackstrap molasses
2 teaspoons grated ginger
½ teaspoon salt
1 tablespoon (15 ml) water

1 tablespoon (15 ml) cider vinegar

½ teaspoon soy sauce

First, sprinkle a teaspoon of tenderizer over one side of the meat, pierce it all over with a fork, flip it over, and repeat with the rest of the tenderizer. Now put the meat in a large resealable plastic bag or in a shallow, nonreactive pan. Mix together everything else and reserve some of the mixture for basting. Pour the rest over the meat. If you're using a resealable plastic bag, press out the air and seal it. Either way, turn the chuck steak over once or twice to make sure it's coated with the marinade. Stash it in the fridge and let it marinate for at least several hours, and overnight is better.

When it's time to cook, get the grill going, setting your gas grill to medium or letting your charcoal get a good coat of ash. Pull your steak out of the marinade and grill it for about 10 minutes per side, basting frequently with the reserved marinade and using a clean utensil each time.

Yield: 6 servings

Each serving will have 3 grams of carbohydrate—again, that's if you consume all of the marinade. I'd count no more than 1 gram of carbohydrate per serving and 24 grams of protein.

Orange Tequila Steak

Here's a Southwestern twist for your steak.

1 pound (455 g) beef steak—Rib eye is my choice, but sirloin or T-bone should do fine.

3 cloves garlic

¼ cup (60 ml) lemon juice

¼ cup (60 ml) lime juice

1½ ounces (45 ml) tequila

1½ teaspoons chili powder

1 tablespoon (1.5 g) Splenda

1½ teaspoons dried oregano

3 tablespoons (45 ml) olive oil

¼ teaspoon orange extract

Throw the steak in a big resealable plastic bag. Mix together everything else, reserving some liquid for basting, and pour the rest into the bag. Seal the bag, pressing out the air as you go. Turn the bag to coat the steak and then throw it in the fridge and let the steak marinate for at least a few hours, and a whole day is fine.

Pull the steak out of the fridge and pour off the marinade. Now you get to decide—outside on the grill or inside in the broiler? Either way, grill or broil your steak fast, close to high heat (but if you're using a charcoal grill, keep down flare-ups; they char, not cook). If your steak is 1¼ inch (3 cm) thick (that's how I have the meat guys cut mine), about 6 to 6½ minutes per side will be right for medium to medium-rare. Baste at least 2 or 3 times with the reserved marinade during cooking—using a clean utensil each time you baste.

Yield: 2 to 3 servings

Assuming 3, each will have 26 g protein; 6 g carbohydrate; 1 g dietary fiber—but this assumes you consume all of the marinade, which you won't. I'd guess no more than 3 g per serving. Analysis does not include any side dishes.

Carne Asada Steak

Carne asada is Spanish for "grilled beef"—well, actually, "meat," but beef is assumed. It's a Mexican and Southwestern specialty. I don't know how authentic my version is, but it sure tastes good, especially with an ice-cold light beer.

2 pounds (910 g) boneless round steak or chuck, 1½ to 2 inches (4 to 5 cm) thick
2 teaspoons meat tenderizer
½ cup (120 ml) red wine vinegar
¼ cup (60 ml) olive oil
2 tablespoons (30 ml) Dana's No-Sugar Ketchup (page 463)
1 tablespoon (15 ml) soy sauce
2 cloves garlic, crushed
2 teaspoons ground or rubbed sage
½ teaspoon salt
1 teaspoon dry mustard
1 teaspoon paprika
2 jalapenos, minced

Sprinkle one side of the meat with 1 teaspoon of the tenderizer and pierce it all over with a fork. Turn it over and treat the other side the same way with the second teaspoon of tenderizer. Put the meat in a large resealable plastic bag or in a shallow, nonreactive pan. Mix together everything else (wash your hands after handling those jalapenos!). Reserve some marinade for basting and pour the rest over the meat. If you're using a bag, press out the air, seal it, and turn it a few times to coat the meat; if you're using a pan, turn the meat over once or twice to coat. Put the meat in the refrigerator and let it marinate for at least several hours—overnight is better—turning it now and then.

When dinnertime rolls around, start your grill and let your charcoal burn down to the well-ashed stage or set your gas grill to medium. Grill your steak for about 10 minutes per side, basting frequently with the reserved marinade. Use a clean utensil each time you baste. If you'd like, you can put the leftover marinade in a microwavable bowl or in a saucepan and either microwave it until it's boiled for a minute or bring it to a boil on the stove and then serve it as a sauce.

Yield: 6 servings

If you do use the leftover marinade as a sauce and eat all of it, each serving will have 3 grams of carbohydrate, and a trace of fiber, for a usable carb count of 3 grams; 29 grams of protein.

Marinated Sirloin

1½ to 2 pounds (680 to 910 g) sirloin steak, 1 inch (2.5 cm) thick
1 cup (240 ml) water
½ cup (120 ml) soy sauce
3 tablespoons (45 ml) Worcestershire sauce
½ medium onion, finely minced
1½ tablespoons (23 ml) balsamic vinegar
½ tablespoon wine vinegar
1½ tablespoons (22.5 ml) lemon juice
1 tablespoon (15 ml) spicy brown or Dijon mustard
2 cloves garlic, crushed

Combine everything but the steak in a large measuring cup or bowl with a pouring lip. This is your marinade.

Place the steak in a large, resealable plastic bag, pour in the marinade, and seal the bag. Place it in a flat pan (in case the bag springs a leak) and stick the whole thing in the fridge for at least several hours or overnight if you have the time.

About 15 minutes before you're ready to cook, remove your steak from the bag and preheat the broiler or grill. Broil or grill it to your liking.

Yield: Figure at least 4 servings from a 1½-pound (680 g) steak, and 5 or 6 servings from a 2-pounder (910 g).

There are a few grams of carbs in the marinade, but since you discard most of it, there's less than 1 gram of carbohydrates added to each serving, no fiber, and no protein. Each serving of steak has no carbohydrates, no fiber, and about 25 grams of protein.

Smoky Marinated Steak

This has a subtle but great smoky flavor that really enhances the meat.

1 pound (455 g) T-bone steak at least 1 inch (2.5 cm) thick (Sirloin or rib eye would do too.)

1 tablespoon (15 ml) liquid smoke flavoring (Most big grocery stores carry this.)

1 teaspoon salt or Vege-Sal

1 clove garlic, crushed

1 dash pepper

1 teaspoon olive oil

⅛ teaspoon onion powder

¼ cup (60 ml) water

Put the steak in a resealable plastic bag. Mix together everything else, reserving some marinade for basting. Pour the rest into the bag and seal, pressing out the air as you go. Turn the bag once or twice to coat and throw the steak in the fridge for a few hours at least, and a day won't hurt a bit.

When dinnertime rolls around, preheat the broiler. Pull out the steak and pour off the marinade. Broil very close to a high broiler—for a steak about 1¼ inches (3 cm), I like about 6 minutes per side, but do it to your liking. Baste halfway through cooking each side, using the reserved marinade and a clean utensil each time.

Yield: 3 servings

Each with 23 g protein; 1 g carbohydrate; trace dietary fiber; 1 g usable carb.

Steak Au Poivre with Brandy Cream

This dish is for black pepper lovers only!

¾ pound (340 g) tender, well marbled steak (such as rib eye or sirloin), ½ to ¾ inch (1 to 2 cm) thick

4 teaspoons coarse cracked pepper

1 tablespoon (14 g) butter

1 tablespoon (15 ml) olive oil

2 tablespoons (30 ml) brandy

2 tablespoons (30 ml) heavy cream

Salt

(continued on page 394)

Place the steak on a plate and sprinkle half of the pepper evenly over it. Using your hands or the back of a spoon, press the pepper firmly into the steak's surface. Turn the steak over and do the same thing to the other side.

Add the butter and oil to a large, heavy skillet over high heat. When the skillet is hot, add the steak. For a ½-inch (1 cm) thick steak, 4½ minutes per side is about right; go maybe 5½ minutes for a ¾-inch (2 cm) thick steak.

When the steak is done on both sides, turn off the heat, pour the brandy over it, and light it on fire.

When the flames die down, remove the steak to a serving platter and pour the cream into the skillet. Stir it around, dissolving the meat juices and brandy into it. Season lightly with salt and pour it over the steak.

Yield: 2 servings

Each with 3 grams of carbohydrates and 1 gram of fiber, for a total of 2 grams of usable carbs and 25 grams of protein.

Platter Sauce for Steak

Make this with the drippings when you're pan-broiling a steak (cooking it in a hot, dry skillet).

2 tablespoons (28 g) butter
1 teaspoon dry mustard
½ teaspoon Worcestershire sauce
½ teaspoon salt or Vege-Sal
½ teaspoon pepper

After pan-broiling a steak, pour off most of the grease. Melt the butter in the pan and then stir in the mustard, Worcestershire sauce, salt, and pepper, stirring it around so you scrape up the nice brown bits from the pan.

Let it bubble a minute, pour it over the hot steak, and serve.

Yield: This is about enough for a 1-pound (455-g) steak

1 gram of carbohydrates, no fiber, and no protein.

Cube Steaks in Gravy

1½ pounds (680 g) cube steaks
1 tablespoon (15 ml) olive oil
1 medium onion, sliced
8 ounces (225 g) sliced mushrooms
3 cups (710 ml) beef broth
1 tablespoon (15 ml) beef bouillon concentrate
Guar or xanthan

In a big, heavy skillet, heat the oil and brown the steaks on both sides.

Put the onion and mushrooms in a slow cooker.

In a bowl, stir the broth and bouillon and pour the mixture over the vegetables. Place the steaks on top. Cover the slow cooker, set it to low, and let it cook for 6 to 7 hours.

When the time's up, remove the steaks and thicken the sauce with guar or xanthan to your liking.

Yield: 6 servings

Each with 29 g protein, 5 g carbohydrate, 1 g dietary fiber, 4 g usable carbs.

Swiss Steak

Here's a no-work version of this old-time favorite.

1 large onion, sliced
3 pounds (1.4 kg) beef round
1 tablespoon (15 ml) beef bouillon concentrate
8 ounces (240 ml) vegetable juice (such as V8)
2 stalks celery, sliced
Guar or xanthan (optional)

Place the onion in a slow cooker. Place the beef on top.

In a bowl, stir the bouillon into the vegetable juice. Pour the mixture over the beef. Scatter the celery on top. Cover the slow cooker, set it to low, and let it cook for 8 to 10 hours.

When the time's up, thicken the juices with guar or xanthan, if desired. Serve over Fauxtatoes (page 209).

Yield: 8 servings

Each with 35 g protein, 3 g carbohydrate, 1 g dietary fiber, 2 g usable carbs. Analysis does not include Fauxtatoes.

Beef Burgundy

This is a handy one-dish company meal. Put it together on a Saturday morning, and it will cook happily by itself all afternoon.

2 pounds (910 g) boneless beef round or chuck, cut into 2-inch (5-cm) cubes
¼ cup (60 ml) olive oil
1 cup (240 ml) dry red wine
¾ teaspoon guar or xanthan
1½ teaspoons salt or Vege-Sal
1 teaspoon paprika
1 teaspoon dried oregano
1 big onion, sliced
8 ounces (225 g) mushrooms, wiped clean with a damp cloth
2 green peppers, cut into chunks

Preheat the oven to 250°F (120°C, or gas mark ½).

Put the oil in a heavy skillet over medium-high heat and brown the beef in the oil.

Put the browned beef in a 10-cup (2.8-L) casserole dish with a lid.

Combine the wine and guar in the blender, blending for 10 seconds or so, and then pour the mixture over the beef.

Add the salt, paprika, oregano, onion, mushrooms, and green peppers to the casserole dish and give it a quick stir. Cover and put it in the oven for 5 hours. When it comes out, you can boil down the liquid a bit in a saucepan to make it thicker, if you like, but it's quite nice just like this.

Yield: 6 generous servings

Each with 8 grams of carbohydrates and 3 grams of fiber, for a total of 5 grams of usable carbs and 25 grams of protein.

Simple Salsa Beef

Here's one of those super-simple dump-and-go recipes. It's great for a day when you didn't get dinner in the slow cooker the night before!

3 pounds (1.4 kg) beef arm pot roast
3 turnips, peeled and cubed
1 pound (455 g) baby carrots
2 cups (520 g) salsa
Guar or xanthan (optional)

Put the turnips and carrots in a slow cooker and place the beef on top. Pour the salsa over everything. Cover the slow cooker, set it to low, and let it cook for 8 to 10 hours.

When the time's up, remove the beef and pull it apart into shreds with two forks. Scoop the vegetables out onto serving plates with a slotted spoon. Pile the beef on top. If desired, thicken the sauce with a little guar or xanthan. Spoon the sauce over the vegetables and beef.

Yield: 8 servings

Each with 26 g protein, 11 g carbohydrate, 3 g dietary fiber, 8 g usable carbs.

New England Boiled Dinner

This is our traditional St. Patrick's Day dinner, but it's a simple, satisfying one-pot meal on any chilly night. If you have carb-eaters in the family, you can add a few little red boiling potatoes, still in their skins.

1 corned beef "for simmering" (about 3 pounds, or 1.4 kg)
6 small turnips (golf ball to tennis ball size)
2 big ribs celery, cut into chunks
2 medium onions, cut into chunks
½ head cabbage
Spicy brown mustard
Horseradish
Butter

Peel the turnips and throw them in into the slow cooker along with the celery and the onions. Set the corned beef on top and add water to cover.

There will be a seasoning packet with the corned beef—dump it into the slow cooker. Put the lid on the slow cooker, set it on low, and leave it alone for 10 to 12 hours. (You can cut the cooking time down to 6 to 8 hours if you set the slow cooker on high, but the low setting yields the most tender results.)

When you come home from work all those hours later, remove the corned beef from the cooker with a fork or some tongs, put the lid back on the slow cooker to retain heat, put the beef on a platter, and keep it someplace warm. Cut the cabbage into big wedges and drop it into the slow cooker with the other vegetables.

Re-cover the slow cooker and turn it up to high. Have a green beer (lite beer, of course) while the cabbage cooks for 30 minutes.

With a slotted spoon, remove all the vegetables and pile them around the corned beef on a platter. Serve with the mustard and horseradish as condiments for the beef and butter for the vegetables.

Yield: 8 servings (and of course, you don't need a thing with it)

Each with 9 grams of carbohydrates and 2 grams of fiber, for a total of 7 grams of usable carbs and 26 grams of protein.

This is easy, but it takes a long time to cook. Do yourself a favor, and assemble it ahead of time.

Maple-Glazed Corned Beef with Vegetables

This is a trifle less traditional but just as good as the New England Boiled Dinner (page 396). The pancake syrup and mustard, plus last-minute glazing under the broiler, give it a new aspect.

5 pounds (2.3 kg) corned beef brisket

6 medium turnips, cut into chunks

2 medium carrots, cut into chunks

1 medium onion, quartered

2 cups (480 ml) water

1 medium head cabbage, cut into wedges

3 tablespoons (45 ml) sugar-free pancake syrup

1 tablespoon (15 ml) brown mustard

Horseradish

Place the turnips, carrots, and onion in your slow cooker. Place the corned beef on top. Scatter the contents of the accompanying seasoning packet over everything and pour the water over the whole thing. Cover the slow cooker, set it to low, and let it cook for 9 to 10 hours, and a bit more won't hurt!

When the time's up, carefully remove the corned beef and put it on a broiler rack, fatty side up. Use a slotted spoon to skim out the vegetables, put them on a platter, cover, and keep in a warm place.

Preheat the broiler.

Place the cabbage in the slow cooker, set it to high, and let it cook for 15 to 20 minutes or until just tender. (Or you can pour the liquid from the pot into a saucepan and cook the cabbage in it on your stovetop, which is faster.)

While the cabbage is cooking, mix together the pancake syrup and the mustard. Spread the mixture over the corned beef, just the side that is up. When the cabbage is almost done, run the corned beef under the broiler for 2 to 3 minutes until glazed.

Transfer the cabbage to the platter with a slotted spoon. Slice the corned beef across the grain and serve immediately with horseradish and mustard.

Yield: 12 servings

Each with 29 g protein, 10 g carbohydrate, 3 g dietary fiber, 7 g usable carbs. (This carb count does not include the polyols in the pancake syrup.)

Beef in Beer

The tea, the beer, and the long, slow cooking make this as tender as can be.

2 pounds (910 g) boneless beef round roast

2 to 3 tablespoons (30 to 45 ml) olive oil

1 medium onion, sliced

(continued on page 398)

1 can (8 ounces, or 225 g) tomato sauce

12 ounces (360 ml) light beer

1 teaspoon instant tea powder

1 can (4 ounces, or 115 g) unsweetened
   mushrooms, drained

2 cloves garlic, crushed

Heat oil in a big, heavy skillet over medium-high heat and sear the beef until it's brown all over. Transfer the beef to a slow cooker.

In the oil left in the skillet, fry the onion for a few minutes and add that to the slow cooker, too.

Pour the tomato sauce and beer over the beef. Sprinkle the tea over it and add the mushrooms and garlic. Cover the slow cooker, set it to low, and let it cook for 8 to 9 hours. This is good served with Fauxtatoes (page 209).

Yield: 6 servings

Each with 28 g protein, 7 g carbohydrate, 2 g dietary fiber, 5 g usable carbs. Analysis does not include Fauxtatoes.

Beef with Asian Mushroom Sauce

Once you have the Hoisin Sauce on hand, this is very quick to put together. The Hoisin Sauce is a snap, and it keeps well in the fridge.

4 pounds (1.8 kg) beef tip roast

4 ounces (115 g) sliced mushrooms

¼ cup (60 ml) Hoisin Sauce (page 464)

2 cloves garlic, minced

½ teaspoon salt

¼ cup (60 ml) beef broth

Guar or xanthan

6 tablespoons (35 g) sliced scallions

Put the mushrooms in a slow cooker and place the beef on top. Spread the Hoisin Sauce over the beef, scatter the garlic and salt over it, and pour in the broth around it. Cover the slow cooker, set it to low, and let it cook for 9 hours.

When the time's up, remove the beef from the slow cooker and put it on a platter. Add guar or xanthan to thicken up the sauce a bit and then pour the sauce into a sauce boat. Slice the beef and serve it with the sauce, topped with the scallions.

Yield: 6 servings

Each with 61 g protein, 4 g carbohydrate, 1 g dietary fiber, 3 g usable carbs.

Peking Slow-Cooker Pot Roast

3 to 5 pound (1.4 to 2.3 kg) beef roast (round,
   chuck, or rump)

5 or 6 cloves garlic

½ cup (120 ml) cider vinegar

½ cup (120 ml) water

1 small onion

1½ cups (360 ml) strong coffee (Instant
   works fine.)

1 teaspoon guar or xanthan

Salt and pepper

At least 24 to 36 hours before you want to actually cook your roast, stick holes in the meat with a thin-bladed knife, cut the garlic cloves into slices, and insert a slice into each hole. Put the garlic-studded roast in a big bowl and pour the vinegar and the water over it. Put it in the fridge and let it sit there for a day or so, turning it over when you think of it so the whole thing marinates.

On the morning of the day you want to serve the roast, drain off the marinade and put the roast in the slow cooker. Thinly slice the onion and put it on top of the roast. Pour the coffee over the roast and onion, put on the lid, set the cooker on low, and leave it alone for 8 hours for a smaller roast or up to 10 hours for a larger one.

When you're ready to eat, remove the roast from the cooker carefully because it will now be so tender it's likely to fall apart.

Scoop out 2 cups (480 ml) of the liquid and some of the onions and put them in the blender with the guar. Blend for few seconds and then pour into a saucepan set over high heat. Boil this sauce hard for about 5 minutes to reduce it a bit. Season the sauce with salt and pepper to taste (it's amazing the difference the salt and pepper make here; I didn't like the flavor of this sauce until I added the salt and pepper, and then I liked it a lot) and slice and serve the roast with this sauce.

Yield: If you use a 4-pound (1.8-kg), boneless roast, you'll get 12 servings

Each with 3 grams of carbohydrates, a trace of fiber, and 34 grams of protein.

Warning: Do not try to make this with a tender cut of beef! This recipe will tenderize the toughest cut; a tender one will practically dissolve. Use inexpensive, tough cuts and prepare to be amazed at how fork-tender they get.

Balsamic Pot Roast

Balsamic vinegar and rosemary give this pot roast an Italian accent.

3½ pounds (1.6 kg) beef round, trimmed of fat
2 tablespoons (30 ml) olive oil
1 large onion, sliced
2 cloves garlic, crushed
1 cup (240 ml) beef broth
1 teaspoon beef bouillon concentrate
¼ cup (60 ml) balsamic vinegar
½ teaspoon dried rosemary, ground
1 cup (240 g) canned diced tomatoes
Guar or xanthan

In a big, heavy skillet, sear the beef in the oil until browned all over. Transfer the beef to a slow cooker. Scatter the onion and garlic around the beef.

In a bowl, stir together the broth, bouillon, vinegar, and rosemary. Pour the mixture over the beef. Pour the tomatoes on top. Season with pepper. Cover the slow cooker, set it to low, and let it cook for 8 hours.

When the time's up, remove the beef with tongs and place it on a serving platter. Scoop the onions out with a slotted spoon and pile them around the roast. Thicken the juice left in the slow cooker with guar or xanthan and serve it with the beef.

Yield: 8 servings

Each with 42 g protein, 5 g carbohydrate, trace dietary fiber, 5 g usable carbs.

Ginger Beef

This is my favorite thing to do with a pot roast. It has a bright flavor full of tomato, fruit, and ginger.

3- to 4-pound (1.4- to 1.8-kg) boneless chuck
   or round roast, about 2 inches (5 cm) thick
3 tablespoons (45 ml) olive oil
1 small onion
1 clove garlic, crushed
1 can (14½ ounces, or 410 g) diced tomatoes
1 tablespoon (1.5 g) Splenda
1 teaspoon ground ginger
¼ cup (60 ml) cider vinegar

Place the oil in a large, heavy skillet and brown the roast in it over medium-high heat. When both sides are well-seared, add the onion, garlic, and tomatoes.

In a bowl, stir the Splenda and ginger into the vinegar and add that mixture to the skillet, stirring to combine.

Cover the skillet, turn the heat to low, and let the whole thing simmer for about 1¼ hours. Serve with the vegetables piled on top.

Yield: A 3-pound (1.4-kg) roast should yield at least 6 servings

Each with 6 grams of carbohydrates and 1 gram of fiber, for a total of 5 grams of usable carbs and 47 grams of protein.

Yankee Pot Roast

This old-time favorite is just as good as you remember.

2½- to 3-pound (1.1- to 1.4-kg) boneless
   chuck roast
¼ cup (60 ml) olive oil
1¾ cups (420 ml) water, divided
1 medium onion, sliced
1 large rib celery, sliced
2 small turnips, cut into chunks
1 medium carrot, sliced
½ cup (30 g) chopped fresh parsley
4 ounces (115 g) mushrooms, thickly sliced
1 teaspoon liquid beef bouillon concentrate
½ teaspoon guar or xanthan gum

Put the oil in a Dutch oven over medium heat and sear the roast in the oil until it's dark brown all over. Remove the roast from the Dutch oven.

Put ¼ cup (60 ml) of the water and the sliced onions in the Dutch oven and place the roast directly on top of the onions. Cover the Dutch oven, set the burner to low, and forget about it for 1½ to 2 hours.

Remove the roast again—it'll be very tender and may break a bit—and add 1 cup (240 ml) of the water and the celery, turnips, carrot, parsley, and mushrooms. Put the roast back in on top of the vegetables and cover the Dutch oven. Let it simmer for another 30 to 45 minutes or until the turnip and carrot are soft.

Remove the roast to a serving platter and use a slotted spoon to pile the vegetables over the roast or in a separate bowl, as you prefer.

Put the last ½ cup (120 ml) of water in the blender with the bouillon and guar and blend for 15 seconds or so until all the thickener is dissolved. Scrape the mixture into the Dutch oven and stir it around to thicken the gravy. Pour the gravy over the roast or put it in a gravy boat or pitcher and serve.

Yield: 6 to 8 servings, depending on the size of the roast. A 3-pound (1.4-kg) roast has 8 servings

Each with 5 grams of carbohydrates and 1 gram of fiber, for a total of 4 grams of usable carbs and 28 grams of protein.

Pepperoncini Beef

Pepperoncini are hot-but-not-scorching pickled Italian salad peppers. You'll find these in the same aisle as the olives and pickles. They make this beef very special.

2 to 3 pounds (910 g to 1.4 kg) boneless chuck pot roast
1 cup (120 g) pepperoncini peppers, undrained
½ medium onion, chopped
Guar or xanthan

Place the beef in a slow cooker, pour the peppers on top, and strew the onion over that. Cover the slow cooker, set it to low, and let it cook for 8 hours.

When the time's up, remove the beef, put it on a platter, and use a slotted spoon to scoop out the peppers and pile them on top of the beef. Thicken the juices in the pot with the guar or xanthan. Add salt and pepper to taste and serve the sauce with the beef.

Yield: 6 servings

Each with 24 g protein, 3 g carbohydrate, trace dietary fiber, 3 g usable carbs. (This analysis is for a 2-pound [910-g] roast.)

Sauerbrauten

This classic German pot roast takes advance planning, but it's not a lot of work and yields impressive results. Don't forget the Fauxtatoes (page 209) for that gravy!

4 pounds (1.8 kg) boneless beef round or chuck
1 cup (240 ml) cider vinegar
1 cup (240 ml) water
½ onion, sliced
2 bay leaves
1 teaspoon pepper
¼ cup (6 g) Splenda
2 tablespoons (26 g) bacon grease or oil
¼ teaspoon ground ginger
1 cup (230 g) light sour cream (Use full-fat sour cream if you prefer, but it's no lower carb.)
Guar or xanthan (optional)

Pierce the beef all over with a fork. In a deep, non-reactive bowl (stainless steel, glass, or enamel), combine the vinegar, water, onion, bay leaves, pepper, and Splenda. Place the beef in the marinade and put the bowl in the refrigerator. Marinate the beef for at least 3 days, and 5 or 6 days won't hurt. Turn it over at least once a day, so both sides marinate evenly.

When the time comes to cook your Sauerbrauten, remove the beef from the marinade and pat it dry with paper towels. Reserve the marinade.

In a big, heavy skillet, heat the bacon grease or oil and sear the beef all over. Transfer the beef to a slow cooker.

(continued on page 402)

Scoop the onion and bay leaves out of the marinade with a slotted spoon and put them on top of the beef. Remove 1 cup (240 ml) of the marinade from the bowl and add the ginger to it. Pour this over the beef and discard the remaining marinade. Cover the slow cooker, set it to low, and let it cook for 7 to 8 hours.

When the time's up, remove the beef to a serving plate. Remove the bay leaves. Stir the sour cream into the liquid in the slow cooker and thicken it with guar or xanthan if you think it needs it. Add salt and pepper to taste and serve the sauce with the beef.

Yield: 10 servings

Each with 38 g protein, 3 g carbohydrate, trace dietary fiber, 3 g usable carbs. Analysis does not include Fauxtatoes.

Lone Star Brisket

The Texas BBQ Brisket Sauce on page 472 would be a natural with this.

2 pounds (910 g) beef brisket
1 teaspoon meat tenderizer
½ cup (120 ml) oil
½ cup (120 ml) cider vinegar
1 teaspoon chili powder
2 tablespoons (30 ml) Worcestershire sauce
1 teaspoon Splenda
½ teaspoon pepper
Wood chips or chunks, soaked for at least 30 minutes

Sprinkle one side of the brisket with ½ teaspoon of the tenderizer and pierce the meat all over with a fork. Turn it over and repeat. Put the brisket in a shallow, nonreactive pan.

Mix together the remaining ingredients. Reserve some marinade for basting, pour the rest over the brisket, and turn it once or twice to coat. Let the brisket marinate for several hours at least, and overnight is great.

At least 3 hours before dinner, set up your grill for indirect cooking (put the coals on one side of the grill or leave half the burners off on a gas grill). Add wood chips or chunks. Smoke the brisket for about 3 hours or until tender. Mop the brisket with the reserved marinade every half hour or so, using a clean utensil each time you baste.

Yield: 5 to 6 servings

Assuming 6, each would have 3 grams of carbohydrate if you consumed all the marinade—which you won't. Figure that you'll get no more than 1 gram of carb per serving, not including any finishing sauce you might add; 26 grams of protein.

Bodacious Brined and Barbecued Beef Brisket

Stand back when you say that! Most Americans have tried one form of brined brisket—corned beef. Well, this may be a brined brisket, but it ain't much like corned beef—it's hot and spicy and so yummy that adding sauce would be a sin. Eat it as is!

2 pounds (910 g) beef brisket

2 teaspoons meat tenderizer

2 tablespoons (40 g) kosher salt

1 quart (960 ml) water

1 tablespoon (7.8 g) chili powder

2 tablespoons (3 g) Splenda

2 cloves garlic

1 tablespoon (16.5 g) tomato paste

Bodacious Beef Brisket Rub (page 488)

Bodacious Beef Brisket Beer Mop (page 489)

Wood chips or chunks, soaked for at least
    30 minutes

Put the brisket on a plate, sprinkle one side with 1 teaspoon of the meat tenderizer, and pierce it all over with a fork. Flip it over and do the same to the other side with the remaining teaspoon of tenderizer. Let that sit a minute.

In a flat, shallow, nonreactive container just big enough to hold the brisket, dissolve the salt in the water (using warm water helps). Stir in the chili powder, Splenda, garlic, and tomato paste. Submerge the brisket in the brine—add just a little more water if the brisket isn't totally submerged. Let the brisket brine for 3 to 5 hours.

When brining time is up, pull out the brisket and sprinkle it liberally all over with the Bodacious Beef Brisket Rub. Set up your grill for indirect cooking (put the coals on one side of the grill or leave half the burners off on a gas grill). Add wood chips or chunks and smoke the brisket for a good 3 to 4 hours. Mop with the Bodacious Beef Brisket Beer Mop every half hour to 45 minutes, using a clean utensil each time you baste. When smoking time's up, slice the brisket thin across the grain and serve.

Yield: Figure 6 servings

This was one of the hardest recipes to estimate the correct carb count for. The analysis comes up saying 19 grams of carbohydrate per serving, with 3 grams of fiber, but the vast majority of that is in the brine and the mop. I'm going to say about 6 grams of carb per serving, and I think that's actually high; 28 grams of protein.

Chipotle Brisket

Our tester, who loved this recipe, halved it. You can feel free to do the same.

4 pounds (1.8 kg) beef brisket, cut into pieces
    if necessary to fit into your slow cooker

2 tablespoons (30 ml) olive oil

1 medium onion, thinly sliced

4 stalks celery, thinly sliced

4 cloves garlic, crushed

1 tablespoon (7.2 g) dry mustard

1 tablespoon (5.4 g) dried oregano

1 teaspoon ground cumin

2 teaspoons pepper

1 teaspoon salt or Vege-Sal

1 can (16 ounces, or 455 g) tomato sauce

½ cup (120 ml) beef broth

1 teaspoon beef bouillon concentrate

¼ cup (60 ml) red wine vinegar

½ cup (12 g) Splenda

½ teaspoon blackstrap molasses

2 chipotle chiles canned in adobo sauce

2 bay leaves

Guar or xanthan

(continued on page 404)

In a big, heavy skillet, brown the beef all over in the oil over medium-high heat. Transfer the beef to a slow cooker.

Add the onion and celery to the skillet and sauté until softened. Stir in the garlic, dry mustard, oregano, cumin, pepper, and salt or Vege-Sal and sauté for another minute or two. Transfer the mixture to the slow cooker.

In a blender or food processor, combine the tomato sauce, broth, bouillon, vinegar, Splenda, molasses, and chipotles and blend until smooth.

Put the bay leaves in the slow cooker and pour the sauce over the whole thing. Cover the slow cooker, set it to low, and let it cook for 12 hours.

When the time's up, remove the beef to a platter. Remove the bay leaves and thicken the sauce to taste with guar or xanthan. Serve the sauce over the beef.

Yield: 8 servings

Each with 41 g protein, 8 g carbohydrate, 2 g dietary fiber, 6 g usable carbs.

Good Low-Carb Slow Cooked Short Ribs

This was one of the first recipes I adapted from Peg Bracken's *I Hate To Cook Book*, aka the World's Funniest Cookbook (and also one of the most useful). It was higher carb and wasn't originally a slow cooker recipe, but it adapted well to both!

3 to 4 pounds (1.4 to 1.8 kg) beef short ribs, frozen or thawed
1 can (8 ounces, or 225 g) tomato sauce
¾ cup (180 ml) water
2 tablespoons (30 ml) wine or cider vinegar
¼ cup (60 ml) soy sauce
2 teaspoons Splenda
1 large onion, sliced
Guar or xanthan (optional)

In a bowl, mix together the tomato sauce, water, vinegar, soy sauce, and Splenda.

Put the ribs in the slow cooker. Place the onion on top of the ribs. Pour the sauce over the onion and ribs. Cover the slow cooker, set it to low, and let it cook for 8 to 9 hours. (If you put the ribs in thawed, cut about 1 hour off the cooking time.)

When the time's up, thicken the sauce with guar or xanthan if you prefer. (This recipe gives you tremendously tasty ribs in a thin but flavorful sauce—it's more like a broth. You can thicken it a bit with guar or xanthan, but I rather like it as it is.)

Yield: 7 servings

Each with 61 g protein, 5 g carbohydrate, 1 g dietary fiber, 4 g usable carbs. (This analysis is for 3 pounds [1.4 kg] of ribs. The total carbs will vary with how much of the sauce you eat, because most of the carbs are in there.)

Asian Slow Cooker Short Ribs

Look for black bean sauce in Asian markets or in the international aisle of a big grocery store. You'll only use a little at a time, but it keeps a long time in the fridge and adds authenticity to Asian dishes.

6 pounds (2.7 kg) beef short ribs
3 tablespoons (45 ml) oil
1 stalk celery, chopped
¼ cup (30 g) shredded carrot
½ cup (80 g) chopped onion
2 tablespoons (12 g) grated ginger
6 teaspoons Chinese black bean sauce
3 teaspoons chili garlic paste
3 cloves garlic, crushed
¼ cup (60 ml) soy sauce
1 cup (240 ml) dry red wine
2 cups (480 ml) beef broth
1 teaspoon five-spice powder
1 tablespoon (1.5 g) Splenda
Guar or xanthan

In a big, heavy skillet, brown the ribs all over in the oil. Transfer the ribs to a slow cooker.

Add the celery, carrot, and onion to the skillet and sauté over medium-high heat until they soften and start to brown. Stir in the ginger, black bean sauce, chili garlic paste, and garlic and sauté for another couple of minutes. Now stir in the soy sauce, wine, broth, five-spice powder, and Splenda. Pour the mixture over the ribs. Cover the slow cooker, set it to low, and let it cook for 6 to 7 hours.

When the time's up, transfer the ribs to a platter and scoop the vegetables into a blender with a slotted spoon. Add 2 cups (480 ml) of the liquid and run the blender until the vegetables are puréed. Thicken the sauce to heavy cream consistency with guar or xanthan and serve the sauce with the ribs.

Yield: 12 servings

Each with 35 g protein, 3 g carbohydrate, trace dietary fiber, 3 g usable carbs.

Short Ribs with Wine and Mushrooms

Short ribs are very flavorful, and this is a simple way to make the most of them.

4 pounds (1.8 kg) beef short ribs
2 bay leaves
1 tablespoon (15 ml) Worcestershire sauce
1 tablespoon (15 ml) beef bouillon concentrate
½ cup (120 ml) dry red wine
1 can (8 ounces, or 225 g) mushrooms, drained
Guar or xanthan

Place the ribs in a slow cooker. Add the bay leaves, Worcestershire sauce, and bouillon. Pour the wine over everything. Place the mushrooms on top. Cover the slow cooker, set it to low, and let it cook for 8 to 10 hours.

(continued on page 406)

When the time's up, use a slotted spoon to scoop out the ribs and mushrooms and put them on a platter. There may be a fair amount of grease on the liquid in the pot; it's best to skim it off. Remove the bay leaves and thicken the sauce to taste with guar or xanthan.

Yield: 10 servings

Each with 42 g protein, 1 g carbohydrate, trace dietary fiber, 1 g usable carbs.

Fauxtatoes (page 209) are the ideal side with this, so you'll have something to eat all that gravy on!

Rosemary-Ginger Ribs with Apricot Glaze

Blue Slaw (page 241) or any coleslaw is good with these. Also, feel free to use a full-size slab of ribs—about 6 pounds (2.7 kg) worth—and double the seasonings if you're feeding a family.

1 slab baby back ribs, about 2½ pounds (1.1 kg)

Purchased Rosemary-Ginger Rub (such as Stubb's)

2 tablespoons (40 g) low-sugar apricot preserves

1½ teaspoons spicy brown mustard

1 teaspoon Splenda

1½ teaspoons soy sauce

Sprinkle both sides of the slab of ribs generously with the Rosemary-Ginger Rub. Curl the slab of ribs around and fit it down into your slow cooker. Cover and set the slow cooker on low. Forget about it for 9 to 10 hours. (No, I didn't forget anything. You don't put any liquid in the slow cooker. Don't sweat it.)

When the time's up, preheat the broiler. Mix together the preserves, mustard, Splenda, and soy sauce. Carefully remove the ribs from the slow cooker—they may fall apart on you a bit because they're so tender. Arrange them meaty-side-up on a broiler rack. Spread the apricot glaze evenly over the ribs. Place them under a broiler set on high at least 3 to 4 inches (7.5 to 10 cm) from the heat for 7 to 8 minutes. Serve.

Yield: 2 or 3 servings

Assuming 3 servings, each will have 5 grams of carbohydrates, a trace of fiber, and 38 grams of protein.

Roman Stew

Instead of using the usual Italian seasonings, this was adapted from a historic Roman stew recipe using spices from the Far East. It's unusual and wonderful.

3 pounds (1.4 kg) beef stew meat, cut into 1-inch (2.5 cm) cubes

3 tablespoons (45 ml) olive oil

4 cloves garlic

2 cups (240 g) sliced celery

1 teaspoon salt or Vege-Sal

¼ teaspoon ground cinnamon
¼ teaspoon ground cloves
¼ teaspoon pepper
⅛ teaspoon ground allspice
⅛ teaspoon ground nutmeg
1 can (14½ ounces, or 410 g) diced tomatoes, undrained
½ cup (120 ml) dry red wine
Guar or xanthan (optional)

In a big, heavy skillet, brown the beef in the oil over medium-high heat in a few batches. Transfer the beef to a slow cooker. Add the garlic and celery to the slow cooker and then sprinkle the salt or Vege-Sal, cinnamon, cloves, pepper, allspice, and nutmeg over the beef and vegetables. Pour the tomatoes and the wine over the beef and vegetables. Cover the slow cooker, set it to low, and let it cook for 7 to 8 hours.

You can thicken the pot juices a little if you like with guar or xanthan, but it's not really necessary.

Yield: 8 servings

Each with 44 g protein, 5 g carbohydrate, 1 g dietary fiber, 4 g usable carbs.

Mexican Stew

This Tex-Mex dinner is a simple family-pleaser.

2 pounds (910 g) beef stew meat, cut into 1-inch (2.5-cm) cubes
1 can (14½ ounces, or 410 g) tomatoes with green chiles
½ cup (80 g) sliced onion
1 teaspoon chili powder
1 envelope (1¼ ounces, or 35 g) taco seasoning mix
1 can (15 ounces, or 425 g) black soybeans
½ cup (65 g) sour cream

Put the beef, tomatoes, onion, and chili powder in a slow cooker. Cover the slow cooker, set it to low, and let it cook for 8 to 9 hours.

Stir in the taco seasoning and soybeans. Re-cover the slow cooker, turn it to high, and let it cook for another 20 minutes. Place a dollop of sour cream on each serving.

Yield: 6 generous servings, and it could even serve 8

Each with 46 g protein, 12 g carbohydrate, 5 g dietary fiber, 7 g usable carbs.

Carne all'Ungherese

The original recipe from which I adapted this said it was an Italian version of a Hungarian stew. Whatever it is, it's good!

1½ pounds (680 g) beef stew meat, cut into 1-inch (2.5-cm) cubes
¼ cup (60 ml) olive oil
1 medium onion, chopped
1 green pepper, cut into strips
2 cloves garlic, crushed
1 cup (240 ml) beef broth

(continued on page 408)

1 teaspoon beef bouillon concentrate

1 teaspoon dried marjoram

1 tablespoon (16.5 g) tomato paste

1 tablespoon (6.9 g) paprika

1 tablespoon (30 ml) lemon juice

½ cup (65 g) plain yogurt

In a big, heavy skillet, heat a tablespoon or two (15 to 30 ml) of the oil over medium-high heat. Start browning the stew meat. It will take two or three batches; add more oil as you need it. Transfer each batch of browned meat to a slow cooker as it's done.

When all the meat is browned, put the last of the oil in the skillet, reduce the heat to medium-low, and add the onion. Sauté the onion until it's just softening and add it to the slow cooker. Add the green pepper to the slow cooker.

In a bowl, mix together the garlic, broth, bouillon, marjoram, tomato paste, paprika, and lemon juice, stirring until the bouillon and tomato paste are dissolved. Pour the mixture over the meat and onions. Cover the slow cooker, set it to low, and let it cook for 6 to 7 hours. When the time's up, stir in the yogurt. Serve over Fauxtatoes (page 209).

Yield: 5 servings

Each with 38 g protein, 7 g carbohydrate, 1 g dietary fiber, 6 g usable carbs. (Analysis does not include Fauxtatoes.)

Beef and Zucchini Stew

Don't try adding the zucchini at the beginning, or they'll cook to a mush! Put out some vegetables and dip for the ravening hoards and sip a glass of wine while you're waiting that last hour.

2 pounds (910 g) boneless beef chuck, trimmed of fat and cubed

1 medium onion, sliced

1 large red bell pepper, cut into 1-inch (2.5-cm) squares

1 large green bell pepper, cut into 1-inch (2.5-cm) squares

1 cup (240 ml) no-sugar-added spaghetti sauce (I suggest Hunt's.)

½ cup (120 ml) beef broth

½ teaspoon beef bouillon concentrate

1½ pounds (680 g) zucchini, cut into ½-inch (1.3-cm) slices

Guar or xanthan (optional)

In a slow cooker, combine the beef with the onion and peppers.

In a bowl, stir together the spaghetti sauce, broth, and bouillon. Pour the mixture over the beef and vegetables and stir. Cover the slow cooker, set it to low, and let it cook for 9 hours.

Turn the slow cooker to high, stir in the zucchini, re-cover, and let it cook for 1 more hour. When the time's up, thicken the sauce with guar or xanthan, if needed.

Yield: 6 servings

Each with 27 g protein, 10 g carbohydrate, 3 g dietary fiber, 7 g usable carbs.

Oxtails Pontchartrain

This has a lot of New Orleans elements, including some serious heat, so I named it after Lake Pontchartrain. Oxtails are bony but very flavorful, and they take very well to the slow cooker. If you haven't had oxtails, don't fear them; they're just muscle meat, like a steak or a roast. It's just that there's a high bone-to-meat ratio.

4 pounds (1.8 kg) beef oxtails

3 tablespoons (18 g) Cajun seasoning

2 tablespoons (30 ml) olive oil

3 large banana peppers, sliced

1 medium onion, sliced

1 medium carrot, shredded

2 stalks celery, sliced

1 clove garlic, crushed

1 cup (240 ml) dry red wine

¼ cup (60 ml) brandy

1½ teaspoons dried thyme

3 bay leaves

1 can (14½ ounces, or 410 g) diced tomatoes

2 chipotle chiles canned in adobo sauce, chopped (You can use just one if you'd like to cut the heat a bit.)

Sprinkle the oxtails all over with the Cajun seasoning.

In a big, heavy skillet, heat the oil and brown the oxtails all over. Transfer the oxtails to a slow cooker.

Add the peppers, onion, carrot, celery, and garlic to the skillet and sauté them until they're just softened. Add them to the slow cooker and mix them in with the oxtails.

Pour the wine and brandy in the skillet and stir it around. Stir in the thyme and add the bay leaves, tomatoes, and chipotles. Stir this all up and pour it over the oxtails and veggies. Cover the slow cooker, set it to low, and let it cook for 8 hours. Remove the bay leaves before serving.

Yield: 6 servings

Each with 96 g protein, 13 g carbohydrate, 3 g dietary fiber, 10 g usable carbs.

12

Pork and Lamb

Pork Chops with Mustard Cream Sauce

Here's something good to do with pork chops, now that you're not breading them.

1 pork chop, 1 inch (2.5 cm) thick
Salt or Vege-Sal
Pepper
1 tablespoon (15 ml) olive oil
1 tablespoon (15 ml) dry white wine
1 tablespoon (15 ml) heavy cream
1 tablespoon (15 ml) spicy brown mustard
  or Dijon mustard

Sprinkle salt and pepper on both sides of the chop.

Heat the oil in a heavy skillet over medium heat. Sauté the chop until it's browned on both sides and cooked through. Put the chop on a serving platter and keep it warm.

Put the wine in the skillet and stir it around, scraping all the tasty brown bits off the pan as you stir. Stir in the cream and mustard, blend well, and cook for a minute or two. Pour over the chop and serve.

Yield: 1 serving

2 grams of carbohydrates, a trace of fiber, and about 20 grams of protein.

Simple Spicy Pork Chops

1½ pounds (680 g) pork chops, about 1 inch (2.5 cm) thick
3 tablespoons (45 ml) olive oil
1 clove garlic
1 tablespoon (7.8 g) chili powder
1 teaspoon ground coriander

Start a charcoal fire or preheat a gas grill.

Measure out the olive oil; crush the garlic and stir it into the oil. Rub the chops thoroughly with the garlicky olive oil. Stir the chili powder and coriander together and sprinkle over both sides of the chops. Grill over well-ashed coals or on a gas grill set to medium-low for about 10 minutes per side or until an instant-read thermometer registers 170°F (80°C).

Yield: 3 to 4 servings

Assuming 3 servings, each will have 2 grams of carbohydrate and 1 gram of fiber, for a usable carb count of 1 gram; 35 grams protein.

Italian Herb Pork Chops

1 pork chop, 1 inch (2.5 cm) thick
1 clove garlic, crushed
½ teaspoon dried, powdered sage
½ teaspoon dried, powdered rosemary
Salt or Vege-Sal
2 tablespoons (30 ml) dry white wine

(continued on page 412)

Rub the crushed garlic into both sides of the pork chop.

In a bowl, mix the sage and rosemary together and sprinkle this evenly over both sides of the pork chop as well. Sprinkle lightly with the salt.

Place the chop in a heavy skillet (if you're multiplying this recipe to feed several people, you may well need two skillets) and add water just up to the top edge of the pork chop. Cover the skillet, turn the heat to low, and let the chop simmer for about 1 hour or until the water has all evaporated.

Once the water is gone, the chop will start to brown. Turn it once or twice to get it browned on both sides. (The pork chop will be very tender, so use a spatula and be careful. If it breaks a little, it will still taste great.)

Remove the pork chop to a serving platter and pour the wine into the skillet. Turn up the heat to medium-high and stir the wine around, scraping up the stuck-on brown bits from the pan. Bring this to a boil and let it boil hard for a minute or two to reduce it just a little. Pour this sauce over the pork chop and serve.

Yield: 1 serving

2 grams of carbohydrates, a trace of fiber, and about 23 grams of protein.

Lemon-Ginger Pork Chops

1 pound (455 g) pork chops, 1 inch (2.5 cm) thick

1 tablespoon (6 g) grated ginger

1 tablespoon (15 ml) olive oil

1 tablespoon (15 ml) soy sauce

1 tablespoon (15 ml) dry sherry

1½ teaspoons lemon juice

1 tablespoon (15 ml) water

½ clove garlic, crushed

¼ teaspoon toasted sesame oil

¼ teaspoon Splenda

1 scallion, sliced, including the crisp part of the green shoot

In a large, heavy skillet over medium-high heat, brown the pork chops on both sides in the olive oil. Mix together everything else but the scallion and pour into the skillet. Turn the chops to coat both sides. Cover the pan, turn the heat to low, and let the chops simmer for 30 to 40 minutes. Spoon pan juices over chops and top with a little sliced scallion to serve.

Yield: 3 to 4 servings

Assuming 3, each will have 24 g protein; 1 g carbohydrate; trace dietary fiber; 1 g usable carb.

Pork Chops and Sauerkraut

3 pork chops, 1 inch (2.5 cm) thick

3 slices bacon

1 small onion, chopped

1 can (14½ ounces, or 410 g) sauerkraut, drained

2 tablespoons (3 g) Splenda

¼ teaspoon dry mustard

2 tablespoons (30 ml) dry white wine

¼ teaspoon blackstrap molasses

Fry the bacon until just barely crisp in a heavy skillet over medium heat. Drain and set aside.

Pour off all but about 2 tablespoons (30 ml) of the grease and brown the chops in it over medium heat. (You want them to have just a little color on each side.) Remove from the skillet and set aside.

Put the onion, sauerkraut, Splenda, mustard, wine, and molasses in the skillet and stir for a moment to blend. Crumble in the bacon and stir again, just for a moment. Place the chops on top of the sauerkraut mixture, turn the heat to low, and cover the pan. Simmer for 45 minutes.

Yield: 3 servings

Each with 11 grams of carbohydrates and 4 grams of fiber, for a total of 7 grams of usable carbs and 27 grams of protein.

Cherry Chops

An unusual sauce of tart cherries and a crunch of toasted almonds enhance these pork chops. Don't expect this sauce to be cherry-red, though, unless you add a drop or two of food coloring.

4 thin pork chops, about 18 ounces (500 g) total
Salt and pepper
1 tablespoon (15 ml) olive oil
½ cup (55 g) canned tart cherries in water (pie cherries)
1 tablespoon (15 ml) wine vinegar
¼ teaspoon dry mustard
⅛ teaspoon ground cloves
1½ tablespoons (2 g) Splenda
⅛ teaspoon guar or xanthan
⅓ cup (40 g) slivered almonds
½ tablespoon butter

Sprinkle salt and pepper over the chops lightly on both sides and start browning them in the oil in a heavy skillet over medium-high heat. Give them about 5 minutes per side. While that's happening, put the cherries, vinegar, mustard, cloves, Splenda, and guar or xanthan in a blender and purée the whole thing together. (If you'd prefer to keep the cherries whole, you could just mix everything together well. I like it puréed.)

It's time to turn the chops now! While the chops are browning on their second side, start browning the almonds in the butter in a small skillet over medium heat. Stir frequently so they don't burn; you just want a touch of gold. When the almonds are toasted, remove the pan from the heat.

When the second side of the chops is browned—again, after about 5 minutes—pour the cherry sauce over them, turn the heat to medium-low, and cover the skillet with a tilted lid. Let the whole thing simmer for 5 minutes and serve. Scrape the sauce from the skillet over the chops and top each with toasted almonds.

Yield: 4 servings

Each with 6 grams of carbohydrates and 1 gram of fiber, for a total of 5 grams of usable carbs and 22 grams of protein.

Apple-Glazed Pork Chops

Pork and apples are a great combination. Ever since I stopped eating applesauce, I've been looking for a way to have this combination of flavors again!

(continued on page 414)

2 pork chops, 1 inch (2.5 cm) thick (about 8 ounces, or 225 g each)

2 tablespoons (30 ml) olive oil

¼ cup (60 ml) cider vinegar

1½ tablespoons (2 g) Splenda

½ teaspoon soy sauce

1 small onion, thinly sliced

Put the oil in a heavy skillet and brown the pork chops in the oil.

When both sides are brown, stir together the vinegar, Splenda, and the soy sauce and pour the mixture over the chops. Scatter the onion on top.

Cover and turn the heat to low. Let the chops simmer, turning at least once, for 45 minutes or until the pan is almost dry. Serve the chops with the onions and scrape all the nice, syrupy pan liquid over them.

Yield: 2 servings

Each with 8 grams of carbohydrates and 1 gram of fiber, for a total of 7 grams of usable carbs and 36 grams of protein.

Peach-Orange Brined Pork Chops with Herb Rub

4 pork chops, totaling about 1½ pounds (680 g)

1 bottle (16 ounces, or 480 ml) peach-flavored Fruit$_2$O

1 tablespoon (18 g) salt

¼ teaspoon blackstrap molasses

¼ teaspoon orange extract

1 clove garlic

1 tablespoon (15 ml) olive oil

1 teaspoon ground rosemary

½ teaspoon ground or rubbed sage

½ teaspoon dried marjoram

⅛ teaspoon cayenne

In a flat, shallow dish—a large glass casserole dish is perfect—combine the Fruit$_2$O, salt, molasses, and orange extract. Stir until the salt is dissolved. (Heating helps with this—you can open the bottle of Fruit$_2$O and microwave it in a separate bowl for a minute before pouring it in the dish or you can microwave the whole batch of brine, if your dish is microwavable. Neither is essential, it just helps the salt dissolve.) Place the chops in the brine (make sure it's cooled to lukewarm first), make sure they're submerged, and stick the whole thing in the fridge. Let them sit for about 3 hours.

Okay, time to grill your pork. First start your grill heating—set a gas grill to medium-high; with a charcoal grill you'll want to let your coals cook down to a medium heat. Crush the garlic and mix it with the olive oil in a small dish. In another dish combine the rosemary, sage, marjoram, and cayenne. Then pull the chops out of the brine and put them on a plate; discard the brine. Pat the chops dry. Rub them all over with the garlic and olive oil mixture, then the herb mixture.

Grill chops about 12 minutes per side or until there's no pink left in the center and then serve.

Yield: 4 servings

Each serving will have 1 gram of carbohydrate, a trace of fiber, 26 grams of protein.

Pork Chops with Garlic and Balsamic Vinegar

The balsamic vinegar gives these a tangy-sweet flavor.

2 or 3 pork rib chops, 2 inches (5 cm) thick
2 tablespoons (30 ml) olive oil
¾ cup (180 ml) chicken broth
3 tablespoons (45 ml) balsamic vinegar
3 cloves garlic, crushed
¼ teaspoon guar or xanthan

Put the oil in a large, heavy skillet over medium-high heat and sear the chops in the oil until well-browned on both sides. Add the broth, vinegar, and garlic.

Cover the skillet, turn the heat to low, and let the chops simmer for 1 hour. Remove the chops to a serving platter or serving plates and put the liquid from the pan into a blender. Add the guar or xanthan, run the blender for a few moments, and pour the thickened sauce over the chops.

Yield: 2 or 3 servings

Each with 2 grams of carbohydrates, a trace of fiber, and 36 grams of protein.

Gingersnap Pork

Okay, it doesn't really have gingersnaps in it, but it is sweet and spicy and good!

4 thin pork chops, about 18 ounces (500 g) total
1 tablespoon (15 ml) olive oil
½ cup (120 ml) cider vinegar
½ teaspoon pepper
¼ teaspoon ground cloves
1 tablespoon (16.5 g) tomato paste
3 tablespoons (4.5 g) Splenda
2 teaspoons grated ginger
2 teaspoons lemon juice
½ teaspoon salt or Vege-Sal
¼ cup (30 g) finely diced celery, including leaves

In a heavy skillet over medium-high heat, start browning the chops in the oil. While that's happening, put the vinegar, pepper, cloves, tomato paste, Splenda, ginger, lemon juice, and salt in a blender and run it for a second or two to blend.

When the chops are browned on both sides—about 5 minutes per side—pour the sauce over them, scatter the celery over the whole thing, turn the heat to low, and cover with a tilted lid. Let it simmer for 5 minutes and then serve. Don't forget to scrape the extra sauce out of the pan and over the chops!

Yield: 4 servings

Each with 5 grams of carbohydrates, a trace of fiber, and 20 grams of protein.

Polynesian Pork

4 or 5 large pork chops, 1 to 1½ inches (2.5 to 4 cm) thick
½ cup (120 ml) soy sauce
4 cloves garlic, crushed
⅓ cup (8 g) Splenda
½ teaspoon blackstrap molasses
1½ teaspoons grated fresh ginger

Preheat the oven to 325°F (170°C, or gas mark 3).

Put the pork chops in a large resealable plastic bag.

Combine the soy sauce, garlic, Splenda, molasses, and ginger, mixing them in a blender for a second or two if possible.

Reserve some marinade for basting, and pour the rest into the bag with the pork. Seal the bag and let it sit for 20 minutes or so, turning once.

Remove the pork from the marinade. Place the chops in a shallow roasting pan and bake for 60 to 90 minutes or until cooked through. Brush once or twice with the reserved marinade, using a clean utensil each time.

Yield: 4 or 5 servings

If you were to eat all the marinade, each serving would have 7 grams of carbohydrates, but you don't, so figure 2 or 3 grams of carbohydrates, a trace of fiber, and 25 grams of protein.

This marinade works well with a pork roast, too, but of course it will take longer to roast.

Island Pork Steaks

This dish uses caribbean-style seasonings!

1½ (680 g) pounds pork shoulder steaks
1 teaspoon ground allspice
¼ teaspoon ground nutmeg
½ teaspoon dried thyme
⅛ teaspoon cayenne
2 tablespoons (30 ml) olive oil
¼ cup (40 g) chopped onion
¼ cup (60 ml) lime juice
¼ cup (60 ml) chicken broth
1 teaspoon Splenda
3 cloves garlic, minced

Put the pork steaks on a big plate. Mix together the allspice, nutmeg, thyme, and cayenne, and sprinkle the mixture over both sides of the pork. Let the steak sit for 30 to 45 minutes.

Heat the olive oil in a big, heavy skillet over medium heat and throw in the pork steaks. Give them 6 or 7 minutes per side—you want them golden on the outside and just cooked through on the inside. Remove to a plate and cover with a spare pot lid to keep warm.

Throw the onion in the skillet and sauté it until it's just translucent. Add the lime juice, chicken broth, Splenda, and garlic. Turn up the heat and boil the sauce hard until it's reduced by about half. Pour over pork and serve.

Yield: 2 to 3 servings

Assuming 3, each will have 30 g protein; 5 g carbohydrate; 1 g dietary fiber; 4 g usable carbs.

Lemon-Garlic-Jalapeno Pork Steaks

1½ pounds (680 g) pork shoulder steaks
1 whole jalapeno, minced
¼ cup (60 ml) olive oil
2 tablespoons (30 ml) lemon juice
2 cloves garlic, crushed
¼ teaspoon cumin
1 teaspoon adobo seasoning (Look for this in the spice aisle.)

Simply stir together everything but the pork. Put the pork on a plate with a rim—a glass pie plate is ideal. Reserve some marinade for basting and pour the rest over it. Turn the steaks over once or twice to coat and let the steaks sit for at least 30 minutes before grilling.

Grill over a medium charcoal or gas fire, holding down flare-ups with a squirt bottle, for 8 to 10 minutes per side. Baste once or twice during cooking with the reserved marinade, using a clean utensil each time.

Yield: 3 servings

Each serving will have 2 grams carbohydrate, a trace of fiber, and 30 grams of protein.

Apple-Mustard Pork Steaks

I've always loved apples and pork together, and the mustard just makes the whole thing better!

1 pound (455 g) pork shoulder steaks
¼ cup (60 ml) cider vinegar
2 tablespoons (3 g) Splenda
1 clove garlic
2 teaspoons soy sauce
½ teaspoon grated ginger
2 teaspoons spicy brown mustard

Place the pork steaks on a plate with a rim. Mix together everything else, reserving some marinade for basting, and pour the rest over the steaks. Turn the steaks once or twice to coat and let them sit for 30 minutes or so. Meanwhile, get a grill going.

Okay, fire's ready! Grill over a medium gas grill or well-ashed coals for about 8 to 10 minutes per side, basting several times with the reserved marinade and using a clean utensil each time. If you like, you can boil any leftover reserved marinade and pour it over the steaks before serving.

Yield: 2 servings

Each serving will have 5 grams of carbohydrate, a trace of fiber, 30 grams of protein.

Pork-Crusted Pork!

8-ounce (225 g) pork shoulder steak, ½ inch (1.3 cm) thick

⅓ cup (25 g) crushed barbecue-flavor pork rinds

1 to 2 tablespoons (15 to 30 ml) oil

Coat both sides of the pork steak with the crushed pork rinds. (It's easiest to spread the crushed pork rinds on a plate and press each side of the pork steak into them.) Heat the oil in a heavy skillet over medium-high heat and sauté the steak until it's crisp on both sides and cooked through—about 7 minutes per side.

Yield: 1 or 2 servings

There are no carbohydrates or fiber here at all, and the whole steak will have about 45 grams of protein.

Sweet and Sour Pork

This is not exactly authentic, because the pork isn't battered and fried. Still, it tastes great! And it's far lower-carb than Sweet and Sour from a Chinese restaurant. If it feels strange to you not to serve this stir-fry over something, there's no reason not to make some cauliflower "rice" to serve with it.

12 ounces (340 g) boneless pork loin, cut into thin strips

3 tablespoons (45 ml) rice or cider vinegar

1½ tablespoons (2 g) Splenda

3 tablespoons (35 g) canned, crushed pineapple in juice

1 teaspoon soy sauce

¼ teaspoon blackstrap molasses

½ teaspoon minced garlic

3 tablespoons (45 ml) oil

½ medium green pepper, cut into squares

½ medium onion, sliced

Guar or xanthan

Mix together the vinegar, Splenda, pineapple, soy sauce, molasses, and garlic and set it by the stove.

Heat the oil in a wok or large skillet over highest heat. Add the pork and stir-fry until it's half-done. Add the peppers and onions and keep stir-frying. When all the pink is gone from the pork, add the vinegar mixture and stir. Let the whole thing simmer for a couple of minutes, stirring once or twice, until the vegetables are tender-crisp. Thicken the pan juices just a touch with guar or xanthan and serve.

Yield: 2 or 3 servings

Assuming 2 servings, each will have 11 grams of carbohydrates and 1 gram of fiber, for a total of 10 grams of usable carbs and 36 grams of protein.

Each serving also packs 782 mg of potassium!

Mu Shu Pork

I hear from lots of people that they miss Chinese food, so here's a Chinese restaurant favorite, de-carbed. Low-carb tortillas stand in here for mu shu pancakes, and they work fine. If you want to de-carb this even further, just eat it with a fork and forget the tortillas.

8 ounces (225 g) boneless pork loin, sliced across the grain and then cut into matchsticks

3 eggs, beaten

Peanut oil

½ cup (35 g) slivered mushrooms

1 cup (70 g) shredded napa cabbage

3 scallions, sliced

1 cup (50 g) bean sprouts

3 tablespoons (45 ml) soy sauce

2 tablespoons (30 ml) dry sherry

4 low-carb tortillas

Hoisin Sauce (page 464)

First, in a wok or heavy skillet over high heat, scramble the eggs in a few tablespoons of the peanut oil until they're set but still moist. Remove and set aside.

Wipe the wok out if there's much egg clinging to it. Add another ¼ cup (60 ml) or so of peanut oil and heat. Add the pork and stir-fry until it's mostly done. Add the mushrooms, cabbage, scallions, and sprouts, and stir-fry for 3 to 4 minutes. Add the eggs back into the wok and stir them in, breaking them into small pieces. Now add the soy sauce and sherry, and stir.

To serve, take a warmed, low-carb tortilla and smear about 2 teaspoons of Hoisin Sauce on it. Put about a quarter of the stir-fry mixture on the tortilla and wrap it up.

Yield: 2 servings

Each with 11 grams of carbohydrates and 3 grams of fiber, for a total of 8 grams of usable carbs and 27 grams of protein (Analysis does not include low-carb tortillas or hoisin sauce.)

Make sure you have everything cut up and ready to go before you cook, and this recipe will be a breeze.

Chili Lime Pork Strips

This is so good and so versatile! Use the strips for a salad or an omelet or just wrap them up in low-carb tortillas with a little salsa and sour cream.

1 pound (455 g) boneless pork loin

1 to 2 tablespoons (15 to 30 ml) oil

1½ teaspoons chili powder

1 tablespoon (15 ml) lime juice

Slice the pork as thinly as you can into small strips (this is easier if the pork is half-frozen). Heat the oil in a large, heavy skillet over medium-high heat and add the pork. Stir-fry the pork strips until they're nearly done—about 6 to 7 minutes—then stir in the chili powder and lime juice. Continue stirring and cooking for another 3 to 4 minutes. These strips keep well for a few days in a closed container in the fridge.

Yield: 4 servings

Each with 1 gram of carbohydrates, a trace of fiber, and 23 grams of protein.

Ginger Sesame Pork

You can serve this simple stir-fry over Cauliflower Rice (page 212), if you like, but it's nice just as it is.

12 ounces (340 g) boneless pork top loin
2 tablespoons (12 g) grated ginger
4 teaspoons soy sauce
1 teaspoon Splenda
2 teaspoons toasted sesame oil
4 scallions, sliced, including the crisp part of
    the green
2 tablespoons (30 ml) dry sherry
2 cloves garlic, crushed
2 tablespoons (30 ml) peanut oil

Slice the boneless pork loin as thinly as you can—it helps to have it half-frozen.

Mix together everything else in a medium-size bowl. Add the pork, stir to coat, and let it marinate for at least a half an hour.

Over high heat, heat the oil in a heavy skillet or wok. Add the pork with all of the marinade and stir-fry until meat is cooked through, about 4 to 5 minutes. Serve.

Yield: 2 servings

Each with 31g protein; 5 g carbohydrate; 1 g dietary fiber; 4 g usable carbs.

Asian Pork and Cabbage

I know of few dishes that offer so much flavor for so little work.

1 pound (455 g) boneless pork loin
½ head cabbage
1 small onion
Canola or peanut oil for stir-frying
1 tablespoon (15 ml) black bean sauce
1 to 2 tablespoons (16.5 to 33 g) chili
    garlic paste

Slice the pork loin as thin as you possibly can—this is easier if the pork is partially frozen. Slice the cabbage about ½ inch (1.3 cm) thick and cut across it a few times. Thinly slice the onion.

In a wok or large skillet, heat 3 to 4 table-spoons (45 to 60 ml) of oil over highest heat. As soon as it's hot, add the pork and stir-fry for 3 to 5 minutes. Add the cabbage and the onion and continue stir-frying until the cabbage and onion are just tender-crisp. Stir in the black bean sauce and the chili garlic paste and serve.

Yield: 3 servings

Each with 6 grams of carbohydrates and 1 gram of fiber, for a total of 5 grams of usable carbs and 32 grams of protein.

You can find black bean sauce, an Asian condiment, in Asian or international grocery stores or in the Asian section of larger grocery stores. I actually bought mine in the international aisle of Bloomingfoods, my beloved natural food store.

This has some sugar in it, but the amount of flavor it offers for the few carbs it adds is well worth it, to my mind. It keeps well in the fridge, so don't think you have to use it all up quickly.

Artichoke-Mushroom Pork

This is wonderful, and it cooks quite quickly because you pound the pork thin.

1½ pounds (680 g) boneless pork loin, cut into 4 slices across the grain

4 tablespoons (56 g) butter, divided

1 small onion, sliced

1 clove garlic, crushed

8 ounces (35 g) sliced mushrooms

1 can (14 ounces, or 400 g) quartered artichoke hearts, drained

½ cup (120 ml) chicken broth

2 teaspoons Dijon or spicy brown mustard

Put a piece of pork into a heavy resealable plastic bag and pound until it is ¼ inch (6 mm) thick. Repeat for the remaining pieces of pork.

Melt 2 tablespoons (28 g) of the butter in a large, heavy skillet over medium heat and brown the meat on both sides (about 4 minutes per side). You'll have to do them one or two at a time. Set the browned pork on a plate and keep it warm.

Add the rest of the butter to the skillet and add the onion, garlic, and mushrooms. Sauté until the mushrooms and onion are limp. Add the artichokes, chicken broth, and mustard and stir around to dissolve the tasty brown bits on the bottom of the skillet.

Add the pork back into the skillet (you'll have to stack it a bit), cover, and let simmer for about 5 minutes. Serve the pork with the vegetables spooned over the top.

Yield: 4 servings

Each with 6 grams of carbohydrates and 2 grams of fiber, for a total of 4 grams of usable carbs and 25 grams of protein.

If you prefer, you can make this out of 4 pork chops with the bones cut out.

Pork and Provolone with White Wine and Mushrooms

I confess, I came up with this to get rid of extra pork, smoked provolone, and mushrooms I had kicking around my fridge—and it got top marks from my husband! It is definitely worth making again.

2 pounds (910 g) boneless pork loin, in 4 slices about ¾ inch (2 cm) thick

6 ounces (170 g) sliced smoked provolone cheese

1 tablespoon (15 ml) olive oil

1 tablespoon (14 g) butter

½ medium onion, chopped

4 cloves garlic, crushed

2 cups (140 g) sliced mushrooms

1 cup (240 ml) dry white wine

(continued on page 422)

1 teaspoon chicken bouillon concentrate
Guar or xanthan (optional)

You'll need four pieces of pork loin that are roughly the same shape. One piece at a time, put the pork in a heavy resealable plastic bag. Using any heavy blunt instrument that comes to hand (I use a 3-pound dumbbell), pound your pork out until it's between ¼ inch (6 mm) and ½ inch (1.3 cm) thick.

Sandwich the sliced smoked provolone between the pounded pieces of pork, using 3 ounces (85 g) in each of two "pork and cheese sandwiches." Heat the oil and butter in a big, heavy skillet over medium-high heat and lay the pork-and-cheese sandwiches in it. Sauté for about 5 minutes per side or until golden, turning carefully.

When the pork-and-cheese sandwiches are browned on both sides, add the onion, garlic, and mushrooms to the skillet, scattering them around the pork.

Mix the wine and chicken bouillon concentrate together and pour around the pork. Cover, turn heat to low, and simmer for 20 minutes.

When time's up, lift the pork-and-cheese sandwiches out with a spatula, put them on a platter, and cover with a lid to keep warm. Now turn up the heat under the skillet and let the sauce boil hard for about 5 minutes—you want just ½ cup (120 ml) or so of liquid left among the mushrooms and onions. Thicken this a trifle with guar or xanthan if you like, but it's not essential by any means. Scrape the mushrooms, onions, and sauce over the meat and cheese and cut in portions to serve.

Yield: 6 servings

Each with 39 g protein; 4 g carbohydrate; trace dietary fiber; 4 g usable carbs.

Pineapple Glazed Pork Loin

You can double this recipe if you like, but if your skillet's the size of mine, you'll have to cook it in two batches—which, of course, takes twice the time.

¾ **pound (340 g) boneless pork loin, cut about ½ inch (1.3 cm) thick**
1 to 2 tablespoons (15 to 30 ml) olive oil
2 tablespoons (25 g) canned, crushed pineapple in juice
2 teaspoons cider vinegar
2 teaspoons Splenda
1 teaspoon spicy brown or Dijon mustard
½ **teaspoon soy sauce**
1 teaspoon minced garlic or 2 cloves garlic, crushed

First, pound the pork until it's about ¼ inch (6 mm) thick. Heat the oil in a heavy skillet over medium-high heat and sauté the pork, covering it with a tilted lid. Cook it 4 to 5 minutes per side.

While the pork's browning, combine the pineapple, vinegar, Splenda, mustard, soy sauce, and garlic. When the pork is browned on both sides, add this mixture to the skillet. Turn the pork over once or twice to coat. Put the tilted lid back on the pan and cook for 1 to 2 minutes, turn, re-cover the pan, and give it another 1 to 2 minutes. Remove to serving plates and scrape any remaining liquid from the pan over the pork before serving.

Yield: 2 servings

Each with 4 grams of carbohydrates, a trace of fiber, and 22 grams of protein.

Feel free to use thin pork chops, instead.

Orange Pork Loin

Boneless pork loin frequently goes on sale. It's very lean, however, so it's often both bland and dry. Slow cooking takes care of that little problem! Sadly, fresh pumpkin is only available for a couple of months in the autumn, so that's when you'll need to make this dish. Buy a small pumpkin, or you'll have piles of it leftover.

2 pounds (910 g) pork loin
**1 pound (455 g) pumpkin, peeled and cut into
    ½-inch (1.3 cm) cubes**
**1 pound (455 g) rutabaga, cut into ½-inch
    (1.3 cm) cubes**
2 tablespoons (30 ml) olive oil
**2 tablespoons (40 g) low-sugar marmalade or
    orange preserves**
¼ teaspoon orange extract
2 teaspoons Splenda
2 cloves garlic, crushed
½ teaspoon salt
½ cup (120 ml) chicken broth
Guar or xanthan

Put the pumpkin and rutabaga in the bottom of a slow cooker.

In a big, heavy skillet, heat the oil over medium-high heat and brown the pork all over. Put the pork in the slow cooker on top of the pumpkin and rutabaga.

In a bowl, stir together the marmalade, orange extract, Splenda, garlic, salt, and broth. Pour the mixture over the pork. Cover the slow cooker, set it to low, and let it cook for 8 hours.

When the time's up, carefully remove the pork to a platter and use a slotted spoon to pile the vegetables around it. Use guar or xanthan to thicken the liquid in the pot to the consistency of heavy cream. Serve the liquid with the pork and vegetables.

Yield: 6 servings

Each with 34 g protein, 13 g carbohydrate, 2 g dietary fiber, 11 g usable carbs.

Braised Pork with Fennel

This was one of my first great slow-cooking triumphs, and it still ranks as one of the two or three best dishes I've ever cooked in my slow cooker. This is easily good enough to serve to company. By the way, some grocery stores label "fennel" as "anise." It looks like a bulb at the bottom, with celery-like stalks above and feathery foliage. The stems are tough, but the foliage can be chopped up in salads or used as a garnish. It has a wonderful licorice-like taste.

4 pounds (1.8 kg) pork shoulder roast
2 tablespoons (30 ml) olive oil
1 medium onion, sliced
1 bulb fennel, sliced
1 cup (240 ml) cider vinegar

(continued on page 424)

3 tablespoons (4.5 g) Splenda

1 cup (240 ml) canned diced tomatoes, drained

1 cup (235 ml) chicken broth

1 teaspoon chicken bouillon concentrate

2 cloves garlic, crushed

½ teaspoon dried thyme

½ teaspoon red pepper flakes, or to taste

Guar or xanthan

In a big, heavy skillet, sear the pork in the oil over medium-high heat until it's brown all over. (This will take 20 minutes or so.) Transfer the pork to a slow cooker.

Pour off all but about 1 tablespoon (15 ml) of fat from the skillet and reduce the heat to medium-low. Sauté the onion and fennel until they're just getting a little golden. Transfer them to the slow cooker, too.

In a bowl, mix together the vinegar and Splenda. Pour the mixture over the pork. Add the tomatoes.

In a bowl, mix together the broth and bouillon until the bouillon dissolves. Stir in the garlic, thyme, and red pepper. Pour this over the pork. Cover the slow cooker, set it to low, and let it cook for 8 hours.

When the time's up, remove the pork from the slow cooker and place it on a serving platter. Using a slotted spoon, scoop out the vegetables and pile them around the pork. Cover the platter with foil and put it in a warm place.

Ladle the liquid from the slow cooker into a saucepan. Place it over the highest heat and boil it hard for 5 to 7 minutes to reduce the sauce a bit. Add some guar or xanthan to thicken the sauce a little. (You want it to be about the texture of half-and-half, not a thick gravy.) Serve the sauce over the pork and vegetables.

Yield: 6 servings

Each with 41 g protein, 10 g carbohydrate, 2 g dietary fiber, 8 g usable carbs.

Easy Pork Roast

This is basic, which is a strength, not a weakness. It would be a great supper with a big salad.

3 pounds (1.4 kg) boneless pork loin

2 tablespoons (30 ml) olive oil

1 can (8 ounces, or 225 g) tomato sauce

¼ cup (60 ml) soy sauce

½ cup (120 ml) chicken broth

½ cup (12 g) Splenda

2 teaspoons dry mustard

Guar or xanthan (optional)

In a big, heavy skillet, brown the pork on all sides in the oil. Transfer the pork to a slow cooker.

In a bowl, mix together the tomato sauce, soy sauce, broth, Splenda, and dry mustard. Pour the mixture over the pork. Cover the slow cooker, set it to low, and let it cook for 8 to 9 hours.

When the time's up, remove the pork to a serving platter. Thicken the pot liquid, if needed, with guar or xanthan. Serve the juice with the pork.

Yield: 8 servings

Each with 37 g protein, 4 g carbohydrate, 1 g dietary fiber, 3 g usable carbs.

Pork Roast with Apricot Sauce

Here's a fabulous Sunday dinner for the family—with very little work.

2½ pounds (1.1 kg) boneless pork loin
2 tablespoons (30 ml) olive oil
⅓ cup (55 g) chopped onion
¾ cup (180 ml) chicken broth
¼ cup (80 g) low-sugar apricot preserves
1 tablespoon (15 ml) balsamic vinegar
1 tablespoon (15 ml) lemon juice
1 tablespoon (1.5 g) Splenda
Guar or xanthan

In a big, heavy skillet, sear the pork all over in the oil. Transfer the pork to a slow cooker. Scatter the onion around it.

In a bowl, mix together the broth, preserves, vinegar, lemon juice, and Splenda. Pour the mixture over the pork. Cover the slow cooker, set it to low, and let it cook for 7 hours.

When the time's up, remove the pork and put it on a serving platter. Season the juices with salt and pepper to taste. Thicken the juices with guar or xanthan. Ladle the juices into a sauce boat to serve.

Yield: 6 servings

Each with 40 g protein, 5 g carbohydrate, trace dietary fiber, 5 g usable carbs.

Pork Roast with Creamy Mushroom Gravy and Vegetables

Here's a great down-home dinner the family will love!

2½ pounds (1.1 kg) boneless pork loin
½ cup (60 g) sliced carrots
4 ounces (115 g) sliced mushrooms
10 ounces (280 g) frozen cross-cut green beans, unthawed
1 tablespoon (15 ml) beef bouillon concentrate
2 tablespoons (30 ml) water
1 can (14½ ounces, or 410 g) tomatoes with roasted garlic
Guar or xanthan
½ cup (120 ml) heavy cream

Put the pork in the bottom of a slow cooker. Surround the pork with the carrots, mushrooms, and green beans. (Don't bother thawing the green beans, just whack the package hard on the counter before opening that so the beans are all separated.)

In a bowl, dissolve the bouillon in the water. Stir in the tomatoes. Pour the mixture over the pork and vegetables. Cover the slow cooker, set it to low, and let it cook for 8 to 9 hours.

When the time's up, remove the pork and vegetables to a platter. Thicken the juices in the pot with guar or xanthan and then whisk in the cream. Add salt and pepper to taste. Serve the juices with the pork and vegetables.

(continued on page 426)

Yield: 8 servings

Each with 23 g protein, 5 g carbohydrate, 1 g dietary fiber, 4 g usable carbs.

Pork with Cabbage

Need I point out that this recipe is for cabbage lovers?

4 pounds (1.8 kg) boneless pork shoulder roast, trimmed of fat
2 tablespoons (30 ml) olive oil
2 carrots, cut into 1-inch (2.5-cm) pieces
2 cloves garlic, crushed
2 stalks celery, cut ½-inch (1.3-cm) thick
1 envelope (1 ounce, or 28 g) onion soup mix
1½ cups (360 ml) water
1½ pounds (680 g) cabbage, coarsely chopped
Guar or xanthan

In a big, heavy skillet, start browning the pork in the oil.

Place the carrots, garlic, and celery in a slow cooker. Add the soup mix and water.

When the pork is brown all over, put it on top of the vegetables in the slow cooker. Cover the slow cooker, set it to low, and let it cook for 7 hours.

When the time's up, stir in the cabbage, pushing it down into the liquid. Re-cover the slow cooker and let it cook for another 45 minutes to 1 hour.

Remove the pork and put it on a platter. Use a slotted spoon to pile the vegetables around the pork. Thicken the liquid in the slow cooker with guar or xanthan. Add salt and pepper to taste.

Pour the liquid into a sauce boat and serve with the pork and vegetables.

Yield: 8 servings

Each with 31 g protein, 10 g carbohydrate, 3 g dietary fiber, 7 g usable carbs.

Pork with Rutabaga

If you haven't tried rutabaga, you simply must. Also sometimes called a "swede" or a "yellow turnip," rutabaga is similar to a turnip, except that it has an entrancing bitter-sweet flavor. Anyway, it's fun confusing grocery store checkout clerks who can't figure out what that big yellow root is! It's actually delicious to make this with half rutabaga and half a fresh, cubed pumpkin, but it's just not possible to find fresh pumpkin some seasons of the year.

3 pounds (1.4 kg) boneless pork shoulder roast, tied or netted
2½ pounds (1.1 kg) rutabaga, peeled and cubed
½ teaspoon blackstrap molasses
½ cup (12 g) Splenda
¼ teaspoon cayenne
1 clove garlic, minced

Put the rutabaga in the bottom of a slow cooker. Put the pork on top. Drizzle the molasses over the pork and rutabaga.

In a bowl, mix together the Splenda, cayenne, and garlic. Sprinkle the mixture over the pork and rutabaga. Cover the slow cooker, set it to low, and let it cook for 8 to 9 hours.

When the time's up, remove the pork from the slow cooker, cut off the string or net, and slice or pull the pork apart. Serve the pork over the rutabaga with the pot liquid.

Yield: 6 servings

Each with 32 g protein, 16 g carbohydrate, 5 g dietary fiber, 11 g usable carbs.

Pork Stew

This winter-night supper is not only low-carb, but it's quite low-calorie, too. Pork loin is a very lean meat.

2 pounds (1.8 kg) boneless pork loin, cut in 1-inch (2.5-cm) cubes
1 tablespoon (15 ml) olive oil
1 tablespoon (14 g) butter
1 medium onion, sliced ¼-inch (6 mm) thick
4 cloves garlic, crushed
1 cup (130 g) sliced carrot
8 ounces (225 g) sliced mushrooms
2 cans (14-ounce, or 400 ml) chicken broth
1 pinch ground cloves
1 teaspoon salt
¼ teaspoon pepper
Guar or xanthan

Heat the olive oil and the butter in a Dutch oven over medium heat. Add the onion and garlic and sauté for a few minutes. Add the carrot and the next 6 ingredients (through pepper) and stir to combine. Cover, turn the heat to low, and let the whole thing simmer for 90 minutes to 2 hours. Thicken the gravy with guar or xanthan and serve.

Yield: 6 servings

Each with 30 g protein; 7 g carbohydrate; 1 g dietary fiber; 6 g usable carbs.

Curried Pork Stew

This is not terribly authentic, but it's awfully good. Try one of the chutneys (pages 495–496) with this.

1 pound (455 g) boneless pork loin, cubed
½ teaspoon salt
2 tablespoons (12 g) curry powder, divided
1 tablespoon (15 ml) olive oil
1 onion, sliced
2 small turnips, cubed
1 cup (240 ml) canned diced tomatoes
½ cup (120 ml) cider vinegar
2 tablespoons (3 g) Splenda
2 cups (300 g) diced cauliflower

Season the pork with the salt and sprinkle with 1 tablespoon (6 g) of the curry powder. In a big, heavy skillet, heat the oil and brown the pork over medium-high heat.

Place the onion and turnips in a slow cooker. Top with the pork and tomatoes.

In a bowl, stir together the vinegar, Splenda, and the remaining 1 tablespoon (6 g) curry powder. Pour the mixture over the pork. Cover the slow cooker, set it to low, and let it cook for 7 hours.

When the time's up, stir in the cauliflower. Re-cover the slow cooker and cook for 1 more hour or until the cauliflower is tender.

(continued on page 428)

Yield: 6 servings

Each with 17 g protein, 11 g carbohydrate, 3 g dietary fiber, 8 g usable carbs. Analysis does not include chutney.

Pork and "Apple" Stew

The apple flavor here comes from the apple cider vinegar. Our tester, Maria, cut her turnips into apple-slice shapes, and her family thought they were apples! They loved the whole thing.

2 pounds (910 g) pork loin, cut into 1-inch (2.5-cm) cubes
2 medium turnips, cubed
2 medium carrots, cut ½ inch (1.3 cm) thick
1 medium onion, sliced
½ cup (60 g) sliced celery
1 cup (240 ml) apple cider vinegar
3 tablespoons (4.5 g) Splenda
1 cup (240 ml) chicken broth
1 teaspoon chicken bouillon concentrate
1 teaspoon caraway seeds
¼ teaspoon pepper

Combine the pork, turnips, carrots, onion, and celery in a slow cooker.

In a bowl, stir together the vinegar, Splenda, broth, and bouillon. Pour the mixture over the pork and vegetables. Add the caraway seeds and pepper and stir everything. Cover the slow cooker, set it to low, and let it cook for 8 hours.

Yield: 6 servings

Each with 34 g protein, 10 g carbohydrate, 2 g dietary fiber, 8 g usable carbs.

Easy Southwestern Pork Stew

Our tester gave this a "10"—and so did her family!

2 pounds (910 g) boneless pork loin, cut into 1-inch (2.5-cm) cubes
1 medium onion, chopped
3 cloves garlic, crushed
2 teaspoons ground cumin
1 tablespoon (5.4 g) dried oregano
½ teaspoon salt
1 can (15 ounces, or 425 g) black soybeans
1 can (14½ ounces, or 410 g) tomatoes with green chiles
1 cup (240 ml) chicken broth
1 teaspoon chicken bouillon concentrate

Put the onion and garlic in a slow cooker and place the pork on top.

In a bowl, stir together the cumin, oregano, salt, soybeans, tomatoes, broth, and bouillon. Pour the mixture over the pork and vegetables. Cover the slow cooker, set it to low, and let it cook for 8 to 9 hours.

Yield: 6 servings

Each with 34 g protein, 6 g carbohydrate, 1 g dietary fiber, 5 g usable carbs.

Cocido de Puerco

This Mexican-style pork stew is simply marvelous. Do use bony cuts of meat because they're more flavorful—and cheaper, too.

3 pounds (1.4 kg) bony cuts of pork (Meaty pork neck bones are ideal.)
2 tablespoons (30 ml) olive oil
1 clove garlic, crushed
1 large onion, sliced
1 large green pepper, diced
2 medium zucchini, cut into chunks
1 can (14½ ounces, or 410 g) diced tomatoes
2 teaspoons cumin
2 teaspoons dried oregano
½ teaspoon red pepper flakes (optional)

In a heavy skillet over medium-high heat, sear the pork bones in the oil until they're brown all over.

Turn the heat to low and add the garlic, onion, pepper, zucchini, tomatoes, cumin, oregano, and pepper flakes. Cover the skillet and let it simmer for 1 hour.

Yield: About 6 servings, depending on how meaty your bones are

Each with 13 grams of carbohydrates and 4 grams of fiber, for a total of 9 grams of usable carbs and about 35 grams of protein.

Pork Chili

The pumpkin seed meal used to thicken this chili is an authentically Mexican touch.

1½ pounds (680 g) boneless pork loin, cut in ½-inch (1.3-cm) cubes
¾ cup (120 g) chopped onion
4 cloves garlic, crushed
2 tablespoons (30 ml) olive oil
2½ teaspoons chili powder
1 teaspoon ground cumin
1 green pepper, chopped
1 cup (240 ml) chicken broth
¼ cup (60 g) picante sauce
3 chipotle chiles canned in adobo, minced
2 teaspoons adobo sauce from the chili can
¼ cup (60 g) pumpkin seed meal (Grind raw shelled pumpkin seeds in a food processor.)
Salt to taste

In a big heavy skillet or Dutch oven, sauté the onion and garlic in the olive oil until the onions are translucent.

Add everything else except the ground pumpkin seeds and the salt, turn the heat to low, cover the pan, and let the whole thing simmer for 45 minutes to an hour.

Now stir in the pumpkin seed meal and let it simmer another 10 to 15 minutes. Season with salt to taste and serve.

Yield: 3 to 4 servings

Assuming 4, each will have 34 g protein; 11 g carbohydrate; 3 g dietary fiber; 8 g usable carbs.

Pork Slow Cooker Chili

Try this when you want to have people over after the kids' soccer game!

2½ pounds (1.1 kg) boneless pork loin, cut into 1-inch (2.5-cm) cubes
1 tablespoon (15 ml) olive oil
1 can (14½ ounces, or 410 g) tomatoes with green chiles
¼ cup (40 g) chopped onion
¼ cup (30 g) diced green bell pepper
1 clove garlic, crushed
1 tablespoon (7.8 g) chili powder

In a big, heavy skillet, heat the oil and brown the pork all over. Transfer the pork to a slow cooker. Stir in the tomatoes, onion, pepper, garlic, and chili powder. Cover the slow cooker, set it to low, and let it cook for 6 to 8 hours.

Serve this with sour cream and shredded Monterey Jack cheese, if you like, but it's darned good as-is.

Yield: 8 servings

Each with 25 g protein, 3 g carbohydrate, 1 g dietary fiber, 2 g usable carbs.

Apple Cheddar Pork Burgers

What can I say? I think apples and pork are a terrific combination.

1 pound (455 g) boneless pork loin, cut into 1½-inch (4 cm) cubes
½ Granny Smith or other crisp, tart apple, cut into a few chunks (no need to peel it)
¼ medium onion, peeled and cut into a couple of chunks
2 tablespoons (13 g) oat bran
1 egg
½ teaspoon salt or Vege-Sal
2 teaspoons prepared horseradish
2 ounces (56 g) cheddar cheese, shredded

Preheat an electric tabletop grill.

Put the apple, onion, pork, oat bran, egg, salt, and horseradish in a food processor and pulse until the meat is ground and everything is well blended. Add the cheese and pulse just long enough to blend it in—you're trying to keep some actual shreds of cheese in the mixture.

Form into 4 burgers and slap them on the grill. Cook for 7 minutes or until the juices run clear.

Yield: 4 servings

Each with 5 grams of carbohydrates and 1 gram of fiber, for a total of 4 grams of usable carbs and 25 grams of protein.

Ham and Pork Burgers

These are sort of plain and simple, but my husband loves them. This is a good recipe to help you use up leftover ham, should you have any on hand—but of course, you can also buy a chunk of precooked ham at the grocery store.

¾ **pound (340 g) boneless pork loin, cut into chunks**

½ **pound (225 g) cooked ham, cut into chunks**

2 **tablespoons (13 g) oat bran**

2 **tablespoons (30 ml) heavy cream**

1 **egg**

½ **teaspoon pepper**

Preheat an electric tabletop grill.

Plunk the ham, pork loin, oat bran, cream, egg, and pepper in a food processor with the S-blade in place and pulse until the meat is finely ground. Form into 4 burgers and put them in the grill. Cook for 6 to 7 minutes and serve.

Yield: 4 servings

Each with no more than 5 grams of carbohydrates (less, if you use really low-carb ham) and 1 gram of fiber, for a total of no more than 4 grams of usable carbs and 28 grams of protein.

Thai Burgers

Boy, are these good! If you can't find fish sauce, you can substitute soy sauce, and this will still taste fine.

1½ **pounds (680 g) boneless pork loin, cut into chunks**

1½ **teaspoons lemon juice**

1 **tablespoon (16.5 ml) chili garlic paste**

1 **clove garlic or ½ teaspoon minced garlic**

4 **scallions, with the roots and the tops cut off (Leave the crisp part of the green!)**

1 **can (4 ounces, or 115 g) mushrooms, drained**

1 **tablespoon (15 ml) fish sauce**

2 **tablespoons (8 g) fresh cilantro**

3 **tablespoons (45 ml) lime juice**

½ **cup (115 g) mayonnaise**

Preheat an electric tabletop grill.

Put the pork loin, lemon juice, chili garlic paste, garlic, scallions, mushrooms, fish sauce, and cilantro in a food processor with the S-blade in place. Pulse until the meat is finely ground and everything is well combined. Form the mixture into 6 burgers and put them on the grill. Cook for 6 to 7 minutes.

While the burgers are cooking, stir the lime juice (bottled works fine) into the mayonnaise. When the burgers are done, top each one with a dollop of the lime mayonnaise and serve.

Yield: 6 servings

Each with 4 grams of carbohydrates and 1 gram of fiber, for a total of 3 grams of usable carbs and 24 grams of protein.

Luau Burgers

Again, all those ingredients make this look intimidating, but it's really just a matter of assembling everything in the food processor and chopping it together.

1 **pound (455 g) boneless pork loin**

¼ **medium onion, cut into chunks**

½ **green pepper, cut into chunks**

1½ **teaspoons grated ginger**

½ **teaspoon minced garlic or 1 clove garlic, crushed**

1 **tablespoon (15 ml) soy sauce**

1 **egg**

(continued on page 432)

¼ cup (20 g) crushed pork rinds, plain or barbeque flavor

½ teaspoon pepper

½ teaspoon salt

¼ cup (50 g) canned crushed pineapple in unsweetened juice

1 tablespoon (15 ml) tomato sauce

½ teaspoon blackstrap molasses

½ teaspoon Splenda

½ teaspoon spicy brown mustard

Preheat an electric tabletop grill.

Place the pork, onion, pepper, ginger, garlic, soy sauce, egg, pork rinds, pepper, and salt in a food processor with the S-blade in place. (You'll need a full-size food processor; this overwhelmed my little one!) Pulse until the meat is finely ground. Add the pineapple and pulse to mix.

Form into 5 burgers—the mixture will be quite soft—and slap them on the grill. Set a timer for 6 minutes.

While the burgers are cooking, mix together the tomato sauce, molasses, Splenda, and mustard. When the 6 minutes are up, open the grill, spread the tomato sauce mixture evenly over the burgers and then close the grill and cook for 1 more minute. Serve.

Yield: 5 servings

Each with 5 grams of carbohydrates and 1 gram of fiber, for a total of 4 grams of usable carbs and 22 grams of protein.

These are low-calorie, too! They have just 178 calories per serving.

Albondigas

I didn't know whether to put these tasty Mexican meatballs in the pork chapter or the beef chapter! They're great by themselves, or you can serve them over Cauliflower Rice (page 212).

1 pound (455 g) ground pork

1 pound (455 g) ground beef

1 cup (120 g) shredded zucchini

¼ cup (40 g) finely minced onion

2 eggs

½ teaspoon oregano

½ teaspoon pepper

½ teaspoon cumin

1 teaspoon salt or Vege-Sal

1 can (14½ ounces, or 410 g) diced tomatoes, undrained

2 chipotle chiles canned in adobo (or less or more, to taste)

¾ cup (180 ml) chicken broth

In a big mixing bowl, combine the two meats. Add the zucchini, the onion, and the eggs to the meat. Measure in the seasonings. Using clean hands, smoosh everything together until it's all very well combined—in particular, you shouldn't be able to tell where one meat ends and the other begins. Form into meatballs a little smaller than a walnut in its shell. Put on a plate and set in the fridge.

Put the tomatoes in a blender—don't drain them first. Add the chipotles and then blend the whole thing until smooth. Dump this combination into a big, heavy skillet and put it over medium-high heat. When it comes to a boil, turn the heat down and let the sauce simmer for 5 minutes. Stir in the chicken broth and bring the sauce back to a simmer.

Add the meatballs and bring to a simmer a third time. Cover the skillet, let the whole thing simmer for 45 to 50 minutes, and then serve.

Yield: 8 servings

Each with 22 g protein; 5 g carbohydrate; 1 g dietary fiber; 4 g usable carbs. Analysis does not include Cauliflower Rice.

Carnitas

These brown and tender cubes of pork are a Mexican classic. Serve them over a salad or make a simple soft taco by piling your carnitas on a low-carb tortilla.

3 pounds (1.4 kg) pork shoulder, skin and bone removed
Water
1 tablespoon (15 ml) lime juice
2 teaspoons salt

Cut the pork into 1-inch (2.5-cm) cubes and put them in a big, heavy skillet. Add just enough water to barely cover the cubes. Add the lime juice, sprinkle with salt, and bring to a boil. Do not cover the pan.

Turn the heat down to medium-low and let the meat continue to boil until all the water has evaporated.

Turn the heat down even lower and let the meat continue to cook, stirring often, until the meat cubes are browned all over, which may take as long as an hour.

Yield: 6 servings

Each with 29 g protein; 0 g carbohydrate; 0 g dietary fiber; 0 g usable carb. Analysis does not include low-carb tortilla.

Carolina Pulled Pork

In much of the country, spareribs are the favorite part of the pig to barbecue. But in the Carolinas, barbecue means pork shoulder (or sometimes even the whole hog!) smoked for ages until it's tender and juicy. Then the meat is cut or pulled off the bone and combined with one of a few different kinds of sauces, depending on the region. The whole process takes a lot of time (though not a tremendous amount of work), but the results are nothing short of spectacular!

1 pork picnic shoulder, about 4 pounds (1.8 kg)
Oil
Salt and pepper
Barbecue rub of choice (optional)
Wood chips or chunks, soaked for at least 30 minutes

This is way too simple. Set up a grill for indirect smoking (pile all the coals on one side or turn on only half the burners on a gas grill) and add the wood chips or chunks. Then rub the pork shoulder all over with a little oil, sprinkle it with salt and pepper, and sprinkle it liberally with barbecue rub if desired. It's a good idea to insert a meat thermometer into the center of the thickest part of the meat, taking care not to let it touch the bone.

(continued on page 434)

Then put that hunk of pork on the grill, fatty side up, and smoke it for a long, long time—6 to 7 hours. (Don't try simmering this like you might a rack of ribs you wanted to speed up. If you don't have the time, make something else.) Make sure you replace the wood chips or chunks when necessary so that you get plenty of good smoky flavor and take care to keep the temperature between 200°F and 225°F (95°C and 110°C). (Lower isn't disastrous, but it can stretch out your cooking time even further. Higher and your meat will grill, not smoke.) When the internal temperature is between 170°F and 180°F (80°C and 85°C), your pork is done. Take it off the grill and let it rest for 10 minutes before cutting it up.

Okay, 10 minutes are up! Cut or pull the pork off the bone; you can discard the bone. Pull or cut off the outside fat. Then, either chop up the meat or pull it apart with two forks until it's in shreds. Now mix it with about 2/3 cup (160 ml) Piedmont Mustard Sauce (page 469), Eastern Carolina Vinegar Sauce (page 469), or Lexington-Style Barbecue Sauce (page 470).

How to serve your pulled pork? After all, it's usually served on a bun, and we're sure not going to eat it that way. Well, you can just eat it with a fork by itself, of course, and it will be extremely nice. However, since Carolina barbecue sandwiches are usually topped with coleslaw, why not serve yourself a big pile of coleslaw, top it with pulled pork, and eat the two together as a main-dish salad?

Yield: A 4-pound (1.8-kg) shoulder will yield about 6 servings

The carb count will depend on which sauce you choose; the meat itself is pretty much carb-free; 39 grams of protein.

Cajun Barbecued Pork

This dish is hot! It's not for the timid, but the taste is complex and delicious.

4 pounds (1.8 kg) country-style pork ribs
1 batch Cajun Rub (page 490)
1 batch Cajun Rib Mop (page 490)
2/3 cup (160 ml) Cajun Sauce (page 474)
Wood chips or chunks, soaked for at least
   30 minutes

Set up a grill for indirect smoking (pile all the coals on one side or turn on only half the burners on a gas grill) and add the wood chips or chunks. Rub the country-style ribs all over with the Cajun Rub and place them on the grill. Smoke them for 30 to 45 minutes and then start to baste them with the Cajun Rib Mop, using a clean utensil each time, every time you open the grill to add more chips or chunks as the smoke dies down. Smoke for 3 to 4 hours, at least, or until an instant-read thermometer registers 170°F (80°C). Serve with the Cajun Sauce.

Yield: 6 servings

Each serving will have 7 grams of carbohydrate and 1 gram of fiber, for a usable carb count of 6 grams; 36 grams protein.

Chinese Pork

Pork is the most popular meat in China, and this is a de-carbed version of a classic Chinese seasoning. Feel free to do this with spareribs instead.

3 pounds (1.4 kg) country-style pork ribs
½ cup (120 ml) soy sauce
¼ cup (60 ml) sherry
1 clove garlic
2 tablespoons (3 g) Splenda
1 tablespoon (6 g) grated ginger
¼ cup (60 ml) oil

Mix together everything from the soy sauce through the ginger. Put the ribs in a shallow, nonreactive pan or a resealable plastic bag. Reserve some marinade for basting and pour the rest over them. If you're using a bag, press out the air and seal it. Either way, turn the ribs to coat. Stick the ribs in the fridge and let them marinate for at least a few hours.

Okay, marinating time's up. Pour off half the marinade. Put the ribs with the remaining marinade in a heavy-bottomed saucepan and just barely cover with water. Bring to a simmer and simmer the ribs for 45 minutes. When they're getting on toward the end of simmering time, start the grill. Mix the oil with the reserved marinade.

Put the ribs over a medium-low charcoal fire or gas grill and grill slowly over direct heat. Baste often with the marinade-oil mixture, using a clean utensil each time, until quite tender—about another 45 minutes.

Yield: 6 servings

If you consumed all of the marinade, each serving would have 4 grams of carbohydrate, and a trace of fiber. Since you don't, figure closer to 3 grams per serving; 28 grams of protein.

Absolutely Classic Barbecued Ribs

This is what most of us think of when we think "barbecued ribs," and a beautiful thing it is, too.

1 slab pork spare ribs, about 7 pounds (3.2 kg)
½ cup (60 g) Classic Barbecue Rub (page 486), divided
½ cup (120 ml) oil
½ cup (120 ml) water
1 cup (240 grams) Kansas City Barbecue Sauce (page 467)
Wood chips or chunks, soaked for at least 30 minutes

First, fire up that grill! Set it up for indirect smoking (pile all the coals on one side or turn on only half the burners on a gas grill) and add the wood chips or chunks.

Sprinkle the ribs heavily on both sides with the Classic Barbecue Rub. Then, when your grill is hot or your charcoal is well covered with ash, throw the ribs on the grill on the side away from the fire. Smoke them for a good 6 hours at 225°F (110°C), adding wood chips whenever the smoke dies down.

Okay, the ribs are in the hot smoke. Put the oil and water in a small pan or bowl and stir in 2 tablespoons (15 g) of the Classic Barbecue Rub. After the ribs have smoked for about 30 to 45 minutes, use this simple mop to baste them every time you add fresh chips or chunks to the fire. Make sure to use a clean utensil each time you baste. Turn the ribs over every 60 to 90 minutes.

(continued on page 436)

Come the last 20 minutes of your cooking time, baste your ribs well with the Kansas City Barbecue Sauce and put them directly over the fire for 10 minutes per side to crisp them a little. Serve with cold light beer, slaw, extra sauce, and a big roll of paper towels!

Feel free to use this same basic method with any rub and any sauce!

Yield: About 8 to 9 servings

Assuming 8, each will have 10 grams of carbohydrate with 2 grams of fiber, for a usable carb count of 8 grams; 49 grams of protein.

Simple Marinated Ribs

Why is this recipe for a half-slab of ribs? Because there are only two of us in my household, that's why! Feel free to double the marinade and use a whole slab if you like—but you'll want to cut the slab into two pieces so it'll fit into a resealable plastic bag. What with the marinade/mop, these have plenty of flavor without a finishing sauce, but feel free to use one if you really want to.

3 pounds (1.4 kg) pork spareribs—about half a slab
½ cup (120 ml) cider vinegar
1 tablespoon (1.5 g) Splenda
1 tablespoon (15 ml) spicy mustard
½ teaspoon grated ginger
½ cup (120 ml) olive oil
Wood chips or chunks, soaked for at least 30 minutes

Combine everything but the ribs and the oil. Put the ribs in a large resealable plastic bag. Reserve some of the vinegar mixture for basting, pour the rest over it, and seal the bag, pressing out the air as you go. Turn the bag a couple of times to make sure the whole surface of the meat comes in contact with the marinade. Throw the ribs in the fridge and let them marinate all day or even overnight, turning now and then when you open the fridge anyway and think of it.

Six hours before dinner, get a fire going for indirect smoking (pile all the coals on one side or turn on only half the burners on a gas grill) and add the wood chips or chunks. When the fire is ready, mix the reserved marinade and the oil—this is your mopping sauce. Drain and throw the ribs on the grill and smoke them for 5 to 6 hours or until quite tender, basting every 30 to 45 minutes (or when you add more chips or chunks to the fire, as the smoke dies down) with the mop sauce. Use a clean utensil each time you baste.

Yield: 4 servings

Each serving will have 2 grams of carbohydrate and a trace of fiber if you finish the marinade, which you won't—I'd count 1 gram, myself; 36 grams of protein.

Apple-Maple Brined Ribs

Okay, I admit it. This is not a spontaneous recipe; it takes forever! It's quite simple, though, and these ribs taste wonderful with no other seasoning at all. This recipe is for a half-slab, so feel free to double it.

½ slab pork spare ribs, about 4 pounds
    (1.8 kg)
½ cup (145 g) salt
7 cups (1.7 L) hot water
2 cups (480 ml) cider vinegar
½ cup (12 g) Splenda
½ cup (120 ml) sugar-free pancake syrup
1½ teaspoons cracked black pepper
½ cup (120 ml) oil, plus more for ribs
Wood chips or chunks, soaked for at least
    30 minutes

Dissolve the salt in the hot water and then stir in everything else but the ribs. Put the ribs in something shallow, flat, and made of a nonreactive material—you may want to cut the slab into a few pieces to fit it in. Reserve ½ cup (120 ml) of the brine for basting and pour the rest over the ribs, making sure they're submerged at least a little bit. Stash them in the fridge and let them sit for 3 to 4 hours.

Six hours before you want to eat, start the grill for indirect cooking—build a charcoal fire to one side or light only one burner of your gas grill. Pull the ribs out of the brine and pat them dry. Rub the surface of the ribs with a little oil.

When the fire is ready, put the ribs over the side of the grill not over the fire and add soaked wood chips to the fire—apple wood would be especially appropriate, but I've used other chips and gotten good results. Smoke the ribs for a good 6 hours, adding wood chips whenever the smoke dies down.

What do you do with that ½ cup (120 ml) of reserved brine? Mix it with ½ cup (120 ml) oil and use it to baste the ribs while they're smoking, every time you add more chips or chunks. Use a clean utensil each time you baste.

You can add other seasonings or a sauce to these if you like, but I like them with just salt and pepper. The brine/mop adds a lovely flavor of its own and makes these ribs wonderfully juicy!

Yield: 5 to 6 servings

If you consumed all of the brine, you'd get a substantial quantity of carbohydrate (7 or 8 grams) but you discard most of the brine, of course. Count 1 to 2 grams per serving, at most; 32 grams of protein. Analysis does not include polyol sweetened in sugar-free syrup.

Oven Barbecued Ribs

3 pounds (1.4 kg) pork spareribs (about a half
    a slab)
1 tablespoon (6.9 g) paprika
1 teaspoon salt or Vege-Sal
2 teaspoons spicy brown mustard
1 bay leaf
½ teaspoon chili powder
¼ teaspoon cayenne
2 tablespoons (30 ml) Worcestershire sauce
¼ cup (60 ml) cider vinegar
⅓ cup (80 ml) tomato sauce
2 tablespoons (30 ml) Dana's No-Sugar
    Ketchup (page 463)
½ cup (120 ml) water
1 teaspoon lemon juice
2 tablespoons (20 g) minced onion
1 clove garlic, crushed
½ teaspoon blackstrap molasses

(continued on page 438)

In a large, nonreactive saucepan combine everything but the ribs. Stir together, bring to a boil, turn down to a simmer, and let it cook for 10 to 15 minutes.

Preheat the oven to 450°F (230°C, or gas mark 8). While the sauce is cooking, I like to cut in between the ribs about halfway up, but that's optional—it just gives more surface for the sauce to coat! Place the ribs on a broiler pan.

Pour some sauce into a small bowl and paint the ribs thoroughly with the rest of the sauce. Let them roast for 30 minutes. Now turn the oven down to 350°F (180°C, or gas mark 4). Baste the ribs with fresh sauce using a clean utensil, turn them over, and baste the other side. Continue roasting the ribs for 90 minutes, basting every 20 to 30 minutes, and turning them over when you do. Serve with plenty of napkins!

Yield: 3 to 4 servings

Assuming 4, each will have 37 g protein; 8 g carbohydrate; 1 g dietary fiber; 7 g usable carbs—and that's if you use up all the sauce.

Orange Brined Ribs

3 pounds (1.4 kg) country-style pork ribs
16 ounces (480 ml) orange-flavored Fruit$_2$O
1 tablespoon (18 g) salt
2 cloves garlic
⅛ teaspoon blackstrap molasses
1½ teaspoons soy sauce
½ cup (120 ml) olive oil
Wood chips or chunks, soaked for at least
**   30 minutes**

Dissolve the salt in the Fruit$_2$O—heating the Fruit$_2$O a bit will help the salt dissolve. Stir in everything else but the ribs and oil. Set aside ½ cup of the brine for basting and 1 tablespoon (15 ml) of the brine to use in the Orange Rib Glaze (following). Put the ribs in a shallow nonreactive dish and pour the rest of brine over them, making sure the ribs are submerged at least a little bit. Put the whole thing in the fridge and let the ribs soak in the brine for 4 to 5 hours.

Five to six hours before you want to eat, prepare the grill for indirect cooking—build a charcoal fire to one side or light only one burner of your gas grill. When the fire is ready, pull the ribs out and drain them. Pat the ribs dry and rub them with a little oil. Put them on the grill and add soaked wood chips to the fire. Cover the grill and smoke the ribs for 5 to 6 hours, adding more chips or chunks when the smoke dies down.

Combine the ½ cup (120 ml) of reserved brine with ½ cup (120 ml) of oil and use it to mop the ribs every time you add chips or chunks to the fire. Use a clean utensil each time you baste.

I like to coat these with Orange Rib Glaze in the last 20 minutes before they come off the grill, but serve them with whatever sauce or seasoning you like!

Yield: 5 servings

Exclusive of any sauce you might add, these are virtually carb-free! 32 grams of protein.

Orange Rib Glaze

1 tablespoon (15 ml) sugar-free imitation
**   honey**

1 tablespoon (15 ml) reserved orange brine
   from Orange Brined Ribs recipe (preceding)
¼ teaspoon orange extract
½ teaspoon soy sauce
1 clove garlic, crushed
½ teaspoon grated ginger

Simply stir everything together and brush evenly over Orange Brined Ribs in the last 20 minutes of cooking. This is just enough to make a thin glaze over the ribs. It's not enough to spoon over them at the table—but trust me, if you've used the brine and the mop, you'll have plenty of flavor.

Yield: 5 servings

Each serving has 3 grams of carbohydrate, exclusive of the polyols in the imitation honey; a trace of fiber; a trace of protein.

Bourbon Mustard Pork Ribs

No rub or finishing sauce needed—the marinade/baste alone makes these mustardy-tangy-sweet.

1 slab pork spare ribs, about 6 to 7 pounds
   (2.7 to 3.2 kg)
1 cup (240 ml) bourbon
1 cup (240 ml) oil
1 tablespoon (15 ml) molasses
1 cup (240 ml) spicy brown mustard
2 tablespoons (4 g) dried sage
2 teaspoons salt or Vege-Sal
2 teaspoons pepper

1 tablespoon (4 g) dried thyme
1 cup (25 g) Splenda
**Wood chips or chunks, soaked for at least
   30 minutes**

Combine everything but the ribs and the wood chunks. Cut the ribs in two so they'll fit in a pot—use a nonreactive one, only big enough to fit the ribs. Reserve some bourbon mixture for basting, pour the rest over them, and let them marinate for several hours, at least.

Now you get to make a choice: to simmer, or not to simmer? I like to simmer—put the pot over medium-low heat, bring the marinade to a simmer, and let the ribs cook for 25 to 30 minutes.

Either way, set up your grill for indirect smoking (pile all the coals on one side or turn on only half the burners on a gas grill) and add the wood chips or chunks.

If you've simmered your ribs, smoke them for 3 hours. If you haven't, smoke them for 5 to 6 hours. Either way, baste them with the reserved bourbon-mustard marinade every 30 to 45 minutes while they're smoking, using a clean utensil each time. Baste them for the last time at least 15 to 20 minutes before pulling the ribs out of the hot smoke. Replace the wood chips whenever the smoke dies down.

These don't need any sauce at all—just eat them as is.

Yield: 8 servings

If you consumed all the marinade/baste, you'd get 8 grams of carb per serving, with 1 gram of fiber, but you won't consume all of the marinade/baste!

(continued on page 440)

Estimating generously that you'll eat two-thirds of the bourbon-mustard mixture, you'll get 6 grams of carb per serving, with a trace of fiber, and the count may actually be lower than that; 39 grams of protein.

Hoisin Basted Ribs

Another Chinese-influenced version of ribs. You'll have to make the low-carb Hoisin Sauce first, but it's a nice thing to have on hand anyway.

1 slab pork spareribs, about 6 pounds (2.7 kg)
¾ cup (180 ml) Hoisin Sauce (page 464)
¼ cup (60 ml) dry sherry
3 tablespoons (45 ml) sugar-free imitation honey
4 cloves garlic, crushed
1 teaspoon grated ginger
1½ tablespoons (2 g) Splenda
Oil
Salt and pepper

Simmer the ribs first for this one—put them in a pot big enough to hold them and cover them with water. (You can add a little soy sauce and Splenda, if you like.) Bring them to a simmer and let them simmer for 30 to 45 minutes.

While that's happening, get the fire going, especially if you're using charcoal. You'll want the fire medium-low.

Next, put the low-carb Hoisin Sauce, sherry, imitation honey, garlic, and ginger in the blender, and run it until everything is well combined.

Okay, the ribs are done simmering. Pull them out, pat them dry with paper towels, and give them a nice massage with a little oil. Season them with salt and pepper and put them over the fire—we're directly grilling them this time, instead of slow smoking them. Put them meaty-side down, close the grill, and let them cook for 20 minutes. Flip them over, re-close the grill, and let them go another 40 to 45 minutes.

About 20 minutes before cooking time is up, baste the ribs with the Hoisin Sauce mixture and baste them again 10 minutes later. Serve the rest of the sauce at the table.

Yield: 9 servings

Each serving will have 5 grams carbohydrate and a trace of fiber, not including the polyols in the imitation honey; 35 grams protein.

Hot Asian Ribs

This is full-bodied Chinese flavor. If your family loves Chinese spareribs, you have to make this!

3½ pounds (1.8 kg) country-style pork ribs
4 scallions, sliced
¼ cup (60 ml) soy sauce
⅓ cup (8 g) Splenda
1 teaspoon blackstrap molasses
2 tablespoons (30 ml) white wine vinegar
2 teaspoons toasted sesame oil
2 teaspoons lemon juice
½ teaspoon hot sauce
1 clove garlic
½ teaspoon ground ginger
½ teaspoon chili powder
¼ teaspoon red pepper flakes
6 teaspoons Hoisin Sauce (page 464)

Put the ribs in a slow cooker.

In a bowl, mix together the remaining ingredients. Pour the sauce over the ribs. Cover the slow cooker, set it to low, and let it cook for 8 to 9 hours.

Yield: 6 servings

Each with 32 g protein, 4 g carbohydrate, 1 g dietary fiber, 3 g usable carbs.

Key West Ribs

Citrusy barbecue sauce gives this a Florida kind of taste!

3 pounds (1.4 kg) country-style pork ribs
¼ cup (40 g) finely chopped onion
¼ cup (60 ml) low-carb barbecue sauce (from Chapter 13 or purchased)
1 teaspoon grated orange peel
1 teaspoon grated lemon rind
½ teaspoon salt
2 tablespoons (30 ml) white wine vinegar
2 tablespoons (30 ml) lemon juice
2 tablespoons (30 ml) lime juice
1½ tablespoons (2 g) Splenda
⅛ teaspoon orange extract
2 tablespoons (30 ml) olive oil

In a big, heavy skillet, brown the ribs over medium-high heat. Transfer them to a slow cooker.

In a bowl, mix together the remaining ingredients. Pour the mixture over the ribs. Cover the slow cooker, set it to low, and let it cook for 7 to 9 hours. Serve the ribs together with the sauce.

Yield: 6 servings

Each with 26 g protein, 3 g carbohydrate, trace dietary fiber, 3 g usable carbs.

Maple-Spice Country-Style Ribs

My pal Ray Stevens, who has tested many recipes for me, raves about this. It's shaping up to be the recipe by which all other recipes are judged!

3 pounds (1.4 kg) country-style pork ribs
½ cup (120 ml) sugar-free pancake syrup
3 tablespoons (4.5 g) Splenda
2 tablespoons (30 ml) soy sauce
¼ cup (40 g) chopped onion
½ teaspoon ground cinnamon
½ teaspoon ground ginger
½ teaspoon ground allspice
3 cloves garlic, crushed
¼ teaspoon pepper
⅛ teaspoon cayenne

Put the ribs in a slow cooker.

In a bowl, mix together the remaining ingredients. Pour the mixture over the ribs. Cover the slow cooker, set it to low, and let it cook for 9 hours.

Yield: 6 servings

Each with 27 g protein, 2 g carbohydrate, trace dietary fiber, 2 g usable carbs. Analysis does not include polyol sweetened in sugar-free syrup.

Sour Cream Ham Supper

This is another updated, decarbed recipe from Peg Bracken's classic, *The I Hate To Cook Book.*

2 cups (300 g) cooked ham, cut into strips
½ head cauliflower
½ medium onion, diced
2 tablespoons (28 g) butter
8 ounces (225 g) sliced mushrooms
½ cup (115 g) sour cream

Run the cauliflower through the shredding blade of your food processor. Put it in a microwaveable casserole dish, add a couple of tablespoons (30 ml) of water, cover, and cook on high for 6 to 7 minutes.

While the cauliflower is cooking, dice the onion and cut the ham into smallish strips. Melt the butter in a large, heavy skillet over medium heat and sauté the onion, ham, and mushrooms in it, stirring frequently. When the onion is limp and translucent, turn the heat to low and stir in the sour cream. Heat through, but don't let it come to a boil or the sour cream will "crack."

Drain the cauliflower, divide it between 3 plates, and spoon the ham mixture over it.

Yield: 3 servings

Each with 9 grams of carbohydrates and 1 gram of fiber, for a total of 8 grams of usable carbs and 19 grams of protein.

"Honey" Mustard Ham

You may wonder how to roast a ham when you're not going to be around for hours to tend the oven. You use your slow cooker, of course. You'll need a big slow cooker for this.

5 pounds (2.3 kg) fully cooked, bone-in ham
⅓ cup (80 ml) apple cider vinegar
½ cup (12 g) Splenda, divided
1 tablespoon (15 ml) brown mustard
½ teaspoon blackstrap molasses
1 teaspoon water

Place the ham in a slow cooker.

In a bowl, mix together the vinegar and 2 tablespoons (3 g) of the Splenda. Add the mixture to the slow cooker. In the same bowl, mix together the mustard, molasses, remaining Splenda, and water and spread the mixture over the ham. Cover the slow cooker, set it to low, and let it cook for 7 hours.

Yield: 6 servings

Each with 68 g protein, 6 g carbohydrate, trace dietary fiber, 6 g usable carbs.

Ham Kedgeree

Oh boy, you are going to thank me for this recipe the Monday after Easter. This quick and tasty skillet supper, based on a traditional dish from the British occupation of India, will help you use up both leftover ham and hard-boiled eggs! It's good enough that you may find yourself buying precooked ham and boiling up some eggs at other times of year.

2 cups (300 g) ham, cut in ½-inch (1.3-cm) cubes
½ head cauliflower
3 tablespoons (42 g) butter
1 tablespoon (6 g) curry powder
3 tablespoons (30 g) minced onion
4 hard-boiled eggs, coarsely chopped
¼ cup (60 ml) heavy cream
Salt and pepper
¼ cup (15.2 g) chopped fresh parsley

Run the cauliflower through the shredding blade of a food processor. Put it in a microwaveable casserole dish with a lid, add a couple of tablespoons (30 ml) of water, cover, and microwave on high for 6 minutes.

Melt the butter in a large, heavy skillet over low heat and add the curry powder and onion. Sauté them together for 2 to 3 minutes. Add everything else, stir gently but thoroughly (gently so that you don't completely pulverize the hunks of egg yolk), heat through, and serve.

Yield: 4 servings

Each with 19 g protein; 6 g carbohydrate; 1 g dietary fiber; 5 g usable carbs.

Creamy Ham Casserole

I made this up to use the end of a ham I'd slow cooked, and it was a hit with my husband.

2 cups (300g) cooked ham, cubed
1 head cauliflower
1 medium onion, chopped
1 large stalk celery, with leaves

2 cups (480 ml) Carb Countdown dairy beverage
1 cup (240 ml) chicken broth
6 teaspoons guar or xanthan
1 teaspoon dry mustard
1 teaspoon salt or Vege-Sal
½ teaspoon pepper
8 ounces (225 g) Gruyère cheese, shredded

Run the cauliflower through the slicing blade of a food processor. Transfer it to a bowl and replace the slicing disc with the S-blade. Chop the onion and celery fine in the food processor.

With a hand blender or regular blender, blend the Carb Countdown and broth. Add the guar or xanthan and blend it until there are no lumps. Pour the mixture it into a saucepan and heat it over medium-low heat. (If you do have a hand blender, you may as well just dump the Carb Countdown and the chicken broth in the saucepan and use the hand blender to blend in the thickener in the pot to save a little dishwashing.) Stir in the dry mustard, salt or Vege-Sal, and pepper. When the sauce is hot, stir in the cheese, a little at a time, until it's all melted. Turn off the heat.

Spray a slow cooker with nonstick cooking spray. Put in a layer of cauliflower, a lighter layer of onion and celery, and then a generous layer of ham. Repeat these layers until everything's gone and the slow cooker is full. Pour half of the sauce over the top. It won't immediately flow down into the food in the slow cooker, so poke down into it several times with the handle of a rubber scraper or spoon, piercing the layers to the bottom. The sauce will start to seep down. When there's more room on top, pour in the rest of the sauce and

(continued on page 444)

poke down through the layers again. Cover the slow cooker, set it to low, and let it cook for 6 to 7 hours.

Yield: 8 servings

Each with 24 g protein, 5 g carbohydrate, 1 g dietary fiber, 4 g usable carbs.

Ham and Beans Skillet

This is very down-home, which is often a good thing. My husband loves it. You can double this if you like, but the beans will take longer to microwave. Even doubled, though, it's a good, fast supper!

6 ounces (170 g) cooked ham, cut into ½-inch (1.3-cm) cubes
1 tablespoon (28 g or 30 ml) butter or oil
2 cups (300 g) frozen cross-cut green beans
1 tablespoon (13 g) canned, crushed pineapple in juice
1 tablespoon (15 ml) low-carbohydrate barbecue sauce
¼ teaspoon grated ginger
½ teaspoon spicy brown mustard

Start to sauté the ham in the butter or oil over medium heat—you're just browning it a little. While that's happening, put the beans in a microwave-able casserole dish, add a couple of tablespoons (30 ml) of water, cover, and microwave on high for 7 minutes.

When the microwave goes "ding," check that the beans are done; if they're not, stir them and give them another 2 to 3 minutes. When they're just tender, drain them and add them to the browned ham cubes in the skillet. Add the pineapple, barbecue sauce, ginger, and mustard and stir well. Let it cook for just a minute to blend the flavors and then serve.

Yield: 2 servings

Each with 13 grams of carbohydrates and 4 grams of fiber, for a total of 9 grams of usable carbs and 19 grams of protein.

Ham Slice with Mustard Sauce

Ham steak, about 2 pounds (910 g)
2 to 3 tablespoons (30 to 45 ml) oil
½ cup (120 ml) water
3 tablespoons (45 ml) prepared mustard
3 tablespoons (4.5 g) Splenda
¼ teaspoon blackstrap molasses
Salt and pepper

Put the oil in a heavy skillet over medium heat and fry the ham steak until it is golden on both sides. Remove the ham from the skillet, set it on a platter, and keep it warm.

Pour the water into the skillet and stir it around, scraping up all the brown bits from the ham. Stir in the mustard, Splenda, molasses, and salt and pepper to taste. Pour over the ham and serve.

Yield: 5 servings

Each with 2 grams of carbohydrates, a trace of fiber, and 36 grams of protein.

Apple Sausage Burgers

Feel free to make these with turkey sausage, if you prefer.

1½ pounds (680 g) bulk pork sausage, hot or mild
½ medium onion, peeled and cut in a few chunks
½ Granny Smith or other crisp, tart apple, cut into a few chunks (no need to peel it)
1 teaspoon dried thyme
1 teaspoon dried sage
1 teaspoon pepper

Preheat an electric tabletop grill.

Put the onion and apple in a food processor with the S-blade in place and pulse until they're chopped to a medium consistency. Add the sausage, thyme, sage, and pepper and pulse until it's all well-blended.

Form into 4 burgers and put them on the grill. Cook for 7 minutes or until the juices run clear.

Yield: 4 servings

Each with 7 grams of carbohydrates and 1 gram of fiber, for a total of 6 grams of usable carbs and 20 grams of protein.

Italian Sausage with Onions and Peppers

Mmmmmmm! This is like revisiting my childhood in the New York City area!

1¼ to 1½ pounds (570 to 680 g) Italian sausage links, hot or mild
¼ cup (60 ml) olive oil
1½ large green peppers
1 large onion
1 clove garlic

Slice the sausage diagonally into ½-inch (1.3-cm) pieces and sauté it in the olive oil over medium-high heat. Meanwhile, slice the peppers into medium-size strips and slice the onion about ¼ inch (6 mm) thick. When the sausage is about half done, stir in the peppers, onion, and garlic. Cook until the sausage is well done and the onion is limp and translucent. Serve.

Yield: 4 servings

Each with 7 grams of carbohydrates and 1 gram of fiber, for a total of 6 grams of usable carbs and 21 grams of protein.

Country Sausage Skillet Supper

1 pound (455 g) bulk pork sausage, hot or mild
1 small onion, chopped
¾ cup (90 g) shredded cheddar cheese

Crumble the sausage in a heavy skillet over medium heat. As the grease starts to cook out of it, add the onion.

Cook until the sausage is no longer pink and the onion is translucent. Pour off the grease, spread the sausage mixture evenly in the pan, and scatter the cheddar over the top. Cover and return to the heat for a minute or two until the cheese is melted and serve.

Yield: 3 servings

Each with 5 grams of carbohydrates and 1 gram of fiber, for a total of 4 grams of usable carbs and 25 grams of protein.

Feel free to substitute turkey sausage, if you prefer it.

Winter Night Sausage Bake

This one-dish meal is serious down-home comfort food. Feel free to make it with turkey sausage, if you prefer.

1-pound (455 g) roll pork sausage
1 apple

1 medium onion
1½ teaspoons chicken bouillon granules
1 cup (240 ml) water
Guar or xanthan
Salt and pepper to taste
1 batch The Ultimate Fauxtatoes (page 209)

Preheat oven to 350°F (180°C, or gas mark 4).

Slice the pork sausage into patties. Put them in a big, heavy skillet over medium heat. You're going to cook them until they're browned on both sides.

In the meantime, slice the apple and the onion thinly and have them standing by.

When the sausage patties are cooked, lay them in an 8 x 8-inch (20 x 20-cm) baking dish you've sprayed with nonstick cooking spray. Now put the apple and onion slices in the skillet and sauté them in the sausage grease until they're tender and turning golden. Spread the apples and onions on top of the sausage in the baking dish.

Put the chicken bouillon and the water in the skillet and stir it around, scraping up any tasty brown stuff stuck to the skillet. Thicken the whole thing to a not-too-thick gravy consistency with guar or xanthan, season with salt and pepper to taste, and pour this gravy over the sausage, apple, and onion.

Now spread the Ultimate Fauxtatoes in an even layer over the whole thing. Bake for 20 minutes and serve.

Yield: 4 to 5 servings

Assuming 4, each will have 24 g protein; 22 g carbohydrate; 9 g dietary fiber; 13 g usable carbs.

Sausage Skillet Mix-Up

1 pound (455 g) bulk pork sausage, hot
 or mild
1 small onion, chopped
2 ribs celery, chopped
1 green pepper, chopped
1 cup (240 ml) chicken broth
2 teaspoons chicken bouillon powder
2 tablespoons (30 ml) Worcestershire sauce
½ teaspoon pepper
3 cups (450 g) Cauliflower Rice (page 212)

Brown and crumble the sausage in a heavy skillet over medium-high heat. When the sausage is no longer pink, pour off the grease, add the remaining ingredients, and give the mixture a stir.

Turn the heat to low, cover the skillet, and let it simmer for 15 to 20 minutes or until the cauliflower is tender.

Yield: 3 servings

Each with 16 grams of carbohydrates and 4 grams of fiber, for a total of 12 grams of usable carbs and 22 grams of protein.

Greek Meatza

A good recipe deserves a variation! Here's my new, Greek-style version of meat-crust pizza.

2 pounds (910 g) ground lamb
½ medium onion, minced
4 cloves garlic, crushed
1½ teaspoons dried oregano

1 teaspoon salt
½ cup (120 ml) pizza sauce (Ragu makes one
 with no sugar, but read the label!)
10 ounces (280 g) frozen chopped spinach,
 thawed and very well-drained
⅓ cup (35 g) sliced black olives
½ cup (120 ml) canned diced tomatoes, drained
2 cups (240 g) shredded Monterey Jack cheese
1 cup (150 g) crumbled feta cheese

Preheat oven to 350°F (180°C, or gas mark 4).

Plunk the first five ingredients in a large mixing bowl and use clean hands to moosh everything together really well. Pat out into an even layer in a 9 x 13-inch (23 x 33-cm) pan and bake for 20 minutes. Pour off the grease.

Spread the pizza sauce over the meat layer. Spread the spinach evenly over the sauce and then top that with the olives and tomatoes. Spread the two cheeses over that. Turn the broiler to low and broil about 4 inches (10 cm) from the heat for about 6 to 8 minutes or until browned and bubbly.

Yield: 8 servings

Each with 30 g protein; 7 g carbohydrate; 2 g dietary fiber; 5 g usable carbs.

Kofta Burgers

Kofta kebabs are kebabs of curried ground lamb formed around skewers. It seemed to me that it would be easier just to make my seasoned lamb into burgers, so that's what I did.

(continued on page 448)

2 pounds (910 g) ground lamb
1 cup (160 g) minced onion
2 tablespoons curry powder
¼ cup (60 g) plain yogurt
2 cloves garlic, crushed

Just plop everything into a mixing bowl—do make sure your onion is pretty finely minced or your burgers will want to crumble on you—and use clean hands to smoosh it all together until it's well blended. Form into 6 burgers about 1 inch (2.5 cm) thick. Chill them for an hour before grilling; then grill over a medium fire for 7 to 10 minutes per side. Serve with Cucumber-Yogurt Sauce (follows).

Yield: 6 servings

Exclusive of the sauce, each will have 4 grams of carbohydrate and 1 gram of fiber, for a usable carb count of 3 grams; 26 grams protein.

Cucumber-Yogurt Sauce
½ cup (60 g) shredded cucumber
1 cup (230 g) plain yogurt
1 clove garlic, crushed
¼ teaspoon salt
1 pinch ground cumin
1 pinch coriander
4 tablespoons (16 g) chopped cilantro

Plunk the shredded cucumber into a strainer over a bowl or in the sink to let some moisture drain out of it. Open the yogurt and pour off any whey (clear liquid) that's gathered. Dump the yogurt into a bowl and add the garlic, salt, cumin, and coriander. Now go back to the cucumber and press it with clean hands or the back of a spoon to get most of the water out. Add the drained

cucumber into the bowl with the yogurt and stir everything up. Add the cilantro, stir again, and serve with Kofta Burgers or anything curried.

Yield: 6 servings.

Each serving will have 3 grams of carb—actually closer to 2, if you use the GO-Diet's figure of 4 grams per cup of plain yogurt—a trace of fiber, and 2 grams of protein.

Orange Lamb Burgers

Don't bother grinding your own lamb in your food processor; I tried this, and it came out a bit gristly. Buy ground lamb, instead. If you can't find ground lamb at your grocery store, ask the nice meat guy.

1 pound (455 g) ground lamb
¼ large sweet red onion
2 cloves garlic or 1 teaspoon minced garlic
1 teaspoon ground cumin
1½ tablespoons (23 ml) soy sauce
2 teaspoons grated orange zest
2 tablespoons (30 ml) orange juice
2 tablespoons (8 g) chopped cilantro
¼ teaspoon salt
½ teaspoon pepper

Preheat an electric tabletop grill.

Either chop the red onion and the garlic to a medium-fine consistency in a food processor using the S-blade or cut up with a knife. Then put them, the lamb, cumin, soy sauce, orange zest, orange juice, cilantro, salt, and pepper in a big bowl. Using clean hands, smoosh everything together until it's all very well blended. Form the mixture into 4 burgers and put them on the grill. Cook for 7 minutes and serve.

Yield: 4 servings

Each with 3 grams of carbohydrates, a trace of fiber, and 20 grams of protein.

Quick Curried Lamb

I invented this for a quick lunch for my husband one day when there just happened to be a hunk of lamb in the fridge that needed to be used. It was so good, I decided it was worth repeating.

1 pound (455 g) lean lamb, cut in ½-inch (1.3-cm) cubes
3 tablespoons (42 g) butter
1 tablespoon (6 g) curry powder
1 clove garlic
1 large onion
Salt and pepper

Melt the butter in a heavy skillet over medium heat. Add the curry powder and stir for a minute or so.

Add the garlic, onion, and lamb. Sauté, stirring frequently, for 7 minutes or until the lamb is cooked through. Sprinkle with salt and pepper to taste and serve.

Yield: 3 servings

Each with 5 grams of carbohydrates and 1 gram of fiber, for a total of 4 grams of usable carbs and 31 grams of protein.

Lamb Kebabs

This dish is very simple and very Greek. Add a Greek salad, and there's dinner.

2 pounds (910 g) lean lamb, cut into 1-inch (2.5-cm) cubes
½ cup (120 ml) olive oil
¼ cup (60 ml) lemon juice
1 clove garlic, crushed
½ teaspoon dried oregano
2 small onions, quartered

Put the lamb cubes into a large resealable plastic bag.

Mix together the olive oil, lemon juice, garlic, and oregano. Reserve some marinade for basting and pour the rest over the lamb cubes in the bag. Refrigerate it for an hour or two (or overnight, if possible).

When it's time to cook dinner, take out the lamb and pour off the marinade. Thread the lamb chunks on skewers, alternating the pieces of meat with a "layer" or two of the onion. You can grill these, if you like, or broil them 8 inches (20 cm) or so from the broiler. Turn the kebabs while they're cooking and brush once or twice with the reserved marinade using a clean utensil each time. Check for doneness by cutting into a chunk of meat after 10 minutes; they should be done within 15 minutes.

Yield: I get 6 skewers from this

Each with 4 grams of carbohydrates and 1 gram of fiber, for a total of 3 grams of usable carbs and 31 grams of protein.

Middle Eastern Shish Kebabs

Serve this with a cucumber-tomato salad for a Middle Eastern feast.

1½ pounds (680 g) boneless lamb (leg or shoulder)
½ cup (120 ml) olive oil
½ cup (120 ml) red wine vinegar
1 clove garlic, crushed
1 teaspoon ground cumin
1 medium onion
Salt and pepper

Cut the lamb into cubes about 1½ inches (4 cm) square. Put them in a nonreactive bowl or in a large resealable plastic bag. Mix together the olive oil, vinegar, garlic, and cumin. Reserve some marinade for basting and pour the rest over the lamb cubes. If using a bowl, stir to make sure cubes are coated. If using a bag, press out the air, seal the bag, and turn it a few times to coat. Either way, let the lamb marinate for at least several hours. If you're going to use bamboo skewers, this is a good time to put them in water to soak. You'll need 4 skewers.

Okay, dinnertime has rolled around. Get a fire going—you'll want to set a gas grill at medium-low or let charcoal cook down pretty well. While that's happening, let's make kebabs.

Peel the onion and cut it into quarters, then into eighths, and separate it into the individual layers. Drain the lamb cubes. Skewer a lamb cube, then a layer of onion, then another lamb cube, and so forth, filling all four skewers evenly. Sprinkle the kebabs with salt and pepper and throw them on the fire. Grill the skewers slowly. Turn often and baste with the reserved marinade, using a clean utensil each time, until the meat is well done and tender—at least 20 minutes.

Yield: 4 servings

If you consume all the marinade, each serving will have 5 grams of carbohydrate and 1 gram of fiber. Since you don't, I'd count 3 grams per kebab, and 35 grams of protein.

Fiery Indian Lamb and Cauliflower

This is a fairly authentic Indian dish, and it is quite hot! Feel free to halve the red pepper if you like it milder.

1 pound (455 g) lean lamb
4 cloves garlic, crushed
2 teaspoons grated ginger
2 teaspoons red pepper flakes
1½ teaspoons ground cumin
2 teaspoons pepper
2 tablespoons (28 g) butter
1 tablespoon (15 ml) olive oil
1 medium onion, chopped
½ cup (115 g) plain yogurt
½ head cauliflower, in small florets
Salt to taste

Trim the lamb well and cut it into ½- to 1-inch (1.3- to 2.5-cm) cubes.

Put it in a mixing bowl and add the garlic, ginger, red pepper, cumin, and pepper. Stir to coat all the lamb cubes evenly and let the lamb sit in this dry marinade for at least 15 minutes.

Melt the butter in a large, heavy skillet over medium-low heat and add the olive oil. Now add the onion and sauté until it's translucent and turning golden. Stir in the yogurt until smooth. Now add the lamb cubes and stir to coat. Let this cook on low heat until the lamb cubes are no longer pink and all excess water has cooked off the yogurt.

Now add 1 cup (240 ml) water and let the lamb simmer until the liquid is reduced by half and the lamb cubes are quite tender. Stir in the cauliflower, cover, and let the whole thing simmer for 15 minutes or until the cauliflower is tender. Uncover, simmer another 5 minutes to boil off extra liquid, and season with salt to taste. Serve.

Yield: 3 to 4 servings

Assuming 3, each will have 24 g protein; 9 g carbohydrate; 2 g dietary fiber; 7 g usable carbs.

Spanish Skillet Lamb

This authentically Spanish skillet dish is quick, easy, and tasty.

16 ounces (455 g) lamb leg (Cutting up a lamb steak or two is good.)
¼ cup (40 g) chopped onion
2 tablespoons (30 ml) olive oil
2 cloves garlic, crushed
2 teaspoons paprika
2 tablespoons (30 ml) lemon juice

Cut the lamb into strips—make sure it's well trimmed of fat. In a big, heavy skillet over high heat, start sautéing the lamb and onion in the olive oil. When the lamb is getting browned all over, stir in the garlic, paprika, and lemon juice.

Turn the heat to medium-low, cover, and let the whole thing simmer for about 15 minutes—check once or twice to make sure your pan hasn't gone dry and add just a little water if it's threatening to. Serve over Cauliflower Rice (page 212) if you like, but this is just fine the way it is.

Yield: 2 to 3 servings

Assuming 3, each will have 22 g protein; 4 g carbohydrate; 1 g dietary fiber; 3 g usable carbs. Analysis does not include Cauliflower Rice.

Balsamic Lamb Skillet

This dish is rich, different, and good!

1 pound (455 g) lamb leg or shoulder, thinly sliced and cut into strips
½ teaspoon minced garlic or 1 clove garlic, crushed
½ medium onion, sliced
¼ cup (60 ml) olive oil
½ red bell pepper, sliced into small strips
1-pound (455-g) bag triple-washed fresh spinach
¼ cup (60 ml) balsamic vinegar
Salt and pepper
Guar or xanthan
4 tablespoons (35 g) toasted pine nuts

(continued on page 452)

Over high heat, start sautéing the lamb, garlic, and onion in the olive oil. When the pinkness has faded from the lamb, add the red bell pepper.

When the lamb is cooked through and the onion is limp, add the spinach. You may have to add it in two or three batches to keep it from overwhelming your skillet, but it wilts quite quickly. Stir until the spinach is just barely limp. Don't overcook!

Stir in the balsamic vinegar and salt and pepper to taste (I like plenty of pepper in this) and thicken the pan juices with a sprinkle of guar or xanthan, if desired. Top each serving with a tablespoon (9 g) of toasted pine nuts and serve.

Yield: 4 servings

Each with 9 grams of carbohydrates and 4 grams of fiber, for a total of 5 grams of usable carbs and 20 grams of protein.

Mediterranean Leg of Lamb

Lamb makes a wonderful Sunday dinner roast. If you don't want to roast a whole leg of lamb at once because it's a lot of meat, ask the butcher to cut one leg into two roasts. Make half now and freeze the other half for another day.

Leg of lamb, with or without the bone in
1 cup (240 ml) dry red wine
1 cup (240 ml) olive oil, divided
5 cloves garlic, crushed, divided
3 tablespoons (45 ml) lemon juice
1 tablespoon (3.6 g) dried rosemary
1 tablespoon (5.4 g) dried oregano

Place the leg of lamb in a pan large enough to hold it.

Combine the wine, ½ cup (120 ml) of the olive oil, 3 cloves of the garlic, and the lemon juice, rosemary, and oregano. Pour this marinade over the lamb and let the lamb sit in it for at least 5 to 6 hours, turning it from time to time.

When the time comes to cook your lamb, preheat the oven to 425°F (220°C, or gas mark 7). Remove the meat from the marinade and place it on a rack in a roasting pan. Leave the rosemary needles and bits of oregano clinging to it.

Combine the remaining olive oil and cloves of garlic and spoon this mixture over the lamb, coating the whole leg. Position the leg with the fat side up and insert a meat thermometer deep into the center of the thickest part of the meat, but don't let it touch the bone.

When the oven is up to temperature, put the roast in and set the timer for 10 minutes. After 10 minutes, turn the oven down to 350°F (180°C, or gas mark 4) and roast for about 30 minutes per pound of meat or until the meat thermometer registers 170 to 180°F (77 to 82°C). Remove the lamb from the oven and let it sit for 15 to 20 minutes before carving.

Yield: 3 servings per pound

Each with no carbohydrates or fiber to speak of, and about 21 grams of protein. (This sounds low, I know, but remember: Part of that weight is bone.)

Serve this with some Cauliflower Rice (page 212) and make Lamb Gravy to go with your roast lamb by combining the drippings from the lamb roast with 1 cup (240 ml) chicken broth, ¾ teaspoon guar or xanthan, and salt and pepper to taste.

First, skim the fat off of the drippings from the roast. Then pour ½ cup (120 ml) of the chicken broth into the roasting pan with the skimmed drippings and stir it around, scraping up the yummy browned bits from the rack and the bottom of the pan. When most of the stuck-on stuff is dissolved into the broth, put the roasting pan over medium-high heat. Put the rest of the chicken broth in a blender with the guar or xanthan and run the blender for a few seconds to dissolve all of the thickener. Pour the thickened broth into the roasting pan and stir until all the gravy is thickened. (If it gets too thick, add a little more chicken broth; if it's not quite thick enough, let it simmer for a few minutes to cook down.) Season with salt and pepper to taste.

Spice-Rubbed Leg of Lamb with Apricot-Chipotle Glaze

A whole leg of lamb will feed a crowd! If you don't have a crowd, feel free to ask the nice meat guys to cut your leg of lamb in half. Keep the tapered shank end for your roast and make half the rub and glaze. Have the broader end sliced ½-inch (1.3-cm) thick for lamb steaks. I've never been charged for this service!

Leg of lamb, about 8 pounds (3.6 kg)
¼ cup (30 g) paprika
1 tablespoon (6.3 g) ground cumin
1 tablespoon (6.9 g) ground cinnamon
1 tablespoon (1.8 g) ground coriander
2 teaspoons garlic powder
1 teaspoon salt or Vege-Sal
1 teaspoon pepper
2 tablespoons (3 g) Splenda
Apricot-Chipotle Glaze (page 482)

Combine all the spices with the Splenda and stir well. Sprinkle liberally over the leg of lamb, coating the whole surface. Roast at 325°F (170°C, or gas mark 3) for 30 minutes per pound of lamb.

About 30 minutes before cooking time is up, start basting with the Apricot-Chipotle Glaze. Baste two or three times before the cooking time is through. Remove lamb from oven and allow to rest for 10 to 15 minutes before carving. Serve with remaining Apricot-Chipotle Glaze.

Yield: 15 to 16 servings, so invite a crowd

Assuming 15, each will have 35 g protein; 6 g carbohydrate; 1 g dietary fiber; 5 g usable carbs.

Caribbean Slow Cooker Lamb

Lamb and goat are very popular in the Caribbean, and this is my slow cooker interpretation of a Caribbean lamb dish. Look for tamarind concentrate in a grocery store with a good international section. I found it in a medium-size town in southern Indiana, so you may well find it near you! If you can't find it, you could use a tablespoon (15 ml) of lemon juice and a teaspoon of Splenda instead. Your lamb will be less authentically Caribbean-tasting, but it'll still be yummy.

(continued on page 454)

2- to 3-pound section (910 g to 1.4 kg) of a leg
    of lamb

½ medium onion, chopped

½ teaspoon minced garlic or 1 clove garlic,
    crushed

1 teaspoon tamarind concentrate

1 tablespoon (15 ml) spicy brown mustard

1 cup (240 ml) canned diced tomatoes

1 teaspoon hot pepper sauce (preferably
    Caribbean Scotch Bonnet sauce) or more or
    less to taste

Guar or xanthan (optional)

Salt and pepper

Place the lamb in a slow cooker.

In a bowl, stir together the onion, garlic, tamarind, mustard, tomatoes, and hot pepper sauce. Pour the mixture over the lamb. Cover the slow cooker, set it to low, and let it cook for a good 8 hours. When it's done, remove the lamb to a serving platter, thicken the pot juices with the guar or xanthan if it seems necessary, and add salt and pepper to taste.

Yield: 6 servings

Each with 27 g protein, 3 g carbohydrate, 1 g dietary fiber, 2 g usable carbs.

Lamb Shanks in Red Wine

This is a hearty one-pot meal.

5 pounds (2.3 kg) lamb shank (4 shanks)

¼ cup (60 ml) olive oil

2 stalks celery, sliced ½ inch (1.3 cm) thick

2 carrots, sliced ½ inch (1.3 cm) thick

8 cloves garlic, crushed

½ onion, chunked

8 ounces (225 g) sliced mushrooms

1 cup (240 ml) chicken broth

1 cup (240 ml) dry red wine

1 teaspoon beef bouillon concentrate

2 teaspoons pepper

½ teaspoon ground rosemary

2 bay leaves

Guar or xanthan

In a big, heavy skillet, sear the lamb all over in the oil.

Place the celery, carrots, garlic, onion, and mushrooms in a slow cooker.

When the lamb is browned all over, transfer it to the slow cooker on top of the vegetables.

In a bowl, stir together the broth, wine, bouillon, pepper, and rosemary. Pour the mixture over the lamb. Add the bay leaves. (Make sure they land in the liquid!) Cover the slow cooker, turn it to low, and let it cook for 6 hours.

When the time's up, remove the lamb to serving plates. Remove the bay leaves. Using guar or xanthan, thicken the liquid in the slow cooker to the consistency of heavy cream. Ladle the sauce and vegetables over the lamb.

Yield: 6 servings

Each with 59 g protein, 8 g carbohydrate, 2 g dietary fiber, 6 g usable carbs.

Lemon Lamb Shanks

Lemon brings out the best in lamb!

4 pounds (910 g) lamb shank
2 tablespoons (30 ml) olive oil
1 teaspoon lemon pepper
½ teaspoon dry mustard
½ cup (120 ml) chicken broth
1 teaspoon beef bouillon concentrate
½ teaspoon grated lemon peel
2 tablespoons (30 ml) lemon juice
1 teaspoon dried rosemary
2 cloves garlic, crushed
Guar or xanthan

Sear the lamb all over in the oil. Place the lamb in a slow cooker.

In a bowl, mix together the lemon pepper and dry mustard. Sprinkle the mixture evenly over the lamb.

In the same bowl, mix together the broth, bouillon, lemon peel, lemon juice, rosemary, and garlic. Pour the mixture over the lamb. Cover the slow cooker, set it to low, and let it cook for 8 hours.

When the time's up, remove the lamb and thicken up the liquid in the slow cooker a bit with guar or xanthan.

Serve this dish with a salad with plenty of cucumbers and tomatoes!

Yield: 6 servings

Each with 46 g protein, 1 g carbohydrate, trace dietary fiber, 1 g usable carbs. Analysis does not include side dishes.

Seriously Simple Lamb Shanks

Simple is good!

3 pounds (1.4 kg) lamb shank
2 tablespoons (30 ml) olive oil
1 cup (240 ml) chicken broth
1 teaspoon beef bouillon concentrate
2 teaspoons paprika
5 cloves garlic, crushed
Guar or xanthan

Season the lamb all over with salt and pepper. In a big, heavy skillet over medium-high heat, sear the lamb in the oil until it's brown all over. Transfer the lamb to a slow cooker.

In a bowl, mix together the broth and bouillon. Pour the mixture over the lamb. Sprinkle the paprika and garlic over the lamb. Cover the slow cooker, set it to low, and let it cook for 6 to 7 hours.

Remove the lamb with tongs and put it on a serving plate. Pour the liquid in the slow cooker into a 2-cup (480-ml) glass measuring cup and let the fat rise to the top. Skim the fat off and discard. Thicken up the remaining liquid using guar or xanthan. Serve the sauce with the shanks.

Either Cauliflower Rice (page 212) or Fauxtatoes (page 209) would be nice with this, but it's fine with just a simple salad or vegetable side.

Yield: 4 servings

Each with 52 g protein, 2 g carbohydrate, trace dietary fiber, 2 g usable carbs. Analysis does not include side dishes.

About Lamb Steaks

Everyone's heard of lamb chops, but I prefer lamb steaks. I buy a whole leg of lamb and ask the nice meat guy behind the counter to cut two smallish roasts off either end (a perfect size for my two-person household) and slice the rest into steaks between ½ inch (1.3 cm) and ¾ inch (2 cm) thick. These are meatier than lamb chops and generally less expensive, as well. Here are some things to do with lamb steaks—but I suspect they'd all work with chops, too.

Five-Spice Lamb Steak

8 ounces (225 g) lamb leg steak
1 tablespoon (15 ml) oil
1 teaspoon grated ginger
1 clove garlic, crushed
2 tablespoons (30 ml) dry sherry
1 teaspoon five-spice powder
½ teaspoon Splenda
1 teaspoon soy sauce

Slash the edges of the lamb steak to keep it from curling. In a big, heavy skillet over medium heat, start pan-frying the lamb steak in the oil. You'll want to give them about 6 minutes per side.

While that's happening, mix together everything else. When the lamb steak is cooked on both sides, pour this mixture into the skillet. Turn the steak over once or twice to coat and let it cook just another minute or two. Serve with the pan liquid scraped over it.

Yield: 1 to 2 servings

Assuming 1, each will have 33 g protein; 2 g carbohydrate; trace dietary fiber; 2 g usable carbs.

Soy and Sesame Glazed Lamb Steaks

2 lamb steaks, 6 to 8 ounces (170 to 225 g) each, ½ inch (1.3 cm) thick
2 tablespoons (30 ml) olive oil
1 teaspoon minced garlic or 2 cloves garlic, crushed
2 scallions, minced
2 tablespoons (30 ml) soy sauce
1 teaspoon Splenda
6 drops or ¼ teaspoon blackstrap molasses*
2 teaspoons sesame oil

In a heavy skillet, start sautéing the lamb steaks in the oil over high heat. Cook for 5 to 6 minutes per side.

While the lamb is browning, prepare and combine the garlic, scallions, soy sauce, Splenda, molasses, and sesame oil.

Remove the lamb from the skillet, add the soy sauce mixture to the skillet, and stir it a bit.

Replace the lamb in the skillet, turn it once to coat with sauce, and cook it for another 1 to 2 minutes per side. Serve, scraping the liquid from the pan over the lamb steaks.

Yield: 2 servings

Assuming each steak is 6 ounces (170 g), each will have 4 grams of carbohydrates and 1 gram of fiber, for a total of 3 grams of usable carbs and 23 grams of protein.

*I keep my molasses in a squeeze container to make it easy to measure out very small quantities.

Lamb Steak with Walnut Sauce

8 ounces (225 g) lamb leg steak
Salt and pepper
1 tablespoon (15 ml) olive oil
2 tablespoons (20 g) minced onion
2 tablespoons (15 g) chopped walnuts
1 clove garlic
2 tablespoons (7.6 g) chopped parsley
¼ teaspoon dried oregano
¼ teaspoon ground rosemary
2 tablespoons (30 ml) lemon juice

Preheat an electric tabletop grill.

Rub the steak with a little olive oil and sprinkle both sides lightly with salt and pepper. When the grill is hot, put the steak on and set a timer for 5 to 6 minutes.

In a small, heavy skillet over medium-low heat, heat the olive oil and sauté the onion, walnuts, and garlic until the onion is soft. Stir in the parsley, oregano, and rosemary and cook another couple of minutes until the parsley is wilted. Stir in the lemon juice and let it simmer for a minute or so.

By now the lamb steak is done. Pull it out, throw it on a plate, and spoon the walnut sauce over it. Serve.

Yield: 1 to 2 servings

Assuming 1, each will have 37 g protein; 8 g carbohydrate; 2 g dietary fiber; 6 g usable carbs.

Barbecued Lamb Steaks

2 lamb steaks, 6 to 8 ounces each (170 to 225 g), ½ inch (1.3 cm) thick
1 tablespoon plus 1 teaspoon (20 ml) sugar-free ketchup
1 tablespoon plus 1 teaspoon (20 ml) cider vinegar
1 tablespoon plus 1 teaspoon (20 ml) Worcestershire sauce
1 teaspoon spicy brown mustard

Broil the lamb steaks close to the flame for 6 to 7 minutes. While the steaks are cooking, combine the ketchup, vinegar, Worcestershire sauce, and mustard.

Turn the steaks and broil the second side for 3 to 4 minutes. Spoon the sauce over the steaks and broil for another 2 to 3 minutes. Serve.

Yield: 2 servings

Assuming each steak is 6 ounces (170 g), each will have 4 grams of carbohydrates, a trace of fiber, and 23 grams of protein.

Orange-Rosemary Lamb Steak

8 ounces (225 g) lamb leg steak
1 tablespoon (15 ml) olive oil
1½ teaspoons butter
2 tablespoons (30 ml) lemon juice
¼ teaspoon orange extract
1 teaspoon Splenda
½ teaspoon ground rosemary

Slash the edges of the lamb steak to keep it from curling.

Put a big, heavy skillet over medium heat and add the olive oil and butter, swirling them together as the butter melts. Add the lamb steak and cook it about 5 to 6 minutes per side. Remove to serving plate.

While the lamb steak is cooking, stir together the lemon juice, orange extract, and Splenda. When you've removed the steak from the skillet, add the lemon juice mixture and stir it around, scraping up the browned bits from the bottom of the skillet. Stir in the rosemary and let the whole thing simmer for a moment or two. Pour this sauce over the lamb steak and serve.

Yield: 1 to 2 servings

Assuming 1, each will have 32 g protein; 3 g carbohydrate; trace dietary fiber; 3 g usable carbs.

Thyme-Perfumed Lamb Steaks

1 lamb steak (6 to 8 ounces, or 170 to 225 g)
2 teaspoons olive oil
2 teaspoons lemon juice
1 tablespoon (2.4 g) fresh thyme leaves, stripped from their stems.

Rub the lamb steak with the olive oil and then the lemon juice. Cover the lamb with the thyme leaves, letting it sit for at least a couple of hours so the thyme flavor permeates the lamb.

Broil close to the heat for 4 to 5 minutes per side or grill.

Yield: 1 serving

1 gram of carbohydrates, a trace of fiber, and 30 grams or so of protein.

Balsamic-Mint Lamb Steak

8 ounces (225 g) lamb leg steak
2 tablespoons (30 ml) olive oil
¼ teaspoon beef bouillon concentrate
1 tablespoon (15 ml) boiling water
1 tablespoon (15 ml) balsamic vinegar
1 teaspoon chopped fresh mint

Slash the edges of the lamb steak to keep it from curling. Then heat the olive oil over medium-high heat in a big, heavy skillet and start the steak sautéing. You'll want to cook it 5 to 7 minutes per side.

Meanwhile, dissolve the bouillon concentrate in the water and stir in the balsamic vinegar.

When the steak is done to your liking, remove it to a serving plate and pour the bouillion-vinegar mixture into the skillet. Stir it around to dissolve the yummy brown stuff stuck to the skillet and then stir in the mint. Pour this sauce over the steak and serve.

Yield: 1 serving

32 g protein; 1 g carbohydrate; trace dietary fiber; 1 g usable carb.

Curried Lamb Steak

2 lamb steaks, 6 to 8 ounces (170 to 225 g) each, ½ inch (1.3 cm) thick
2 tablespoons (28 g) butter
2 teaspoons curry powder
1 teaspoon minced garlic or 2 cloves garlic, crushed

Melt the butter in large, heavy skillet over medium heat. Add the curry powder and garlic, stir, and add the lamb steak. Cover with a tilted lid and cook for 7 minutes. Turn, re-cover with a tilted lid, and cook for another 7 minutes. Remove the lamb to serving plates, scrape the curry butter over the steaks, and serve.

Yield: 2 servings

Assuming each steak is 6 ounces (170 g), each will have 2 grams of carbohydrates and 1 gram of fiber, for a total of 1 gram of usable carbs and 23 grams of protein.

Cape Town Lamb Steaks

You can use lamb chops instead, but as I mentioned earlier, I like steaks cut from a leg of lamb. When I buy a whole leg, I ask the nice meat guy to slice some steaks from the center, leaving me two small roasts from either end. Since leg of lamb is often as cheap as $1.99 a pound around here, while lamb chops are usually over $4.99 a pound, this is also economical!

1 pound (455 g) lamb leg steaks, about ½ inch (1.3 cm) thick
2 tablespoons (30 ml) Worcestershire sauce
2 tablespoons (30 ml) soy sauce
2 tablespoons (3 g) Splenda
¼ teaspoon blackstrap molasses
1 tablespoon plus 1 teaspoon (9.6 g) dry mustard
1 tablespoon plus 1 teaspoon (20 ml) lemon juice
1 tablespoon plus 1 teaspoon (20 ml) olive oil
2 cloves garlic, crushed
2 teaspoons grated ginger

First get a grill going—set your gas grill to medium to medium-low or let your coals get thoroughly white.

Mix together everything but the steaks. Pour some sauce into a small bowl and brush the steaks liberally with the sauce remaining. Grill for about 7 minutes per side, basting frequently. With the reserved sauce and using a clean utensil. If you like, bring any leftover sauce to a boil (to prevent cross-contamination) and serve with the steaks at the table.

(continued on page 460)

Yield: 2 servings

If you do eat all of the sauce, each serving will have 5 grams of carbohydrate, a trace of fiber, and 33 grams of protein.

Winter Night Lamb Stew

On a raw winter's night, sometimes you just want stew. Here's one with no potatoes, and you can make it in your big skillet.

1½ pounds (680 g) lean lamb stew meat, cut into chunks
3 tablespoons (45 ml) olive oil
1 cup (160 g) chopped onion
1½ cups (225 g) diced turnip
1½ cups (225 g) diced rutabaga
¾ cup (180 ml) beef broth
½ teaspoon guar or xanthan (optional)
½ teaspoon salt or Vege-Sal
¼ teaspoon pepper
1 bay leaf
3 cloves garlic, crushed

Put the oil in a heavy skillet over medium-high heat and brown the lamb in the oil. Add the onion, turnip, and rutabaga.

Put the beef broth and guar in a blender and blend for a few moments. Pour the mixture into the skillet. (If you choose not to use a thickener, just add the broth directly to the skillet.) Add the salt, pepper, bay leaf, and garlic, and stir.

Cover, turn the heat to low, and let simmer for 1 hour. Remove the bay leaf before serving.

Yield: 4 servings

Each with 12 grams of carbohydrates and 3 grams of fiber, for a total of 9 grams of usable carbs and 38 grams of protein.

Lamb Stew Provençal

I turned this recipe over to my sister to test. She's mad for French food, especially from Provence. She gave this the thumbs-up.

3 pounds (1.4 kg) lamb stew meat—shoulder is good, cubed (Have the meat guys cut it off the bone.)
Salt and pepper
3 tablespoons (45 ml) olive oil
1 whole fennel bulb, sliced lengthwise
1 medium onion, sliced lengthwise
4 cloves garlic, crushed
1 bay leaf
1 teaspoon dried rosemary, whole needles
1 can (15 ounces, or 425 g) black soybeans, drained
1 cup (240 ml) beef broth
1 teaspoon chicken bouillon concentrate
½ teaspoon dried basil
½ teaspoon dried marjoram
½ teaspoon dried savory
½ teaspoon dried thyme
Guar or xanthan

Season the lamb with salt and pepper. In a big, heavy skillet, heat the oil and brown the lamb on all sides over medium-high heat.

Place the fennel, onion, and garlic in the bottom of a slow cooker. Add the bay leaf and rosemary. Dump the soybeans on top of that. When the lamb is browned, put it on top of the vegetables.

In a bowl, stir together the broth, bouillon, basil, marjoram, savory, and thyme. Pour the mixture over the lamb. Cover the slow cooker, set it to low, and let it cook for 8 to 9 hours. When it's done, thicken the liquid to the texture of heavy cream with guar or xanthan. Remove the bay leaf before serving.

Yield: 8 servings

Each with 41 g protein, 8 g carbohydrate, 4 g dietary fiber, 4 g usable carbs.

Irish Stew

I came up with this for St. Patrick's Day, and it's amazing. The Ketatoes mix gives it a true potato flavor, while keeping the carb count remarkably low. This takes time, but not that much work—so make it on a day when you're hanging around the house getting chores done.

2 pounds (910 g) leg of lamb, cut in 1 inch (2.5 cm) cubes
2 large turnips, cut in ½ inch (1.3 cm) cubes
½ head cauliflower, cut in ½ inch (1.3 cm) cubes or chunks
3 medium onions, sliced
½ cup (25 g) Ketatoes mix
Salt and pepper

Water to cover
½ teaspoon chicken bouillon concentrate
½ teaspoon beef bouillon concentrate
Guar or xanthan

You'll need the meat and vegetables all cut up before you do anything else; make sure the lamb cubes are well trimmed of all fat. Spray a Dutch oven or large, heavy soup pot with nonstick cooking spray.

Now, put a layer of mixed turnip and cauliflower in the bottom of the pot. Add a layer of onion. Scatter 2 tablespoons (6 g) of the Ketatoes mix over that and then put in a layer of cubed lamb. Season the lamb with salt and pepper. Now repeat the layers two more times, at which point you should be out of meat and vegetables.

Pour cold water over everything to just barely cover. Put a lid on the pot and set it over the lowest possible heat. Let it simmer for 2 hours.

Take the lid off and stir in the chicken and beef bouillon concentrate. Now, continue to simmer over lowest heat, uncovered, for another 2 hours or so—you're cooking down the gravy a little.

Finally, using a whisk and guar or xanthan, thicken up the gravy. Add salt and pepper to taste and then serve.

Yield: 8 servings

Each with 29 g protein; 13 g carbohydrate; 5 g dietary fiber; 8 g usable carbs.

13

Sauces and Seasonings

Dana's No-Sugar Ketchup

Ketchup is an essential ingredient in so many recipes, but store-bought ketchup usually has so much sugar. Recently, commercially-made low-carb ketchup has been appearing in the grocery stores. If you can get this, do so because food manufacturers can get ingredients the home cook cannot, so store-bought low-carb ketchup is lower in carbs than this. If you can't find low-carb ketchup, however, this is easy to make, tastes great, and is about half the carbs of regular ketchup. Be aware that recipes in this book that list ketchup as an ingredient are analyzed for this homemade version, so if you use commercial low-carb ketchup, the carb counts will be a tad lower.

1 can (6 ounces, or 170 g) tomato paste
⅔ cup (160 ml) cider vinegar
⅓ cup (80 ml) water
⅓ cup (8 g) Splenda
2 tablespoons (20 g) minced onion
2 cloves garlic
1 teaspoon salt
⅛ teaspoon ground allspice
⅛ teaspoon ground cloves
⅛ teaspoon pepper

Put everything in a blender and run it until the onion disappears. Scrape it into a container with a tight lid and store it in the refrigerator.

Yield: Makes roughly 1½ cups (360 ml), or 12 servings of 2 tablespoons (30 ml)

Each with 1 g protein, 5 g carbohydrate, 1 g fiber, 4 g usable carbs.

Stir-Fry Sauce

If you like Chinese food, make this up and keep it on hand. Then you can just throw any sort of meat and vegetables in your wok or skillet and have a meal in minutes.

½ cup (120 ml) soy sauce
½ cup (120 ml) dry sherry
2 cloves garlic, crushed, or 1 teaspoon minced garlic
2 tablespoons (12 g) grated fresh ginger
2 teaspoons Splenda

Simply combine everything and store in a tightly sealed container in the refrigerator.

Yield: Makes 1 cup (240 ml). Use about 1½ to 2 tablespoons (23 to 30 ml) per serving of stir-fry.

Each serving contains 2 grams of carbohydrates, no fiber, and no protein.

Thai Peanut Sauce

½ teaspoon hot sauce
1 tablespoon (6 g) grated ginger
1 clove garlic, crushed
2 scallions, sliced, including the crisp part of the green
⅓ cup (85 g) natural peanut butter
⅓ cup (80 ml) coconut milk (You can find this in cans in Asian markets or grocery stores with good international sections.)
2 tablespoons (30 ml) fish sauce (nam pla or nuoc mam)

(continued on page 464)

1½ tablespoons (23 ml) lime juice
2 teaspoons Splenda

Put everything in a blender or in a food processor with the S-blade in place and process until smooth.

Yield: Makes roughly 1 cup (240 ml), or 8 servings of 2 tablespoons (30 ml) each

4 grams of carbohydrate per serving, and 1 gram of fiber, for a usable carb count of 3 grams; 3 grams of protein.

Not-Very-Authentic Peanut Sauce

This is inauthentic because I used substitutes for such traditional ingredients as lemongrass and fish sauce. I wanted a recipe that tasted good but could be made without a trip to specialty grocery store.

1 piece of fresh ginger about the size of a walnut, peeled and thinly sliced across the grain
½ cup (130 g) natural peanut butter, creamy
½ cup (120 ml) chicken broth
1½ teaspoons lemon juice
1½ teaspoons soy sauce
¼ teaspoon hot pepper sauce
1 large or 2 small cloves garlic, crushed
1½ teaspoons Splenda

Put all the ingredients in a blender and run it until everything is well combined and smooth. If you'd

like it a little thinner, add another tablespoon (15 ml) of chicken broth.

Yield: About 2 cups, or 16 servings

Each with 2 grams of carbohydrates, a trace of fiber, and 2 grams of protein.

Hoisin Sauce

This Chinese sauce is usually made from fermented soybean paste, which has tons of sugar in it. Peanut butter is inauthentic, but it tastes quite good here.

¼ cup (60 ml) soy sauce
2 tablespoons (32 g) creamy natural peanut butter
2 tablespoons (3 g) Splenda
2 teaspoons white vinegar
1 clove garlic, crushed
2 teaspoons toasted sesame oil
⅛ teaspoon Chinese five-spice powder

Put all the ingredients in a blender and run it until everything is smooth and well combined. Store in a snap-top container.

Yield: Roughly ⅓ cup (80 ml)

Each 1 tablespoon (15 ml) serving contains 2 grams of carbohydrates, a trace of fiber, and 2 grams of protein.

Of course, this sauce is essential for Mu Shu Pork (page 418)—or Mu Shu anything, for that matter—but it's also good for dipping plain chicken wings in.

Duck Sauce

What are you going to eat duck sauce on, now that you're not eating egg rolls? Well, Crab and Bacon Bundles (page 77), for one thing. It's good with chicken, too. This does have the sugar that's in the peaches, of course, but not all the added sugar of commercial duck sauce. And it tastes better, too.

1 bag (1 pound, or 455 g) unsweetened frozen peaches or 2½ to 3 cups (500 to 600 g) sliced, peeled fresh peaches
½ cup (120 ml) water
2 tablespoons (30 ml) cider vinegar
2 tablespoons (3 g) Splenda
¼ teaspoon blackstrap molasses
⅛ teaspoon salt
1 teaspoon soy sauce
1 clove garlic, crushed

Put all the ingredients in a heavy-bottomed saucepan and bring them to a simmer. Cook, uncovered, until the peaches are soft (about 30 minutes).

Purée the duck sauce in a blender, if you like, or do what I do: simply mash the sauce with a potato masher or a fork. (I like the texture better this way.)

Yield: About 2 cups (480 ml)

Each 2 tablespoon (30 ml) serving has 3 grams of carbohydrates and 1 gram of fiber, for a total of 2 grams of usable carbs and no protein.

It's best to freeze this if you're not going to use it up right away.

Teriyaki Sauce

It's good on chicken, beef, fish—just about anything!

½ cup (120 ml) soy sauce
¼ cup (60 ml) dry sherry
1 clove garlic, crushed
2 tablespoons (3 g) Splenda
1 tablespoon (6 g) grated fresh ginger

Simply combine all ingredients.

Yield: Makes just over ¾ cup (180 ml)

About 3 g carbohydrate per tablespoonful.

Looing Sauce

This is a Chinese sauce for "red cooking." You stew things in it, and it imparts a wonderful flavor to just about any sort of meat.

2 cups (480 ml) soy sauce
1 star anise
½ cup (120 ml) dry sherry (The cheap stuff is fine.)
4 tablespoons (6 g) Splenda
1 tablespoon (6 g) grated fresh ginger
4 cups (960 ml) water

Combine the ingredients well and use the mixture to stew things in. After using Looing Sauce, you can strain it and refrigerate or freeze it to use again, if you like.

(continued on page 466)

Yield: 6½ cups (1.5 L) of looing sauce, or plenty to submerge your food in

In the whole batch there are about 50 grams of usable carbohydrates, but only a very small amount of that is transferred to the foods you stew in it.

Star anise is available in Oriental markets, and my natural food store carries it too. It actually does look like a star, and it's essential to the recipe. Don't try to substitute regular anise.

Cocktail Sauce

You'll need this for the Easy Party Shrimp (page 76)!

½ cup (120 ml) Dana's No-Sugar Ketchup
    (page 463) or purchased low-carb ketchup
2 teaspoons prepared horseradish
¼ teaspoon hot pepper sauce
1 teaspoon lemon juice

Combine all ingredients in a bowl and mix well.

Yield: Makes about ½ cup (120 ml)

The whole batch contains 5 g protein, 36 g carbohydrate, 6 g dietary fiber, 30 g usable carbs. Good thing you'll be sharing it! You can drop this carb count considerably by using commercially-made low-carb ketchup.

Cheese Sauce

Try this over broccoli or cauliflower. It's wonderful!

½ cup (120 ml) heavy cream
¾ cup (90 g) shredded cheddar cheese
¼ teaspoon dry mustard

In a heavy-bottomed saucepan over the lowest heat, warm the cream to just below a simmer.

Whisk in the cheese about 1 tablespoon at a time, only adding the next tablespoonful after the last one has melted. When all the cheese is melted in, whisk in the dry mustard and serve.

Yield: Enough to sauce 1 pound (455 g) of broccoli or cauliflower, or about 4 servings of sauce

Each with 1 gram of carbohydrates, no fiber, and 6 grams of protein.

Low-Carb Steak Sauce

¼ cup (60 ml) Dana's No-Sugar Ketchup
    (page 463)
1 tablespoon (15 ml) Worcestershire sauce
1 teaspoon lemon juice

Combine well and store in an airtight container in the fridge.

Yield: 5 servings of 1 tablespoon (15 ml)

Each with 2.25 grams of carbohydrates, a trace of fiber, and a trace of protein.

Reduced-Carb Spicy Barbecue Sauce

1 clove garlic, crushed

1 small onion, finely minced

¼ cup (56 g or 60 ml) butter or oil

4 tablespoons (6 g) Splenda

1 teaspoon salt or Vege-Sal

1 teaspoon dry mustard

1 teaspoon paprika

1 teaspoon chili powder

½ teaspoon black pepper

2 teaspoons blackstrap molasses

1½ cups (360 ml) water

¼ cup (60 ml) cider vinegar

1 tablespoon (15 ml) Worcestershire sauce

1 tablespoon (15 g) prepared horseradish

1 can (6 ounces, or 170 g) tomato paste

1 tablespoon (15 ml) liquid smoke flavoring
    (such as the one made by Colgin)

In a saucepan, cook the garlic and onion in the butter or oil for a few minutes.

Stir in the Splenda, salt, mustard, paprika, chili powder, and pepper. Add in the molasses, water, vinegar, Worcestershire sauce, and horseradish, and stir to combine. Let the mixture simmer for 15 to 20 minutes.

Whisk in the tomato paste and liquid smoke and let the sauce simmer another 5 to 10 minutes.

Let the mixture cool, transfer it to a jar with a tight-fitting lid, and store in the refrigerator.

Yield: About 2⅔ cups (640 ml) of sauce

Each 2 tablespoon (30 ml) serving has 3 grams of carbohydrates and 1 gram of fiber, for a total of 2 grams of usable carbs and no protein.

If you're wondering whether it's worth it to make your own barbecue sauce from scratch, chew on this for a moment: Your average commercial barbecue sauce has between 10 and 15 grams of carbs per 2-tablespoon (30-ml) serving—and do you know anyone who ever stopped at 2 tablespoons of barbecue sauce?

Kansas City Barbecue Sauce

This is what most of us think of when we think of barbecue sauce: tomato-y, spicy, and sweet. It's unbelievably close to a top-flight commercial barbecue sauce—and my Kansas City-raised husband agrees. If you like a smoky note in your barbecue sauce, add 1 teaspoon of liquid smoke flavoring to this.

2 tablespoons (28 g) butter

1 clove garlic

¼ cup (40 g) chopped onion

1 tablespoon (15 ml) lemon juice

1 cup (240 g) Dana's No-Sugar Ketchup
    (page 463)

⅓ cup (8 g) Splenda

1 tablespoon (15 ml) blackstrap molasses

2 tablespoons (30 ml) Worcestershire sauce

1 tablespoon (7.8 g) chili powder

1 tablespoon (15 ml) white vinegar

1 teaspoon pepper

¼ teaspoon salt

(continued on page 468)

Just combine everything in a saucepan over low heat. Heat until the butter melts, stir the whole thing up, and let it simmer for five minutes or so. That's it!

Yield: Roughly 1¾ cups (420 g), or 14 servings of 2 tablespoons (30 ml) each

Each serving will have 7 g carbohydrate, with 1 g fiber, for a usable carb count of 6 g; 1 g protein.

Cranberry Barbecue Sauce

The cranberries make this a natural with poultry, but it's good with pork, too.

½ cup (120 ml) Dana's No-Sugar Ketchup (page 463)
1 tablespoon (15 ml) cider vinegar
1 tablespoon (15 ml) spicy brown mustard
1 tablespoon (15 ml) Worcestershire sauce
3 tablespoons (4.5 g) Splenda
1 clove garlic
¼ small onion, cut in hunks
¼ cup (25 g) fresh cranberries
1 dash salt
1 dash pepper

This one starts in your food processor. Dump everything into the food processor with the S-blade in place and purée until the cranberries disappear.

Scrape the mixture out of the food processor into a saucepan and bring to a simmer over low heat. Let it simmer, stirring now and then, for just a few minutes. Thin with a little water if needed.

Yield: About 1 cup (240 ml), or 8 servings of 2 tablespoons (30 ml) each

4 grams of carbohydrate, with 1 gram of fiber, for a usable carb count of 3 grams; a trace of protein.

Memphis Sweet Sauce

The obvious choice for ribs seasoned with Memphis Rub (page 487) and mopped with the Memphis Mop (page 488)! It's the mustard that makes this a Memphis-style sauce.

1 tablespoon (16.5 g) tomato paste
3 tablespoons (45 ml) water
¼ cup (60 ml) Dana's No-Sugar Ketchup (page 463)
2 tablespoons (30 ml) spicy brown mustard
1 tablespoon (15 ml) Worcestershire sauce
1 tablespoon (28 g) butter
½ teaspoon lemon juice
1 tablespoon (1.5 g) Splenda
¼ teaspoon blackstrap molasses
1 teaspoon paprika
1 teaspoon seasoned salt
1 clove garlic

Measure everything into a nonreactive saucepan and whisk it together. Bring to a simmer over low heat and simmer for 5 minutes or so.

Yield: Makes roughly 1 cup (240 ml), or 8 servings of 2 tablespoons (30 ml) each

4 grams of carbohydrate per serving, with 1 gram of fiber, for a usable carb count of 3 grams; 1 gram protein.

Memphis Mustard Barbecue Sauce

This tasty Memphis-style barbecue sauce is one of the lowest-carb sauces in this book, and it packs a serious mustard note. Enjoy!

½ cup (120 ml) white vinegar
¼ cup (60 ml) yellow mustard
2 tablespoons (20 g) minced onion
½ tablespoon paprika
2 tablespoons (33 g) tomato paste
2 cloves garlic
¼ teaspoon cayenne
¼ teaspoon pepper
¼ teaspoon salt
2 teaspoons Splenda

Just measure everything into a nonreactive saucepan, whisk it together, bring it to a simmer, and let it simmer for 5 minutes or so. That's it!

Yield: Makes about 1 cup (240 ml), or 8 servings of 2 tablespoons (30 ml) each

3 grams of carbohydrate each, with 1 gram of fiber, for a usable carb count of just 2 grams; 1 gram protein.

Piedmont Mustard Sauce

This bright-yellow sauce, heavy on the mustard but with no tomato at all, is typical of the Piedmont region of North Carolina. It's typically used on pulled pork, but it would be good on any barbecued pork, I think.

½ cup (120 ml) yellow mustard
2 tablespoons (30 ml) lemon juice
2 tablespoons (3 g) Splenda
1 tablespoon (15 ml) white vinegar
¼ teaspoon cayenne

Just combine everything in a saucepan and simmer for 5 minutes over low heat.

Yield: Makes roughly ¾ cup (180 ml), or 6 servings of 2 tablespoons (30 ml) each

2 grams of carbohydrate per serving, with 1 gram of fiber, for a usable carb count of just 1 gram; 1 gram of protein.

Eastern Carolina Vinegar Sauce

This is the traditional eastern Carolina sauce for pulled pork. I'd never had anything like this before researching this book, but it's delicious! It's just sweetened vinegar with a good hit of hot pepper. Try it!

½ cup (120 ml) cider vinegar
1½ tablespoons (2 g) Splenda
¼ teaspoon blackstrap molasses
1 teaspoon red pepper flakes
¼ teaspoon cayenne

Combine all ingredients and stir together.

Yield: 6 servings

2 grams of carbohydrate and a trace of fiber, for a usable carb count of 2 grams; a trace of protein.

Lexington-Style Barbecue Sauce

This is your third choice for what to mix into your Carolina pulled pork—mostly vinegary, but with a tomato note.

1 cup (240 ml) cider vinegar
¾ cup (180 ml) Dana's No-Sugar Ketchup (page 263)
3 tablespoons (4.5 g) Splenda
½ teaspoon salt
½ teaspoon red pepper flakes
⅛ teaspoon cayenne

Combine everything in a nonreactive saucepan over low heat and stir together well. Bring to a simmer and let it cook for 15 minutes or so. That's it!

Yield: Makes roughly 1¾ cups (420 ml), or 14 servings of 2 tablespoons (30 ml) each

6 grams of carbohydrate with 1 gram of fiber, for a usable carb count of 5 grams; 1 gram protein.

Bourbon-Molasses Barbecue Sauce

Bourbon-based sauces are particularly popular on pork ribs, but they're also good on chicken.

¼ cup (40 g) minced onion
1 tablespoon (15 ml) oil
½ cup (120 ml) red wine vinegar

1 teaspoon blackstrap molasses
1 cup (240 ml) Dana's No-Sugar Ketchup (page 263)
¼ cup (6 g) plus 1 tablespoon (1.5 g) Splenda
2 tablespoons (30 ml) water
¼ cup (60 ml) bourbon

In a nonreactive saucepan, sauté the onion in the oil for 4 or 5 minutes. Stir in everything else and let it all simmer for 5 minutes or so.

Yield: Makes about 2 cups (480 ml), or 16 servings of 2 tablespoons (30 ml) each

5 grams carbohydrate, 1 gram fiber, for a usable carb count of 4 grams; a trace of protein.

Alabama White Sauce

This is unlike any other kind of barbecue sauce—it's mayonnaise-based, and when you baste chicken with it during smoking, it creates an amber color and a mellow flavor.

½ cup (120 g) mayonnaise
3 tablespoons (45 ml) white wine vinegar
1 teaspoon spicy brown mustard
½ teaspoon Creole Seasoning (page 485 or purchased)
1 clove garlic, crushed
1 teaspoon prepared horseradish

Just whisk everything together and use to baste chicken or as a finishing sauce. However, unlike with many other sauces, this sauce cannot be boiled. Make sure you set part of the sauce aside to use as a finishing sauce before you use the rest for basting.

Yield: Makes about ⅔ cup (160 ml), or 6 servings of 2 tablespoons (30 ml) each

1 gram of carbohydrate, a trace of fiber, and a trace of protein.

Lone Star Beef Sauce

Forget pork! In Texas, barbecue means beef, and lots of it. The typical barbecue cut for Texans is brisket, but I like this sauce on beef ribs. Especially if they've been rubbed with the Big Bad Beef Rib Rub (page 488)!

1 cup (240 ml) Dana's No-Sugar Ketchup (page 463)
2 tablespoons (30 ml) white vinegar
2 tablespoons (30 ml) oil
1½ teaspoons blackstrap molasses
1 tablespoon (15 ml) sugar-free imitation honey
2 tablespoons (3 g) Splenda
1½ teaspoons Worcestershire sauce
1½ teaspoons lemon juice
1 teaspoon pepper
1 clove garlic
¼ teaspoon cayenne

Stir everything together in a saucepan and let it simmer over low heat for five minutes or so.

Yield: Makes roughly 1½ cups (360 ml), or 12 servings of 2 tablespoons (30 ml) each

6 grams of carbohydrate per serving, with 1 gram of fiber, for a usable carb count of 5 grams; 1 gram of protein. Carb count does not include polyol in sugar-free honey.

Five-Spice Barbecue Sauce

This is the obvious choice if you want a finishing sauce to go with something you've seasoned with the Five-Spice Rub and Mop (pages 489–490). It's good on anything, though!

¾ cup (180 ml) Dana's No-Sugar Ketchup (page 463)
½ cup (120 ml) light beer
⅓ cup (80 ml) cider vinegar
1½ tablespoons (2 g) Splenda
¼ teaspoon molasses
1 tablespoon (15 ml) Worcestershire sauce
1 clove garlic
1 teaspoon cumin
¾ teaspoon five-spice powder

Combine everything in a nonreactive saucepan and let it simmer for 5 minutes or so.

Yield: Makes roughly 1¾ cup (420 g), or 14 servings of 2 tablespoons (30 ml) each.

3 grams of carbohydrate, with a trace of fiber, and a trace of protein.

Texas BBQ Brisket Sauce

This is a classic Texas-style barbecue sauce, and it's killer on a slow-smoked hunk of brisket.

2 tablespoons (28 g) butter

½ cup (80 g) minced onion

1 clove garlic, crushed

1 cup (240 ml) Dana's No-Sugar Ketchup (page 263)

1 tablespoon (7.8 g) chili powder

¼ cup (6 g) Splenda

½ teaspoon molasses

2 tablespoons (30 ml) lemon juice

1 tablespoon (15 ml) wine vinegar

2 teaspoons Worcestershire sauce

1 teaspoon liquid smoke flavoring (such as the one made by Colgin)

1 teaspoon yellow mustard

½ teaspoon salt

½ teaspoon pepper

¼ teaspoon cayenne

Melt the butter in a nonreactive saucepan and sauté the onion and garlic for 4 or 5 minutes. Add everything else, whisk it smooth, and bring to a simmer over low heat. Let the whole thing simmer for 5 minutes or so. It's hot! It's wonderful, too, especially on beef.

Yield: Makes about 2 cups (480 ml), or 16 servings of 2 tablespoons (30 ml) each

4 grams of carbohydrate per serving, with 1 gram of fiber, for a usable carb count of 3 grams.

North-South-East-West Barbecue Sauce

This is perhaps the most unusual barbecue sauce in this book—and one of the best. The flavor is evenly balanced between maple, orange, bourbon, and cayenne, giving it flavors from virtually every region of the country. It's wonderful on pork or chicken.

2 tablespoons (28 g) butter

2 tablespoons (20 g) minced onion

½ cup (120 ml) bourbon

½ cup (120 ml) Dana's No-Sugar Ketchup (page 463)

¼ cup (60 ml) cider vinegar

¼ teaspoon orange extract

¼ cup (60 ml) sugar-free pancake syrup

1 tablespoon (15 ml) blackstrap molasses

2 tablespoons (3 g) Splenda

1 tablespoon (15 ml) Worcestershire sauce

¼ green pepper, minced

¼ teaspoon cayenne

In a nonreactive saucepan over low heat, melt the butter and sauté the onion for 5 minutes or so. Add everything else, stir it up, and bring it to a simmer. Let it cook for 7 to 10 minutes.

Yield: Makes roughly 1 cup (240 ml), or 8 servings of 2 tablespoons (30 ml) each

8 grams of carb, with 1 gram of fiber, for a usable carb count of 7 grams. This count does not include the polyols in the sugar-free pancake syrup.

Apricosen und Horseradish BBQ Sauce

My German-descended husband named this one. It's very fruity! It's especially good on poultry, but try it on pork as well.

½ jalapeno
⅓ cup (110 grams) low-sugar apricot preserves
2 tablespoons (30 ml) bourbon
2 tablespoons (30 ml) lime juice
1 tablespoon (15 ml) cider vinegar
2 tablespoons (30 ml) Dana's No-Sugar Ketchup (page 463)
1½ teaspoons soy sauce
2 teaspoons Splenda
¼ teaspoon blackstrap molasses
1 teaspoon Worcestershire sauce
1 tablespoon (10 g) minced onion
2 cloves garlic
½ teaspoon ginger
1 dash salt
1 dash pepper
2 teaspoons prepared horseradish

Mince the jalapeno (don't forget to wash your hands afterward!). Measure everything into a nonreactive saucepan and whisk together well. Turn heat to low and bring to a simmer. Let simmer for 5 to 10 minutes.

Yield: 8 servings of 2 tablespoons (30 ml) each

6 grams carbohydrate, with a trace of fiber, and a trace of protein.

Florida Sunshine Tangerine Barbecue Sauce

The name of this sauce is partly from the tangerine note, which is unusual and delicious, but it's also from the fact that this sauce is at least as hot as the Florida sun! It is especially good on poultry.

1 12-ounce (360-ml) can Diet-Rite tangerine soda
¼ cup (6 g) Splenda
1 tablespoon (7.8 g) chili powder
2 teaspoons black pepper
1 teaspoon ginger
1 teaspoon dry mustard
1 teaspoon onion salt
4 cloves garlic, crushed
½ teaspoon cayenne
½ teaspoon coriander
½ teaspoon red pepper flakes
1 whole bay leaf
½ cup (120 ml) cider vinegar
1 tablespoon (15 ml) sugar-free imitation honey
1 tablespoon (15 ml) Worcestershire sauce
¾ cup (180 ml) Dana's No-Sugar Ketchup (page 463)

Pour the soda into a nonreactive saucepan and turn the heat under it to medium-low. While that's heating, measure the other ingredients into the sauce. By the time you get to the ketchup, it

(continued on page 474)

should be simmering. Whisk everything together until smooth and let it simmer over lowest heat for 10 to 15 minutes.

Yield: Makes about 3 cups (710 ml), or 24 servings of 2 tablespoons (30 ml) each

Only 3 grams of carb per serving, with a trace of fiber, a trace of polyols, a trace of protein.

Sweet Spice Islands Sauce

This is for use with the Sweet Spice Islands Rub (page 493), of course!

2 tablespoons (28 g) butter
¼ cup (40 g) minced onion
1 clove garlic, crushed
⅓ cup (80 ml) Dana's No-Sugar Ketchup
   (page 463)
1 tablespoon (15 ml) cider vinegar
1 tablespoon (15 ml) lemon juice
1 tablespoon (15 ml) Worcestershire sauce
1 tablespoon (15 ml) sugar-free imitation
   honey
1 tablespoon (1.5 g) Splenda
1 tablespoon (7 g) Sweet Spice Islands Rub
   (page 493)

Melt the butter over lowest heat in a nonreactive saucepan and sauté the onion and garlic in it for 4 or 5 minutes. Whisk in everything else, bring to a simmer, and let it cook for 5 minutes or so.

Yield: Makes a little over 1 cup (240 ml), or about 9 servings of 2 tablespoons (30 ml) each

9 grams of carbohydrate per serving, but 2 grams of that are the polyols in the imitation honey, and 1 gram is fiber, so count 6 grams of usable carb; 1 gram protein.

Cajun Sauce

This is the most complicated sauce in this book to make, but it's marvelous and makes quite a lot. It's also quite hot—you could mellow it a bit by leaving out the cayenne, I suppose, but then it wouldn't really be Cajun would it?

1 small onion
½ small green bell pepper
2 celery ribs
3 cloves garlic
2 tablespoons (30 ml) olive oil
1 can (14 ounces, or 420 ml) chicken broth
⅔ cup (160 ml) cider vinegar
3 tablespoons (49.5 g) tomato paste
5 tablespoons (75 ml) spicy mustard
3 tablespoons (4.5 g) Splenda
¼ teaspoon blackstrap molasses
2 tablespoons (30 ml) Dana's No-Sugar
   Ketchup (page 463)
½ teaspoon chili powder
½ teaspoon cayenne

Chop the onion, pepper, and celery fairly fine—feel free to use a food processor for this; I did! Crush the garlic, too.

In a big saucepan with a heavy bottom over medium heat, heat the olive oil and add the chopped vegetables. Sauté them until everything is soft. Now stir in everything else, turn the heat down, and let the whole thing simmer for 15 to 20 minutes. Spoon over pork—preferably pork you've rubbed with Cajun Seasoning (page 484) and mopped with Cajun Rib Mop (page 490)!

Yield: Makes about 1 quart (960 ml), or about 16 servings of ¼ cup (60 ml) each, though you may eat more!

Each serving will have 4 grams of carbohydrate and 1 gram of fiber, for a usable carb count of 3 grams; 1 gram protein.

Polynesian Sauce

If a luau is what you're dreaming of, try this sauce! It's great on pork of any kind.

¼ cup (66 g) tomato paste
¼ cup (60 ml) canned crushed pineapple in juice
¼ cup (60 ml) white vinegar
1 tablespoon (15 ml) soy sauce
2 tablespoons (3 g) Splenda
5 tablespoons (75 ml) water
¼ teaspoon blackstrap molasses

Combine everything in a saucepan and simmer over low heat for 5 minutes.

Yield: Makes a little over 1 cup (240 ml), or 8 servings of 2 slightly generous tablespoons (30 ml) each

5 grams of carbohydrate per serving, with 1 gram of fiber, for a usable carb count of 4 grams; 1 gram of protein.

Sweet and Spicy Mustard Sauce

If you like honey-mustard dressing, give this barbecue sauce a try.

½ cup (120 ml) spicy brown mustard
¼ cup (6 g) Splenda
½ teaspoon blackstrap molasses
⅛ teaspoon instant coffee crystals
1 teaspoon Worcestershire sauce
1 teaspoon hot sauce
2 tablespoons (30 ml) water

Just whisk everything together in a nonreactive saucepan over low heat. Bring it to a simmer and let it cook just a few minutes to blend the flavors.

Yield: Makes just under 1 cup (240 ml), or about 7 servings of 2 tablespoons (30 ml) each

3 grams of carb per serving, with a trace of fiber, and 1 gram of protein.

Apricot White Wine Sauce

Unlike the Apricosen und Horseradish BBQ Sauce (page 473), this has no tomato note—just apricot, wine, and all those wonderful spices. Like

(continued on page 476)

the Apricosen sauce, this is especially good on poultry!

6 tablespoons (120 g) low-sugar apricot preserves
⅓ cup (80 ml) white wine
¼ medium onion
¼ teaspoon ginger
¼ teaspoon cayenne
⅛ teaspoon allspice
¼ cup (16 g) tarragon
¼ teaspoon turmeric
⅛ teaspoon cardamom
3 tablespoons (45 ml) Dijon or spicy brown mustard

Measure everything into a nonreactive saucepan and whisk together well. Simmer on low for 5 to 10 minutes.

Yield: Roughly 1¼ cups (300 ml), or 10 servings of 2 tablespoons (30 ml) each

5 grams carbohydrate, with a trace of fiber, and 1 gram of protein.

Easy Remoulade Sauce

This is good on anything fishy or seafoodlike.

1 cup (230 g) mayonnaise
2 tablespoons (30 ml) spicy brown or Dijon mustard
2 tablespoons (30 ml) lemon juice

1 teaspoon dried tarragon, crumbled
2 tablespoons (17 g) capers, drained and chopped a bit

Just stir everything up and you're good to go!

Yield: Makes about 1⅓ cups (320 ml), or 5 servings of just under ¼ cup (60 ml) each

Each serving has 1 gram of carbohydrates, a trace of fiber, and 1 gram of protein.

Cilantro Chimichurri

This amazingly flavorful herb sauce is wonderful over a grilled steak, especially one that you've seasoned with something a bit hot and spicy.

1 bunch cilantro
5 cloves garlic
2 tablespoons (30 ml) lime juice
½ small red onion, cut in a few hunks
½ teaspoon red pepper flakes
⅔ cup (160 ml) olive oil

Chop up the cilantro enough to fit it in your food processor with the S-blade in place. Add everything else but the olive oil and pulse until everything's fairly finely minced. Scrape the resulting incredibly fragrant mixture into a bowl and whisk in the olive oil. Spoon over a grilled steak or anything else you can think of!

Yield: Makes 6 servings of roughly 2 tablespoons (30 ml)

Each serving will have 3 grams of carbohydrate, with a trace of fiber, and a trace of protein.

Chipotle Sauce

This is essential for Chipotle Cheeseburgers (page 363), but it's great on a grilled chicken breast, too as a dip for lightly cooked, chilled asparagus.

¾ cup (180 g) mayonnaise
3 chipotle chiles canned in adobo
2 tablespoons (30 ml) Dana's No-Sugar
 Ketchup (page 463)

Measure the mayonnaise into a bowl. Chop up the chipotles quite fine and stir into the mayonnaise along with the ketchup.

Yield: 6 servings of 1 generous tablespoon (15 ml) each

1 gram of carbohydrate per serving, with a trace of fiber, 1 gram protein.

Mustard-Horseradish Dipping Sauce

I came up with this to dip some stuffed mushrooms in, but it's very versatile.

½ cup (120 g) mayonnaise
2 teaspoons spicy brown mustard
1 teaspoon prepared horseradish
½ teaspoon Splenda
1 teaspoon white vinegar

Simply mix everything together. It's good for dipping most anything—chicken bites, vegetables, or whatever you've got.

Yield: About 6 servings

Each with trace protein; trace carbohydrate; trace dietary fiber; no usable carb.

"Honey" Mustard Dipping Sauce

This is great with the fried Chicken Tenders (page 309) or with a simple chicken breast or pork chop.

¼ cup (60 ml) mayonnaise
2 tablespoons (30 ml) spicy mustard
1 teaspoon Splenda

Simply combine everything and you're all set.

Yield: Makes a little more than ⅓ cup (about 70 ml), or enough for about 4 people eating Chicken Tenders.

Each serving has 1 gram of carbohydrates, no fiber, and 1 gram of protein.

Apricot Ginger Dipping Sauce

This is also great with Chicken Tenders (page 309)—or anything else you might use the "Honey"

(continued on page 478)

Mustard Dipping Sauce on. But it tastes a lot different.

¼ cup (60 ml) mayonnaise
1½ tablespoons (30 g) low-sugar apricot
    preserves
1 teaspoon grated ginger
¼ teaspoon minced ginger or ½ clove garlic,
    crushed
½ teaspoon Splenda
¾ teaspoon soy sauce

Simply combine everything and you are dare.

Yield: Makes just under ¹/₃ cup (about 70 ml), or enough for about 4 people eating Chicken Tenders

Each serving has 3 grams of carbohydrates, with a trace of fiber and protein.

Asian Dipping Sauce

This is perfect with the Lettuce Wraps (page 348), but it's also good with Chicken Tenders (page 309), or whatever you have on hand.

¼ cup (6 g) Splenda
¼ cup (60 ml) water
2 tablespoons (30 ml) soy sauce
2 tablespoons (30 ml) rice vinegar
2 tablespoons (30 ml) Dana's No-Sugar
    Ketchup (page 463) or commercial sugar-
    free ketchup
1 tablespoon (15 ml) lemon juice

¼ teaspoon toasted sesame oil
2 teaspoons dry mustard
2 teaspoons chili garlic paste

Just assemble everything in a blender and run it until everything's well combined. If you don't use it all up at once, keep in a tightly sealed container in the fridge and it will last a week, at least.

Yield: Makes roughly ¾ cup (180 ml), or 6 servings of 2 tablespoons (30 ml) each

Each serving has 3 grams of carbohydrates, a trace of fiber, and 1 gram of protein.

Nuoc Cham

This sweet-tart-spicy dipping sauce is purely Vietnamese, and it's absolutely wonderful! Once you try this, you'll think of all sorts of ways to use it.

2 tablespoons (30 ml) fish sauce
2 tablespoons (30 ml) lime juice
1½ teaspoons rice vinegar
3 tablespoons (4.5 g) Splenda
½ teaspoon minced garlic or 1 clove garlic,
    crushed
1 teaspoon chili garlic paste

Simply combine everything in a small dish—that's it!

Yield: About ⅓ cup (80 ml), or 4 or 5 servings

Assuming 4 servings, each will have 4 grams of carbohydrates, a trace of fiber, and a trace of protein. (And approximately 15 metric boatloads of flavor!)

Aioli

This is basically just very garlicky mayonnaise. It's good on all kinds of vegetables and on fish, too.

4 cloves garlic, crushed very thoroughly
1 egg
¼ teaspoon salt
2 tablespoons (30 ml) lemon juice
½ to ⅔ cup (120 to 160 ml) olive oil

Put the garlic, egg, salt, and lemon juice in a blender. Run the blender for a second and then pour in the oil in a very thin stream, like you would when making mayonnaise. Turn off the blender when the sauce is thickened.

Yield: About 1 cup (240 ml), or 8 servings of 2 tablespoons (30 ml)

Each with 1 gram of carbohydrates, only a trace of fiber, and 1 gram of protein.

Chili Lime Mayo

¼ cup (60 ml) mayonnaise
2 teaspoons lime juice
¼ teaspoon chili paste
2 teaspoons minced cilantro

Just stir everything together and serve over anything Asian or Mexican.

Yield: 4 servings of 1 tablespoon (15 ml)

Each with trace protein; trace carbohydrate; trace dietary fiber; 0 g usable carb.

Hollandaise for Sissies

This is an easy sauce for asparagus, artichokes, broccoli, or whatever you like.

4 egg yolks
1 cup (230 g) sour cream
1 tablespoon (15 ml) lemon juice
½ teaspoon salt or Vege-Sal
Dash hot pepper sauce or other hot sauce

You'll need either a double boiler or a heat diffuser for this—it needs very gentle heat. If you're using a double boiler, you want the water in the bottom hot but not boiling. If you're using a heat diffuser, use the lowest possible heat under the diffuser.

Put all the ingredients in a heavy-bottomed saucepan or in the top of a double boiler. Whisk everything together well. Let it heat through and serve it over vegetables or whatever you like.

Yield: 6 to 8 servings

Each with 2 g carbohydrate, a trace fiber, and 3 g protein in each.

Curried Mock Hollandaise

Oh man, this is the bomb with artichokes or asparagus! This is a variation of the Hollandaise for Sissies recipe (page 479).

(continued on page 480)

4 egg yolks
1 cup (230 g) sour cream
1 tablespoon (15 ml) lemon juice
½ teaspoon salt or Vege-Sal
1 teaspoon curry powder
2 cloves garlic, crushed

You'll need either a double boiler or a heat diffuser for this—it needs very gentle heat. If you're using a double boiler, you want the water in the bottom hot but not boiling. If you're using a heat diffuser, use the lowest possible heat under the diffuser.

Put all the ingredients in a heavy-bottomed saucepan or the top of a double boiler. Whisk everything together well, let it heat through, and serve with vegetables.

Yield: 6 servings

Each with 3 g protein; 3 g carbohydrate; trace dietary fiber; 3 g usable carbs.

Adobo Sauce

This traditional Mexican seasoning is great with chicken.

3 cloves garlic
1 teaspoon salt
¾ teaspoon cumin
1 teaspoon oregano
½ teaspoon pepper
¾ cup (180 ml) lime juice
¼ teaspoon orange extract

Just measure everything and whisk it together. Use it to marinate and baste chicken.

Yield: Makes just over ¾ cup (180 ml), or enough to marinate 1 good-sized cut-up chicken

Assuming 5 servings, each will have 4 grams of carbohydrate, with a trace of fiber and protein—if you manage to consume all the marinade, which you won't.

Tequila Lime Marinade

⅓ cup (80 ml) lime juice (Bottled is fine.)
⅓ cup (80 ml) water
3 tablespoons (45 ml) tequila
1 tablespoon (1.5 g) Splenda
1 tablespoon (15 ml) soy sauce
2 cloves garlic, crushed.

Combine the ingredients and store in the refrigerator until ready to use.

Yield: Roughly ¾ cup (180 ml)—enough for a dozen boneless, skinless chicken breasts or a couple of pounds of shrimp

In the whole batch there are 13 grams of carbohydrates and 1 gram of fiber, for a total of 12 grams of usable carbs and no protein, but since you drain most of the marinade off, you won't get more than a gram or two of carbs total.

Marco Polo Marinade

This marinade is named after its combined Italian and Chinese influences. It's wonderful for steak, but try it on chicken, too! It's also good on vegetables.

1 cup (240 ml) bottled Italian salad dressing
¼ cup (60 ml) soy sauce
2 teaspoons grated ginger
2 tablespoons (3 g) Splenda
4 drops blackstrap molasses

Just measure everything and stir it together. Use it to marinate or season whatever you like!

Yield: 1¼ cups (300 ml), or 5 servings of ¼ cup (60 ml)

1 g protein; 6 g carbohydrate; trace dietary fiber; 6 g usable carbs. However, you can drop this lower by using a seriously low-carb Italian dressing—and anyway, since you use this as a marinade, you're unlikely to consume anything like ¼ cup (60 ml) of this at a time.

Beer-Molasses Marinade

It's great for ribs or kind of any pork!

1½ (360 ml) cups water
12-ounce (360-ml) can light beer
1 teaspoon blackstrap molasses
¼ cup (6 g) Splenda
1 tablespoon (4.2 g) dried thyme

1 tablespoon (18 g) salt
1 whole bay leaf
½ teaspoon pepper

Combine everything in a nonreactive bowl or pan. Marinate the meat in a big resealable plastic bag or shallow pan large enough to hold the meat. Either way, let it marinate for several hours before cooking. Don't forget to discard the bay leaf.

Yield: Makes about 3 cups (710 ml)—double it if you need to

18 grams of carbohydrate in the whole batch, with 2 grams of fiber, for a usable carb count of 16 grams; 1 gram protein. But remember, this is a marinade, so you won't consume anything like the whole batch. I'd count only 1 or 2 grams of carb per serving.

Jerk Marinade

Jerk is a Jamaican way of life. Make it with one pepper if you want it just nicely hot or with two peppers if you want it traditional—also known as take-the-top-of-your-head-off hot.

1 or 2 Scotch Bonnet or habanero peppers, with or without seeds and ribs (the hottest parts)
½ small onion
3 tablespoons (45 ml) oil
1 tablespoon ground (5.7 g) allspice
2 tablespoons (12 g) grated fresh ginger
1 tablespoon (15 ml) soy sauce
1 teaspoon dried thyme
1 bay leaf, crumbled

(continued on page 482)

¼ teaspoon cinnamon

1 tablespoon (1.5 g) Splenda

2 cloves garlic, crushed

Put all the ingredients in a food processor with the S-blade in place and process until the mixture is fairly smooth. (You'll get a soft paste that looks like mud but smells like heaven!) Smear this over the meat of your choice and let it sit for a day before cooking. Remember to always wash your hands after handling hot peppers!

Yield: Enough for about 4 servings of meat

Each serving serving of Jerk Marinade adds 4 grams of carbohydrates and 1 gram of fiber, for a total of 3 grams of usable carbs and no protein.

If you just can't take the heat, you can chicken out and use a jalapeño or two instead of the habaneros or Scotch Bonnets, and your jerk marinade will be quite mild, as these things go. But remember: There is no such thing as a truly mild jerk sauce.

Apricot-Chipotle Glaze

I invented this for my Easter leg of lamb, but there's no reason you can't use it on pork and chicken, too—anywhere you want a hit of sweet-and-hot flavor.

½ cup (80 g) minced red onion

¼ cup (60 ml) canola oil

4 cloves garlic, crushed

½ cup (120 ml) red wine vinegar

½ cup (160 g) low-sugar apricot preserves

2 chipotle chiles canned in adobo

5 tablespoons (7.5 g) Splenda

2 tablespoons (30 ml) lemon juice

In a saucepan, sauté the onion in the oil until it's soft. Add the garlic and vinegar and whisk in the preserves. Bring to a simmer and let cook for 5 minutes or so.

Let it cool for a few minutes and then pour the glaze into a blender and add the chipotles, Splenda, and lemon juice. Whirl until the chipotles are ground up. Use to baste meat or poultry that's roasting or grilling.

Yield: 12 to 14 servings

Assuming 14, each will have trace protein; 4 g carbohydrate; trace dietary fiber; 4 g usable carbs.

Maple-Orange Ham Glaze

It's common to glaze a roasting ham with brown sugar, honey, or the like—but we all know what that does to the carb count! Here's a glaze that'll impress your family and friends, while leaving your diet intact.

½ cup (120 ml) sugar-free pancake syrup

¼ cup (60 ml) lemon juice

1 teaspoon Splenda

¼ teaspoon orange extract

1 tablespoon (15 ml) brown mustard

1 tablespoon (14 g) butter

Simply combine everything in a small saucepan over low heat and simmer for five minutes. Use to baste a ham during the last hour of roasting time. You can also use this to glaze a ham steak for a much quicker supper!

Yield: Enough for a good-sized ham

The whole batch has 2 g protein; 6 g carbohydrate; trace dietary fiber; 6 g usable carbs. Carb count does not include the polyols in the sugar-free pancake syrup.

Taco Seasoning

Many store-bought seasoning blends include sugar or cornstarch—my food counter book says that several popular brands have 5 grams of carb in 2 teaspoons! This is very easy to put together, and it tastes great. It's even cheaper than the premixed stuff.

2 tablespoons (15.6 g) chili powder
1½ tablespoons (9.5 g) cumin
1½ tablespoons (9.5 g) paprika
1 tablespoon (7.2 g) onion powder
1 tablespoon (8.4 g) garlic powder
⅛ teaspoon cayenne pepper (mild) or
    ¼ teaspoon cayenne (a bit hotter)

Simply combine all ingredients, blending well, and store in an airtight container. Use 2 tablespoons (18 g) of this mixture to 1 pound (455 g) of ground beef, ground turkey, or chicken.

Yield: This makes about 8 tablespoons (70 g), or 4 batches' worth

Using 2 tablespoons (18 g) of this seasoning will add just under 2 g carbohydrate to a 4-ounce (115 g) serving of taco meat.

Dana's Chicken Seasoning

This is wonderful sprinkled over a chicken breast before grilling or as a table seasoning for any poultry. (It's also great sprinkled over whole or cut-up chicken before roasting.)

3 tablespoons (55 g) salt
1 teaspoon paprika
1 teaspoon onion powder
1 teaspoon garlic powder
1 teaspoon curry powder
½ teaspoon black pepper

Combine all the ingredients thoroughly and store in a salt shaker or the shaker from an old container of herbs. Simply sprinkle over chicken before roasting; I use it to season at the table, as well.

Yield: Makes just over ¼ cup (30 g)

In the whole recipe there are only 7 grams of carbohydrates and 1 gram of fiber, for a total of 6 grams of usable carbs and no protein—so the amount of carbohydrates in the teaspoon or so you sprinkle over a piece of chicken is negligible.

Cajun Seasoning

This sprinkle-on seasoning will liven up chops, steaks, chicken, fish—just about anything!

2½ tablespoons (17.3 g) paprika
2 tablespoons (36 g) salt
2 tablespoons (16 g) garlic powder
1 tablespoon (6.3 g) black pepper
1 tablespoon (7.2 g) onion powder
1 tablespoon (5.4 g) cayenne pepper
1 tablespoon (3.4 g) dried oregano
1 tablespoon (4.2 g) dried thyme

Combine all the ingredients thoroughly and keep in an air-tight container.

Yield: Makes ⅔ cup (70 g)

In this whole recipe there are 37 grams of carbohydrates and 9 grams of fiber, for a total of 28 grams of usable carbs and no protein. Considering how spicy this is, you're unlikely to use more than a teaspoon or two at a time. One teaspoon has 1 gram of carbohydrates, a trace of fiber, and no protein.

Jerk Seasoning

Sprinkle this over chicken, pork chops, or fish before cooking for an instant hit of hot, sweet, spicy flavor.

1 tablespoon (5 g) onion flakes
2 teaspoons ground thyme
1 teaspoon ground allspice
¼ teaspoon ground cinnamon

1 teaspoon black pepper
1 teaspoon cayenne pepper
1 tablespoon (7.2 g) onion powder
2 teaspoons salt
¼ teaspoon ground nutmeg
2 tablespoons (3 g) Splenda

Combine all the ingredients and store in an air-tight container.

Yield: Makes about ⅓ cup (30 g)

If you use 1 teaspoon, it will have 1 gram of carbohydrates, a trace of fiber, and no protein.

Adobo Seasoning

Adobo is a popular seasoning in Latin America and the Caribbean. It's available at many grocery stores in the spice aisle or the international aisle, but if you can't find it, it sure is easy to make.

10 teaspoons (28 g) garlic powder
5 teaspoons dried oregano
5 teaspoons pepper
2½ teaspoons paprika
5 teaspoons (30 g) salt

Simply measure everything into a bowl, stir, and store in a lidded shaker jar.

Yield: A little over ½ cup (70 g), or about 48 servings of ½ teaspoon

Each with trace protein; 1 g carbohydrate; trace dietary fiber; 1 g usable carb.

Creole Seasoning

Creole seasoning is great when you want to add a hit of spicy-hot flavor to pork, chicken, seafood—or just about anything, actually. You can buy it premade, but you know how food manufacturers are—you have to keep an eye out for added sugar. It's easy to stir some up on your own.

2 tablespoons (35 g) salt
3 teaspoons garlic powder
3 teaspoons onion powder
3 teaspoons paprika
3 teaspoons dried thyme
2 teaspoons cayenne pepper
1½ teaspoons pepper
1½ teaspoons dried oregano
2 bay leaves
½ teaspoon chili powder

Put everything in a food processor or blender, crumbling the bay leaf as you put it in. Run until the bay leaf is pulverized and everything is evenly mixed. Pour into a lidded shaker jar for storage.

Yield: ½ cup (70 g) or 48 servings of ½ teaspoon

Trace protein; 1 g carbohydrate; trace dietary fiber; 1 g usable carb.

Many-Pepper Steak Seasoning

This adds real zing to a steak without covering up the flavor. Make this up, keep it in a shaker, and you'll be ready to cook a really special steak at a moment's notice.

1 tablespoon (9 g) onion powder
3 tablespoons (27 g) garlic powder
3 tablespoons (21 g) paprika
1 tablespoon (3 g) oregano
1½ tablespoons (9 g) pepper
2 teaspoons lemon pepper
1 teaspoon cayenne—or more if you like it really hot!

Simply combine everything well and put it in a shaker. Sprinkle liberally over both sides of a steak before broiling or grilling.

Yield: This is enough to season 12 to 15 steaks

Assuming 15 steaks, each will have 3 grams of carbohydrates and 1 gram of fiber, or for a total of 2 grams of carbs to a whole steak—and that steak is likely to be 2 or more servings, so figure 1 gram per serving—and no fiber or protein.

New Orleans Gold

This is hot and spicy New Orleans seasoning! It's good on chicken, steak, pork, seafood—heck, anything but ice cream.

2½ tablespoons (15.8 g) paprika
1 tablespoon (18 g) salt
2 tablespoons (16.8 g) garlic powder
1 tablespoon (6.3 g) pepper
1 tablespoon (7.2 g) onion powder
1 tablespoon (5.4 g) cayenne
1 tablespoon (5.4 g) dried oregano
1 tablespoon (4.2 g) dried thyme
1½ teaspoons dried basil
1½ teaspoons celery seed

(continued on page 486)

Combine the ingredients in a food processor with the S-blade attachment and run for thirty seconds.

Yield: 54 servings of 1 teaspoon

Each with trace protein; 1g carbohydrate; trace dietary fiber; 1 g usable carb.

Italian Seasoned Crumbs

Use this the way you would packaged Italian seasoned crumbs—to "fill" meatballs or "bread" chicken or chops. To get pork rind crumbs, just run a bag of pork rinds through your food processor.

1 cup (80 g) pork rind crumbs
½ teaspoon dried parsley
½ teaspoon dried oregano
¼ teaspoon garlic powder
¼ teaspoon onion powder
¼ teaspoon Splenda

Yield: Makes 1 cup (85 g), or 8 servings of 2 tablespoons (10 g)

Each with 7 g protein; trace carbohydrate; trace dietary fiber; so call it 0 usable carb.

Classic Barbecue Rub

As the name suggests, this is the rub that cries "classic barbecue!" It makes a great combo with the Kansas City Barbecue Sauce (page 467), but use it with any sauce—and on any meat!

¼ cup (6 g) Splenda
1 tablespoon (12 g) seasoned salt
1 tablespoon (8.4 g) garlic powder
1 tablespoon (12 g) celery salt
1 tablespoon (7.2 g) onion powder
2 tablespoons (12.6 g) paprika
1 tablespoon (7.8 g) chili powder
2 teaspoons pepper
1 teaspoon (2 g) lemon pepper
1 teaspoon sage
1 teaspoon mustard
½ teaspoon dried thyme
½ teaspoon cayenne

Combine everything, stir well, and store in a shaker. Sprinkle heavily over just about anything, but especially over pork ribs and chicken.

Yield: Makes just over ⅔ cup (100 g), or roughly 12 tablespoons

3 g carbohydrate, with 1 g fiber, for a usable carb count of 2 g; 1 g protein.

Herb Chicken Rub

This rub has the herbs we traditionally associate with poultry—sage, thyme, and the like. Consider seasoning a chicken with this rub and the matching mop and then using one of the fruity barbecue sauces—the Cranberry Barbecue Sauce (page 468) or the Apricot White Wine Sauce (page 476), perhaps.

1½ teaspoons poultry seasoning
1½ teaspoons garlic salt
1 teaspoon dry mustard
1 teaspoon ground ginger
1 teaspoon Splenda

Just measure everything into a small dish and stir it together.

Yield: Enough rub for 1 good-sized chicken

The whole batch has just 1 gram of carbohydrate, with a trace of fiber.

Herb Chicken Mop

This mop is for use with the Herb Chicken Rub, of course!

1 teaspoon Herb Chicken Rub (page 486)
¼ cup (60 ml) olive oil
¼ cup (60 ml) chicken broth

Just combine everything and use to baste chicken during indirect cooking.

Yield: Makes about ½ cup (120 ml)

The whole batch has only a trace of carbohydrate, and you won't use it all up mopping your chicken. Call this one free.

Memphis Rub

3 tablespoons (18 g) paprika
1 tablespoon (12 g) seasoned salt
1 tablespoon (6.3 g) pepper

1½ teaspoons garlic powder
1½ teaspoons cayenne
1½ teaspoons dried oregano
1½ teaspoons dry mustard
1½ teaspoons chili powder

Just mix everything together and use on ribs, pork chops, or even chicken. Mop with the Memphis Mop (page 488) and finish with one of the Memphis-style sauces!

Yield: Makes 7½ tablespoons, or about 7 servings

4 grams of carb per serving, with 1 gram of fiber, for a usable carb count of 3 grams; 1 gram protein.

Memphis "Dry Sauce"

This is really a rub, but the recipe I adapted this from called it a dry sauce. Who am I to argue?

½ cup (12 g) Splenda
½ teaspoon blackstrap molasses
1 tablespoon (7.8 g) chili powder
1 tablespoon (6.3 g) black pepper
1 tablespoon (9 g) dry mustard
3 teaspoons garlic powder
1 tablespoon (6.3 g) paprika
1 teaspoon celery salt
1 teaspoon onion powder

Just combine everything in a food processor or blender until the molasses is distributed—for

(continued on page 488)

some odd reason, I find a blender works better for this. Then sprinkle over pork or chicken before smoking.

Yield: Makes roughly ⅔ cup (60 g), or 12 servings of 1 tablespoon (5 g) each

3 grams of carbohydrate and 1 gram of fiber, for a usable carb count of 2 grams; a trace of protein.

Memphis Mop

This is one of the most complex mopping sauces in this book, and just looking at the ingredients, you can see it's going to add loads of flavor to your 'cue!

1 cup (240 ml) water
2 tablespoons (3 g) Splenda
½ teaspoon blackstrap molasses
1 cup (240 ml) wine vinegar
2 tablespoons (30 ml) Worcestershire sauce
½ teaspoon chili powder
½ teaspoon hot pepper sauce
2 tablespoons (30 ml) canola oil
1 clove garlic

Just whisk everything together in a nonreactive bowl or pan and mop away!

Yield: Makes roughly 2¼ cups (540 ml)

7 grams of carbohydrate in the whole batch, which you won't use up even if you do 2 slabs of ribs. We're talking well under 1 extra gram of carbohydrate per serving.

Big Bad Beef Rib Rub

I'd never had beef ribs before I made them with this rub, and I was an instant convert!

2 tablespoons (3 g) Splenda
2 tablespoons (16 g) DiabetiSweet or other polyol sweetener
2 tablespoons (36 g) garlic salt
2 tablespoons (16.8 g) garlic powder
2 tablespoons (12.6 g) paprika
2 teaspoons chili powder
½ teaspoon ground ginger
½ teaspoon onion powder
½ teaspoon ground coriander
½ teaspoon cayenne

This is extremely simple: Just put everything in a bowl and stir it together. Sprinkle generously over beef ribs before barbecuing.

Yield: Roughly ¾ cup (90 g), or 12 tablespoons

Each tablespoonful will have 3 grams of carbohydrate, exclusive of polyols, and 1 gram of fiber, for a usable carb count of 2 grams; 1 gram protein.

Bodacious Beef Brisket Rub

4 tablespoons (25 g) paprika
1 tablespoon (6.3 g) pepper
2 tablespoons (3 g) Splenda
2 teaspoons chili powder

2 teaspoons onion powder

2 teaspoons garlic powder

½ teaspoon cayenne (optional, if you like your food really fiery—but this has plenty of heat without it)

Stir everything together. Save a tablespoon for the mop use and the rest to sprinkle liberally over your brined brisket.

Yield: Makes about 8 servings of 1 tablespoon each

4 grams of carbohydrate, 1 gram of fiber, 1 gram protein.

Bodacious Beef Brisket Beer Mop

1 12-ounce (360-ml) can or bottle light beer (Michelob Ultra, Miller Lite, or Milwaukee's Best Light are the lowest carb—and Milwaukee's Best Light is the cheapest!)

½ cup (120 ml) cider vinegar

¼ cup (60 ml) olive oil

2 cloves garlic, crushed

¼ onion, minced

1 tablespoon (15 g) Worcestershire sauce

1 tablespoon Bodacious Beef Brisket Rub (page 488)

Stir everything together and use to mop your brisket while it's smoking.

Yield: Makes enough to mop 1–2 briskets (but rarely will you use up the entire batch in the course of cooking).

14 grams of carbohydrate, 1 gram of fiber (in entire batch). But since you won't use the entire batch, and a 4-pound brisket will serve at least 8 people, no one will get more than a couple of grams of carbohydrate.

Five-Spice Beef Rub

Wow—This is sort of sweet and Chinese-y. I invented this for beef ribs, but there's no law that says you can't use it on brisket or even on a steak.

2 tablespoons (16.2 g) five-spice powder

2 tablespoons (36 g) garlic salt

1 tablespoon (1.5 g) Splenda

Simply combine everything and stir well. Sprinkle over beef ribs before barbecuing—but set aside 1 ½ teaspoons of the rub first to make the Five-Spice Beef Mop (page 490).

Yield: Makes 5 tablespoons (but then, you'd figured that out already, right?)

Each tablespoonful will have 2 grams of carbohydrate and 1 gram of fiber, for a usable carb count of 1 gram; 0 grams protein.

Five-Spice Beef Mop

1 ½ teaspoons Five-Spice Beef Rub (page 489)

½ cup (120 ml) oil

(continued on page 490)

½ cup (120 ml) water

1 teaspoon blackstrap molasses

Stir everything together and use to mop beef you've first seasoned with Five-Spice Beef Rub.

Yield: This makes 1 cup (240 ml), or plenty for a slab or two of beef ribs, a brisket, or what have you.

4 grams of carbohydrate in the whole batch, and there's no way you'll consume anything like the whole batch. I'd call this one free, carb-wise. 0 grams protein.

Cajun Rub

2 tablespoons (35 g) celery salt

2 tablespoons (13 g) pepper

2 tablespoons (3 g) Splenda

1½ teaspoons garlic powder

2 teaspoons dried thyme

1 teaspoon ground sage

2 teaspoons cayenne

¼ teaspoon blackstrap molasses

This rub needs to be made in a blender to distribute that sticky molasses throughout the mixture. Put everything but the molasses in your blender. Turn the blender on and while it's running drizzle in the ¼ teaspoon molasses. Turn off the blender and sprinkle the rub heavily on pork ribs before barbecuing.

Yield: Makes 5 servings

Each serving will have 5 grams of carbohydrate and 1 gram of fiber, for a usable carb count of 4 grams; 1 gram protein.

Cajun Rib Mop

½ cup (120 ml) cider vinegar

½ cup (120 ml) olive oil

1 tablespoon (15 ml) Worcestershire sauce

½ teaspoon cayenne

Simply combine everything and use to mop pork ribs every 30 to 45 minutes while barbecuing.

Yield: Makes just over 1 cup (240 ml)

10 grams of carbohydrate in the batch, with a trace of fiber and a trace of protein. But you won't actually eat more than 1 tablespoon (15 ml) or so of the mop with a serving, so I'd say no more than 1 gram of carbohydrate per serving.

Wasabi Baste

This is good on any kind of fish or seafood.

2 teaspoons wasabi paste (Buy this in tubes in Asian markets or in grocery stores with a good international section.)

1½ tablespoons (2 g) Splenda

¼ teaspoon blackstrap molasses

2 tablespoons (30 ml) dry sherry

2 tablespoons (30 ml) lime juice

6 tablespoons (90 ml) soy sauce

¼ teaspoon sesame oil

Just stir everything together and baste away.

Yield: A little over ½ cup (120 ml), or enough to baste one darned big salmon, inside and out, as I have reason to know. Figure at least 8 servings.

Each serving will have 2 grams of carbohydrate, a trace of fiber, and 1 gram protein.

Amazing Barbecue Rub

It's the sweetness and the celery undertone that really set this rub apart. It's one of my favorites on pork or chicken.

½ cup (12 g) Splenda
1 teaspoon molasses
3 tablespoons (36 g) celery salt
2 tablespoons (24 g) seasoned salt
2 tablespoons (14.4 g) onion powder
1 tablespoon (8.4 g) garlic powder
1 tablespoon (7.8 g) chili powder
1 tablespoon (6.3 g) pepper
½ teaspoon cayenne
¼ teaspoon cloves, ground
1 whole bay leaf

Simply combine everything and stir well.

Yield: 18 servings of 1 tablespoon each

3 grams of carbohydrate, with a trace of fiber, and a trace of protein.

Bourbon Maple Mop

¼ cup (60 ml) oil
¼ cup (60 ml) water

2 tablespoons (30 ml) bourbon
1 tablespoon (15 ml) sugar-free pancake syrup
1 teaspoon barbecue spice or Classic Barbecue Rub (page 486)

Simply combine all ingredients in a nonreactive bowl or saucepan and stir.

Yield: Enough for a slab or two of ribs.

Not counting the polyols in the sugar-free pancake syrup, there's only a trace of carbohydrate in the whole batch. No fiber, no protein.

Curry Rub

I invented this for poultry, but it would be good on lamb, too!

1 tablespoon (6 g) curry powder
1½ teaspoons onion salt
1½ teaspoons garlic salt
1 teaspoon celery salt

Just combine everything and sprinkle it on chicken, lamb, or what have you. This is just about enough for 1 chicken of about 3½ to 4 pounds (1.6 to 1.8 kg), so feel free to double, triple, or quadruple this recipe, if you like.

Yield: This whole batch—2 tablespoons plus 1 teaspoon worth

Contains 6 grams of carbohydrate, of which 4 grams are fiber, for 2 grams of usable carb. So, if you figure that 1 chicken will serve 5 people, each will get less than ½ gram carbohydrate. 1 gram protein in the whole batch.

Peppery Lamb Rub

2 tablespoons (12.6 g) pepper
1 tablespoon (1.5 g) Splenda
1 tablespoon (18 g) salt or Vege-Sal
1 tablespoon (8.4 g) garlic powder
¼ teaspoon allspice
¼ teaspoon molasses

Put everything but the molasses in a blender. Turn on the blender, drizzle in the molasses, and let everything blend for 30 seconds. Stop the blender and stir the mixture down from the sides if needed.

Yield: Makes about 5 tablespoons (40 g) of rub

Each will have 3 grams of carbohydrate and 1 gram of fiber, for a usable carb count of 2 grams; 1 gram protein.

Lamb Mop

½ cup (120 ml) light beer
¼ cup (60 ml) oil
3 tablespoons (45 ml) vinegar
2 tablespoons (30 ml) Worcestershire sauce
1 tablespoon (8 g) Peppery Lamb Rub
  (page 492)

Just measure everything into a nonreactive bowl or saucepan and stir it up.

Yield: Makes about 1 cup (240 ml)

13 grams of carb and 1 gram of fiber for the whole batch, but you won't end up consuming anything like all of this. I'd doubt very much whether you'll end up with more than 2 grams per serving from this mop.

Dixie Belle Rub

This Southern-style rub is particularly good on pork or chicken.

2 tablespoons (12.6 g) pepper
2 tablespoons (12.6 g) paprika
2 tablespoons (3 g) Splenda
2 teaspoons salt
1 tablespoon (7.2 g) dry mustard
1 teaspoon cayenne
2 teaspoons garlic powder

Just stir everything together and rub on ribs, a pork shoulder, chicken, or what have you!

Yield: Make ½ cup (60 g), or 8 tablespoons

Each serving will have 3 grams of carbohydrate and 1 gram of fiber, for a usable carb count of 2 grams; 1 gram protein.

Southern Sop

The perfect southern mopping sauce to use with your Dixie Belle Rub.

½ cup (120 ml) cider vinegar
½ tablespoon pepper
1 teaspoon salt
1 teaspoon Worcestershire sauce
1 teaspoon paprika
1 tablespoon (8 g) Dixie Belle Rub (page 492)
¼ cup (60 ml) water
¼ cup (60 ml) oil

Just combine everything and use to baste meat or chicken during smoking.

Yield: Makes a little over 1 cup (240 ml), or plenty for your ribs or shoulder or whatever you're barbecuing

14 grams of carbohydrate in the whole batch, with 2 grams of fiber, for a usable carb count of 12 grams; 1 gram of protein. However, you won't use all of this sauce, even for a couple of slabs of ribs, and a couple of slabs will serve 15 to 20 people. Figure that each diner will get no more than 1 to 2 grams of usable carb from this mop.

Sweet Spice Islands Rub

Allspice, ginger, and cloves set this rub apart from the pack. I like this on pork, but it would be great on chicken or duck—lamb, too. You'll need to have Classic Barbecue Rub on hand, of course.

¼ cup (6 g) Splenda
2 tablespoons (16 g) Classic Barbecue Rub (page 486)
1 tablespoon (12 g) seasoned salt
¼ teaspoon allspice
⅛ teaspoon ginger
⅛ teaspoon clove, ground
¼ teaspoon cayenne
½ teaspoon black pepper

Just stir everything together and rub on whatever you feel like barbecuing!

Yield: Makes about 7 servings of 1 tablespoon each

2 grams of carbohydrate, a trace of fiber, and a trace of protein.

Spicy Citrus Butter

This is good melted over grilled fish or seafood, chicken, vegetables, or even a steak. Actually, it's hard to think of what it's not good on!

6 tablespoons (84 g) butter
2 jalapeños
2 tablespoons (3 g) Splenda
2 tablespoons (30 ml) lemon juice
½ teaspoon orange extract

Have the butter at room temperature. Put it in the food processor with the S-blade in place. Seed the jalapeños and whack each one into several pieces; dump them into the food processor and then wash your hands! Add everything else; then run the food processor until the jalapeños are finely minced. Scoop a dollop over your food, hot off the grill.

If you'd like to use this as a baste, you can do it this way, instead: Put the butter in a saucepan over the lowest possible heat. Seed the jalapeños and mince them as fine as you can. Add them to the butter and wash your hands. As the butter liquefies, whisk in the Splenda, lemon juice, and orange extract. Keep it warm on a corner of your grill (not over direct heat) and use it to baste fish fillets, seafood, or chicken breasts.

Yield: Makes 8 servings of a little over 1 tablespoon each

1 gram of carbohydrate, a trace of fiber, and a trace of protein.

Chipotle Garlic Butter

This is easy, and it gives a huge hit of flavor to anything you use it on. Melt it over a steak or use it to baste grilled vegetables or fish—you'll find endless ways to use this!

¼ pound (115 g) butter at room temperature
2 chipotle chiles canned in adobo
1 clove garlic, crushed

Just plunk everything into a food processor with the S-blade in place and run the processor until everything is well combined.

Yield: 8 servings of just over 1 tablespoon each

A trace of carbohydrate, a trace of fiber, and a trace of protein.

Cranberry Sauce

This is unbelievably easy and it's good with roast chicken or turkey—as though you needed to be told!

½ teaspoon plain gelatin (optional)
1 cup (240 ml) water
1 bag (12 ounces, 340 g) fresh cranberries
1 cup (25 g) Splenda

Combine water, cranberries, and Splenda in a saucepan over medium-high heat. (If you're using the gelatin, dissolve it in ½ cup [120 ml] of the water and then add it to the cranberries and Splenda in a saucepan over medium-high heat.) Bring the mixture to a boil and boil it hard until the cranberries pop. Keep it in a tightly covered jar in the fridge.

Yield: Roughly 2 cups (480 ml)

Each 2 tablespoon (30 ml) serving will have 4 grams of carbohydrates and 1 gram of fiber, for a total of 3 grams of usable carbs.

Fresh cranberries are available only in fall, but they freeze beautifully. Just stick them in a plastic bag in the freezer and pull them out when you need them.

Slow Cooker Cranberry Sauce

I like to have cranberry sauce on hand for those occasions when I don't want to do much cooking. It adds interest to plain roasted chicken (or even store-bought rotisseried chicken.) It's easy to do, and this makes plenty!

24 ounces (670 g) cranberries
1 cup (240 ml) water
2 cups (50 g) Splenda

Simply combine everything in a slow cooker and give it a stir. Cover the slow cooker, set it to low, and let it cook for 3 hours.

This won't be as syrupy as commercial cranberry sauce because of the lack of sugar. If this bothers you, you can thicken the sauce with guar or xanthan, but I generally leave mine as-is.

This makes quite a lot, so divide it between three or four snap-top containers and store it in the freezer. This way, you'll have cranberry sauce on hand whenever you bring home a rotisseried chicken!

Yield: Makes about 2¾ cups (660 ml), or 22 servings of 2 tablespoons (30 ml)

Each with trace protein, 4 g carbohydrate, 1 g dietary fiber, 3 g usable carbs.

Cranberry Chutney

Think of this as cranberry sauce with a kick. It's good with any curried poultry even with plain old roast chicken.

1 bag (12 ounces, or 340 g) cranberries
1 cup (240 ml) water
½ cup (12 g) Splenda
2 cloves garlic, crushed
1 tablespoon (5.1 g) pumpkin pie spice
⅛ teaspoon salt

Combine all the ingredients in a saucepan over medium heat, bring it to a boil, and boil until the cranberries pop (7 to 8 minutes).

Yield: Roughly 2 cups (480 ml)

Each 2 tablespoon (30 ml) serving will have just over 3 grams of carbohydrates and 1 gram of fiber, for a total of 2 grams of usable carbs and only a trace of protein.

This recipe improves if you let the boiled mixture sit for a while before serving. Try it with a little cinnamon, too.

Green Tomato Chutney

Most chutneys are full of sugar, so I invented my own—now I plant extra tomatoes in the summer to have enough to make this. It's wonderful with anything curried.

4 quarts (2.9 kg) green tomatoes, cut into chunks
3 cups (710 ml) apple cider vinegar
1 whole ginger root, sliced into very thin rounds
5 or 6 cloves garlic, thinly sliced
1 tablespoon (5 g) whole cloves
5 or 6 sticks whole cinnamon
½ cup (12 g) Splenda
1 tablespoon (15 ml) blackstrap molasses
3 teaspoons stevia/FOS blend

Combine all the ingredients in a large stainless steel or enamel pot—no iron, no aluminum. (This is an acidic mixture, and if you use iron or aluminum you'll end up with your chutney chock full of iron, which will turn it blackish, or aluminum, which simply isn't good for you.) Simmer on low for 3 to 4 hours. Store in tightly closed containers in the refrigerator.

Yield: Roughly 2 quarts (1.9 L)

Each 2 tablespoon (30 ml) serving will have 5 grams of carbohydrates and 1 gram of fiber, for a total of 4 grams of usable carbs and no protein.

(continued on page 496)

There are two things you need to know when buying and cooking with ginger. The first is that a whole ginger is also called a "hand" of ginger. The second is that you should always cut ginger across the grain, not along it, or you'll end up with woody ginger.

Major Grey's Chutney

Major Grey's chutney is not a brand but a type, and it's the most popular kind of chutney in the United States—maybe in the world. But I'm afraid it's usually loaded with sugar. This version isn't, of course! I also substituted peaches for the mangoes you usually find in Major Grey's chutney—peaches are a whole lot easier to find. Go ahead and use frozen unsweetened peach slices in this. It'll save you lots of time and trouble, and since you're going to cook them, the difference in texture won't matter in the end.

2 pounds (910 g) peach slices
1/3 cup (35 g) paper-thin ginger slices
1 1/2 cups (37 g) Splenda
3 cloves garlic
1 teaspoon red pepper flakes
1 teaspoon cloves
1 1/2 cups (360 ml) cider vinegar
Guar or xanthan

Put everything in a large, nonreactive saucepan and stir to combine. Bring to a boil, turn the heat to low, and simmer for 1 1/2 to 2 hours. Thicken a bit with guar or xanthan if you like and store in an airtight container in the fridge.

Yield: 1 quart (960 ml), or 32 servings of 2 tablespoons (30 ml)

Each with trace protein; 4 g carbohydrate; 1 g dietary fiber; 3 g usable carbs.

Easy Orange Salsa

1/2 cup (115 g) salsa
1/4 teaspoon orange extract
2 teaspoons Splenda

Just measure everything into a bowl, stir, and serve.

Yield: 4 servings of 2 tablespoons (30 ml)

Each with trace protein; 2 g carbohydrate; 1 g dietary fiber; 1 g usable carb.

Simple No-Sugar Pickle Relish

24 ounces (670 g) sour pickle spears
1 cup (160 g) chopped onion
1/3 cup (8 g) Splenda
1/2 teaspoon celery seed
1/2 teaspoon mustard seed
2 tablespoons (30 ml) cider vinegar
Guar or xanthan

Open the jar of pickle spears and pour off the liquid into a nonreactive saucepan. Throw the chopped onion into the pickle liquid and stir in the Splenda, celery seed, and mustard seed.

Bring to a simmer, turn to low, and let the whole thing simmer for 20 to 30 minutes.

In the meantime, cut the pickle spears into 3 to 4 chunks each and throw them into a food processor with the S-blade in place.

When the onions are done simmering, pour the contents of the saucepan into the food processor. Add the cider vinegar. Pulse the food processor until everything's chopped to about the consistency of commercial pickle relish. Thicken it up a bit with a little guar or xanthan to make up for the lack of syrupiness and pour the whole thing back into the pickle jar. Store in the fridge and use as you would commercial pickle relish.

Yield: 3 cups (710 ml), or 24 servings of 2 tablespoons (30 ml)

Each with trace protein; 1 g carbohydrate; trace dietary fiber; 1 g usable carbs.

14

Sweets

Butter Cookies

1 cup (225 g) butter

8 ounces (225 g) cream cheese

¼ cup plus 1 tablespoon (7.5 g) Splenda, divided

1 egg

2 cups (160 g) sifted soy powder

½ teaspoon baking powder

½ teaspoon ground cinnamon

Use an electric mixer to cream the butter and cream cheese together until well blended and soft. Add ¼ cup Splenda (6 g) and cream until completely combined. Beat in the egg.

Sift the soy powder and then sift again with the baking powder (to combine the baking powder with the soy powder and to break up any lumps in the baking powder). Sift the combined powders into the mixing bowl with the butter mixture and mix to make a soft dough.

Chill the dough for several hours in a covered container or wrapped in foil; this will make it easier to handle.

When the dough is chilled, preheat the oven to 375°F (190°C, or gas mark 5). Make small balls of the dough and place them on an ungreased cookie sheet.

Mix remaining 1 tablespoon (1.5 g) of Splenda with the cinnamon on a small plate or saucer. Take a flat-bottomed glass, measuring cup, or something similar (I use an old scoop from a jar of protein powder) and butter the bottom. Then dip the buttered cup in the cinnamon and Splenda and use it to press the cookies flat. (You'll need to dip your "pressing glass" in the cinnamon and Splenda for each cookie, but you won't have to rebutter the bottom each time. The butter just keeps the cup from sticking to the cookies and puts yummy cinnamon and Splenda on each one!)

Bake for about 9 minutes, checking at 8 minutes to make sure the bottoms aren't browning too fast. The cookies are done when the bottoms are just starting to brown.

Yield: About 6 dozen

Each with 1 gram of carbohydrates, a trace of fiber, and 1 gram of protein.

Don't butter the cookie sheet or spray it with nonstick cooking spray. Why not? These cookies are so rich, they practically float on the butter that cooks out of them. I had no trouble with them sticking—I had trouble with them sliding around the cookie sheet while they were baking! I call them The Incredible Migrating Cookies. Hopefully your cookie sheets are flatter and your oven more level than mine.

Peanut Butter Cookies

I can't tell these from my mom's peanut butter cookies!

½ cup (115 g) butter, at room temperature

½ cup (12 g) Splenda

2 tablespoons plus 1 teaspoon (19 g) stevia/ FOS blend

1 tablespoon (15 ml) blackstrap or dark molasses

1 egg

(continued on page 500)

1 cup (260 g) natural peanut butter (Creamy is best.)
½ teaspoon salt
½ teaspoon baking soda
½ teaspoon vanilla
1 cup (80 g) soy powder
2 tablespoons (15 g) oat bran

Preheat the oven to 375°F (190°C, or gas mark 5).

Use an electric mixer to beat the butter until creamy. Add the Splenda, stevia/FOS blend, and molasses and beat again until well combined.

Beat in the egg, peanut butter, salt, baking soda, and vanilla. Beat in the soy powder and oat bran.

Butter or spray cookie sheets with nonstick cooking spray. Roll the dough into small balls and place them on the sheets. Use the back of a fork to press the balls of dough flat, leaving those traditional peanut butter cookie crisscross marks. Bake for 10 to 12 minutes.

Yield: About 4½ dozen cookies

Each with 2.3 grams of carbohydrates and 1 gram of fiber, for a total of 1.3 grams of usable carbs and 2 grams of protein.

Almond Cookies

These are crumbly and delicate but very delicious!

1 cup (225 g) butter, at room temperature
1 cup (25 g) Splenda
1 egg
1 cup (260 g) smooth almond butter
½ teaspoon salt
½ teaspoon baking soda

1½ cups (200 g) vanilla whey protein powder
2 tablespoons (30 ml) water
30 whole, shelled almonds

Preheat the oven to 375°F (190°C, or gas mark 5).

Use an electric mixer to beat the butter until smooth and fluffy. Add the Splenda and beat again, scraping down the sides of the bowl until very well combined.

Beat in the egg and then add the almond butter, salt, and baking soda.

Beat in the protein powder about ½ cup (65 g) at a time.

Add the water and beat until everything is well combined.

Use a measuring tablespoon to scoop heaping tablespoons of dough onto greased cookie sheets (each cookie should be made of about 2 tablespoons of dough). Press an almond into the center of each cookie. Bake for 10 to 12 minutes or until the cookies just begin to brown around the edges.

Yield: 2½ dozen nice big cookies

Each with 3.5 grams of carbohydrates and 0.5 grams of fiber, for a total of 3 grams of usable carbs and 4 grams of protein.

Sesame Cookies

½ cup (115 g) butter
1 cup (25 g) Splenda
1 egg
1 cup (240 g) tahini (roasted sesame butter)
½ teaspoon salt

½ teaspoon baking soda
1½ cups (200 g) vanilla whey protein powder
¼ cup (30 g) sesame seeds

Preheat the oven to 375°F (190°C, or gas mark 5).

Use an electric mixer to beat the butter and Splenda together until smooth and fluffy. Beat in the egg, mixing well, and then the tahini, again mixing well.

Add the salt and baking soda and then beat in the protein powder ½ cup (65 g) at a time. Beat in the sesame seeds last.

Spray a cookie sheet with nonstick cooking spray and drop the dough onto it by spoonfuls. Bake for 10 to 12 minutes or until golden.

Yield: About 4½ dozen cookies

Each with 2 grams of carbohydrates, a trace of fiber, and 6 grams of protein.

Mom's Chocolate Chip Cookies

With this recipe, I assume the title of Low-Carb Cookie God.

1 cup (225 g) butter, at room temperature
1½ cups (38 g) Splenda
1½ teaspoons blackstrap molasses
2 eggs
1 cup (125 g) ground almonds
1 cup (130 g) vanilla whey protein powder
¼ cup (25 g) oat bran
1 teaspoon baking soda

1 teaspoon salt
1 cup (125 g) chopped walnuts or pecans
12 ounces (340 g) sugar-free chocolate chips

Preheat the oven to 375°F (190°C, or gas mark 5). If you haven't ground your almonds yet, now would be a good time to do that as well.

Use an electric mixer to beat the butter, Splenda, and molasses until creamy and well blended. Add the eggs, one at a time, and beat well after each addition.

In a separate bowl, stir together the ground almonds, protein powder, oat bran, baking soda, and salt. Add this mixture about ½ cup (65 g) at a time to the Splenda mixture, beating well after each ½-cup addition until it's all beaten in. Stir in the nuts and chocolate chips.

Spray a cookie sheet with nonstick cooking spray and drop the dough by rounded tablespoons onto it. These cookies will not spread and flatten as much as standard chocolate chip cookies, so if you want them flat, flatten them a bit now.

Bake for 10 minutes or until golden. Cool on baking sheets for a couple minutes and then remove to wire racks to cool completely.

Yield: About 4½ dozen cookies

Each with 3 grams of carbohydrates, a trace of fiber, and 5 grams of protein. (This carbohydrate count does not include the polyols used to sweeten the sugar-free chocolate, since it remains largely undigested and unabsorbed.)

If you can't get sugar-free chocolate chips, you need to make some from sugar-free chocolate bars. Break 7 or 8 of the bars (1.3 to 1.5 ounces, or 36 to 42 g each) into three or four pieces each and place the pieces in a food processor with the

S-blade in place. Pulse the food processor until the chocolate bars are in pieces about the same size as commercial chocolate morsels and set them aside until you're ready to use them.

Gingersnaps

So crisp and gingery-cinnamony, these cookies are nothing short of extraordinary.

¼ cup (55 g) butter
½ cup (120 ml) coconut oil
1 cup (25 g) Splenda
¼ cup (50 g) polyol sweetener
1 tablespoon (15 ml) blackstrap molasses
1 egg
1 cup (125 g) almond meal
1 cup (130 g) vanilla whey protein powder
¼ cup (25 g) gluten
2 teaspoons baking soda
½ teaspoon salt
1 teaspoon ground ginger
2 teaspoons cinnamon
½ teaspoon ground cloves

Preheat oven to 350°F (180°C, or gas mark 4).

Using an electric mixer, beat the butter, coconut oil, Splenda, polyol sweetener, blackstrap molasses, and egg together until mixture is creamy and fluffy.

Beat in the almond meal, vanilla whey protein powder, and gluten, then the baking soda, salt, and spices.

The dough will be fairly soft but cohesive. Scoop scant tablespoons of dough onto ungreased cookie sheets, shaping a bit with your fingers to make little balls.

Flatten balls slightly with the back of a spoon or your fingers. Keep in mind when placing cookies on sheets that they will spread some—I find that 10 per sheet is about right.

Bake for about 7 to 9 minutes or until cookies are just getting golden around the edges. Cool on wire racks and store in an airtight container.

Yield: About 42 cookies

Each with 7 g protein; 2 g carbohydrate; trace dietary fiber; 2 g usable carbs. Carb count does not include polyol sweetener.

Hazelnut Shortbread

Do you love Walker's Shortbread cookies? Meet their new low-carb replacement.

2 cups (270 g) hazelnuts
1 cup (225 g) butter, at room temperature
½ cup (12 g) Splenda
1 egg
½ teaspoon salt
¼ teaspoon baking powder
1 cup (130 g) vanilla whey protein powder
2 tablespoons (30 ml) water

Preheat the oven to 325°F (170°C, or gas mark 3).

Grind the hazelnuts to a fine meal with a food processor. Set aside.

Use an electric mixer to beat the butter until it's fluffy. Add the Splenda and beat well again. Beat in the egg, combining well.

Sprinkle the salt and baking powder over the top of the mixture and add half of the ground hazelnuts. Beat them in, add the rest of the hazelnuts, and beat again.

Beat in the vanilla whey protein powder and then the water to make a soft, sticky dough.

Line a shallow baking pan (a jelly roll pan is best, and mine is 11½ × 15½ inches [29 × 39 cm]) with baking parchment and turn the dough out onto the parchment. Cover it with another piece of parchment and press the dough out into an even layer covering the whole pan. (The pressed dough should be about ¼ inch [6 mm] thick.)

Peel off the top sheet of parchment and score the dough into squares using a pizza cutter or a knife with a straight, thin blade. Bake for 25 to 30 minutes or until golden. You'll need to rescore the lines before removing the shortbread from the pan. Use a straight up-and-down motion, and the shortbread will be less likely to break outside the score lines.

Yield: 4 dozen cookies

Each with 1.5 grams of carbohydrates, a trace of fiber, and 1 gram of protein.

Coconut Shortbread

½ cup (115 g) butter, at room temperature
½ cup (120 ml) coconut oil
3 tablespoons (4.5 g) Splenda
1½ cups (200 g) vanilla whey protein powder
1 cup (70 g) finely shredded, unsweetened coconut
2 tablespoons (30 ml) water

Preheat oven to 375°F (190°C, or gas mark 5).

Using an electric mixer, beat together the butter, coconut oil, and Splenda until light and creamy. Beat in the protein powder, coconut, and water, in that order, scraping down the sides of the bowl several times to make sure everything is well blended.

Line a jelly roll pan with baking parchment and turn the dough out onto it. Place another sheet of baking parchment on top and press the dough out into a thin, even sheet. Use a sharp knife, or better yet a pizza cutter, to score the dough into small rectangles. Bake for 7–10 minutes or until golden. Cool and break apart.

Yield: 4 dozen cookies

Each with 1 gram of carbohydrates, a trace of fiber, and 6 grams of protein.

Hermits

Hermits are an old-fashioned cookie with a chewy texture and a brown-sugar-spicy flavor.

½ cup (115 g) butter
¾ cup (18 g) Splenda
¼ cup (50 g) polyol sweetener
2½ teaspoons blackstrap molasses
1 egg
½ cup (120 ml) buttermilk
¾ cup (90 g) almond meal
¼ cup (25 g) wheat gluten
⅓ cup (40 g) vanilla whey protein powder
¾ teaspoon cinnamon

(continued on page 504)

½ **teaspoon ground cloves**
¼ **teaspoon baking soda**
⅓ **cup (50 g) currants**
¼ **cup (30 g) chopped pecans**

Preheat oven to 350°F (180°C, or gas mark 4).

In a large mixing bowl beat the butter until soft with an electric mixer.

Add the Splenda, polyol, and blackstrap molasses and beat until light and creamy. Beat in the egg and the buttermilk.

In a separate bowl, combine the almond meal, gluten, protein powder, cinnamon, cloves, and baking soda. Stir them together to distribute the ingredients.

Add the dry ingredients to the butter mixture in three or four additions, beating well and scraping down the sides of the bowl when needed. Now add the currants and pecans and mix just enough to blend.

Drop the batter by spoonfuls onto greased cookie sheets, keeping in mind that they spread. Bake for 12 to 15 minutes or until just starting to darken around the edges. Cool on wire racks and store in a tightly lidded container.

Yield: About 40 cookies

Each with 4 g protein; 2 g carbohydrate; 2 g usable carbs. Carb count does not include polyol sweetener

I've used currants instead of the traditional raisins in the hermits because they're little and therefore distribute more evenly through the dough—to me, they taste like raisins anyway. If your currants are sort of dry, put them in a small bowl and pour a little boiling water over them before you start.

Then drain them right before you add them. And if you can't get currants, you could use raisins. I'd suggest snipping each one into two or three pieces before adding them, or you're likely to end up with just one or two raisins per cookie.

Pecan Sandies

Peggy Witherow sent me a recipe for Pecan Sandies that she wanted de-carbed, and this is the result.

1 cup (225 g) butter, at room temperature
1 cup (25 g) Splenda
1 egg
1½ cups (200 g) vanilla whey protein powder
1½ cups (185 g) chopped pecans
½ teaspoon salt

Preheat the oven to 325°F (170°C, or gas mark 3).

Beat the butter and Splenda together until light and creamy. Beat in the egg, mixing well. Then beat in the protein powder, pecans, and salt.

Spray a cookie sheet with nonstick cooking spray. Form the dough into balls about the size of a marble and flatten them slightly on the cookie sheet. Bake for 10 to 15 minutes or until golden.

Yield: 4½ dozen cookies

Each with 2 grams of carbohydrates, a trace of fiber, and 5 grams of protein.

Oatmeal Cookies

OMG—These are so good!

1 cup (240 ml) coconut oil
1 cup (225 g) butter, at room temperature
1½ cups (38 g) Splenda
1 teaspoon molasses
2 eggs
1 cup (125 g) ground almonds
1 cup (130 g) vanilla whey protein powder
½ teaspoon salt
1 teaspoon baking soda
1 teaspoon cinnamon
1 cup (80 g) rolled oats
1 cup (125 g) chopped pecans

Preheat the oven to 350°F (180°C, or gas mark 4).

With an electric mixer, beat together the coconut oil, butter, and Splenda until well combined, creamy, and fluffy.

Beat in the molasses and eggs, combining well. Beating the ground almonds, protein powder, salt, and baking soda, scraping down the sides of the bowl a few times and making sure the ingredients are well combined.

Beat in the cinnamon, rolled oats, and pecans.

Spray a cookie sheet with nonstick cooking spray and drop dough onto it by the scant tablespoonful, leaving plenty of room for spreading. Bake for 10 minutes or until golden. Transfer the cookies carefully to wire racks to cool.

Yield: About 5 dozen outrageously good cookies

Each with 3 grams of carbohydrates, a trace of fiber, and 4 grams of protein.

Nut Butter Balls

The high-carb version of this recipe has been around for decades under various names, including Russian Teacakes, of all things. They're a cookie my mom has made every Christmas as far back as I can remember.

1 cup (125 g) almond meal
¾ cup (90 g) vanilla whey protein powder
2 tablespoons (15 g) wheat gluten
1 cup (225 g) butter, softened
⅓ cup (8 g) Splenda
2 tablespoons (25 g) polyol sweetener
½ teaspoon salt
1 teaspoon vanilla
1½ cups (190 g) pecans, finely chopped
6 ounces (170 g) sugar-free dark chocolate, finely chopped

First measure and stir together the almond meal, protein powder, and gluten. Have this standing by.

Using an electric mixter, beat the butter with the Splenda and polyol sweetener until very creamy and fluffy. Beat in the salt and vanilla.

Now beat in the almond meal mixture, about a third at a time.

Finally, beat in the chopped pecans and chopped chocolate. Chill the dough for at least a few hours.

Preheat oven to 350°F (180°C, or gas mark 4). Using clean hands, make balls about 1½ inches (3.75 cm) in diameter and place on ungreased cookie sheets. Bake for 10 to 12 minutes. While still warm, sift just a little extra Splenda over the tops of the cookies to make them look spiffy (if you wait till they cool, none of it will stick!).

Yield: Makes about 50 cookies

Each with 5 g protein; 2 g carbohydrate; trace dietary fiber; 2 g usable carbs. Carb count does not include polyol, either added or in the sugar-free chocolate.

Chocolate Walnut Balls

These are great to make around Christmastime when high-carb temptations abound.

½ cup (115 g) butter, at room temperature
2 ounces (55 g) cream cheese
½ cup (12 g) Splenda
2 tablespoons (16 g) stevia/FOS blend
1 egg
1 teaspoon vanilla extract
1½ cups (120 g) sifted soy powder
¼ teaspoon salt
1½ teaspoons baking powder
2 ounces (55 g) unsweetened baking chocolate
½ cup (65 g) chopped walnuts

Preheat the oven to 375°F (190°C, or gas mark 5).

With an electric mixer, cream the butter and cream cheese until soft and well combined, then the Splenda and stevia/FOS blend. Add the egg and the vanilla and beat until well combined.

Sift the soy powder and then resift it with the salt and baking powder. Add the powders to the butter mixture. (It's easier to beat it in if you add it one-half at a time.)

Melt the chocolate and beat that in and then add the nuts. Mix well.

Butter or spray cookie sheets with nonstick cooking spray. Roll the dough into small balls and place them on the sheets. Bake for 8 to 10 minutes.

Yield: About 40 cookies

Each with 2 grams of carbohydrates and 1 gram of fiber, for a total of 1 gram of usable carbs and 1 gram of protein.

Cocoa-Peanut Logs

This very simple recipe is an adaptation of a recipe using Cocoa Krispies that was around back in the '60s.

4 sugar-free dark chocolate bars (about 1.5 ounces [42 g] each) or 6 ounces (170 g) sugar-free chocolate chips
½ cup (130 g) natural peanut butter (salted is best)
4 cups (115 g) crisp soy cereal (like Rice Krispies, only made from soy)

Over very low heat (preferably using a double boiler or a heat diffuser), melt the chocolate and the peanut butter. Blend well. Stir in the cereal until it's evenly coated.

Coat a 9 × 11-inch (23 × 28-cm) pan with nonstick cooking spray or line it with foil. Press the cereal mixture into the pan and chill for at least a few hours. Cut into squares and store in the refrigerator until ready to serve.

Yield: About 3 dozen logs

Each with 1.5 grams of carbohydrates, a trace of fiber, and about 5 grams of protein. (This does not include the polyols in the chocolate. And remember, those polyols have to be eaten in moderation, or you'll be in gastric distress!)

Chocolate Dips

The high-carb version of this cookie is part of my earliest memories—my mother makes them for Christmas every year, and they're a favorite with everyone. They really dress up a holiday cookie plate, too!

1⅓ cups (160 g) vanilla whey protein powder
1 cup (125 g) almond meal
2 tablespoons (15 g) gluten
½ teaspoon salt
½ cup (115 g) butter, softened
½ cup (120 ml) coconut oil
⅓ cup (8 g) Splenda
2 tablespoons (25 g) polyol sweetener
1 teaspoon vanilla
½ cup (50 g) oat bran
2 tablespoons (30 ml) water
Dipping Chocolate (page 552)

Preheat oven to 325°F (170°C, or gas mark 3).

In one bowl, combine the protein powder, almond meal, gluten, and salt and stir together.

In another bowl, use an electric mixer to beat the butter and coconut oil together. When they're combined, beat in the Splenda and polyol sweetener until the mixture is creamy and fluffy. Beat in the vanilla.

Now beat in the protein powder mixture, adding it in two or three batches. Finally, beat in the oat bran and then the water.

You'll have a stiff, somewhat crumbly dough. Use clean hands to form little logs about 1½ inches (3.75 cm) long and the diameter of a thumb (unless your fingers are huge!), pressing them together well. Bake on ungreased cookie sheets for 25 to 30 minutes. Cool before dipping into the Dipping Chocolate. Dip one end of each cookie in the chocolate. Place on waxed paper to cool.

Yield: At least 36

Assuming 36, each will have 9 g protein; 3 g carbohydrate; trace dietary fiber; 3 g usable carbs. Carb count does not include polyol sweetener.

Great Balls of Protein!

You may recognize this updated version of an old health food standby.

1 jar (16 ounces, or 455 g) natural peanut butter, oil and all
2 cups (260 g) vanilla whey protein powder
Splenda, saccharine, stevia, or whatever sweetener you prefer (optional)
Sesame seeds (optional)
Unsweetened shredded coconut (optional)
Sugar-free chocolate bars (optional)
Unsweetened cocoa powder (optional)
Splenda (optional)

(continued on page 508)

Thoroughly combine the peanut butter with the protein powder. (I find that working in about ⅓ cup (45 g) of the protein powder at a time is about right.) This should make a stiff, somewhat crumbly dough.

Work the sweetener of your choice (if using) into the dough. My whey protein powder is sweetened with stevia, and I find that that's enough sweetener for me. But if you want your Great Balls of Protein to be sweeter, simply add sweetener. (If you're using stevia, dissolve it in a couple of tablespoons [30 ml] of water and sprinkle it evenly over the mixture before working it in, or it's not likely to spread throughout the mixture very well. Actually, it's best to sprinkle any sweetener evenly before combining it with a mixture this thick.)

Roll into balls about 1 inch (2.5 cm) in diameter.

It's nice to coat these with something. If you like sesame seeds, you can toast them by shaking them in a dry, heavy skillet over medium heat until they start popping and jumping around the pan and then roll the balls in them while they're still warm. You could roll them in coconut, if you prefer; most natural food stores carry it unsweetened and shredded. Again, you can toast it lightly in a dry frying pan and add a little Splenda. Or you could melt sugar-free chocolate bars and dip your Balls of Protein in chocolate—although it would probably be simpler to chop them up and mix them in. Another option is to roll them in unsweetened cocoa mixed with a little Splenda.

Yield: About 50 balls

Each with 3 grams of carbohydrates, a trace of fiber, and 10 grams of protein. (Analysis does not include coatings for balls.)

This is easiest to make if you have a powerful stand mixer or a heavy-duty food processor. If you don't, don't try to use a smaller appliance—you'll only burn it out and destroy it! Rather than dooming your old mixer, just roll up your sleeves, scrub your hands, and dive in.

Espresso Chocolate Chip Brownies

A friend posted the original version of this recipe—definitely not low carb—online. (Thanks, Robin!) I couldn't resist the challenge. They're wonderful!

1 cup (25 g) Splenda
½ cup (65 g) vanilla whey protein powder
¼ cup (30 g) almond meal
½ cup (45 g) unsweetened cocoa powder
1 tablespoon (12 g) instant coffee crystals (regular or decaf, as you prefer)
½ teaspoon salt
½ cup (115 g) butter
2 large eggs
¼ cup (60 ml) water
6 ounces (170 g) sugar-free chocolate chips or sugar-free dark chocolate bars, chopped to chocolate chip–size in the food processor

Preheat oven to 350°F (180°C, or gas mark 4).

Put Splenda, protein powder, almond meal, cocoa, instant coffee crystals, and salt in a food processor with the S-blade in place. Pulse to combine. Add the butter and pulse until the butter is "cut in"—well combined with the dry ingredients. Turn out into a bowl. Mix in the eggs, one at a time, beating well with a whisk after each. Then beat in the water. Finally, stir in the chocolate chips or chopped-up chocolate bars. Spray an 8 × 8-inch (20 × 20-cm) pan with nonstick cooking spray and spread the batter evenly in the pan. Bake for 15 to 20 minutes—do not overbake! Cool and cut into squares.

Yield: I made 25 small brownies from this—I like to have the option of having a little something, and if I want more, I can always have two.

If you do, indeed, make 25, each brownie will have 3 g carbohydrate and 1 g fiber, for a usable carb count of 2 g; 3 g protein.

Yield: If you prefer, you can make 16 bigger brownies

At 4 g carb each, and 1 g fiber, for a usable carb count of 3 g, with 4 g protein. Carb count does not include polyol sweetener in the sugar-free chocolate.

Dana's Brownies

2 ounces (55 g) bitter chocolate
8 ounces (225 g) butter
½ cup (100 g) polyol sweetener
½ cup (12 g) Splenda
2 eggs
½ cup (65 g) vanilla whey protein powder
1 pinch salt

Preheat oven to 350°F (180°C, or gas mark 4).

In the top of a double boiler or in a saucepan over a heat diffuser set on lowest possible heat, melt the chocolate and the butter together. Stir until they're well combined. Scrape this into a mixing bowl.

Add the polyol sweetener and stir well and then stir in the Splenda. Next, beat in the eggs, one at a time. Stir in the vanilla whey protein powder and salt.

Pour into an 8 × 8-inch (20 × 20-cm) baking pan you've sprayed well with nonstick cooking spray. Bake for 15 to 20 minutes. Do not overbake! Cut into 12 bars and let cool in the pan. Store in a tightly covered container in the refrigerator.

Yield: 12 servings

Each with 9 g protein; 2 g carbohydrate; 1 g dietary fiber; 1 g usable carb. Carb count does not include polyol sweetener.

Zucchini-Carrot Cake

About 1¼ cups (170 g) hazelnuts
2 eggs
½ cup (120 ml) oil
½ cup (120 ml) yogurt
⅔ cup (17 g) Splenda
½ cup (65 g) vanilla whey protein powder
1 teaspoon baking soda
½ teaspoon salt
1½ teaspoons cinnamon

(continued on page 510)

¼ teaspoon nutmeg

¾ cup (45 g) shredded zucchini

¼ cup (30 g) shredded carrot

Preheat the oven to 350°F (180°C, or gas mark 4).

In a food processor with the S-blade in place, use the pulse control to grind the hazelnuts to a mealy consistency. (You want 1½ cups of ground hazelnuts when you're done, and for some inexplicable reason they seem to actually grow a little rather than shrink a little when you grind them.) Set the ground hazelnuts aside.

In a large mixing bowl, whisk the eggs until well blended. Add the oil, yogurt, ground hazelnuts, Splenda, protein powder, baking soda, salt, cinnamon, and nutmeg, mixing well after each addition. (It's especially important that the baking soda be well distributed through the mixture.) Add the zucchini and carrots last, mixing well.

Thoroughly coat a ring mold or bundt pan with nonstick cooking spray and turn the batter into it. (If you sprayed your pan ahead of time, give it another shot just before adding the batter. And don't expect the batter to fill the pan to the rim; it fills my bundt pan about halfway.)

Bake for 45 minutes and turn out gently onto a wire rack to cool.

Yield: 8 generous servings

Each with 8 grams of carbohydrates and 2 grams of fiber, for a total of 6 grams of usable carbs and 16 grams of protein.

This doesn't need a darned thing—it's simply delicious exactly the way it is. If you wish to gild the lily, however, you could top it with whipped topping, pumpkin cream, or cream cheese frosting. This cake, by the way, makes a fabulous breakfast, and since it's loaded with protein and good fats, it should keep you going all morning.

Adam's Chocolate Birthday Cake

I made a low-carb feast for my friend Adam's birthday, and this was the cake. It's not a layer cake, it's a snack-type cake: dense, moist, and fudgy—a lot like brownies. It's easy, too, because it needs no frosting, tasting great just as it is.

1 cup (125 g) finely ground hazelnuts

½ cup (65 g) vanilla whey protein powder

3 tablespoons (17 g) unsweetened cocoa powder

1 teaspoon baking soda

1 cup (25 g) Splenda

½ teaspoon salt

5 tablespoons (75 ml) oil (peanut, sunflower, canola, or whatever)

1 tablespoon (15 ml) cider vinegar

1 cup (240 ml) cold water

Preheat the oven to 350°F (180°C, or gas mark 4).

In a bowl, combine the hazelnuts, protein powder, cocoa, baking soda, Splenda, and salt and stir them together quite well. (Make sure there are no lumps of baking soda!)

Spray a 9 × 9-inch (23 × 23-cm) baking dish with nonstick cooking spray and place the hazelnut mixture in it. Make two holes in this mixture. Pour the oil into one, the vinegar into the other, and the water over the whole thing. Mix with a spoon or fork until everything's well combined. Bake for 30 minutes.

Yield: 9 servings

Each with 7 grams of carbohydrates and 1 gram of fiber, for a total of 6 grams of usable carbs and 12 grams of protein.

Italian Walnut Cake

This traditional Italian cake is a clear demonstration that a few simple ingredients properly combined can yield extraordinary results. If it takes you a few days to eat up all of your Italian Walnut Cake, the Splenda on top will melt, leaving a glazed look instead of powdery whiteness, but it will still taste wonderful. This would be fabulous with a simple cup of espresso.

12 ounces (340 g) walnuts
½ cup (100 g) polyol sweetener, divided
4 eggs
1 pinch cream of tartar
¾ cup (18 g) Splenda
2 teaspoons lemon zest
1 pinch salt
2 tablespoons (3 g) extra Splenda for topping

Preheat oven to 350°F (180°C, or gas mark 4). Spray a 9-inch (23-cm) springform pan with nonstick cooking spray and line the bottom with a circle of baking parchment or a reusable Teflon pan liner.

Put the walnuts in a food processor with the S-blade in place. Pulse until the nuts are chopped medium-fine. Add 2 tablespoons (25 g) of the polyol sweetener to the nuts and pulse until nuts are finely ground but not oily. (Don't overprocess. You don't want nut butter!)

Separate the eggs. Since even the tiniest speck of egg yolk will cause the whites to stubbornly refuse to whip, do yourself a big favor and separate each one into a small dish or cup before adding the white to the bowl you plan to whip them in! Then, if you break one yolk, you've only messed up that white. Put the whites in a deep, narrow mixing bowl and put the yolks in a larger mixing bowl.

Add the pinch of cream of tartar to the whites and use an electric mixer (not a blender or food processor!) to whip the egg whites until they stand in stiff peaks. Set aside.

In a larger bowl, beat the yolks with the rest of the polyol sweetener and the ¾ cup (18 g) Splenda until the mixture is pale yellow and very creamy—at least 3 to 4 minutes. Beat in the lemon zest and the salt.

Stir the ground walnuts into the yolk mixture—you can use the electric mixer, but the mixture will be so thick, I think a spoon is easier. When that's well combined, use a rubber scraper to gently fold in the egg whites one-third at a time, incorporating each third well before adding the next. When all the egg whites are folded in, gently pour batter into the prepared pan.

(continued on page 512)

Bake for 45 minutes. Sprinkle top with the 2 additional tablespoons (3 g) Splenda while the cake is hot and then let cool before serving. Cut in thin wedges to serve.

Yield: 12 servings

Each with 9 g protein; 4 g carbohydrate; 1 g dietary fiber; 3 g usable carbs. Carb count does not include polyol sweetener.

Gingerbread

I've always loved gingerbread and this is as good as any high-carb gingerbread I've ever had! Don't worry about that zucchini; it completely disappears, leaving only moistness behind.

1 cup (125 g) ground almonds (or ²/₃ cup raw almonds finely ground in a food processor)
½ cup (65 g) vanilla whey protein powder
1 teaspoon baking soda
½ teaspoon salt
2½ teaspoons ground ginger
½ teaspoon ground cinnamon
½ cup (12 g) Splenda
½ cup (120 ml) plain yogurt
¼ cup (60 ml) oil
1 teaspoon blackstrap molasses
1 egg
2 tablespoons (30 ml) water
½ cup (65 g) shredded zucchini

Preheat the oven to 350°F (180°C, or gas mark 4).

In a mixing bowl, combine the almonds, protein powder, baking soda, salt, ginger, cinnamon, and Splenda and mix them well.

In a separate bowl or measuring cup, whisk together the yogurt, oil, molasses, egg, and water. Pour into the dry ingredients and whisk until everything is well combined and there are no dry spots. Add the zucchini and whisk briefly to distribute evenly.

Spray an 8 × 8-inch (20 × 20-cm) baking pan with nonstick cooking spray and pour the batter into it. Bake for 30 minutes or until a toothpick inserted in the middle comes out clean.

Yield: 9 servings

Each with 9 grams of carbohydrates, a trace of fiber, and 17 grams of protein.

Try serving this with Whipped Topping (page 552).

Chocolate Cheesecake

You'll be surprised how good a cheesecake you can make from cottage cheese! It's high in protein, too.

2 cups (450 g) cottage cheese
2 eggs
½ cup (115 g) sour cream
2 ounces (55 g) unsweetened baking chocolate, melted
¼ cup (6 g) Splenda
1 Hazelnut Crust (page 522) or Simple Almond Crust (page 522), prebaked in a large, deep pie plate

Preheat the oven to 375°F (190°C, or gas mark 5).

Put the cottage cheese, eggs, and sour cream in a blender. Run the blender, scraping down the sides now and then, until this mixture is very smooth. Add the melted chocolate and Splenda, and blend again.

Pour into the prebaked crust. Place the cake on the top rack of the oven and place a flat pan of water on the bottom rack. Bake for 40 to 45 minutes.

Cool and then chill well before serving. Serve with whipped cream.

Yield: 12 servings

Each with 7 grams of carbohydrates and 2 grams of fiber, for a total of 5 grams of usable carbs and 16 grams of protein. (Analysis includes the crust but not the whipped cream.)

Cheesecake to Go with Fruit

This lemon-vanilla cheesecake is wonderful with strawberries, blueberries, cherries—any fruit you care to use. It also makes a nice breakfast.

2 cups (450 g) cottage cheese
2 eggs
½ cup (115 g) sour cream
¼ cup (32 g) vanilla whey protein powder
¼ cup (6 g) Splenda
Grated rind and juice of 1 fresh lemon
1 teaspoon vanilla extract

1 Hazelnut Crust (page 522) or Simple Almond Crust (page 522), prebaked in a large, deep pie plate

Preheat the oven to 375°F (190°C, or gas mark 5).

Put the cottage cheese, eggs, sour cream, protein powder, Splenda, lemon rind and juice, and vanilla extract in a blender and blend until very smooth.

Pour into the prebaked crust. Place the cake on the top rack of the oven and place a flat pan of water on the bottom rack. Bake for 30 to 40 minutes. Cool and then chill well before serving.

Yield: 12 servings

Each with 8 grams of carbohydrates and 2 grams of fiber, for a total of 6 grams of usable carbs and 21 grams of protein. (Analysis includes crust.)

Serve this cheesecake with the fruit of your choice. I like to serve it with thawed frozen, unsweetened strawberries, blueberries, or peaches mashed coarsely with a fork and sweetened slightly with Splenda. If you use 1½ cups (450 g) of frozen strawberries with 2 tablespoons (3 g) Splenda for the whole cake, you'll add 2 grams of carbohydrates per slice, plus a trace of fiber and a trace of protein. Use 1½ cups (235 g) sour cherries—you can get these canned, with no added sugar—and sweeten them with ¼ cup (6 g) Splenda, and you'll add 3 grams per slice. I'm lucky enough to have a sour cherry tree, and cherry cheesecake is one of the joys of early summer around here!

Lime Cheesecake with Ginger Almond Crust

Using Neufchâtel cheese in this cheesecake gives a lower calorie count without increasing the carb count, and it still gives a superb flavor and texture.

16 ounces (455 g) Neufchâtel or cream cheese, softened
½ cup (12 g) Splenda
2 eggs
½ cup (115 g) plain yogurt or sour cream
Juice and grated rind of 1 lime
½ teaspoon vanilla extract
Ginger Almond Crust (page 524)

Preheat oven to 325°F (170°C, or gas mark 3).

With an electric mixer, beat the Neufchâtel or cream cheese until smooth and fluffy. Beat in the Splenda, eggs, and yogurt, in that order, beating well after each addition. Scrape down the sides of the bowl often with a rubber scraper. Now, beat in the lime juice, rind, and vanilla extract. Pour into prepared crust. Put a flat container of water on the floor of the oven and then put your cheesecake on the oven shelf. Bake for about 45 minutes or until only the very center of the cake jiggles a little when you shake it. Chill well before serving.

Yield: 8 to 10 servings

Assuming 8, each will have 11 grams of carbohydrate, with 3 grams of fiber, for a usable carb count of 8 grams; 15 grams protein. (Analysis includes Ginger Almond Crust.)

Margarita No-Bake Cheesecake

I saw Emeril make a margarita cheesecake on his show one night, and I had to decarb it the very next day! It's fabulous. You can make this with cream cheese and sour cream, if you like, for added richness or with Neufchâtel cheese and plain yogurt for a lower calorie count with no increase in carbs.

1½ tablespoons (10.4 g) unflavored gelatin
1 cup (25 g) Splenda
¾ cup (180 ml) boiling water
1½ pounds (680 g) cream cheese or Neufchâtel cheese, softened
1 cup (230 g) sour cream or plain yogurt
¼ cup (60 ml) lime juice
2 teaspoons grated lime rind
½ teaspoon orange extract
¼ cup (60 ml) tequila
Sweet-and-Salty Almond Crust (page 523)

Combine the gelatin and Splenda in a saucepan and pour the boiling water over them. Stir over low heat until the gelatin is completely dissolved. Turn off the heat.

Put the softened cream cheese or Neufchâtel cheese in a mixing bowl and beat with an electric mixer until very soft and creamy. (If you have a stand mixer, you can start the cheese beating before you dissolve the gelatin and just leave the mixer mixing on its own.) When the cheese is very smooth and creamy, add the sour cream or yogurt and beat that in well, scraping down the sides of the bowl as needed. Next, beat in the lime juice, grated lime rind, orange extract, and tequila. Go back to the saucepan of gelatin. It should still be liquid! If it's not, you'll need to heat it again, gently. Beat the gelatin mixture into the cheese mixture and make sure everything is very well combined. Pour into the Sweet-and-Salty Almond Crust and chill for at least 4 or 5 hours, and overnight is better.

Run a knife around the cake between the cake and the rim of the springform pan before removing the rim. Slice with a thin-bladed knife—dipping the knife in hot water before each slice is a good idea, although not essential.

Garnish with paper-thin slices of lime, strips of lime zest, or both.

Yield: 12 servings

Each serving will have 11 grams of carbohydrate and 2 grams of fiber, for a usable carb count of 9 grams, and 12 grams of protein. (Analysis includes crust.)

Sunshine Cheesecake

This has a lovely, creamy texture and a bright, sunshiney orange flavor. Using the stevia/FOS blend keeps the carb count very low.

1 cup (225 g) cottage cheese
1 package (8 ounces, 225 g) cream cheese, softened
1 cup (230 g) sour cream
4 eggs
Grated rind of 1 orange
1 tablespoon (15 ml) orange extract
1 tablespoon plus 1 teaspoon (10 g) stevia/ FOS blend
2 tablespoons (30 ml) lemon juice
Tiny pinch salt
1 Hazelnut Crust (page 522) or Simple Almond Crust (page 522), prebaked in a springform pan

Preheat oven to 325°F (170°C, or gas mark 3).

Put the cottage cheese, cream cheese, sour cream, eggs, orange rind, orange extract, stevia, lemon juice, and salt in a blender and run the blender until everything is well-blended and a bit fluffy.

Pour into the prebaked crust. Place the cake on the top rack of the oven and place a flat pan of water on the bottom rack. Bake for 50 minutes. The cheesecake will still jiggle slightly in the center when you take it out. Cool and then chill well before serving.

Yield: 12 servings

Each with 8 grams of carbohydrates and 2 grams of fiber, for a total of 6 grams of usable carbs and 17 grams of protein. (Analysis includes crust.)

This is wonderful with sugar-free chocolate syrup. Many grocery stores carry it; it's worth your while to try to find it.

Blackbottomed Mockahlua Cheesecake

You'll have to make yourself some Mockahlua before you can make this. What better incentive could you have?

(continued on page 516)

FOR THE BLACKBOTTOM LAYER:

3 sugar-free dark chocolate bars (about 1.5 ounces [42 g] each)

¼ cup (60 ml) heavy cream

1 Simple Almond Crust (page 522), prebaked in a springform pan

FOR THE MOCKAHLUA FILLING:

3 packages (8 ounces [225 g] each) cream cheese, softened

¾ cup (18 g) Splenda

¾ cup (175 g) sour cream

1 tablespoon (15 ml) vanilla extract

4 eggs

⅓ cup (80 ml) Mockahlua (page 46)

Preheat the oven to 325°F (170°C, or gas mark 3).

To make the blackbottom layer: Over the lowest possible heat, melt the chocolate bars (preferably in a heat diffuser or a double boiler to keep the chocolate from burning). When the chocolate is melted, stir in the cream, blending well. Pour over the crust and spread evenly.

To make the Mockahlua filling: In large bowl, use an electric mixer to beat the cream cheese until smooth, scraping down the sides of the bowl often. Beat in the Splenda and sour cream and mix well. Beat in the vanilla and eggs, one by one, beating until very smooth and creamy. Beat in the Mockahlua last and mix well.

Pour the filling into the chocolate-coated crust. Place the cake in the oven and place a pie pan of water on the rack below it or on the floor of the even. Bake for 1 hour.

Cool in the pan on a wire rack. Chill well before serving.

Yield: 12 servings

Each with 10 grams of carbohydrates and 2 grams of fiber, for a total of 8 grams of usable carbs and 18 grams of protein. (Analysis includes crust, but omits the polyols in the sugar-free chocolate.)

Chocolate Chocolate Chip Cheesecake

This cake happened because I found a bottle of white chocolate sugar-free coffee flavoring syrup on sale at a discount store. My brain immediately cried, "Cheesecake!" Feel free to use cream cheese and full-fat sour cream, if you prefer—you'll raise the calorie count but not the carb count.

Crisp Chocolate Crust (page 521, but see instructions below)

24 ounces (680 g) Neufchâtel cheese

¾ cup (180 ml) white chocolate sugar-free coffee-flavoring syrup (such as Da Vinci)

3 eggs

½ cup (115 g) light sour cream

5 ounces (140 g) sugar-free dark chocolate

Preheat oven to 325°F (170°C, or gas mark 3).

Make the Crisp Chocolate Crust first, only this time make it in a 9-inch (23-cm) springform pan. You won't be able to build it all the way up the sides, but be sure you cover the seam around the bottom of the pan and press the crust mixture firmly in place. Prebake crust for 5 minutes. Remove from oven and let it cool a bit while you make the filling.

In a big mixing bowl, use an electric mixer to beat the Neufchâtel cheese and white chocolate syrup together until very smooth and creamy—scrape down the sides of the bowl often during this process.

Now beat in the eggs, one at a time, then the light sour cream. Turn off the mixer for the next step.

With a knife or using the S-blade in your food processor, chop the sugar-free dark chocolate into little chunks about the size of mini-chips. Add to the cheese mixture and beat in. Pour the filling into the prepared crust.

Put a pan of water on the floor of the oven. Now place the cake on the rack above it and bake for 50 to 60 minutes. Cool and then chill before slicing.

Yield: 12 servings

Each with 13 g protein; 7 g carbohydrate; 3 g dietary fiber; 4 g usable carbs. Analysis includes crust.

Butter-Pecan Cheesecake

All you butterscotch fans are going to love this one.

FOR THE PECAN COOKIE CRUST:
½ **cup (115 g) butter, softened**
½ **cup (12 g) Splenda**
¾ **cups (90 g) vanilla whey protein powder**
¾ **cups (90 g) chopped pecans**
½ **teaspoon salt**

FOR THE BUTTERSCOTCH FILLING:
3 **packages (8 ounces [225 g] each) cream cheese, softened**
¾ **cup (18 g) Splenda**
¾ **cup (98 g) sour cream**
2 **teaspoons butter flavoring**
1 **tablespoon (15 ml) vanilla extract**
1 **tablespoon (15 ml) blackstrap molasses**
4 **eggs**

Preheat the oven to 325°F (170°C, or gas mark 3).

To make the crust: Beat the butter and Splenda together until light and creamy. Then beat in the protein powder, pecans, and salt. Spray a springform pan with nonstick cooking spray and press the crust evenly and firmly into the bottom of the pan, plus just far enough up the sides to cover the seam at the bottom. Bake for 12 to 15 minutes until lightly golden. Set aside to cool while you make the filling.

To make the filling: In a large bowl, use an electric mixer to beat the cream cheese until smooth, scraping down the sides of the bowl often. Next, beat in the Splenda and the sour cream and mix well. Beat in the butter flavoring, vanilla, and molasses; add the eggs one by one, beating until very smooth and creamy.

Pour the mixture into the crust. Place the cake in the oven and place a pie pan of water on the oven rack below it or on the floor of the oven. Bake for 1 hour.

Cool in the pan on a wire rack. Chill well before serving.

Yield: 12 servings

(continued on page 518)

Each with 9 grams of carbohydrates and 1 gram of fiber, for a total of 8 grams of usable carbs and 18 grams of protein. (Analysis includes crust.)

For a nice touch, decorate this with some pretty pecan halves.

Grasshopper Cheesecake

If you're a mint chocolate chip ice cream fan, this is your cheesecake! Chocolate extract can be a little hard to find, but it's worth it for this. If you can only find "flavoring," not extract (you'll know because flavorings are in teeny little bottles), keep in mind that these are far more concentrated, so taste as you go.

FOR THE CHOCOLATE LAYER:
3 sugar-free dark chocolate bars (about 1.5 ounces [42 g] each)
¼ cup (60 ml) heavy cream
1 Simple Almond Crust (page 522) or Hazelnut Crust (page 522), prebaked in a springform pan

FOR THE GRASSHOPPER FILLING:
3 packages (8 ounces [225 g] each) cream cheese, softened
¾ cup (18 g) Splenda
¾ cup (90 g) sour cream
¾ teaspoon peppermint extract
1½ tablespoons (23 ml) chocolate extract
1 or 2 drops green food coloring (optional, but pretty)
4 eggs

Preheat oven to 325°F (170°C, or gas mark 3).

To make the chocolate layer: In the top of a double boiler over hot water (or in a heavy-bottomed saucepan over the lowest possible heat), melt the chocolate and whisk in the cream until smooth. Spread this mixture evenly over the crust and set aside.

To make the filling: In a large bowl, use an electric mixer to beat the cream cheese until smooth, scraping down the sides of the bowl often. Beat in the Splenda and the sour cream and mix well. Beat in the peppermint and chocolate extracts, food coloring (if using), and eggs, one by one, beating until very smooth and creamy.

Pour the mixture into the chocolate-coated crust. Place the cake in the oven and place a pie pan of water on the oven rack below it or on the oven floor. Bake for 1 hour.

Cool in the pan on a wire rack. Chill well before serving.

Yield: 12 servings

Each with 9 grams of carbohydrates and 2 grams of fiber, for a total of 7 grams of usable carbs and 18 grams of protein. (Analysis includes crust, but omits the polyols in the sugar-free chocolate.)

Mochaccino Cheesecake

This cheesecake is extraordinary, as good as any dessert I ever had in a restaurant. This alone is a good enough reason to go buy a large, round slow cooker and an 8-inch (20-cm) springform pan to fit into it! It's also a good excuse to make some Mockahlua, but who needs an excuse to do that?

16 ounces (455 g) light cream cheese or Neufchâtel cheese, softened

1 egg

¼ cup (60 ml) heavy cream

½ cup plus 2 tablespoons (50 g) unsweetened cocoa powder

½ cup (12 g) Splenda

¼ cup (60 ml) Mockahlua (page 46)

2 tablespoons (30 ml) brewed coffee

Crisp Chocolate Crust (page 521), prebaked into an 8-inch (20-cm) springform pan

Using an electric mixer, beat together the cream cheese, egg, and cream until quite smooth. (You'll need to scrape down the sides of the bowl several times.) Now beat in the cocoa powder, Splenda, Mockahlua, and coffee. When it's all well blended and very smooth, pour into the crust. Cover the springform pan tightly with foil, squeezing it in around the rim.

Take a big sheet of foil, at least 18 inches (46 cm) long, and roll it into a loose cylinder. Bend it into a circle and place it in the bottom of a slow cooker. (You're making a rack to put the pan on.) Pour ¼ inch (6 mm) of water in the bottom of the slow cooker and then put the pan on the donut of foil. Cover the slow cooker, set it to high, and let it cook for 3 to 4 hours.

Turn off the slow cooker, uncover, and let cool for at least 20 to 30 minutes before you try to remove the pan from the slow cooker. Chill well before serving.

It's nice to make the Whipped Topping (page 552), with a little Mockahlua in it, to serve on top of this, but it's hardly essential.

Yield: 12 servings

Each with 11 g protein, 10 g carbohydrate, 4 g dietary fiber, 6 g usable carbs. (Analysis includes Crisp Chocolate Crust. You could cut this into eight, more generous servings if you'd like.)

New York–Style Cheesecake

You can top this with fruit if you like, but it's mighty good just as it is.

"Graham" Crust (page 524)

1 pound (455 g) light cream cheese or Neufchâtel cheese, softened

½ cup (115 g) light sour cream

2 eggs

½ cup (12 g) Splenda

2 teaspoons vanilla extract

1 pinch salt

Prepare the "Graham" Crust and let it cool.

Using an electric mixer, beat the cheese, sour cream, and eggs until they're very smooth. (You'll need to scrape down the sides of the bowl at least a few times.) Now beat in the Splenda, vanilla extract, and salt. Pour into the waiting crust. Cover the pan tightly with foil, squeezing it in around the rim.

Take a big sheet of foil, at least 18 inches (45 cm) long, and roll it into a loose cylinder. Bend it into a circle and place it in the bottom of a slow cooker. (You're making a rack to put the pan on.) Pour ¼ inch (6 mm) of water into the

(continued on page 520)

slow cooker and then put the pan on the donut of foil. Cover the slow cooker, set it to high, and let it cook for 3 to 4 hours.

Turn off the slow cooker, uncover, and let cool for at least 20 to 30 minutes before you try to remove the pan from the slow cooker. Chill well before serving.

Yield: 12 servings

Each with 8 g protein, 6 g carbohydrate, 2 g dietary fiber, 4 g usable carbs. (Analysis includes graham crust. You could cut this into eight, more generous servings if you'd like.)

Peanut Butter Cheesecake

You can certainly eat this plain, but I'd likely top it with some sugar-free chocolate sauce. Sorbee makes one that's available in my grocery store, or you could order some from a low-carb online retailer. Or you could make some from the recipe on page 551. Or for that matter, you could melt 6 to 8 ounces (170 to 225 g) of your favorite sugar-free chocolate bars and swirl them into the peanut butter batter before baking. The possibilities are endless!

Crisp Chocolate Crust (page 521) or "Graham" Crust (page 524)
16 ounces (455 g) light cream cheese or Neufchâtel cheese, softened
½ cup (115 g) light sour cream
1 egg

¾ cup (200 g) natural peanut butter (Salted is better than no-salt-added, here.)
⅔ cup (16 g) Splenda
½ teaspoons blackstrap molasses

Have the crust made and standing by.

Using an electric mixer, beat the cream cheese or Neufchâtel, sour cream, and egg until they're very smooth. (You'll want to scrape down the sides of the bowl several times.) Now beat in the peanut butter, Splenda, and molasses. When the mixture is very smooth and well blended, pour it into the crust. Cover the pan tightly with foil, squeezing it in around the rim.

Take a big sheet of foil, at least 18 inches (45 cm) long, and roll it into a loose cylinder. Bend it into a circle and place it in the bottom of a slow cooker. (You're making a rack to put the pan on.) Pour ¼ inch (6 mm) of water into the slow cooker and then put the pan on the donut of foil. Cover the slow cooker, set it to high, and let it cook for 3 to 4 hours.

Turn off the slow cooker, uncover, and let cool for at least 20 to 30 minutes before you try to remove the pan from the slow cooker. Chill well before serving.

Yield: 12 servings

Each with 13 g protein, 10 g carbohydrate, 4 g dietary fiber, 6 g usable carbs. (Analysis includes Crisp Chocolate Crust. Analysis does not include any chocolate sauce or melted chocolate you might add! You could cut this into eight, more generous servings if you'd like.)

Pie Crust

Because rolling this pie crust out doesn't work well, you'll have to settle for one-crust pies. But that's lots better than no-crust pies! I'm very pleased with how the texture of this crust worked out; it's brittle and flaky, just like a pie crust should be.

½ cup (60 g) almond meal
⅓ cup (40 g) rice protein powder
¼ cup (25 g) wheat gluten
1 pinch baking powder
½ teaspoon salt
⅓ cup (80 ml) coconut oil, chilled
1 tablespoon (14 g) butter, chilled
3 tablespoons (45 ml) ice water

Put the almond meal, rice protein powder, gluten, baking powder, and salt in a food processor with the S-blade in place. Add the coconut oil and the butter and pulse the food processor until the shortening is cut into the dry ingredients—it should be sort of mealy in texture.

Do use ice water, not just cold water (I put an ice cube in a cup, cover it with water, and let the water sit for a minute). Now add 1 tablespoon (15 ml) of this water to the dough, pulse the food processor briefly and then repeat 2 more times with the other 2 tablespoons (30 ml) of water.

I find that pressing this crust into place works better than rolling it out. Dump out the dough into a 9-inch (23-cm) pie plate and press it into place evenly across the bottom and up the sides; then crimp the top rim, if you want to be spiffy about it.

You can now bake the pie shell empty and use it for any recipe that calls for a prebaked pie shell or you can fill and bake it according to any recipe that calls for an unbaked pie shell. If you want to prebake the pie shell, preheat your oven to 450°F (230°C, or gas mark 8). Prick the bottom of the pie shell all over with a fork and then add a layer of dried beans, marbles, or clean, round pebbles—this is to keep the pie shell from buckling. Bake for 10 minutes, take it out of the oven, and remove the beans, marbles, or pebbles, dealing gingerly with any that may have embedded themselves a bit. Return the crust to the oven for another 3 to 5 minutes and then cool and fill.

Yield: 8 servings

Each with 15 g protein; 3 g carbohydrate; 1 g dietary fiber; 2 g usable carbs.

Crisp Chocolate Crust

1½ cups (225 g) almonds
¼ cup (6 g) Splenda
2 squares bitter chocolate, melted
3 tablespoons (42 g) butter, melted
2 tablespoons (15 g) vanilla whey protein powder

Preheat oven to 325°F (170°C, or gas mark 3).

Using the S-blade of a food processor, grind the almonds until they're the texture of corn meal. Add the Splenda and pulse to combine. Pour in the melted chocolate, then the melted butter, and run the processor until they're evenly distributed—you may need to stop the processor and run the

(continued on page 522)

tip of a knife blade around the outer edge to get everything to combine properly. Then add the protein powder and pulse again to combine.

Pour out into a 10-inch (25-cm) pie plate you've coated with nonstick cooking spray. Press firmly and evenly into place. Bake for 8 minutes. Cool before filling.

Yield: 10 servings

Each with 7 g protein; 6 g carbohydrate; 3 g dietary fiber; 3 g usable carbs.

Chocolate Cookie Crust

1½ cups (225 g) almonds
5 tablespoons (70 g) butter, melted
⅓ cup (40 g) vanilla whey protein powder
¼ cup (60 ml) Splenda
¼ cup (30 g) unsweetened cocoa powder
2 tablespoons (30 ml) water

Preheat oven to 325°F (170°C, or gas mark 3).

Put the almonds in a food processor with the S-blade in place. Run the processor until the almonds are finely ground. Add the butter, protein powder, Splenda, and cocoa and pulse the food processor until everything is well mixed.

Add the water and pulse until you have a soft, sort of sticky mass.

Pour this into a 10-inch (25-cm) pie plate you've sprayed well with nonstick cooking spray and press evenly into place, building all the way up the sides. Bake for 7 to 10 minutes or until set. Cool before filling.

Yield: 12 servings

Each serving will have 5 grams of carbohydrate and 3 grams of fiber, for a usable carb count of 2 grams; 6 grams protein.

Hazelnut Crust

This is a great substitute for a graham cracker crumb crust with any cheesecake. And I think it tastes even better than the original.

1½ cups (225 g) hazelnuts
⅓ cup (40 g) vanilla whey protein powder
4 tablespoons (56 g) butter, melted

Preheat the oven to 350°F (180°C, or gas mark 4).

Put the hazelnuts in a food processor with the S-blade in place. Pulse the processor until the hazelnuts are ground to a medium-fine texture. Add the protein powder and butter and pulse to combine.

Spray a pie plate or springform pan, depending on which your recipe specifies, with nonstick cooking spray and press this mixture firmly and evenly into the pan. Don't try to build the crust too high up the sides, but if you're using a springform pan, be sure to cover the seam around the bottom and press the crust into place firmly over it.

Place the crust in a preheated oven on the bottom rack and bake for 12 to 15 minutes or until lightly browned and slightly pulling away from the sides of the pan. Remove the crust from the oven and let it cool while you make the filling.

Yield: 12 servings

Assuming 12 slices of cheesecake, this crust will add to each slice 4 grams of carbohydrates and 1 gram of fiber, for a total of 3 grams of usable carbs and 10 grams of protein.

Simple Almond Crust

1½ cups (225 g) almonds
¼ cup (30 g) vanilla whey protein powder
¼ cup (56 g) butter, melted

Preheat oven to 350°F (180°C, or gas mark 4).

Using a food processor with the S-blade in place, grind the almonds to a consistency similar to cornmeal. Add the protein powder and butter; pulse to combine well. Turn out into a pie plate you've sprayed with nonstick cooking spray and press firmly and evenly into place, building up around sides. Bake for 12 to 15 minutes or until edges are starting to brown lightly. Remove from oven and cool.

Yield: 8 servings

Each serving will have 6 grams of carbohydrate and 3 grams of fiber, for a usable carb count of 3 grams; 7 grams protein.

Sweet-and-Salty Almond Crust

To use with Margarita Cheesecake (page 514), Emeril made his crust with crushed pretzels to get that salty note so characteristic of margaritas.

We're not going to use pretzels, so I came up with this crust instead. It's great with the margarita-flavored filling!

1½ cups (225 g) almonds
⅓ cup (40 g) vanilla whey protein powder
¼ cup (6 g) Splenda
¼ cup (56 g) butter, melted
1 tablespoon (15 g) kosher salt (I like kosher salt for this because the larger grains make a real contribution.)

Preheat oven to 325°F (170°C, or gas mark 3). Have on hand a 9-inch (23-cm) springform pan assembled and well sprayed with nonstick cooking spray.

Put the almonds in a food processor with the S-blade in place. Run the food processor until the almonds are ground. Add the protein powder and Splenda and pulse to mix. You may need to open the processor and run a knife around the bottom edge of the bowl to get everything into the path of the blade. Now, turn the processor on and pour in the butter while it's running. Let everything blend—and once again, you may need to do the knife-around-the-bottom-edge-of-the-processor trick. When the butter is evenly distributed, turn off the processor. Add the kosher salt and pulse the processor just enough to distribute the salt throughout the mixture.

Press firmly into the prepared pan, making sure you cover the seam around the bottom—but don't expect to be able to build it all the way up the sides. Bake for about 10 minutes or until lightly golden and cool before filling.

Yield: 12 servings

(continued on page 524)

4 grams of carbohydrate, and 2 grams of fiber, for a usable carb count of 2 grams; 8 grams protein.

Cinnamon Almond Crust

1½ cups (225 g) almonds
⅓ cup (40 g) vanilla whey protein powder
2 tablespoons (3 g) Splenda
½ teaspoon cinnamon
¼ cup (56 g) butter, melted

Preheat oven to 325°F (170°C, or gas mark 3).

Put the almonds in a food processor with the S-blade in place. Run the food processor until the almonds are ground medium-fine. Add the protein powder, Splenda, and cinnamon and pulse the processor to blend. Turn the processor on and pour in the butter—if needed, stop the food processor, run a knife around the bottom to make sure everything mixes evenly, put the lid back on, and process a little more.

Spray a 10-inch (25-cm) pie plate with nonstick cooking spray. Turn the almond mixture into the pie plate and press firmly and evenly into place, building it up the side about 1 inch (2.5 cm). Bake for 8 to 10 minutes or until turning golden. Cool before filling.

Yield: 8 servings

Each serving will have 6 grams carbohydrate and 3 grams fiber, for a usable carb count of 3 grams; and 8 grams protein.

Ginger Almond Crust

1½ cups (225 g) almonds
¼ cup (30 g) vanilla whey protein powder
1 teaspoon ground ginger
2 tablespoons (3 g) Splenda
¼ cup (56 g) butter, melted

Preheat oven to 325°F (170°C, or gas mark 3).

Put the almonds in a food processor with the S-blade in place. Run the processor until the almonds are ground medium-fine. Add the protein powder, ginger, and Splenda and pulse to combine. Add the butter, and pulse to combine—you may need to run a knife around the bottom of the food processor to make sure everything gets combined.

Press firmly into a 10-inch (25-cm) pie plate or springform pan you've sprayed with nonstick cooking spray, building up the sides about 1 inch (2.5 cm)—if you're using a springform pan, make sure you cover the seam at the bottom. Bake for 8 to 10 minutes or until it just barely turns golden.

Yield: 8 to 10 servings

Assuming 8, each will have 5 grams of carbohydrate and 2 grams of fiber, for a usable carb count of 3 grams; 6 grams protein.

"Graham" Crust

Wheat germ and wheat bran give this a "graham" flavor.

1¼ cups (190 g) almonds
2 tablespoons (14 g) wheat germ

2 tablespoons (14 g) wheat bran

3 tablespoons (4.5 g) Splenda

1 pinch salt

6 tablespoons (84 g) butter, melted

Preheat the oven to 325°F (170°C, or gas mark 3).

Put the almonds in a food processor with the S-blade in place. Run it until they're ground to about the texture of cornmeal. Add the wheat germ, wheat bran, Splenda, and salt and pulse to combine. Now turn on the processor and pour in the butter, running the processor until everything's well combined. (You may need to stop the processor and run a knife around the bottom edge to make sure all the dry ingredients come in contact with the butter.)

Turn this mixture out into an 8-inch (20-cm) springform pan you've sprayed with nonstick cooking spray. Press firmly into place. Bake for 10 to 12 minutes or until just turning gold around the edges. Cool before filling.

Yield: 12 servings

Each with 3 g protein, 4 g carbohydrate, 2 g dietary fiber, 2 g usable carbs.

No-Sugar-Added Cherry Pie Filling

Our tester Ray Stevens made this when he couldn't find the Lucky Leaf cherry low-carb pie filling. It's very, very simple.

1 can (14.5 ounces, or 410 g) sour cherries packed in water

½ cup (12 g) Splenda

2 teaspoons guar or xanthan

Red food coloring (optional)

Open the can of cherries and dump the whole thing, water and all, into a bowl. Stir in the Splenda and thickener, plus 4 to 6 drops of red food coloring if you want a pretty color. Let stand 5 minutes before using.

Yield: 6 to 8 servings

Assuming 6, each will have 1 g protein; 6 g carbohydrate; 1 g dietary fiber; 5 g usable carbs.

Strawberry Cheese Pie

This is a killer company dessert! Feel free to use cream cheese instead, if you prefer—your carb count will remain about the same, though your calorie count will be higher.

FOR THE CHEESE LAYER:

8 ounces (225 g) Neufchâtel cheese, softened (or regular or light cream cheese)

2 tablespoons (30 ml) heavy cream

1 tablespoon (1.5 g) Splenda

½ teaspoon vanilla extract

Pie Crust, prebaked (page 520)

FOR THE STRAWBERRY LAYER:

1 pound (455 g) frozen, unsweetened straw-berries

1 cup (240 ml) water

¼ cup (6 g) Splenda

(continued on page 526)

2 tablespoons (30 ml) lemon juice

2 teaspoons unflavored gelatin

To make the cheese layer: Using an electric mixer, beat the Neufchâtel cheese, heavy cream, 1 tablespoon (1.5 g) Splenda, and the vanilla together until very smooth and fluffy. Smooth evenly over the bottom of the prebaked pie shell.

To make the strawberry layer: Put the strawberries, water, the ¼ cup (6 g) Splenda, and lemon juice in a nonreactive saucepan. Bring to a boil, then turn down to low, and let it simmer until the strawberries are soft. Use a whisk to coarsely mash the strawberries. Now, stir with the whisk in a circle while you sprinkle the gelatin over the surface of the strawberry mixture, a little at a time. (You're trying to make sure that all the gelatin dissolves thoroughly, instead of leaving chewy little gelatin "seeds" in your finished pie.) Turn the heat off and let the strawberry mixture cool until it's getting syrupy. Pour or spoon the mixture over the cream cheese layer and then put the pie in the fridge for at least several hours before serving.

Yield: 8 servings

Each with 20 g protein; 10 g carbohydrate; 2 g dietary fiber; 8 g usable carbs.

Here's my confession: This actually makes a little too much strawberry mixture to fit in the pie shell, but I hate the idea of having a few leftover frozen strawberries just hanging around. So I pour the extra strawberry stuff into a custard cup and chill it for a gelatin dessert. But if you prefer, you could use an ounce or two less cheese instead to make room for the extra strawberries.

Chocolate Raspberry Pie

This is fairly simple, but it looks terribly elegant, what with the chocolate-brown crust and the deep pink filling. It's yummy, too. It's best to make this for an occasion where it will all get eaten up. The leftovers will still taste great, but they will look less and less impressive as days in the fridge go by.

1 package (4-serving size) sugar-free raspberry-flavored gelatin

1 tablespoon (15 ml) lemon juice

1¼ cups (300 ml) boiling water

1 pint (475 ml) no-sugar-added vanilla ice cream, softened (I used Breyer's Carb Smart.)

Crisp Chocolate Crust (page 521)

Maltitol-Splenda Chocolate Sauce (page 551)

In a large mixing bowl, combine the sugar-free raspberry gelatin with the lemon juice and boiling water. Stir until gelatin is completely dissolved. Now stir in the softened low-carb vanilla ice cream. Stick the bowl in the fridge for a few minutes until the mixture is thickened a bit but not set and pour into the Crisp Chocolate Crust. Chill for at least several hours, and overnight is a good idea.

Serve with the Maltitol-Splenda Chocolate Sauce or with Sugar-Free Chocolate Sauce (page 551).

Yield: 8 servings

Each with 8 g protein; 8 g carbohydrate; 4 g dietary fiber; 4 g usable carb. Analysis includes crust. Carb count does not include the polyol sweetener in the ice cream or chocolate sauce.

Easy Key Lime Pie

Tester Julie calls this "Yummy, light, and summery." She also says it couldn't be easier to make!

1½ cups (225 g) almonds
¼ cup (30 g) vanilla whey protein powder
⅓ cup (8 g) Splenda
1 teaspoon ground ginger
4 tablespoons (56 g) butter, melted
2 packages (4-serving size each) sugar-free lime gelatin
2 cups (480 ml) boiling water
2 limes, grated zest and juice
1 pint (475 ml) no-sugar-added vanilla ice cream (I use Breyer's Carb Smart.)
1 cup (240 ml) heavy cream, chilled
1 tablespoon (10 g) vanilla sugar-free instant pudding mix

Preheat your oven to 325°F (170°C, or gas mark 3).

In a food processor with the S-blade in place, grind the almonds fine. Add the protein powder, the Splenda, and the ground ginger and pulse to mix. Now add the butter and pulse until everything's blended. Turn the mixture out into a 9-inch (23-cm) pie plate you've sprayed with nonstick cooking spray. Press firmly into place, building up the sides, and bake for 12 minutes or until golden. Cool before filling.

In a big mixing bowl, dissolve the gelatin in the boiling water. Add the grated lime zest and the juice. Now stir in the ice cream until the ice cream is melted and the mixture is smooth. Chill until the mixture is thickened but not set.

Spoon the lime mixture into the prepared crust. Chill until firm. In the meantime, whip the cream with the pudding mix until you have whipped topping—but don't overbeat, or you'll get butter! Serve the pie with the whipped topping.

Yield: 8 servings,

Each with 14 g protein; 9 g carbohydrate; 3 g dietary fiber; 6 grams usable carbs. Analysis does not include polyol sweeter in sugar-free ice cream.

Coconut Cream Pie

This is my decarbed version of the old-time favorite!

FOR THE PIE:
1½ cups (225 g) almonds
¼ cup (30 g) vanilla whey protein powder
3 tablespoons (4.5 g) Splenda
4 tablespoons (56 g) butter, melted
1⅓ cups (95 g) Angel-Type Coconut (page 553), divided
2⅔ cups (640 ml) Carb Countdown dairy beverage
1½ packages (3.4 ounces, or 95 g each) vanilla sugar-free instant pudding mix

FOR THE WHIPPED TOPPING:
1 cup (240 ml) heavy cream, chilled
1 tablespoon (10 g) vanilla sugar-free instant pudding mix

(continued on page 528)

Preheat oven to 325°F (170°C, or gas mark 3).

To make the pie: In a food processor using the S-blade, grind the almonds fine. Add the protein powder and Splenda and pulse to combine. Now add the butter and pulse until it's all well mixed. Turn this out into a 9-inch (23-cm) pie plate you've sprayed with nonstick cooking spray. Press firmly into place, building up the sides. Bake for 12–15 minutes or until starting to turn golden. Cool before filling.

Put ⅔ cup (45 g) of the Angel-Type Coconut in the pie shell, spreading evenly. Set aside.

Pour the Carb Countdown into a mixing bowl and add the 1½ packages pudding mix. Whisk until smooth, about 2 minutes. Pour over the coconut in the pie shell. Chill for at least 1 hour.

While the pie is chilling, stir the remaining coconut in a dry skillet over medium heat until it's touched with gold. Set aside to cool.

To make the whipped topping: Using an electric mixer, whip the heavy cream with the 1 tablespoon of pudding mix until you have whipped topping (then turn off the mixer fast! You don't want vanilla butter!). Spread over the pie and top with the toasted coconut before serving.

Yield: 10–12 servings.

Assuming 12, each will have 11 g protein; 9 g carbohydrate; 3 g dietary fiber; 6 grams usable carbs.

Peanut Butter Silk Pie

This pie is incredible, decadent, outrageous, utterly scrumptious. This is a real special-occasion dessert and a surefire crowd pleaser.

FOR THE CRUST:

1¼ cups (190 g) shelled raw hazelnuts

4 tablespoons (56 g) butter, melted

½ cup (65 g) vanilla-flavored whey protein powder

FOR THE CHOCOLATE LAYER:

4 sugar-free dark chocolate bars (about 1.5 ounces [42 g] each)

5 tablespoons (75 ml) heavy cream

¼ teaspoon instant coffee crystals

FOR THE PEANUT BUTTER SILK LAYER:

1 package (8 ounces, or 225 g) cream cheese, softened

1 cup (25 g) Splenda

1 cup (260 g) creamy natural peanut butter

1 tablespoon (14 g) butter, melted

1 teaspoon vanilla extract

1 cup (240 ml) heavy cream

Preheat the oven to 325°F (170°C, or gas mark 3).

To make the crust: Use the S-blade in a food processor to grind the hazelnuts to a meal. Add the butter and protein powder and pulse until well combined. Spray a large pie plate with nonstick cooking spray and press the hazelnut mixture firmly into the bottom of the pie plate (it won't build up the side very far). Bake for 10 to 12 minutes or until lightly browned. Remove from the oven to cool.

To make the chocolate layer: Melt the chocolate over the lowest possible heat since chocolate burns very easily. (If you have a double boiler or a heat diffuser, this would be a good time to use it!) Whisk in the cream and coffee crystals, and continue stirring until the crystals disappear. Spread this mixture evenly over the bottom of the hazelnut crust.

To make the peanut butter silk layer: Use an electric mixer to beat the cream cheese, Splenda, peanut butter, butter, and vanilla together until creamy.

In a separate bowl, whip the heavy cream until stiff. Turn the mixer to the lowest setting and beat the whipped cream into the peanut butter mixture one-third at a time.

Spread the peanut butter filling gently over the chocolate layer and chill. (This is best made a day in advance to allow plenty of time for chilling.)

Yield: 10 generous servings

Each with 12 grams of carbohydrates and 2 grams of fiber, for a total of 10 grams of usable carbs and 20 grams of protein. Carb count does not include the polyol in the sugar-free chocolate.

Peanut Butter and Jelly Pie

I invented this for my peanut butter-obsessed husband, who adored it.

FOR THE JELLY LAYER:
1 cup (120 g) raspberries (fresh, or frozen with no sugar)
2 tablespoons (30 ml) water
3 tablespoons (4.5 g) Splenda

FOR THE PEANUT BUTTER LAYER:
1 package (4-serving size) sugar-free vanilla instant pudding mix
1 cup (240 ml) heavy cream
1 cup (240 ml) water
1 cup (260 g) natural peanut butter

½ **teaspoon blackstrap molasses**
⅛ **teaspoon salt**
Cinnamon Almond Crust (page 523)

To make the jelly layer: Put the raspberries, 2 tablespoons (30 ml) water, and Splenda in a saucepan over medium-low heat and bring to a simmer. Stir until the berries are quite soft and mash up with a fork. Turn off heat and set aside.

To make the peanut butter layer: With an electric mixer, beat the pudding mix with the heavy cream and water until smooth and starting to thicken. Beat in peanut butter, molasses, and salt, scraping down the sides of the bowl as needed, until everything is well combined and very smooth.

Spread the raspberry mixture evenly over the bottom of the prepared Cinnamon Almond Crust. Spoon the peanut butter mixture evenly over the raspberry layer. Chill for at least several hours, and overnight is better.

Yield: 8 servings

Each serving will have 16 grams of carbohydrate and 6 grams of fiber, for a usable carb count of 10 grams; 17 grams protein—which means you can legitimately have a slice for breakfast, if you want to. (Analysis includes Cinnamon Almond Crust.)

Peanut Butter Cup Pie

This is so easy! And who doesn't love chocolate and peanut butter?

(continued on page 530)

1 package (4-serving size) sugar-free instant chocolate pudding mix

2 tablespoons (11 g) unsweetened cocoa powder

1 cup (240 ml) heavy cream

1 cup (240 ml) water

¾ cup (195 g) natural peanut butter (I used creamy.)

1 Simple Almond Crust (page 522)

In a large bowl, combine the pudding mix and cocoa powder. Pour in the heavy cream and water and beat with an electric mixer to combine well. Then beat in the peanut butter until everything's well combined. Pour mixture into cooled crust, scraping it all out of the bowl with a rubber scraper. Spread evenly in crust and chill.

Yield: 8 servings

Each serving will have 12 grams of carbohydrate and 4 grams of fiber, for a usable carb count of 8 grams; 14 grams of protein. (Analysis includes Simple Almond Crust.)

Pumpkin Pie with Pecan Praline Crust

I'm very proud of this recipe. Serve it at Thanksgiving Dinner, and no one will guess it's made without sugar.

FOR THE CRUST:

2 cups (300 g) shelled raw pecans

¼ teaspoon salt

2½ tablespoons (4 g) Splenda

1½ teaspoons blackstrap molasses

4 tablespoons (56 g) butter, melted

2 tablespoons (30 ml) water

FOR THE PUMPKIN PIE FILLING:

1 can (15 ounces, or 420 ml) pumpkin

1½ cups (360 ml) heavy cream

3 eggs

¾ cup (18 g) Splenda

½ teaspoon salt

2 teaspoons blackstrap molasses

1 tablespoon (6 g) pumpkin pie spice

Preheat the oven to 350°F (180°C, or gas mark 4).

To make the crust: Put the pecans and salt in a food processor with the S-blade in place. Pulse until the pecans are chopped to a medium consistency. Add the Splenda, molasses, and butter and pulse again until well blended. Add the water and pulse again until well combined. At this point, you'll have a soft, sticky mass.

Spray a 10-inch (25-cm) pie plate with nonstick cooking spray or butter it well. Pour the pecan mixture into it and press firmly in place, all over the bottom and up the sides by 1½ inches (3 cm) or so. Try to get it an even thickness with no holes, and if you wish, run a finger or a knife around the top edge to get an even, nice-looking line. Bake for about 18 minutes. Cool.

Increase the oven temperature to 425°F (220°C, or gas mark 7).

To make the filling: Combine the pumpkin, heavy cream, eggs, Splenda, salt, molasses, and spice in a bowl and whisk together well. Pour into the prebaked and cooled pie shell. Bake for 15 minutes, lower the oven temperature to 350°F (180°C, or gas mark 4), and bake for an additional 45 minutes. Cool and serve with whipped cream.

Yield: 8 servings

Each with 14 grams of carbohydrates and 4 grams of fiber, for a total of 10 grams of usable carbs and 6 grams of protein. Analysis does not include whipped cream.

Wondering how many carbs you're really saving by making your pumpkin pie from scratch? A lot—especially when you consider that a slice of Mrs. Smith's frozen pumpkin pie has 37 grams of usable carbs, well over three times as much as my version!

Brownie Mocha Fudge Pie

1 batch Dana's Brownies (page 509, but see instructions)

4 teaspoons instant coffee granules, divided

2 cups (480 ml) well-chilled heavy cream, divided

3 tablespoons (30 g) sugar-free instant vanilla pudding mix, divided

1½ cups (360 ml) Carb Countdown dairy beverage or half-and-half

3 tablespoons (45 ml) Mockahlua (page 46), divided

2 packages (4-serving-size) sugar-free instant chocolate pudding mix

Make the brownies, adding 2 teaspoons of instant coffee granules. Instead of baking in an 8 × 8-inch (20 × 20-cm) pan, use a 10-inch (25-cm) pie plate you've sprayed well with nonstick cooking spray. Let the brownie crust cool thoroughly before starting on the filling.

Pour 1 cup (240 ml) of the heavy cream into a small, deep mixing bowl, and add 1½ tablespoons (15 g) of the sugar-free vanilla instant pudding powder. Using a whisk or an electric mixer, whip until well thickened (but don't go overboard and make sweet vanilla butter!). Set this aside for a moment.

In another mixing bowl, dissolve 1 teaspoon of the instant coffee granules in the Carb Countdown dairy beverage and stir in 2 tablespoons (30 ml) of the Mockahlua. Now add the sugar-free instant chocolate pudding mix and beat with an electric mixer for a minute or two until very smooth and thick. Add the whipped cream you made. Turn the mixer to its very lowest setting and beat the whipped cream into the pudding mixture until everything is just combined. Spread this mixture over the brownie crust.

Okay, you need your cream-whipping bowl again—don't bother to wash it, though you'll want to wash the beaters. Pour the last tablespoon (15 ml) of Mockahlua and the last teaspoon of coffee granules into the bowl, and dissolve the coffee granules in the Mockahlua. Now add the second cup (240 ml) of heavy cream and the second 1½ tablespoons (15 g) of vanilla instant pudding powder.

Whip until thickened (again, don't overbeat and get butter). Spread this coffee whipped cream over the pudding layer and chill well—at least a few hours. Decorate with bitter chocolate shavings, if you like.

Yield: 12 servings

Each with 11 g protein; 8 g carbohydrate; 1 g dietary fiber; 7 g usable carbs. Analysis does not include polyol sweetener.

Layered Chocolate-and-Vanilla Decadence

I adapted this recipe, and my sister, Kim, tested it for me one night when she was having company. She said that they threatened to eat the whole thing—and it makes a lot! This is a good choice if you want to take a dessert to a gathering.

FOR THE CRUST:
1¼ cups (190 g) pecans
1 cup (130 g) vanilla whey protein powder
½ cup (12 g) Splenda
½ cup (115 g) melted butter
FOR THE LAYERS:
2½ cups (600 ml) heavy cream, chilled
2½ tablespoons (25 g) sugar-free instant vanilla pudding mix
8 ounces (225 g) cream cheese, softened
½ cup (12 g) Splenda
2½ cups plus 2 tablespoons (630 ml) Carb Countdown dairy beverage, divided
1 package (6-serving size) sugar-free instant chocolate pudding mix

Preheat oven to 350°F (180°C, or gas mark 4).

To make the crust: Chop the pecans in a food processor, add the other crust ingredients, and pulse to blend thoroughly. Pour into a 9 × 13-inch (23 × 33-cm) baking pan; press down to make firm so that it covers the bottom. Bake for 15 minutes. Let cool.

To make the layers: While the crust is cooling, whip the heavy cream and the vanilla pudding mix with you electric mixer. Set aside.

In another bowl, beat the cream cheese, Splenda, and 2 tablespoons (30 ml) of Carb Countdown dairy beverage together until smooth. Fold in a little less than half of the whipped cream. Spread cream cheese mixture over the crust.

In the same bowl from which you've removed the cream cheese mixture, mix the package of chocolate pudding mix with 2½ cups (600 ml) of Carb Countdown dairy beverage. Beat until smooth and creamy and beginning to thicken. Spread over the top of the cream cheese layer.

Put the pan in the refrigerator to set. Store the leftover whipped cream in the refrigerator. After about 2½ to 3 hours, spread the remaining whipped cream over the top of the pudding as the top layer. Chill for at least another hour. Serve.

Yield: About 12 to 16 servings

Assuming 16 servings, each will have 15 g protein; 7 g carbohydrate; 1 g dietary fiber; 6 g usable carbs.

Mud Pie

Frozen coffee pie with a chocolate crust and chocolate sauce—What's not to like? This has a mild coffee flavor, but feel free to add more instant coffee granules—tasting as you go—if you like it more intense. Also feel free to use decaf if you, like me, have trouble sleeping if you have caffeine after dinner!

2 packages (4-serving size) sugar-free vanilla instant pudding mix
1 cup (240 ml) water
1 cup (240 ml) heavy cream

3 tablespoons (9 g) instant coffee crystals

2 cups (280 g) sugar-free vanilla ice cream, softened (but not melted!)

Chocolate Cookie Crust (page 521)

1 batch Sugar-Free Chocolate Sauce (page 551)

Put the pudding mix, water, and heavy cream in a large mixing bowl and beat with an electric mixer until well blended. Beat in the coffee crystals, then the softened ice cream. Beat just long enough to get everything mixed together and then pour half of the filling into the prepared Chocolate Cookie Crust. Top with half of the chocolate sauce. Add the rest of the filling and top with the remainder of the sauce.

Stash the pie in the freezer for at least several hours. Then take it out about 15 to 20 minutes before you serve it to let it soften a bit (but not thaw!).

Yield: 12 servings (I know that sounds like a lot, but I've tried serving bigger slices, and people get too full!)

Each serving will have 9 grams of carbohydrate and 3 grams of fiber, for a usable carb count of 6 grams. Analysis includes chocolate cookie crust out not the polyol in the sugar-free chocolate sauce.

German Chocolate Pie

My tester Julie claims that the true name of this recipe is "OH SWEET MOTHER OF ALL THAT IS HOLY, THIS IS LIKE A SYMPHONY IN MY MOUTH!" and rates it a 15 on the 1 to 10 scale. She also says it looks "gorgeous!" I hope you like it just as much!

FOR THE CRUST:

1 cup (70 g) Angel-Type Coconut (page 553)

1 cup (125 g) finely chopped pecans

6 tablespoons (84 g) butter, melted

⅓ cup (40 g) vanilla whey protein powder

3 tablespoons (4.5 g) Splenda

FOR THE FILLING:

4 ounces (115 g) cream cheese, softened

1 package (4-serving size) sugar-free chocolate instant pudding

1 package (4-serving size) sugar-free vanilla instant pudding

2¾ cups (660 ml) Carb Countdown dairy beverage

½ cup (35 g) Angel-Type Coconut

FOR THE TOPPING:

½ cup (35 g) Angel-Type Coconut

½ cup (65 g) chopped pecans

2 tablespoons (28 g) butter

1 teaspoon vanilla

3 tablespoons (4.5 g) Splenda

½ cup (120 ml) heavy cream, chilled

Preheat oven to 325°F (170°C, or gas mark 3).

To make the crust: Combine all the crust ingredients well. Turn out into a 10-inch (25-cm) pie plate you've sprayed with nonstick cooking spray and press firmly into place, building all the way up the sides. Bake for 12–15 minutes or until it browns a little. Let cool before filling.

(continued on page 534)

To make the filling: Beat the cream cheese until smooth. Now beat in the two pudding mixes and the Carb Countdown and then fold in the coconut. Spread this in the pie shell.

To make the topping: In a big skillet over medium-low heat, sauté the the coconut and pecans in the butter until the coconut is golden. Stir in the vanilla and the Splenda and let the mixture cool. Now scatter it evenly over the pie. Chill the pie for several hours.

Whip the cream and use it to decorate the pie before serving.

Yield: 8–12 servings.

Assuming 12, each will have 10 g protein; 10 g carbohydrate; 2 g dietary fiber; 8 grams usable carbs.

Gingered Melon

This is light and elegant—and people following a low-fat diet can eat it, too.

½ ripe cantaloupe
½ ripe honeydew
⅓ cup (80 ml) lime juice
2 tablespoons (3 g) Splenda
1 teaspoon grated fresh ginger

Peel the cantaloupe and honeydew and cut it into bite-sized chunks, or if you have a melon baller, cut balls from it. Place in a serving dish.

Combine the lime juice, Splenda, and ginger. Pour over the melon, toss, and serve.

Yield: 8 servings

Each with 12 grams of carbohydrates and 1 gram of fiber, for a total of 11 grams of usable carbs and 1 gram of protein.

Strawberries in Wine

This is simple and simply delicious.

8 ounces (225 g) fresh strawberries
½ cup (120 ml) burgundy wine
1 tablespoon (1.5 g) Splenda
Cinnamon stick

Hull the strawberries and slice or cut them into quarters.

Mix the wine and the Splenda and pour the mixture over the berries. Add the cinnamon stick and refrigerate, stirring from time to time, for at least 12 hours (but 2 days wouldn't hurt!).

Yield: 4 servings

Each with 8 grams of carbohydrates and 3 grams of fiber, for a total of 5 grams of usable carbs and 1 gram of protein.

Broiled Grapefruit

This is a classic sort of recipe.

½ grapefruit
½ teaspoon butter (optional)
Splenda
A touch of blackstrap molasses, if you like
Ground cinnamon (optional)

Loosen the sections of the grapefruit by running a sharp, thin-bladed knife around each one. Sprinkle with the sweetener of your choice, plus cinnamon if you like, and broil a few inches (7.5 cm) from the flame for 10 minutes.

Yield: 1 serving

10.4 grams of carbohydrates and 1.4 grams of fiber, for a total of 9 grams of usable carbs from the grapefruit. Splenda has 0.5 grams of carbohydrates per teaspoon. Blackstrap has 1 gram of carbohydrates per ¼ teaspoon—and it's so strong-flavored you won't want to use more than this!

Some people like to cut the white core out and put butter in there.

Figs with Gorgonzola

It doesn't get any simpler or more elegant than this.

4 fresh, medium figs
¼ cup (30 g) crumbled Gorgonzola
½ cup (60 g) chopped walnuts

Slice the figs in half, spread each half with a tablespoon of Gorgonzola, and sprinkle with ½ tablespoon chopped walnuts.

Yield: 4 servings of 2 halves

Each with 12 grams of carbohydrates and 2 grams of fiber, for a total of 10 grams of usable carbs and 9 grams of protein.

Note: Some people like to broil the figs for a few minutes first.

Rhubarb Flummery

Because it's so sour, rhubarb is low-carb. This is a simple, old-fashioned dessert.

1 pound (455 g) frozen rhubarb
½ cup (12 g) Splenda
½ cup (120 ml) water
⅛ teaspoon orange extract
Guar or xanthan

Place the rhubarb in a slow cooker and stir in the Splenda, water, and orange extract. Cover the slow cooker, set it to low, and let it cook for 5 to 6 hours.

When the time's up, the rhubarb will be very soft. Mash it with a fork to a rough pulp. Thicken the sauce to a soft pudding consistency with guar or xanthan and serve hot or cold.

This dessert is great with a little heavy cream or Whipped Topping (page 552).

Yield: 6 servings

Each with trace protein, 4 g carbohydrate, 1 g dietary fiber, 3 g usable carbs. Analysis does not include whipped topping.

Grandma's Peach Cobbler

Well, Grandma's version was a lot higher-carb than this! This is a charming, old-fashioned dessert.

4 cups (800 g) sliced peaches
¼ cup plus 1 tablespoon (7.5 g) Splenda, divided
¼ cup (50 g) polyol sweetener
1 tablespoon (15 ml) lemon juice
8 tablespoons (115 g) butter, divided
½ cup (60 g) almond meal
½ cup (65 g) vanilla whey protein powder
2½ teaspoons baking powder
1 teaspoon salt
½ cup (120 ml) heavy cream

Preheat oven to 375°F (190°C, or gas mark 5). Spray an 8 × 8-inch (20 × 20-cm) baking pan with nonstick cooking spray.

In a mixing bowl, combine the sliced peaches (I use unsweetened frozen peach slices, which saves lots of time and trouble, and since they're going to be cooked, it makes no difference in the final texture), ¼ cup (6 g) Splenda, polyol sweetener, and lemon juice. Toss everything together and spread evenly in the pan. Dot with 2 tablespoons (30 g) of the butter.

In another mixing bowl (or use the same one if you like), combine the almond meal, protein powder, baking powder, the remaining 1 tablespoon (1.5 g) Splenda, and the salt. Stir together to evenly distribute ingredients.

Melt the remaining 6 tablespoons (85 g) of butter. Stir the butter into the cream. Pour into the dry ingredients and mix with a few swift strokes of your whisk or a spoon—you just want to stir enough to ensure that there are no pockets of dry ingredients lurking.

Spread the batter evenly over the peaches and bake for 30 minutes or until the crust is crisp and evenly golden brown. Serve warm.

Yield: 9 servings

Each with 14 g protein; 13 g carbohydrate; 2 g dietary fiber; 11 g usable carbs. Carb count does not include polyol sweetener.

Variation: Grandma's Blueberry Cobbler. Swap 4 cups (580 g) fresh blueberries or 4 cups (620 g) unsweetened frozen blueberries for the peaches, and follow the recipe as directed.

Yield: 9 servings

Each with 13 g protein; 13 g carbohydrate; 2 g dietary fiber; 11 g usable carbs.

Speedy Low-Carb Peach Melba

This is a short-cut, no-sugar-added version of a very famous dessert—and it's scrumptious! You can use fresh peaches in this, if you'd prefer, but unlike the frozen ones, you'll have to peel and slice them, which takes longer.

2 cups (500 g) frozen, sliced, no-sugar-added peaches
¼ cup (60 ml) lemon juice, divided
¼ teaspoon orange extract
½ cup (12 g) Splenda

1 cup (110 g) raspberries—fresh or frozen with no sugar added

4 tablespoons (30 g) toasted slivered almonds (optional)

Don't bother to thaw the frozen peaches. Put them in a microwaveable bowl, mix together 2 tablespoons (30 ml) of the lemon juice, the orange extract, and half of the Splenda and pour it over them. Cover (I just lay a plate on top) and microwave on high for 5 to 7 minutes or until tender.

While the peaches are poaching, put the raspberries, the remaining 2 tablespoons (30 ml) of lemon juice, and the remaining Splenda in a food processor with the S-blade in place. Pulse a few times until everything is puréed together.

When the peaches are done, divide between 4 small serving dishes and divide the raspberry sauce between them. Sprinkle each dish with a tablespoon of almonds, if desired. Serve.

Yield: 4 servings

Each with 17 grams of carbohydrates and 4 grams of fiber, for a total of 13 grams of usable carbs and 1 gram of protein. Add the optional almonds and each serving has 19 grams of carbohydrates and 5 grams of fiber, for a total of 14 grams of usable carbs and 3 grams of protein.

This also has a mere 68 calories, every one of them nutritious.

Now, this is not the traditional way to serve Peach Melba—the traditional way would include a scoop of vanilla ice cream. You could do this, of course, using one of the no-sugar-added ice creams, or Atkins Endulge, but since this is already in the upper range of the low-carb recipe spectrum, I'd probably only do this for a very special occasion. You could also serve this with vanilla yogurt and add only about 2.5 grams of carbs per ½ cup (120 ml) of yogurt.

Tip: Feel free to make the raspberry sauce all by itself—it's great over melon, stirred into plain yogurt, or as an elegant quick dessert when combined with no-sugar ice cream.

Peaches with Butterscotch Sauce

These are delectable. You can serve them as is, with a little heavy cream, with Whipped Topping (page 552), or with a scoop of low-carb vanilla ice cream.

1 pound (455 g) frozen, unsweetened, sliced peaches

2 teaspoons lemon juice

⅓ cup (8 g) Splenda

2 tablespoons (30 ml) sugar-free imitation honey

½ teaspoon blackstrap molasses

2 tablespoons (30 ml) heavy cream

¼ teaspoon cinnamon

2 tablespoons (28 g) butter, melted

Guar or xanthan

Place the peaches in a slow cooker. (I didn't even bother to thaw mine.)

In a bowl, stir together the lemon juice, Splenda, honey, molasses, cream, cinnamon, and butter. Pour the mixture over the peaches. Cover

(continued on page 538)

the slow cooker, set it to low, and let it cook for 6 hours.

Thicken the sauce to a creamy consistency with a little guar or xanthan and serve hot.

Yield: 6 servings

Each with 1 g protein, 9 g carbohydrate, 2 g dietary fiber, 7 g usable carbs. (Analysis does not include polyols or toppings.)

Strawberries with Balsamic Vinegar

This is so light and flavorful! These are good without the cream cheese sauce, too.

2 pounds (910 g) strawberries
¼ cup (6 g) plus 2 teaspoons Splenda, divided
¼ cup (60 ml) balsamic vinegar
4 ounces (115 g) cream cheese, softened
4 tablespoons (60 g) plain yogurt

Remove the green hulls from the strawberries and halve them—if you have some really huge berries, quarter them. Place in a glass, plastic, or stainless steel mixing bowl. Sprinkle ¼ cup (6 g) Splenda over the berries and toss to coat. Now sprinkle on the balsamic vinegar and stir again. Stash the bowl in the fridge for at least a few hours, and a whole day would be fine.

Using an electric mixer, beat the cream cheese, yogurt, and remaining 2 teaspoons Splenda together until very smooth—you can do this in advance, too, if you'd like.

Simply spoon the berries into pretty dessert dishes and drizzle some of the balsamic vinegar syrup in the bottom of the bowl over each serving. Top each serving with a dollop of the cream cheese sauce and serve.

Yield: 8 servings

Each with 2 g protein; 9 g carbohydrate; 3 g dietary fiber; 6 g usable carbs.

Strawberries with Orange Cream Dip

This will look fancy if you serve it on a pretty chip-and-dip tray. It's good finger food for a party. You can drop the calorie count on this without increasing the carb count by using light (but not fat-free!) sour cream.

1 package (4-serving size) sugar-free instant
**   vanilla pudding**
1 cup (230 g) sour cream
1½ cups (360 ml) heavy cream
2 teaspoons grated orange zest
2 pounds (910 g) strawberries

Using an electric mixer, beat the pudding mix, sour cream, heavy cream, and orange zest together until smooth and fluffy. Put in the bowl of a chip-and-dip tray, surround with whole strawberries, and serve.

Yield: 10 servings

Each with 11 g protein; 15 g carbohydrate; 4 g dietary fiber; 11 g usable carbs.

Strawberry Crunch Parfait

In their book *The GO-Diet*, Drs. Goldberg and O'Mara explain that plain yogurt has far fewer carbs than the label would indicate because most of the lactose in the milk has been converted to lactic acid by the yogurt bacteria. Accordingly, they say that we can count just 4 grams of carbohydrates per cup (230 g) of plain yogurt. Reading this, I added yogurt back to my low-carb diet, and it's never caused weight gain or rebound hunger for me, so I think Goldberg and O'Mara are right! This recipe is so versatile—it makes a great dessert, a phenomenal quick breakfast, or a delicious and nutritious snack. Enjoy!

3 ripe strawberries

1 tablespoon plus ¼ teaspoon (0.1 g) Splenda, divided

¾ cup (170 g) plain yogurt

½ teaspoon vanilla extract

2 tablespoons (15 g) Cinnamon Splenda Nuts (page 553), chopped a bit, or 2 tablespoons low-carb commercial granola-like product

Cut the green hulls off the strawberries and slice them thinly into a dish. Sprinkle them with ¼ teaspoon of the Splenda and stir.

Combine the yogurt with the vanilla extract and the remaining tablespoon (1.5 g) of Splenda, stirring well. Spoon over the strawberries. Top with the nuts or granola and devour!

Yield: 1 serving

Using the GO-Diet's carb count of 4 grams of carbohydrates per cup (230 g) of plain yogurt, this has 12 grams of carbohydrates and 3 grams of fiber, for a total of 9 grams of usable carbs and 10 grams of protein.

Feel free to substitute ¼ cup (35 g) blueberries, blackberries, raspberries, or even diced peaches. Make this in a clear glass dish or even layer it in a parfait glass, and it'll look pretty enough for company.

Strawberry Cups

This is a good make-ahead company dessert, and it's a really beautiful color.

1 cup (240 ml) water

1 package (4-serving size) sugar-free lemon gelatin

10 ounces (280 g) frozen unsweetened strawberries, partly thawed

1 cup (240 ml) heavy cream, divided

½ teaspoon vanilla extract

1 teaspoon Splenda (if desired)

Bring the water to a boil. Put the gelatin and boiling water in a blender and whirl for 10 to 15 seconds to dissolve the gelatin. Add the strawberries and whirl again, just long enough to blend in the berries.

Put the blender container in the refrigerator for 10 minutes or just until the mixture starts to thicken a bit.

Add ¾ cup (180 ml) of the heavy cream and run the blender just long enough to mix it all in (10 to 15 seconds). Pour into 5 or 6 pretty little dessert cups and chill. Whip the remaining ¼ cup (60 ml) of cream with the vanilla and a teaspoon of Splenda (if using), to garnish.

(continued on page 540)

Yield: About 5 servings

Each with 6 grams of carbohydrates and 1 gram of fiber, for a total of 5 grams of usable carbs and 3 grams of protein.

Mixed Berry Cups

For you raspberry and blackberry lovers, here's a quick and tasty dessert.

1 package (4-serving size) sugar-free raspberry gelatin
1 cup (240 ml) boiling water
2 teaspoons lemon juice
Grated rind of ½ orange
¾ cup (100 g) frozen blackberries, partly thawed
1 cup (240 ml) heavy cream, divided
½ teaspoon vanilla extract
1 teaspoon Splenda (optional)

Put the gelatin, water, lemon juice, and orange rind in a blender and whirl for 10 to 15 seconds to dissolve the gelatin. Add the blackberries and blend again, just long enough to mix in the berries.

Put the blender container in the refrigerator for 10 minutes or just until the mixture starts to thicken a bit. Add ¾ cup (180 ml) heavy cream and run the blender just long enough to mix it all in (10 to 15 seconds). Pour into 5 or 6 pretty little dessert cups and chill.

Whip the remaining ¼ cup (60 ml) of cream with vanilla and Splenda (if using) to garnish.

Yield: 5 servings

Each with 5 grams of carbohydrates and 1 gram of fiber, for a total of 4 grams of usable carbs and 2 grams of protein.

Black Forest Parfaits

This has too many carbs for you to want to eat it on a regular basis, but it's great for a company dinner or a holiday. It's really pretty, too.

1 (4-serving size) package sugar-free instant chocolate pudding mix
2 cups (480 ml) Carb Countdown dairy beverage
1 cup (240 ml) heavy cream, chilled
1 tablespoon (10 g) sugar-free instant vanilla pudding mix
1 tablespoon (14 g) butter
½ cup (60 g) almond meal
½ cup (35 g) shredded coconut
2 tablespoons (11 g) cocoa powder
2 tablespoons (25 g) polyol sweetener
1 batch No-Sugar-Added Cherry Pie Filling (page 525)

Mix the chocolate pudding mix with the Carb Countdown dairy beverage and stir with a whisk for 2 minutes or until thickened. Set aside.

Pour the chilled heavy cream into a deep mixing bowl. Add the vanilla instant pudding mix and use an electric mixer to whip until cream is stiff—do not overbeat, or you'll get sweetened vanilla butter! (Also do not try to do this step in a blender or food processor. It simply will not work.)

Scoop out 1½ cups (360 ml) of the whipped cream and add to the bowl with the chocolate pudding; fold in with a rubber scraper.

In a medium skillet, melt the butter and add the almond meal, coconut, cocoa powder, and polyol sweetener. Stir over medium heat for about five minutes or until toasted. Remove from heat.

Okay, we're on the home stretch. Get out 6 pretty dessert dishes—preferably clear parfait glasses so that everyone can see the layers. Spoon half of the chocolate mixture into the bottom of the dessert dishes and then top with half the coconut mixture and half the cherry mixture. Repeat the layers, reserving just a couple of teaspoons of the coconut mixture. There should be just enough whipped cream left in the bowl to put a little dollop on top of each serving. Sprinkle the reserved little bit of coconut on top of that and chill for at least a few hours before serving.

Yield: 6 servings

Each with 10 g protein; 17 g carbohydrate; 2 g dietary fiber; 15 g usable carbs. Carb count does not include polyol sweetener.

Coeur a la Crème

This is a classic French dessert, traditionally made in a heart-shaped mold. Coeur a la Crème molds are hard to come by, but you can buy a regular 2-cup (480-ml) heart-shaped mold and stick three or four holes in it with a nail, which is what I did. Serve with fresh strawberries or Strawberry Sauce (see page 550) for a truly beautiful Valentine's Day dessert.

2 packages (8 ounces, or 225 g each) cream cheese, softened
2 tablespoons (3 g) Splenda
3 tablespoons (45 ml) heavy cream
2 tablespoons (30 g) sour cream
¼ teaspoon salt

Use an electric mixer to beat the cream cheese until it's very creamy. Beat in the Splenda, heavy cream, sour cream, and salt, mixing very well.

Line the mold with a double layer of dampened cheesecloth and pack the cheese mixture into it, pressing it in well. Place the mold on a plate to catch any moisture that drains out and chill for at least 24 hours.

Yield: 8 servings

Each with 2 grams of carbohydrates, no fiber, and 5 grams of protein. Analysis does not include toppings.

Warning: This is not a quick dessert to whip up before your sweetheart comes over. You need to start making this dessert at least 24 hours in advance to give it plenty of time to chill.

Maria's Flan

My childhood friend Maria found me on the Internet a couple of years ago, and we got together. Her mom is Colombian, so Maria had grown up eating flan, a traditional Latin American dessert. Here's the version we came up with together.

(continued on page 542)

FOR THE SYRUP:

2 tablespoons (3 g) Splenda

1 teaspoon blackstrap molasses

2 tablespoons (30 ml) water

FOR THE CUSTARD:

1 cup (240 ml) heavy cream

1 cup (240 ml) half-and-half

6 eggs

1 teaspoon vanilla extract

Pinch of nutmeg

Pinch of salt

2/3 cup (17 g) Splenda

Preheat the oven to 350°F (180°C, or gas mark 4).

To make the syrup: Combine the Splenda, molasses, and water, stirring until the lumps are gone. Spray a glass pie plate with nonstick cooking spray and pour the mixture into it, spreading it over the bottom. Microwave for 2 minutes on medium power. (You could substitute the sugar-free syrup of your choice for this syrup; just use 2 to 3 tablespoons [30 to 45 ml].)

To make the custard: Whisk together well the heavy cream, half-and-half, eggs, vanilla, nutmeg, salt, and Splenda and pour the mixture over the syrup in the pie plate.

Place the pie plate carefully in a large, flat baking dish and pour water around it, not quite up to the rim of the pie plate. Put the baking pan with the pie plate in its water bath in the oven. Bake for 45 minutes or until a knife inserted in the center comes out clean.

Cool and cut the flan into wedges. Traditionally, each piece is served inverted on a plate with the syrup on top.

Yield: 8 generous servings

Each with 5 grams of carbohydrates, no fiber, and 6 grams of protein.

Mocha Custard

1 cup (240 ml) boiling water

1 ounce (28 g) unsweetened baking chocolate

1 rounded (1 g) teaspoon instant coffee crystals

1 cup (240 ml) heavy cream

3 eggs

1/3 cup (8 g) Splenda

A pinch of salt

Preheat the oven to 300°F (150°C, or gas mark 2).

Put the boiling water in a blender container and drop in the chocolate. Let it sit for 5 minutes or so.

Add the coffee crystals, heavy cream, eggs, Splenda, and salt and blend for a minute or so.

Spray a 1-quart (960-ml) casserole dish with nonstick cooking spray and pour the mixture into it. (If you prefer, pour into individual custard cups.)

Place the casserole dish or custard cups in a larger pan filled with hot water and place the entire thing in the oven. Bake for 1 hour and 20 minutes.

Cool and then chill well before serving. (The chilling makes a big difference in the texture.)

Yield: 4 generous servings

Each with 6 grams of carbohydrates and 1 gram of fiber, for a total of 5 grams of usable carbs and 6 grams of protein.

Apricot Custard

Don't go increasing the quantity of apricot preserves here. They're the biggest source of carbs. This dessert is yummy, though!

⅓ cup (105 g) low-sugar apricot preserves

2 tablespoons (30 ml) lemon juice

⅔ cup plus 2 teaspoons (17 g) Splenda, divided

1½ cups (360 ml) Carb Countdown dairy beverage

½ cup (120 ml) heavy cream

4 eggs

½ teaspoon almond extract

1 pinch salt

Whisk together the preserves, lemon juice, and 2 teaspoons (1 g) of the Splenda. Spread over the bottom of a 6-cup (1.4-L) glass casserole dish you've sprayed with nonstick cooking spray. Set aside.

Whisk together the Carb Countdown, cream, eggs, remaining ⅔ cup (16 g) Splenda, almond extract, and salt. Pour into the prepared casserole dish gently so as not to mix in the apricot preserves.

Place the casserole dish in a slow cooker. Pour water around the casserole to within 1 inch (2.5 cm) of the rim. Cover the slow cooker, set it to low, and let it cook for 4 hours.

When the time's up, turn off the slow cooker, uncover it, and let it cool until you can remove the casserole dish without risk of scalding. Chill well before serving.

Yield: 6 servings

Each with 7 g protein, 7 g carbohydrate, trace dietary fiber, 7 g usable carbs.

Chocolate Fudge Custard

This really is dense and fudgy. It's intensely chocolatey, too.

1 cup (240 ml) Carb Countdown dairy beverage

3 ounces (85 g) unsweetened baking chocolate

⅔ cup (16 g) Splenda

1 cup (240 ml) heavy cream

½ teaspoon vanilla extract

1 pinch salt

6 eggs, beaten

In a saucepan over the lowest possible heat (use a double boiler or heat diffuser if you have one), warm the Carb Countdown with the chocolate. When the chocolate melts, whisk the two together and then whisk in the Splenda.

Spray a 6-cup (1.4-L) glass casserole dish with nonstick cooking spray. Pour the cream into it and add the chocolate mixture. Whisk in the vanilla extract and salt. Now add the eggs, one by one, whisking each in well before adding the next one.

Put the casserole dish in a slow cooker and pour water around it, up to 1 inch (2.5 cm) of the top rim. Cover the slow cooker, set it to low, and let it cook for 4 hours.

Then turn off the slow cooker, remove the lid, and let the water cool enough so it won't scald you before removing the casserole dish. Chill the custard well before serving.

Yield: 6 servings

Each with 10 g protein, 6 g carbohydrate, 2 g dietary fiber, 4 g usable carbs.

Southeast Asian Coconut Custard

I adapted this from a carb-y recipe in another slow cooker book. Maria, who tested it, says it's wonderful and also has a Latino feel to it. Look for shredded unsweetened coconut in Asian markets and natural food stores.

¼ cup (60 ml) sugar-free imitation honey
½ teaspoon blackstrap molasses
2½ teaspoons grated ginger, divided
1 tablespoon (15 ml) lime juice
14 ounces (390 ml) coconut milk
⅔ cup (16 g) Splenda
¼ teaspoon ground cardamom
½ cup (120 ml) Carb Countdown dairy beverage
½ cup (120 ml) heavy cream
½ teaspoon vanilla extract
4 eggs
½ cup (35 g) shredded unsweetened coconut

Spray a 6-cup (1.4-L) glass casserole dish with nonstick cooking spray. Put the honey and molasses in the casserole dish. Cover the casserole dish with plastic wrap or a plate and microwave on high for 2 minutes. Add 1½ teaspoons of the ginger and the lime juice and stir. Set aside.

In a mixing bowl, combine the coconut milk, Splenda, cardamom, remaining 1 teaspoon ginger, Carb Countdown, cream, vanilla extract, and eggs. Whisk until well combined. Pour into the casserole dish. Cover the casserole dish with foil and secure it with a rubber band.

Put the casserole dish in a slow cooker and pour water around it to within 1 inch (2.5 cm) of the rim. Cover the slow cooker, set it to low, and let it cook for 3 to 4 hours.

Turn off the slow cooker, uncover, and let it cool until you can lift out the casserole dish without scalding your fingers. Chill overnight.

Before serving, stir the coconut in a dry skillet over medium heat until it's golden. Remove the custard from the fridge and run a knife carefully around the edge. Put a plate on top and carefully invert the custard onto the plate. Sprinkle the toasted coconut on top.

Yield: 8 servings

Each with 5 g protein, 5 g carbohydrate, 2 g dietary fiber, 3 g usable carbs. Carb count does not include polyol sweetener in the sugar-free honey.

Maple Custard

This is for all you maple fans out there, and I know you are legion!

1½ cups (360 ml) Carb Countdown dairy beverage
½ cup (120 ml) heavy cream
⅓ cup (80 ml) sugar-free pancake syrup
⅓ cup (8 g) Splenda
3 eggs
1 pinch salt
1 teaspoon vanilla extract
½ teaspoon maple extract

Simply whisk everything together and pour the mixture into a 6-cup (1.4-L) glass casserole dish you've sprayed with nonstick cooking spray. Put the casserole dish in a slow cooker and pour water around it to within 1 inch (2.5 cm) of the rim. Cover the slow cooker, set it to low, and let it cook for 4 hours.

When the time's up, turn off the slow cooker, remove the lid, and let it sit until the water is cool enough so that you can remove the casserole dish without risk of scalding. Chill well before serving.

Yield: 6 servings

Each with 6 g protein, 2 g carbohydrate, 0 g dietary fiber, 2 g usable carbs. (Counts do not include polyols in pancake syrup.)

Maple-Pumpkin Custard

This is very much like the filling of a pumpkin pie without the crust. The pecans add a little textural contrast.

15 ounces (420 g) canned pumpkin
1 cup (240 ml) Carb Countdown dairy beverage
½ cup (120 ml) heavy cream
⅓ cup (80 ml) sugar-free pancake syrup
⅓ cup (8 g) Splenda
½ teaspoon maple flavoring
3 eggs
1 pinch salt
1 tablespoon (5.1 g) pumpkin pie spice
⅓ cup (35 g) chopped pecans
1½ teaspoons butter
Whipped Topping (page 552)

In a mixing bowl, preferably one with a pouring lip, whisk together the pumpkin, Carb Countdown, cream, pancake syrup, Splenda, maple flavoring, eggs, salt, and pumpkin pie spice.

Spray a 6-cup (1.4-L) glass casserole dish with nonstick cooking spray. Pour the custard mixture into it. Place it in a slow cooker. Now carefully fill the space around the casserole dish with water up to 1 inch (2.5 cm) from the rim. Cover the slow cooker, set it to low, and let it cook for 3 to 4 hours.

Remove the lid, turn off the slow cooker, and let it cool until you can remove the casserole dish without scalding your fingers. Chill the custard for at least several hours.

Before serving, put the pecans and butter in a heavy skillet over medium heat and stir them for 5 minutes or so. Set aside. Also have the Whipped Topping made and standing by. Serve the custard with a dollop of Whipped Topping and 1 tablespoon (6 g) of toasted pecans on each serving.

Yield: 6 servings

Each with 7 g protein, 10 g carbohydrate, 3 g dietary fiber, 7 g usable carbs. Carb count does not include polyol sweetener in sugar-free syrup.

Slow Cooker Maple Pumpkin Pudding

This is a great dessert for any of you pumpkin pie freaks out there!

(continued on page 546)

15 ounces (420 g) canned pumpkin

1 cup (240 ml) Carb Countdown dairy
beverage

3 eggs

¼ cup (60 ml) sugar free pancake syrup

½ cup (12 g) Splenda

1 tablespoon (5.1 g) pumpkin pie spice

½ teaspoon maple flavoring

½ cup (65 g) chopped pecans—toasted

Cinnamon

This is simple: Combine everything but the pecans and cinnamon in a mixing bowl and whisk together well. Spray a 1½-quart (1.4-L) casserole dish or other heat-proof dish that fits into your slow cooker with nonstick cooking spray. Pour the pumpkin mixture into the casserole dish. Now put the casserole dish in your slow cooker and carefully pour water around it to within 1 inch (2.5 cm) of the rim.

Cover, set the slow cooker to high, and let it cook for 4 hours. When the time's up, turn off the pot, uncover it, and let the whole thing cool until you can remove the casserole dish without scalding your fingers. You can chill this or serve it warm. Either way, scatter those toasted pecans over each serving and dust each with just a little cinnamon. You can also add whipped cream if you like, but it's not essential.

Yield: 6 servings,

Each with 7 g protein; 10 g carbohydrate; 3 g dietary fiber; 7 g usable carbs. Carb count does not include polyol sweetener in sugar-free syrup. Analysis does not include whipped cream.

Lemon-Vanilla Custard

Don't save this just for dessert—it makes a lovely breakfast, too.

1 cup (240 ml) heavy cream

1 cup (240 ml) half-and-half

3 eggs

⅓ cup (8 g) Splenda

1 teaspoon lemon extract

½ teaspoon vanilla extract

2 tablespoons (16 g) vanilla-flavored whey
protein powder

Pinch of salt

Grated rind of ½ lemon

Preheat the oven to 300°F (150°C, or gas mark 2).

Put all the ingredients in a blender and blend well.

Spray a 1-quart (960-ml) casserole dish with nonstick cooking spray and pour the mixture into it. (If you prefer, use individual custard cups.) Place the casserole dish or custard cups in a larger pan filled with hot water and place the entire thing in the oven. Bake for 2 hours. Cool and chill well.

Yield: 4 generous servings

Each with 8 grams of carbohydrates, a trace of fiber, and 13 grams of protein.

Lemon Mousse Cup

This is pretty darned simple, but it's delicious, with a sunny lemon flavor.

1 package (4-serving size) sugar-free lemon gelatin

¾ cup (180 ml) boiling water

3 ounces (85 g) Neufchâtel cheese or light cream cheese, softened

½ cup (120 ml) cold water

1 teaspoon grated lemon rind

¾ cup (180 ml) heavy cream

2 teaspoons sugar-free vanilla instant pudding mix

2 tablespoons (15 g) almond meal

½ teaspoon polyol sweetener

Put the gelatin and the boiling water in a blender and run it for a minute or so to dissolve the gelatin. Cut the Neufchâtel cheese into chunks, add it to the blender, and run the blender again until the mixture is smooth, about 1 more minute. Now add the cold water and the grated lemon rind and run it one more time to blend.

Pour the gelatin mixture from the blender jar into a mixing bowl and stick it in the fridge. You're going to chill it until it's just starting to thicken a bit.

Use an electric mixer to whip the heavy cream with the vanilla pudding mix until you have a good, thick whipped topping. (Don't overbeat, or you'll get vanilla butter!)

When the gelatin is starting to thicken, fold ½ cup (40 g) of the whipped topping gently into it until everything is well blended. Pour into four pretty dessert dishes. Put the dessert dishes and the leftover whipped topping in the fridge. Let the mousse chill for at least a couple of hours.

Sometime before dinner, stir the almond meal with the polyol sweetener in a skillet over medium heat until it just gets a hint of golden color. Remove from heat.

When dessert time rolls around, top each serving of mousse with a little of the leftover whipped topping and 1½ teaspoons of the toasted almond meal and serve.

Yield: 4 servings

Each with 7 g protein; 4 g carbohydrate; trace dietary fiber; 4 g usable carbs. Carb count does not include polyol sweetener.

Sugar-Free Chocolate Mousse to Die For!

This is the very first low-carb dessert I came up with, and it still blows people away.

1 package (4-serving size) chocolate sugar-free instant pudding mix

1 package (10 ounces, or 280 g) soft tofu

1 heaping tablespoon (6 g) unsweetened cocoa powder

¼ to ½ teaspoon instant coffee crystals (use more if you like mocha flavoring.)

1 to 1½ cups (240 to 360 ml) heavy whipping cream, chilled

(continued on page 548)

Use an electric mixer to beat the pudding mix, tofu, cocoa powder, and coffee crystals until very smooth.

In a separate bowl, whip the cream until just about stiff.

Turn the mixer to its lowest setting, blend in the pudding mixture, and turn off the mixer—quickly. (If you over-beat, you'll end up with chocolate butter.)

Yield: Made with 1 cup (240 ml) of heavy cream, you'll get 6 servings

Each with 8 grams of carbohydrates and 1 gram of fiber, for a total of 7 grams of usable carbs and 5 grams of protein. Made with 1½ cups (360 ml) of heavy cream, your yield increases to at least 7 servings, each with 7.5 grams of carbohydrates and just under 1 gram of fiber, for a total of about 6.5 grams of usable carbs and 4 grams of protein. (I like this made with the smaller amount of cream, for a sturdier texture, but I know folks who like it with the larger amount, for a fluffier texture. It's your choice.) Carb count does not include polyol sweetener.

Variation: Sugar-Free Vanilla Mousse to Die For! Here's one for those non-chocoholics out there: Just use sugar-free vanilla instant pudding mix and a teaspoon of vanilla extract and omit the cocoa powder and the coffee crystals.

Yield: 6 or 7 servings

Made with 1 cup (240 ml) of cream, you'll get 6 servings, each with 7 grams of carbohydrates, a trace of fiber, and 4 grams of protein. Made with 1½ cups (360 ml) of cream, you'll get 7 servings, each with 6.5 grams of carbohydrates, a trace of fiber, and 4 grams of protein.

Better Than S-X!

The Jell-O company invented this quite spectacular special-occasion dessert, which I had to alter in numerous ways to make it fit for low carbers. They're responsible for the name, too. Cryptic, isn't it? Better than the Sox? Better than playing the sax? Better than any other six desserts? Who knows? Since the nice folks at Jell-O came up with the original recipe (though the chocolate sauce was my idea!), it would be nice to use their sugar-free pudding to make this.

FOR CRUST:
1½ cups (225 g) almonds
3 tablespoons (40 g) polyol sweetener
3 tablespoons (4.5 g) Splenda
½ cup (115 g) butter, melted
½ cup (75 g) pecan halves

FOR FILLING:
8 ounces (225 g) cream cheese, softened
3 cups (720 ml) Carb Countdown dairy beverage, divided
2 (4-serving-size) packages sugar-free instant vanilla pudding mix
1 batch Angel-Type Coconut (page 553)
1 batch Maltitol-Splenda Chocolate Sauce (page 551) or Sugar-Free Chocolate Sauce (page 551)

FOR TOPPING:
1½ cups (360 ml) heavy cream, chilled
1½ tablespoons (15 g) sugar-free instant vanilla pudding mix

Preheat oven to 350°F (180°C, or gas mark 4).

To make the crust: Put the almonds in a food processor with the S-blade in place and run it until they're fairly finely ground. Add the polyol and Splenda and pulse to combine.

Now pour in the melted butter and the pecan halves and pulse until the butter is melted in and the pecans are chopped medium-fine.

Spray a 9 × 13-inch (23 × 33-cm) pan with nonstick cooking spray. Dump the almond mixture into it and press it firmly and evenly into place. Bake for 12 to 15 minutes or until golden. You'll want a little time for this to cool before you put the filling on top.

To make the filling: Beat the softened cream cheese until it's smooth. Beat in ½ cup (120 ml) of the Carb Countdown dairy beverage. Now add the 2 packages of pudding mix and the rest of the Carb Countdown. Beat for about 2 minutes, scraping down the sides of the bowl often. Now beat in 1 cup (70 g) of the Angel-Type Coconut. Spread this mixture over the crust.

Spread the Maltitol-Splenda Chocolate Sauce over the pudding layer.

To make the topping: Whip the cream with the 1½ tablespoons (15 g) of vanilla pudding mix, making whipped topping. Spread this over the chocolate layer.

Take the remaining coconut and stir it in a dry skillet over medium heat until it acquires just a touch of gold. Sprinkle the toasted coconut evenly over the whipped topping. Chill for at least 2 hours before serving.

Yield: 12 servings

Each with 10 g protein; 14 g carbohydrate; 4 g dietary fiber; 10 g usable carbs. Carb count does not include polyol sweetener.

Helen's Chocolate Bread Pudding

Helen was my dad's mom, and this was our family's traditional Christmas dessert the whole time I was growing up. People have threatened to marry into the family to get the secret recipe, but since this is the decarbed version, it's not secret! It is still high-carb enough that you'll want to save it for a special occasion, though.

2 cups (480 ml) half-and-half

1 cup (240 ml) heavy cream

1 cup (240 ml) water

6 slices "lite" white bread (5 grams of usable carbs per slice or less—the squishiest you can find)

3 ounces (84 g) unsweetened baking chocolate

²/₃ cup (16 g) Splenda

2 eggs, beaten

1 teaspoon vanilla extract

Pinch salt

Preheat the oven to 375°F (190°C, or gas mark 5).

Combine the half-and-half, cream, and water in a medium saucepan over medium heat and bring it just up to a simmer.

While it's heating, spray a large casserole dish with nonstick cooking spray, tear the bread into small bits, and put them in the dish. Pour the hot half-and-half mixture over the bread and let it sit for 10 minutes.

(continued on page 550)

Melt the chocolate and add it to the bread mixture; it's good to use a little of the hot cream to rinse out the pan you melted the chocolate in so you get all of it. Stir well. Now stir in the Splenda, eggs, vanilla, and salt, mixing very well. Bake for 1 hour or until firm. Serve with Not-So-Hard Sauce (page 549).

Yield: 8 servings

Each with 12 grams of carbohydrates and just over 1 gram of fiber, for a total of 11 grams of usable carbs and 7 grams of protein.

Not-So-Hard Sauce

Traditional hard sauce is made with sugar, butter, and egg, plus vanilla, rum, or brandy, and when it's refrigerated it gets quite hard—hence the name. However, with Splenda instead of sugar, my hard sauce just didn't work—it fell apart in little globs. I added cream cheese, and it all came together, but it doesn't get quite so hard when refrigerated, which is why this is Not-So-Hard Sauce. It still tastes great, though!

1 cup (25 g) Splenda
5 tablespoons (70 g) butter, softened
⅛ teaspoon salt
1 teaspoon vanilla extract
1 egg
1 ounce (28 g) cream cheese, softened
Nutmeg

Use an electric mixer to beat the Splenda and butter together until well blended. Beat in the salt, vanilla extract, and egg. At this point, you'll be sure you've made a dreadful mistake.

Beat in the cream cheese and watch the sauce smooth out! Mix very well, until light and fluffy. Pile the Not-So-Hard Sauce into a pretty serving dish, sprinkle it lightly with nutmeg, and refrigerate until well chilled.

Yield: About 1 cup (240 ml), or a 2 tablespoon (30 ml) serving of sauce for each serving of Helen's Chocolate Bread Pudding (page 549)

Each serving will have 3 grams of carbohydrates, no fiber, and 1 gram of protein.

Strawberry Sauce

Traditionally, Coeur a la Crème (page 541) is served with fresh strawberries, but I make this for Valentine's Day. Since I'm generally not impressed with the quality of the fresh strawberries I can get in February, I'd rather use frozen.

1 bag (1 pound, or 455 g) frozen, unsweetened strawberries, thawed
1 tablespoon (15 ml) lemon juice
2 or 3 tablespoons (3 to 4.5 g) Splenda

Simply pour the strawberries and any liquid in the package into a bowl and stir in the lemon juice and Splenda. Mash the strawberries a little with a fork, if you'd like; I like mine fairly chunky.

Yield: 8 servings

Each with 6 grams of carbohydrates and 1 gram of fiber, for a total of 5 grams of usable carbs and only a trace of protein.

Fast Strawberry-Orange Sauce

This is especially nice for spiffing up a simple dessert for company, using up strawberries threatening to go bad in the refrigerator, or just because it's Tuesday.

½ cup (55 g) strawberries—fresh, or frozen with no sugar added, thawed
1 tablespoon (1.5 g) Splenda
¼ teaspoon orange extract

Assemble the ingredients in a food processor and purée. Serve over sliced melon or sugar-free ice cream or stir it into plain yogurt.

Yield: About ⅓ cup (80 ml), or 3 servings

Each with 2 grams of carbohydrates and 1 gram of fiber, for a total of 1 gram of usable carbs and a trace of protein.

Maltitol-Splenda Chocolate Sauce

I actually think that chocolate sauce made with only maltitol is a little better than this, but this version is less likely to cause digestion problems. Anyway, maltitol makes Splenda look cheap! Do use maltitol, not any of the other polyols, in this recipe. When I tried isomalt and erythritol in chocolate sauce, they turned grainy on me as they cooled. Maltitol makes a sauce with an excellent texture.

½ cup (120 ml) water
2 ounces (55 g) bitter chocolate
¼ cup (50 g) maltitol
¼ cup (6 g) Splenda
3 tablespoons (42 g) butter
¼ teaspoon vanilla
Guar or xanthan

Put the water and the chocolate in a 4-cup (960-ml) glass measuring cup and microwave on high for 45 to 60 seconds. Stir and microwave for another 30 seconds or until chocolate is melted.

Stir in the maltitol and microwave on high for 1 minute. Stir and microwave on high for 1 more minute. Stir in the Splenda, butter, and vanilla—keep stirring until the butter is melted. If you find the chocolate sauce a trifle thin or if you find that a little of the butter refuses to be incorporated into the sauce, use just a tiny bit of guar or xanthan to thicken further. Serve right away or store in a closed container in the fridge.

Yield: 1 cup (240 ml), or 8 servings of 2 tablespoons (30 ml)

Each with 1 g protein; 2 g carbohydrate; 1 g dietary fiber; 1 g usable carb. Carb count does not include maltitol.

Sugar-Free Chocolate Sauce

This is as good as any sugar-based chocolate sauce you've ever had, if I do say so myself.

(continued on page 552)

Which I do. Don't try to make this with Splenda, it won't work—the polyol sweetener somehow makes the water and the chocolate combine. It's either chemistry or magic, or some darned thing.

⅓ cup (80 ml) water
2 ounces (55 g) bitter baking chocolate
½ cup (100 g) maltitol
3 tablespoons (42 g) butter
¼ teaspoon vanilla

Put the water and bitter chocolate in a large glass measuring cup and microwave on high for 1 to 1½ minutes or until chocolate is melted. Stir in the maltitol and microwave on high for another 3 minutes, stirring halfway through. Stir in the butter and vanilla and it's ready to serve (or make into a pie!).

Yield: Makes roughly 1 cup (240 ml), or 8 servings of 2 tablespoons (30 g)

Each 2 g carbohydrate and 1 g fiber, not including the maltitol, for a usable carb count of 1 g; 1 g protein.

This worked beautifully with maltitol. However, when I tried to make it with erythritol, it started out fine but crystallized and turned grainy as it cooled—though it would still have been okay used hot over ice cream, it wouldn't have worked for the frozen pies in this chapter.

Dipping Chocolate

12 ounces (340 g) sugar-free dark chocolate
2 tablespoons (30 ml) sugar-free imitation honey or 2 tablespoons (25 g) polyol sweetener
2 tablespoons (30 ml) heavy cream
¼ cup plus 1 tablespoon (75 ml) water

In a double boiler over hot but not boiling water, melt the chocolate. Stir in the sugar-free imitation honey, the cream, and the water. Keep hot over water while dipping cookies, fruit, or what have you.

Yield: It's hard to know how many things you're going to dip!

But assuming you make 36 Chocolate Dip cookies (page 507), or dip three dozen strawberries, the dip will add to each of them trace protein; trace carbohydrate; trace dietary fiber; no usable carbs. Carb count does not include polyols in the sugar-free chocolate.

Cream Cheese Frosting

This is my sister's recipe. It's good on the Zucchini-Carrot Cake (page 509) or the Gingerbread (page 511).

¾ cup (180 ml) heavy cream, chilled
1 package (8 ounces, or 225 g) cream cheese, softened
½ cup (12 g) Splenda
1 teaspoon vanilla

Whip the heavy cream until it's stiff.
    In a separate bowl, beat the cream cheese until very smooth and then beat in the Splenda and vanilla. Turn the mixer to its lowest speed and blend in the whipped cream. Then turn off the mixer, quick!

Yield: 9 servings

Each with 3 grams of carbohydrates, no fiber, and 2 grams of protein.

Whipped Topping

This has a wonderful flavor and texture.

1 cup (240 ml) heavy cream, well chilled
1 tablespoon (10 g) vanilla sugar-free instant pudding powder

Simply whip them together until the cream is stiff. The pudding adds a very nice texture and helps the whipped cream "stand up." It also adds a slightly vanilla/sweet flavor to the cream, of course.

Yield: This makes about 2 cups (480 ml), or 16 2 tablespoon (30 ml) servings

Each with only a trace carbohydrate, no fiber, and a trace protein.

This is incredible with berries as a simple but elegant dessert. I like to serve strawberries and whipped cream in my nice chip-and-dip dish—it looks so pretty! And it makes the whole thing engagingly informal. This whipped topping is also great on any dessert and terrific on Irish coffee!

Angel-Type Coconut

You'll need this to make the extraordinary dessert we call Better Than S-X (page 548) and several others in this book! You could use it over fresh fruit, for that matter, or anywhere you think a little coconut might be nice.

3 tablespoons (40 g) polyol sweetener
⅓ cup (80 ml) boiling water
2 cups (140 g) shredded coconut meat

In a medium-size mixing bowl, dissolve the polyol sweetener in water. Stir in the coconut, making sure the coconut is evenly damp. Cover the bowl and let it sit for 10 to 15 minutes.

Yield: 2 cups (180 g), or 16 servings of 2 tablespoons each

Each with trace protein; 2 g carbohydrate; 1 g dietary fiber; 1 g usable carb. Carb count does not include polyol sweetener.

Cinnamon Splenda Nuts

This is a nice little nibble to pass around with coffee.

2 tablespoons (28 g) butter
1 cup (120 g) shelled walnuts, pecans, or a combination of the two
1½ to 2 tablespoons (2 to 3 g) Splenda
½ teaspoon cinnamon

Melt the butter in a heavy skillet over medium heat and then add the nuts. Cook for 5 to 6 minutes, stirring from time to time. Turn off the heat and immediately sprinkle the Splenda and cinnamon over the top and stir to distribute. (If

(continued on page 454)

you wait for the nuts to cool, the Splenda doesn't stick nearly so well.) I like these best warm, although they're still quite nice when cooled.

Yield: 4 or 5 servings (remember, this is just a nibble)

Assuming 4 servings, each will have 5 grams of carbohydrates and 2 grams of fiber, for a total of 3 grams of usable carbs and 5 grams of protein.

Easy Low-Carb Fudge

This recipe had a very special tester—my 7-year-old friend Austin McIntosh. He gives this recipe a 10. His mom, Julie, who helped, says it's quite easy to do and really is doable for kids, especially since no heat is involved. She also says it's good without the nuts, too!

1 pound (455 g) cream cheese, softened
2 ounces (55 g) bitter chocolate, melted
½ cup (12 g) Splenda
1 teaspoon vanilla extract
½ (65 g) cup chopped walnuts or pecans

Beat the cream cheese until smooth and then beat in the chocolate, Splenda, and vanilla. Stir in the chopped nuts.

Line an 8 × 8-inch (20 × 20-cm) pan with foil and smooth the cream cheese mixture into it. Chill well and then cut in squares. Store in the fridge

Yield: 64 1-inch (2.5-cm) squares

Each with 1 g protein; 1 g carbohydrate; trace dietary fiber; 1 gram carbohydrate.

Peach Ice Cream

This isn't dirt-low in carbs, but it's astonishingly delicious, with a fabulous, creamy texture. If you make only one frozen dessert from this book, make this one.

16 ounces (480 ml) peach-flavored Fruit$_2$O
1 tablespoon (7 g) unflavored gelatin
2 cups (400 grams) sliced peaches (Unsweetened frozen peach slices work great.)
¼ cup (60 ml) lemon juice
⅓ cup (8 g) Splenda
2 cups (480 ml) heavy cream, chilled
3 tablespoons (30 g) sugar-free vanilla pudding mix

Pour the Fruit$_2$O into a nonreactive saucepan and turn the heat underneath to medium-low. Sprinkle the gelatin over the top. Stir with a whisk as the mixture heats, making sure all the gelatin dissolves.

Add the peaches, lemon juice, and Splenda to the gelatin mixture and simmer for about 10 minutes or until the peaches are just getting tender. Transfer the mixture to a blender (this assumes your blender can take the heat—if it can't, let the mixture cool a bit first) and pulse the blender a few times—you want to leave some small chunks of peach, rather than puréeing everything completely smooth.

Let the peach mixture cool until it's room temperature—it should be syrupy but not gelled for the next step.

Pour the chilled heavy cream into a large mixing bowl and add the pudding mix. Whip with an electric mixer until the cream stands in soft peaks. Turn the mixer to low and beat in the peach/gelatin mixture. Beat only long enough to get everything blended and then turn off the mixer.

Pour the whole thing into an ice cream freezer. (This actually was a bit too much mixture for my freezer, so we had to eat the little bit left over unfrozen. This was not a hardship.) Freeze according to the directions that come with the freezer and then serve.

If you have leftover Peach Ice Cream, let it soften at room temperature for at least 15 minutes before serving—it's likely to be unappealingly hard straight out of the freezer.

Yield: Makes about 1½ quarts (1.4 L), or roughly 10 servings, assuming you're using self-restraint, which is actually a bad bet.

Assuming you manage to share, and not pig out, each serving will have about 10 grams of carbohydrate, with 1 gram of fiber, for a usable carb count of 9 grams; 2 grams protein.

Vanilla Frozen Custard

This is so rich and delicious! The polyols in this help to keep it from freezing like a rock—which it would if you used Splenda instead. Try serving it with the Sugar-Free Chocolate Sauce (page 551).

6 eggs
2 cups (480 ml) half-and-half
½ cup (100 g) polyol sweetener
3 tablespoons (45 ml) sugar-free imitation honey
¼ teaspoon salt

2 cups (480 ml) whipping cream, chilled
1 tablespoon (15 ml) vanilla extract

In a medium saucepan, beat together the eggs, half-and-half, sweetener, honey, and salt. Cook over low heat, stirring constantly (don't quit or you'll get very rich scrambled eggs!), until the mixture is thick enough to coat a metal spoon and has reached at least 160°F (75°C).

Cool quickly by setting the pan in ice or cold water and stirring until it's just barely warm—this prevents trapped steam from making the custard watery. Cover and refrigerate until thoroughly chilled, at least 1 hour.

When you're ready to freeze the custard, use an electric mixer to whip the cream with the vanilla until it stands in soft peaks. Turn the mixer to low and beat in the custard, running the mixer just enough longer to blend well. Pour the mixture into the ice cream freezer and freeze according to the directions that came with the freezer; then serve.

Yield: Makes between 1½ and 2 quarts (1.4 to 1.9 L), or 10 servings, at least!

Assuming 10 servings, each will have 8 grams of carbohydrate, not counting polyols; 6 grams protein.

Lime-Vanilla Sherbet

In Ray Bradbury's extraordinary novel *Dandelion Wine*, the characters, visiting an ice cream parlor, choose the unusual flavor "Lime-Vanilla Ice."

(continued on page 556)

Consider this my tribute to one of the greatest American novels of the twentieth century.

1 package (4-serving size) sugar-free lime gelatin
2 cups (480 ml) boiling water
Juice and grated rind of 1 lime
5 tablespoons (7.5 g) Splenda
2 cups (460 g) plain yogurt
¼ cup (30 g) vanilla whey protein powder
2 teaspoons vanilla extract

If your blender can take the heat, combine the gelatin and boiling water in the blender container and whir to dissolve the gelatin. If your blender can't take the heat, stir the two together in a heatproof container until the gelatin is completely dissolved and then let the mixture cool to the point where your blender can handle it but the whole thing is still liquid. Pour it into the blender and turn it on to a low speed. Add the other ingredients, one at a time, adding the yogurt in several additions to avoid overwhelming the blender.

When everything's well blended, let the whole thing cool until it's starting to get really syrupy. Pour into an ice cream freezer and freeze according to the directions.

Yield: 8 servings

Each serving will have 5 grams of carbohydrate, a trace of fiber, and 5 grams of protein.

Lime-Honeydew-Ginger Ice

This is light, refreshing, and brilliant green.

1 package (4-serving size) sugar-free lime gelatin
2 cups (480 ml) boiling water
2 cups (310 g) honeydew melon, cubed
1½ tablespoons (9 g) grated ginger
Juice and grated rind of 1 lime

Assuming that you have a blender that can deal with boiling water, put the gelatin and the boiling water in your blender and whirl until the gelatin is completely dissolved. If your blender won't take the heat, whisk the water and the gelatin together in a bowl instead until the gelatin is completely dissolved. Let it cool to a temperature your blender can take before you do the next step.

If you've used a bowl to dissolve your gelatin, pour it into the blender now, turn it on, and add the honeydew, a few chunks at a time. When the honeydew is all puréed, add the ginger and lime juice, let it whirl another couple of seconds, and then turn off the blender.

Put the blender container in the fridge and chill until it's starting to thicken up. Pour it into an ice cream freezer and follow the directions until the mixture is frozen; then serve. Or you can do this in traditional granita form, which is to freeze it in a shallow pan and scrape it with a fork every 20 to 30 minutes as it freezes to separate the crystals.

You can just pour this into dessert cups and let it chill as a gelatin dessert instead, if you prefer.

Yield: 8 servings

Each serving will have 4 grams of carb, a trace of fiber, and a trace of protein.

Lemon Sherbet

This recipe is low-carb, low-fat, low-calorie—and delicious!

1 package (4-serving size) sugar-free lemon gelatin
2 cups (480 ml) boiling water
2 cups (460 g) plain yogurt
2 teaspoons lemon extract
3 tablespoons (4.5 g) Splenda
¼ cup (30 g) vanilla whey protein powder

Put the gelatin powder in a blender and add the water. Blend for 20 seconds or just long enough to dissolve the gelatin.

Add the other ingredients and blend well. Put the blender container in the refrigerator and let it chill for 10 to 15 minutes. Take it out and blend it again for about 10 seconds, chill it for another 10 to 15 minutes, and then give it another quick blend it when it's done chilling.

Pour the sherbet mixture into a home ice cream freezer and freeze according to the directions.

Yield: 8 servings of ½ cup (120 ml)—but just try to eat only ½ cup! Just try!

Each serving has 2.5 grams of carbohydrates (if you use the GO-Diet figure of 4 grams of carbs in a cup of plain yogurt); even if you go with the count on the label, this only has 4 grams of carbohydrates per serving, no fiber, and 9 grams of protein.

Orange Sherbet

Isn't orange everybody's favorite flavor of sherbet?

1 package (4-serving) sugar-free orange gelatin
2 cups (480 ml) boiling water
2 cups (460 g) plain yogurt
5 tablespoons (7.5 g) Splenda
¼ cup (30 g) vanilla whey protein powder
2 tablespoons (30 ml) lemon juice
Juice and grated rind of 1 orange

If your blender can take the heat, combine the gelatin and boiling water in the blender container and whir to dissolve the gelatin. If your blender can't take the heat, stir the two together in a heatproof container until the gelatin is completely dissolved and then let the mixture cool to the point where your blender can handle it but the whole thing is still liquid. Pour it into the blender and turn it on to a low speed. Add the other ingredients, one at a time, adding the yogurt in several additions to avoid overwhelming the blender.

When everything's well blended, let the whole thing cool until it's starting to get really syrupy. Pour into an ice cream freezer and freeze according to the directions.

Yield: 8 servings

Each serving will have 5 grams of carbohydrate, a trace of fiber, and 5 grams protein.

INDEX